Ischemic Heart Disease

Ischemic Heart Disease

A Rational Basis for Clinical Practise
and Clinical Research

Attilio Maseri, M.D.

Institute of Cardiology
Catholic University of
the Sacred Heart
Rome, Italy

Churchill Livingstone
New York, Edinburgh, London, Melbourne, Tokyo

Library of Congress Cataloging-in-Publication Data

Maseri, Attilio.
    Ischemic heart disease / Attilio Maseri.
       p.   cm.
    Includes bibliographical references and index.
    ISBN 0-443-07910-2
    1. Coronary heart disease. I. Title.
    [DNLM: 1. Myocardial Ischemia. WG 300 M396i 1995]
  RC685.C6M354   1995
  616.1′23—dc20
  DNLM/DLC
  for Library of Congress   95-17707
                                              CIP

Distributed in the United Kingdom by Churchill Livingstone, Robert Stevenson House, 1–3 Baxter's Place, Leith Walk, Edinburgh EH1 3AF, and by associated companies, branches, and representatives throughout the world.

Accurate indications, adverse reactions, and dosage schedules for drugs are provided in this book, but it is possible that they may change. The reader is urged to review the package information data of the manufacturers of the medications mentioned.

The Publishers have made every effort to trace the copyright holders for borrowed material. If they have inadvertently overlooked any, they will be pleased to make the necessary arrangements at the first opportunity.

Acquisitions Editor: *Lucy Gardner and Allan Ross*
Production Editor: *Bridgett L. Dickinson*
Production Supervisor: *Laura Mosberg Cohen*
Cover Design: *Paul Moran*

Printed in the United States of America

First published in 1995   7 6 5 4 3 2 1

To our son, Filippo

Preface

Cardiologists of my generation have witnessed some dramatic progress in the treatment of ischemic syndromes as a result of a more precise understanding of its various pathogenetic mechanisms. However, the same clinical syndrome and even the same pathogenetic mechanism can have different etiologic components and, therefore, the average benefit provided by new forms of treatment may not apply equally to all eligible patients. Identification of the varied etiologic components, genetically and environmentally determined, which concur to cause, or to provide protection from, the various ischemic syndromes, will be a major challenge for the next generation of cardiologists.

During the past 25 years of clinical and research activities that have been devoted entirely to patients with ischemic heart disease (IHD), time and again I have wrongly disbelieved a patient's clinical history simply because it did not fit into a traditionally accepted pattern. Thus, in 1984 I began to reexamine thoroughly the generally accepted paradigms about IHD, in an effort to reconcile clinical observations with pathophysiologic, histopathologic and epidemiologic studies. Now, some 10 years later, my work on this book, which is far from perfect, is finished only because my search for a coherent picture of IHD has come to a natural break.

Consensus conferences and the results of megatrials are now determining standards of practice for the "average" patient suffering from any given ischemic syndrome, by providing physicians with appropriate guidelines and, at the same time, also providing them with a means of defense against criticism and accusations of malpractise. Yet, until the 1950s, it was standard practise to confine patients with acute myocardial infarction to strict bed rest for 3 weeks, and until as recently as the late 1970s the only "respectable" cause of angina was critical, flow-limiting organic coronary stenoses.

The variable relation between risk factors, coronary atherosclerosis, ischemic manifestations and individual responses to treatment, so commonly observed in clinical practice, is due largely to the multiplicity of mechanisms that can cause the same clinical ischemic syndrome. Varied mechanisms of disease imply varying prognoses and varying management strategies: they can be identified only by attentive, open-minded clinical research and, once identified, should be studied in depth at the cellular and molecular levels.

As I have tried to provide a rational basis for both clinical practise and clinical research, the book should be read starting from the first, introductory, chapter. The beginning of each chapter and each section outline the most fundamental principles, which, for readers with specific interest, are subsequently expanded. Conclusive remarks are depicted in italics, whilst those of lesser importance are set in small print areas bound by horizontal lines.

This book is dedicated to all physicians wishing to develop and expand their knowledge on how best to adapt available guidelines to individual patients under their care, and to all investigators eager to identify and "search" their own clinical questions, rather than only "re-search" details of established paradigms in previous publications. It is not my intention to replace old paradigms with new ones, but to offer an open-minded approach to problem solving whereby physicians and investigators progressively gain confidence in their own findings also when not fitting into traditionally accepted schemes.

Attilio Maseri, M.D.

Acknowledgments

This book is a tribute to all the teachers who have guided me in clinical medicine and research, and to all the colleagues who have shared with me throughout the years clinical duties and the excitement of research.

I am deeply indebted to all my colleagues, far too numerous to mention individually, who over the past 10 years, but especially during the last few months, have discussed critically with me, and helped complete, the various chapters.

I wish to thank Andrew Porter and Manlio Fabrucci for preparing the illustrations and Ms. Heather Russell for her editorial services, but this book would never have seen the end had it not been for the competence, total dedication, and patience of my secretary, Vanessa.

It is to Francesca, my wonderful supportive wife, that I owe the serenity of my every day life, the courage to undertake this ambitious task and the strength to complete it. Whenever in doubt about major decisions I have been able to count on her good sense; when depressed I could always count on her encouragement. She has been my "musa inspiratrice."

Attilio Maseri, M.D.

Contents

General concepts of ischemic heart disease

INTRODUCTION

This introductory chapter is intended to offer an overview of ischemic heart disease (IHD), outlining its many complexities. It is the recognition of these complexities that indicates the need for a review of the physiologic and pathophysiologic principles presented in the following chapters. This is basic to an understanding of the varied causes of IHD and hence to a more effective management of the clinical syndromes.

Ischemic diseases of the heart comprise four clinical syndromes caused by myocardial ischemia:

a. angina pectoris
b. acute myocardial infarction (MI)
c. chronic postischemic cardiac failure
d. sudden ischemic cardiac death (SICD).

As each of these four syndromes may occur in succession in some patients, they are usually considered as varied manifestations of a progressively worsening single disease of the coronary arteries, i.e. "atherosclerotic coronary artery disease," that has a long preclinical course and a certain "threshold" above which its manifestations begin to develop. This traditional view, developed during the 1950s and 1960s on the basis of information then available, is still widely accepted today.[1] Yet, in ischemic coronary syndromes, the fundamental problem is myocardial ischemia, without which no ischemic syndromes would occur. This view was proposed originally in two classic textbooks of clinical cardiology, one by Goldberger[2] and the other by Wood,[3] who used, respectively, the terms "coronary heart disease" and "ischemic heart disease." Subsequently, however, general attention has focused more and more on the chronic coronary atherosclerotic background than on myocardial ischemia and its outcome.

A considerable body of evidence, gathered during the last two decades, and based on both a cross-sectional view of ischemic syndromes and a longitudinal view of the mode of first presentation of IHD, its course, and its outcome, suggests that this traditional view is valid only as a crude first approximation.

The time has come, therefore, to consider separately all the major pathogenetic components of IHD that are responsible for the chronic atherosclerotic background, the acute ischemic stimuli, and the cardiac response to the ischemic insult.

1

A CROSS-SECTIONAL VIEW

In each ischemic syndrome the most obvious features are similar in spite of the multiplicity of underlying causes. Anginal pain is the same, regardless of whether myocardial ischemia is caused by an excessive increase in myocardial demand, coronary thrombosis, coronary artery spasm, or small vessel dysfunction (see Chs 14, 15, and 16). The signs and consequences of MI are also similar regardless of whether it was caused by coronary thrombosis, embolism, or spasm and regardless of the actual causes of thrombotic occlusion (see Chs 9 and 21). Chronic postischemic cardiac failure may result from a very severe left ventricular dysfunction or from an intense neurohumoral activation occurring in the presence of moderate cardiac dysfunction (see Ch. 23). Sudden ischemic cardiac death may result from fatal arrhythmias triggered by potentially reversible ischemic episodes or by acute necrosis, or from fatal arrhythmias occurring only in the presence of postinfarction scarring (see Chs 10 and 24).

For these reasons angina pectoris, MI, SICD, and chronic postischemic cardiac failure should be considered as merely clinical syndromes, like, for instance, anemia. The diagnosis of anemia was once considered to be adequate until it was appreciated that there were many possible causes of a reduced blood hemoglobin content; nowadays "anemia" is an incomplete diagnosis until its actual cause can be specified. In the same way, the diagnosis of angina pectoris, MI, chronic postischemic cardiac failure, or SICD will remain incomplete diagnoses until all their pathogenetic and etiologic components can be specified.

THE MODE OF FIRST PRESENTATION OF IHD

The commonest form of first clinical presentation of IHD is unheralded and dramatic. The Framingham Study showed that MI, SICD, or acute coronary insufficiency were the first presenting events in about 70% of men and 50% of women. These epidemiologic data concur with the clinical observation that about 65% of patients presenting with their first MI had no previous symptoms of IHD (see Ch. 11).

These unpredicted and startling events are not related to the subclinical development of critical (i.e. flow-limiting) coronary stenoses. A low-grade residual infarct-related stenosis is often found after thrombolysis, not only in patients suffering their first MI but also in unselected cases. Preinfarction angiograms do not allow the identification of the infarct-related artery which, usually, has only nonflow-limiting stenoses that often are milder than those present in other arteries. Conversely, the coronary angiograms of patients presenting with uncomplicated chronic stable angina often show more severe and more extensive atherosclerosis than the angiograms of those in whom the very first manifestation of IHD was an unheralded acute MI (see Ch. 8).

If ischemic events were only the consequence of a slow, gradually progressive narrowing of the lumen of coronary arteries, the expected initial clinical manifestation of IHD would be angina occurring during unusual effort, followed by a gradual, slow, progressive impairment of exercise tolerance.

THE COURSE OF IHD

Chronic stable effort-induced angina may last for years with no evolutive tendency, even when angiography shows multiple critical stenoses and, sometimes, even in spite of their progression to total occlusion. In contrast, although unstable angina is characterized by a similar or lesser degree of severity of coronary atherosclerosis than the stable type, it may evolve into MI or SICD (see Chs 16–20).

Among patients suffering their first MI, only about 35% previously had either unstable or chronic stable angina. In survivors of MI, totally asymptomatic periods of several years are frequently observed; similarly, patients presenting with recent-onset angina, or even chronic stable angina, often have long asymptomatic periods. In the Framingham Study, remissions of at least 2 years were observed in 32% of men and 44% of women with recent-onset angina and in 14% of men and 19% of women with chronic stable angina. As discussed in Chapters 9, 11, and 13, the variable course of IHD cannot be explained simply by the progression and regression of coronary stenoses or by the development of collaterals.

Thus, the waxing and waning of ischemic stimuli, on a variable and variably deteriorating atherosclerotic background, plays the major part in determining the course of IHD.

THE OUTCOME OF IHD

Mortality from IHD increases exponentially with age, so that about 80% of total mortality from IHD occurs in individuals over the age of 65, yet both the extent and severity of coronary atherosclerosis reach a plateau at the age of 60 (see Ch. 8). The progressive increase in IHD mortality rates is related not only to a greater incidence of new cases of infarction occurring in the elderly, but also to a much larger number of fatalities. In the Gruppo Italiano per lo Studio della Sopravvivenza nell'Infarto Miocardico-2 (GISSI-2) study, hospital mortality rates in the 9730 patients who had suffered their first MI increased about 16-fold (largely because of cardiac rupture), in patients aged 80 years and over compared with those aged up to 40 years, in spite of a similar prevalence of a previous history of chronic stable angina (about 20%) and a lower average estimated infarct size in the older age-group. Moreover, mortality rates were consistently higher in women, than in men, at all ages (see Ch. 10).

The unpredictable development of fatal arrhythmias, and the progressive increase in the heart's vulnerability to MI with increasing age and the higher mortality rates in women, represent examples of the varying responses of the heart to ischemic insults. These responses, therefore, represent major components of the outcome of IHD above and beyond the progressive development of the atherosclerotic background and of acute ischemic stimuli.

THE THREE MAJOR PATHOGENETIC COMPONENTS
OF ISCHEMIC SYNDROMES

As argued above, effort in the past has been directed predominantly toward finding a single cause for angina pectoris, MI, and SICD. The impetus to find a clearly identifiable culprit reflects the natural human inability to live with major complex problems without providing a plausible explanation, and has led to considerable shortcuts being taken along the route of the search from predisposing and etiologic factors, through pathophysiologic mechanisms, and thence to clinical syndromes.

The time has come to search for the major missing links between atherosclerosis and ischemic syndromes, rather than continuing to focus in greater and greater depth only on the mechanisms of atherosclerosis.

Thus, from the first-generation approach in which coronary atherosclerosis is considered to be the common background against which ischemic syndromes are assumed to occur—largely at random once a critical threshold has been reached—we should now proceed to a second-generation and novel approach. This is based on the consideration that the manifestations and outcome of IHD are determined not only by the *chronic atherosclerotic background* but, to a major extent, also by *multiple acute stimuli* that cause transient or persistent myocardial ischemia, and by the *heart's response* to ischemia (see Fig. 1). These *three major patho-*

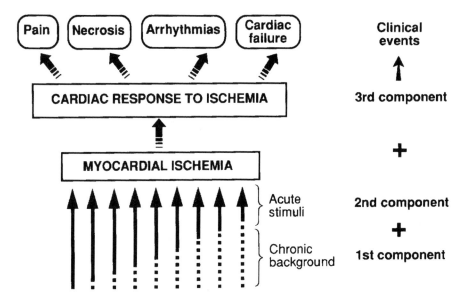

Fig. 1 Cross-sectional view of IHD: the three major pathogenetic components of IHD. The variable severity of *coronary atherosclerosis* (represented by dashed vertical lines) may result from various types of intimal injury and from a variable combination of smooth muscle cell proliferation and lipid and ground substance deposition, as well as from fibrinogen and fibrin deposition and from thrombus organization. *Stimuli* that may suddenly reduce regional coronary blood flow, transiently or persistently, causing coronary constriction, thrombosis, or both are represented by solid lines. Weaker stimuli may be sufficient to cause ischemia in the presence of a severe atherosclerotic background; flow-limiting stenoses can reduce coronary flow reserve and cause ischemia when the increase in myocardial demand is excessive. The *response of the heart* to ischemic insults in terms of the development of collateral blood flow, anginal pain, ischemia, necrosis, heart failure, and fatal arrhythmias may also vary considerably.

These three pathogenetic components contribute to cause the four major ischemic syndromes and to determine their outcome. Of these components of IHD, undoubtedly the most important is the development of ischemic stimuli. The chronic atherosclerotic background, together with the response of the heart, become relevant only because they can predispose to or modulate the effects of ischemic stimuli.

genetic components of IHD, with their individual etiologic and pathogenetic components, concur to cause the four major ischemic syndromes and to determine their outcome.

The *chronic atherosclerotic background* lesions in the coronary arteries may have a variable composition, extent, and origin and, before the age of 70, they are more common in men than in women. These lesions could be caused not only by different varieties of noxious stimuli, acting either chronically over several years or acutely over much shorter periods, but also by different local and systemic responses to the injury. They may also have a different ischemic potential, depending on the nature of the noxious stimuli and on the vasomotor and hemostatic response (see Ch. 8).

The various *acute ischemic stimuli* may cause myocardial ischemia when they are transient and necrosis when they are persistent. Although most often developing in the presence of a chronic atherosclerotic background, the actual triggers of such stimuli are largely unknown. In patients with chronic stable angina, stimuli are "stable" because they recur chronically without causing a sudden interruption of coronary blood flow (CBF) and have no detectable evolutive tendency. Such stimuli are represented by an excessive increase in myocardial demand in the presence of flow-limiting coronary stenoses, or by dynamic coronary constriction at the site of a stenosis or in small distal vessels. In patients with unstable angina, stimuli are "unstable" because they appear suddenly, wax and wane, and have the tendency to cause coronary thrombosis and vasoconstriction leading to sudden transient or persistent interruption of CBF and MI or SICD. Furthermore, in MI the stimuli that lead to sudden persistent coronary occlusion and thrombosis are multiple (see Ch. 9).

The *cardiac response to ischemic stimuli* manifests clinically with the following:

a.   ischemic cardiac pain
b.   myocardial necrosis
c.   acute cardiac failure
d.   cardiac arrhythmias.

The response is determined not only by the severity, duration, and extent of myocardial ischemia, but also by collateral development and function and by neurohumoral and biologic factors, which play a major part in determining the age and gender-related responses to MI and the susceptibility to malignant arrhythmias.

These three pathogenetic components concur to produce the variable longitudinal picture of IHD, in which ischemic cardiac death may occur not only in symptomatic patients, but also unexpectedly in those who are in a totally quiescent phase, or in previously asymptomatic individuals (see Fig. 2A, B).

CONCLUSIONS

Given the multiplicity of mechanisms that combine to cause ischemic syndromes and to determine their outcome, it is obvious that not all individuals are susceptible to the same risk factors (see Ch. 12), and that not all patients with similar syndromes may require the same management. This state of affairs has profound implications for both clinical practise and clinical research.

Cardiologists and physicians should consider possible individual differences among patients, rather than merely the similarities that allow their classification into traditionally established syndromes. They should apply informed pathophysiologic reasoning, as well as personal experience, when adapting information gleaned from published diagnostic, prognostic, and therapeutic studies, to individual patients.

Clinical investigators should try to identify homogeneous subsets of patients with similar pathogenetic and etiologic components, in order to study the various factors involved in the

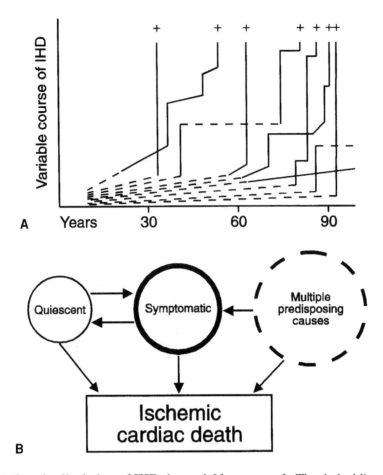

Fig. 2 Longitudinal view of IHD: its variable course. A. The dashed lines indicate the chronic atherosclerotic background accumulating at variable, often irregular, rates as a result of exposure to different stimuli over varying periods of time. The continuous lines indicate the onset and progression of symptoms, most often occurring suddenly, and the crosses signs indicate mortality from IHD. **B.** Symptomatic phases develop in the presence of a variable, composite predisposing background that formed either gradually or in occasional bouts. They are often followed by totally quiescent phases with no symptoms or signs of spontaneous or inducible ischemic episodes. During these phases, treatment is obviously only intended to improve prognosis. Mortality from IHD may occur not only in symptomatic patients, but also suddenly or following myocardial infarction, with no recurrence of symptoms in quiescent phases, and as the first manifestation of IHD in individuals with a predisposing background still too imprecisely known.

development of the atherosclerotic background, the multiple ischemic stimuli, and the variable cardiac responses to the ischemic insult.

The new framework of IHD presented above is intended to set the stage in the search for the relative roles of the multiple etiologic components, as well as of the genetically and environmentally determined predisposing, precipitating and protecting factors of ischemic syndromes. The identification of homogeneous subsets of patients with the same pathogenetic and etiologic components is essential when attempting to capitalize on the research capabilities offered by the rapidly expanding developments that are taking place in cellular and molecular biology. Old and new established facts, like the tesserae of a mosaic or like the pieces in a jigsaw puzzle, should be assembled in order to form a comprehensive picture of IHD; the gaps in our knowledge should generate further questions, so that subsequent new hypotheses can be advanced to fit the facts more closely and thus clarify, rather than distort, the final picture.

REFERENCES

1. Fuster V, Badimon L, Badimon JJ, Chesebro JH. The pathogenesis of coronary artery disease and the acute coronary syndromes. New Engl J Med 1992;*326:*310.
2. Goldberger E. Heart Disease. Lea & Febiger, Philadelphia, 1951.
3. Wood P. Diseases of the Heart and Circulation. Eyre & Spottiswoode, London, 1956.

Physiologic principles

CHAPTER

1

Elements of cardiovascular biology

INTRODUCTION

The explosive development of knowledge in the field of cellular and molecular biology is providing a more profound understanding of the mechanisms of cellular and subcellular stimuli and responses, and of their pathologic alterations. The rapid accumulation of more precise information regarding the cellular and subcellular disruption of myocardial and vascular function calls for the delineation of a general framework against which new information can be seen in perspective. In whole organisms, specific biologic dysfunctions of cells, enzymes, receptors and intracellular transduction are often compensated for by changes in other systems, thus preserving function to a great extent. A brief review of vascular and cellular biology and of the blood/vessel-wall interaction is useful in order to achieve a better understanding of the physiologic regulation of blood perfusion and myocardial function, and of their adaptation to pathologic conditions.

This chapter outlines, with broad brushstrokes, the fundamental principles involved in:

a. the maintenance of a dynamic equilibrium of the constituents of the body and of individual organs and tissues
b. inter- and intracellular signaling
c. the biology of the vessel wall and myocardium
d. the blood/vessel-wall interaction in thrombus formation.

1.1 DYNAMIC EQUILIBRIUM OF BODY CONSTITUENTS

In common with all body tissues, the blood vessels and the heart evolve during differentiation and growth to reach a state of development that is maintained at a virtually constant level throughout adult life. The adult state is attained when the genetic program of non-replicating cells is set at the mature phenotype. This apparent steady state of organs and tissues in adult life is the result of a continuous process of turnover of ions, molecules, macromolecules, cell components, and, for most tissues (but not for the myocardium), also of individual cells. The various constituents of the body, cell components, and cells turn over at widely different rates, but for each the rate of replacement precisely balances the rate of removal or breakdown. This is akin to the number of soldiers in a battalion, which remains constant although a certain number are continuously replaced by others.

11

The turnover of ions and of inorganic, organic, and diffusible molecules is determined by their exchange through food intake, body metabolism, and excretion, as well as by exchange among intravascular, extravascular, extracellular, and intracellular compartments.

The turnover of cell components and cell replication is controlled by genetic programing. In response to physiologic or pathologic stimuli, genetic programing allows cells to adapt their structure and function continuously in response to functional requirements: the cell can increase or decrease turnover and replication rates and can also modify the phenotypic expression and hence cellular composition and function. Continuing the analogy of tissues and organs with a battalion, the type of soldiers, their training, and rate of turnover can be changed by modifying the selection process, training program, and length of service in the batallion according to functional needs. Impaired genetic programing represents a possible source not only of the general alterations in the structure and function of organs and tissues caused by a gene mutation present from birth but also of abnormality or death of individual mature cells, when their own individual genetic material is damaged by chemical or physical agents or by the wear and tear related to cellular aging. Mitochondrial DNA abnormalities in individual myocardial cells have been found to increase markedly with age and to be associated with defects in protein replication and, ultimately, with cell dysfunction and death.[1]

1.1.1 Dynamic equilibrium of exchangeable ions and molecules

The concentration of ions and diffusible compounds can differ very considerably between extracellular and intracellular compartments as well as within the cytosol and among intracellular organelles. The concentration differences between compartments outside and within cells are maintained by a balanced rate of exchange through passive diffusion along concentration gradients and through various active transport systems.

Ions and diffusible molecules, introduced with food or produced by metabolic processes, tend to equilibrate with those already present in the various compartments. Any ion and molecule of a given species has the same probability of exchanging with others of the same species in adjacent compartments.

The use of radioactive and nonradioactive tracers is based on this principle. Tracer substances behave exactly as the substances to be traced, thus providing information on rates of exchange and turnover among compartments. Following intravenous injection, nondiffusible labeled molecules remain almost entirely confined to the intravascular space for a few minutes (5–10 min for albumin). Thus, after mixing uniformly with the blood volume in the vascular bed, they enable it to be measured. Conversely, the initial distribution of diffusible extravascular tracers such as water, potassium, or thallium is flow dependent: immediately after the intravenous injection of such tracers, the amount taken up by each organ and tissue is proportional to blood flow as they diffuse along the concentration gradient into the extravascular space and into cells, but as the concentration of the tracer increases in the interstitial fluid, it begins to diffuse back into the bloodstream. If the extraction of the tracer during the first pass is complete, measurement taken before significant back-diffusion into the bloodstream permits measurement of the fraction of cardiac output perfusing each organ. This principle is straightforward for flow indicators trapped in the microvasculature that do not recirculate, such as microspheres. It also applies to some extent to diffusible tracers with very high initial extraction such as water, potassium tracers, and ammonia, but only up to flow values about double the basal values.

1.1.2 Turnover and expression of cell components

The various structural and functional components of adult cells such as ion channels and receptors, intracellular organelles, and enzymes, although apparently constant, are continuously renewed, each at its own rate. Maintenance of the normal structure and physiologic function of the heart and blood vessels is not attributable to inactivity of genetic processes once the cells have reached their state of terminal differentiation: it results from the constancy of the mechanisms that continuously regulate the expression of genes encoding the many proteins that constitute the cells and interstitial matrix. In normal conditions it is such constancy that ensures that the various components of cell membranes, intracellular organelles, and enzymes are regularly replaced with new ones having exactly the same characteristics. When functional conditions change, it is this continuous process of renovation that affords a means of switching the production of structural and functional components of cells and interstitium, by changes in gene expression, to suit the new demands better.

Thus, the adaptation of the heart and blood vessels to new physiologic stimuli and pathologic states is regulated by changes in the expression of genes. In the heart, such changes can induce, for example, a gradual transition in receptor expression, in isoforms of contractile proteins, in Na^+/K^+-ATPase, and in the proportion of myofibrillar elements and their geometric rearrangement, in response to stimuli such as pressure and volume overload, and cardiac failure. In blood vessels they can induce changes in membrane receptors and channels, growth factor expression, and intracellular organelles in response to sustained increments of pressure and flow. Hence, cellular hyperplasia, hypertrophy, and various modifications can develop as adaptations to stress and injury. The expression of cell type-specific protein isoforms that allow these structural and functional diversities to occur derives from two broad mechanisms:

a. selection of a particular gene among the members of a multigene family for expression under particular conditions
b. generation of isoforms from a single gene by DNA rearrangement and alternative pre-mRNA splicing.

The latter is prevalent in the contractile genes of the myocardium and is regulated at the transcriptional level.[2] For example:

1. In the heart, in response to sustained pressure overload, the expression of genes controlling sarcomere renewal is modified to increase the number of sarcomeres in parallel.[3] Thus cardiac hypertrophy is achieved by increasing the thickness of myocardial cells. In contrast, in volume overload the programing of sarcomere renewal is predominantly modified to increase their number in series. Thus, under these circumstances, cardiac hypertrophy is achieved by increasing the length of myocardial cells.
2. In myocardial cells the proportion of fast (α) and slow (β) myosin heavy chain changes with age as well as with work overload.[4]
3. Myocardial ischemia increases both β[5] and α[6] adrenergic receptors, activates all gene expression of heat-shock proteins (which seem to have a broad protective effect against cellular injury)[7] and increases the production of the interstitial cell matrix.[8]
4. Vascular smooth muscle cells (SMCs) proliferate in the media in response to increased blood pressure; they also migrate into the intima and proliferate in response to a variety of noxious stimuli.[9]

Both the type and magnitude of the structural and functional changes depend on the intensity of the stimuli and on gene expression. Withdrawal of the stimuli may cause gene expression to revert to the previous mode, but some structural changes, once induced, may be partly or totally irreversible.

■ *Understanding the mechanisms that control gene expression could lead to therapeutic manipulation of the response of the heart and blood vessels to injury or abnormal working conditions and, eventually, to gene therapy.* ■

1.1.3 Cellular multiplication and renewal

In the adult organism, cell multiplication occurs from a proliferative cell phenotype. This phenotype:

a. can be constantly present in a specific form such as blood cell precursors (erythroblasts, myeloblasts, megakaryocytes)
b. can be reacquired by other types of cells such as smooth muscle and endothelial cells when they dedifferentiate, or by tumor cells
c. can be lost permanently after reaching the mature phenotype, as in neural and myocardial cells.

Tissues such as vascular endothelium and smooth muscle, in which cells can differentiate into a proliferative phenotype, are constantly renewed by replacement of cells that have completed their life span or have died because of tissue damage.

For example, endothelial cells have a life span of several years, but following endothelial denudation, proliferation of surrounding endothelial cells covers the denuded area within days. The life span of SMCs is of the order of years. Upon appropriate stimuli, they can migrate into the intima and multiply there, as their gene expression is modified in response to intracellular signaling and they acquire the proliferative phenotype from the adult contractile phenotype.

Tissues such as the myocardium that have lost the ability to reacquire the proliferative phenotype are renewed constantly by replacement of their structural and functional components.

1.2   INTER- AND INTRACELLULAR SIGNALING

The function of cells within an organ or tissue of the body is coordinated to provide optimal physiologic function; in turn, the function of various organs and tissues is coordinated to optimize the physiologic needs of the body. Generally, signals are carried by agonists that interact with cells, by binding to specific receptors. Following agonist binding to receptors, the signal is transduced in the cell membrane and within the cell by regulatory proteins and second messengers.

1.2.1   Intra- and interorgan cellular signaling

Communication between organs and tissues is provided by electrochemical and chemical signals carried, respectively, by nerves and by the bloodstream; that among cells within the same organ or tissue can be achieved by intercellular signaling. Cellular coordination (within organs and tissues) is provided by chemical agonists reaching the cells via the interstitial fluid. Myocardial cells and, to a lesser extent, vascular SMCs can be coordinated by both chemical and electrical signaling. Agonists reaching individual cells can be:

a. released by nerve terminals (neurotransmitters)
b. carried by the bloodstream from other organs and tissues (endocrine function)
c. produced by some cells of the organ or tissue (autacoids) acting on other cells of the
    same organ or tissue (paracrine function) or on the same cells (autocrine function)
    (see Fig. 1.1).

Autacoids are vasoactive molecules (locally produced in tissues and acting on the same
tissues) such as histamine, 5-hydroxytryptamine (5-HT), kinins, prostaglandins,
leukotrienes, and endothelial-derived relaxing and constricting factors.
    The agonists that bind to receptors are as diverse as amines (e.g. catecholamines, sero-
tonin), nucleosides (e.g. adenosine) or nucleotides, peptides (e.g. neuropeptides), and lipids
(e.g. prostaglandins) and their release may be triggered or prevented by nervous impulses,
by other agonists or by physical or chemical stimuli.

1.2.2 Receptor–agonist interaction

The term "receptor" refers to a protein molecule or molecular complex that is capable of
recognizing and binding specific transmitter substances and that, as a consequence of such
binding, produces a biologic effect. Receptors for neurotransmitters, for most humoral
transmitters, and for most drugs are located on the cell membrane, but receptors for gluco-

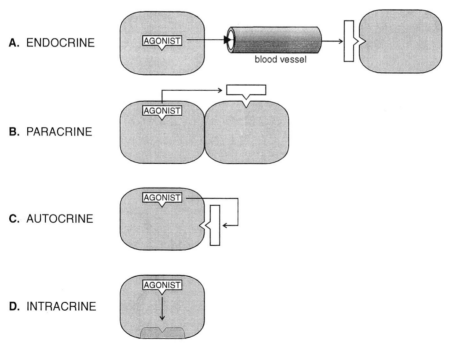

Fig. 1.1 Pathways of humoral intercellular signaling. A. The agonist enters the
circulation and produces its effects on the cells of target organs located at a distance
(endocrine function). **B.** After secretion, the agonist acts on receptors located on adjacent cells (paracrine function). **C.** After release, the agonist acts on receptors located
on the same cell (autocrine function). **D.** The agonist may also act within the cell of
origin (intracrine function). Hormones are secreted in the circulation and have an
endocrine function; autacoids have both paracrine and autocrine functions.

corticoids are located in the cytosol and those for thyroid hormones are located in the nucleus. Binding of the agonist (first messenger) to the receptor on the cell membrane produces the biologic effect by interacting with intermediary guanine nucleotides and G-proteins. These link the extracellular signal to membrane-bound effectors that may act as intracellular second messengers.

The receptor binds not only the specific agonist, but also a number of chemically related compounds that do not necessarily either have the same affinity for the receptor or produce identical changes in the activity of the cell. For example, the affinity for α- and β-adrenergic receptors varies considerably for a series of agonists (isoproterenol: only β, epinephrine: $\beta > \alpha$, norepinephrine: $\alpha < \beta$ in the periphery and $\beta < \alpha$ in the heart, phenylephrine: only α). The biologic effect of the same type of receptor binding to the same transmitter may be excitatory or inhibitory, depending on the type of cell on which the receptor is located, i.e. on its coupling to regulatory proteins. Receptor stimulation can be regulated at three main levels:

a. the number of receptors can vary, over a period of several minutes or hours (e.g. during ischemia—see below)
b. the affinity of the receptor for the transmitter can vary
c. the number of receptors available to the transmitter can be reduced by antagonists, which compete for the binding site with the transmitter but which, once bound, either produce no effect (no biologic intrinsic activity; complete antagonism) or have a lesser effect (partial agonism).

When agonists have the same intrinsic activity, their effects depend on the affinity of the agonist for the receptor. Antagonists, once bound, can be displaced by the agonist (competitive binding) or, less often, can occupy the site permanently (non-competitive binding) (see Fig. 1.2A, B).

On the basis of the degree of affinity for specific agonists and antagonists, subtypes of vascular and cardiac receptors for a variety of agonists have been identified that have different biologic effects and tissue distribution. Information on the tissue distribution and biologic effects of most vascular and myocardial receptors in humans is still scanty.

The biologic effect of receptor stimulation is then determined by the coupling of receptors with their transduction systems.

1.2.3 Intracellular signal transduction

Binding of agonists to membrane receptors generally activates G-proteins that reside in the cell membrane and couple several hormone receptors to ion channels and enzymes.[10]

Fig. 1.2 Relation between cellular response and agonist concentration. A. Agonists with a high affinity for the receptor produce their action at lower concentrations than agonists with a low affinity. The relation between agonists and effect is dose dependent and is described by a sigmoid curve. (The affinity is indicated by the ED_{50}, which is the dose that produces 50% maximum response.) Agonists with a high intrinsic activity produce a greater *maximal* response than agonists with a low intrinsic activity. Receptor ligands without an intrinsic activity block the receptor without producing a biologic effect. **B.** When blockers compete reversibly with the agonist for binding with the receptor (competitive binding), the dose–response curve of the agonist is progressively displaced to the right by higher doses of receptor blocker. Thus the relation between agonists and blockers is also dose dependent.

Curve	Affinity	Intrinsic activity
a	high	high
b	high	low
c	low	high
d	low	low

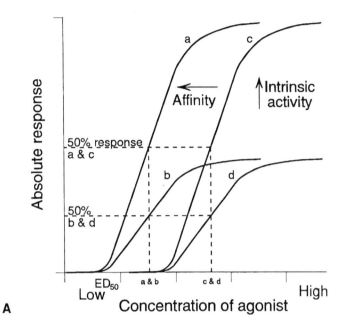

A

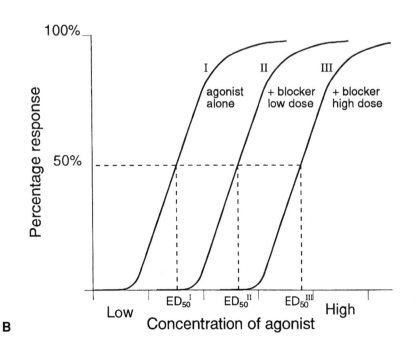

B

17

Various G-proteins have been identified, each coupling a receptor to a different intracellular enzyme or to an ion channel and each composed of three subunits (α, β, and γ). Upon binding of the agonist to the receptor, the α subunits of the G-protein bind to an effector system. One of the best-characterized transmitter–receptor interactions is that for β-adrenergic receptors (it can serve as a general example of receptor function and modulation); these receptors produce biologic effects by increasing the activity of adenylate cyclase, with a consequent increase in cyclic adenosine monophosphate (cAMP), which then acts as an intracellular stimulus (second messenger) for a number of reactions.

Desensitization of adrenergic receptors is not associated initially with reduction of receptor number, but with uncoupling between agonist–receptor binding and the stimulation of adenylate cyclase;[11] however, the synthesis of β-adrenergic receptors is reduced by chronic exposure to high doses of catecholamines (down-regulation)[12] and increased by hyperthyroidism (up-regulation), and the number of α and β receptors can increase rapidly following acute myocardial ischemia.[5,6]

Other G-protein–receptor interactions activate guanylate cyclase, with a consequent increase in cyclic guanosine monophosphate (cGMP); receptors for both angiotensin II and growth factors couple to phospholipase C, which generates inositol-1,4,5-triphosphate (IP_3) and diacylglycerol.[13]

1.3 BIOLOGY OF THE VESSEL WALL

The structural components of the vessel wall evolve during growth in order to perform specific functions in different segments of the vascular tree, arranged both in series and in parallel. Major differences in series are:

a.   the systolic expansion of the aorta and other elastic arteries, which can accommodate part of the stroke volume during systole
b.   the conductive function of muscular arteries, which can vary their caliber in proportion to flow
c.   the resistive function of arterioles, which can regulate organ blood flow
d.   the distributive function of capillaries, which can insure adequate blood–tissue delivery of oxygen
e.   the capacitance and conductive function of venules and veins, which enables blood to return to the heart under low distending pressure (see Ch. 3).

Some of the major differences in parallel are:

a.   the kidney circulation, with high basal flow rate and small variations in other physiologic conditions
b.   the skeletal muscle circulation, with a very low resting flow rate but major increases during work
c.   the coronary circulation, with high resting flow rate and major increases during work
d.   the skin circulation, with very low flow rate when body heat needs to be preserved and high flow when it needs to be dispersed.

■ *Such functional differentiation of blood vessels is likely to be associated with different biologic characteristics and different vasomotor and hemostatic responses. In addition, animal species that have developed specific functional vascular adaptations may exhibit different segmental and organ biologic, vasomotor and hemostatic responses. For these reasons, experimental findings in one type of vessel or in one species may not apply to other types of vessels or to other species.* ■

Within these limitations, a broad range of functions is largely common to the endothelial lining and vascular smooth muscle, which are the components of the wall that have received the greatest amount of attention in recent years. In elastic and muscular arteries (which are the site of atheroma formation) the possible importance of the adventitia, with its resident cells, of the blood supply and drainage, via vasa vasorum and lymphatics, has received scant attention.

1.3.1 Endothelial lining

In adults, endothelial cells occupy an area of about 1000 m² and weigh about 100 g. Until recently, the endothelium was considered to be merely an electronegative, passive barrier preventing contact of fluid and cellular elements of blood with the subendothelial matrix, thus preserving blood fluidity. It subsequently became apparent that mature endothelial cells have major (largely common) biologic functions; these include:

a. a metabolic function
b. a trophic function for the intimal and medial layers
c. a sensor–effector function for vasomotor control
d. an anticoagulant function.[14,15]

These functions may be variably represented in different types of vessels and in young, mature and senescent vessels. They can be altered, not only where there is endothelial denudation by injury (or freshly regenerated endothelium), but also by activation of the endothelium caused by inflammatory or immune stimuli.

Metabolic function

Endothelial cells have several metabolic properties, as follows:

1. They synthesize vasoactive compounds and adhesive molecules and synthesize and bind hemostatic factors (see below).
2. They contain angiotensin-converting enzyme which
   a. catalyzes the formation of angiotensin II from its inactive precursor angiotensin I
   b. inactivates bradykinin (a potent vasodilator).
3. They transport serotonin (5-HT) and adenosine intracellularly, both of which are then metabolized by monoamine oxidase and adenosine deaminase.
4. They contain angiotensinases, which inactivate angiotensin II.
5. They bind lipoprotein lipase, which is synthesized by SMCs and macrophages and which hydrolyzes very-low-density lipoproteins and chylomicrons.

These metabolic properties are not present equally in all endothelial cells: for example, arterial endothelial cells bind twice as much insulin as venous endothelial cells; angiotensin-converting enzymes and other enzymes are more active in pulmonary than in other systemic vessels.

Trophic function

Endothelial cells produce various types of collagen, as well as fibronectin, elastin, laminin, and mucopolysaccharides, which constitute the basement membrane and the normal inter-cellular intimal matrix. They can also produce collagenases capable of digesting the various types of collagen and thus of remodeling basement membranes. Like SMCs, activated endothelial cells can also produce cellular growth factors that stimulate smooth muscle and endothelial cell proliferation (see 1.3.2); they also secrete heparan sulfates that are heparin-like inhibitors of smooth muscle growth.

Vasoactive function

Endothelial cells produce vasoactive autacoids with paracrine function on SMCs (see Fig. 1.3A, B). These include:

a.   one or more endothelial-derived relaxing factor(s) (EDRF[s])
b.   prostacyclin (PGI$_2$)
c.   endothelin

EDRFs. EDRFs are released not only in response to a large number of agonists but also in response to pulsatile stretching and to wall shear stress; thus, blood vessels dilate, reducing their wall shear stress and resistance to flow when flow increases (see Chs 4 and 5).

In a variety of vessels and species, stimulation of normal endothelium by acetylcholine and by a variety of agonists triggers the release of a vasodilator substance, termed "endothelial-derived relaxing factor" by Furchgott and Zawadski.[16] This substance has a half-life of only a few seconds, which is curtailed by hemoglobin and methylene blue and prolonged by super-oxide dismutase. NO was shown to mimic closely these properties of EDRF and selective blockade of NO synthesis by a specific metabolic inhibitor blocks the effects of EDRF.[17] Thus, NO,[18] or an NO carrier molecule L-nitrosocysteine,[19] can be identified as an EDRF. NO is syn-thesized from L-arginine and synthesis is inhibited by metabolic arginine antagonists such as L-*N*-monomethyl-L-arginine (LNMMA). The release of NO is triggered by the interaction of a variety of agonists with specific receptors and the signal transduction from the receptor to the release of NO may differ. It is dependent on intracellular Ca^{2+} but is not reduced by Ca^{2+} antag-onists. NO is also synthesized by inflammatory cells and cells of the nervous system.[15] The mechanism of the vasodilator action of NO is similar to that of exogenous nitrovasodilator: it activates soluble guanylate cyclase with consequent production of cGMP.

There is strong evidence that NO exerts a tonic vasodilator effect on blood vessels, in that infusion of LNMMA causes hypertension in experimental animals and reduces blood flow in the human forearm, both effects being reversed by arginine.[20,21]

Under some conditions and in some vessels, endothelial cells can also release a different type of EDRF—endothelial-derived hyperpolarizing factor (EDHF)[22]—which causes smooth muscle relaxation by hyperpolarizing the cell membrane through the opening of potassium channels (see Ch. 5).

PGI$_2$. PGI$_2$ is a prostaglandin discovered a few years before EDRF: it has powerful vasodilator effects, it inhibits platelet aggregation by increasing cAMP activity,[15] and, together with thromboxane A$_2$ and leukotrienes, it is produced from arachidonic acid (AA) (see Fig. 1.4). Its half-life in plasma is about 10 s and it is broken down to 6-keto-prostaglandin F1α. PGI$_2$ generation is stimulated by pulsatile pressure and by bradykinin, thrombin, 5-HT, and platelet-derived growth factor (PDGF), which activate the enzyme phospholipase A. Its physiologic action is that of a local hormone rather than a circulating one; however, unlike NO, it does not have an obvious tonic hemodynamic effect, as block-ade of its synthesis by aspirin or indomethacin does not appreciably influence blood pres-sure, flow, or vasomotor tone. Thromboxane A$_2$, although generated in platelets and inflam-matory cells from the same precursor as PGI$_2$, has opposite effects of vasoconstriction and platelet aggregation.

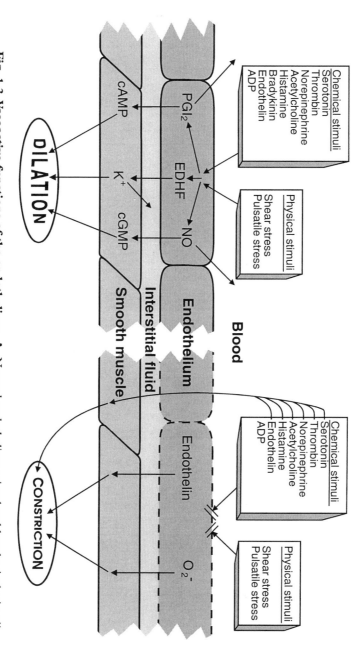

A NORMAL ENDOTHELIUM   **B** ACTIVATED ENDOTHELIUM

Fig. 1.3 Vasoactive functions of the endothelium. A. Normal endothelium stimulated by physical stimuli and by a variety of agonists produces vasodilator substances. In the presence of normal endothelium, the indirect vasodilator effect of substances such as serotonin and acetylcholine prevails at low doses and the direct vasoconstrictor effect prevails at high doses. EDHF, endothelial-derived hyperpolarizing factor; PGI_2, prostacyclin. **B.** Activated endothelium produces vasoconstrictor substances and leaves the direct smooth muscle constrictor action of some agonists unopposed.

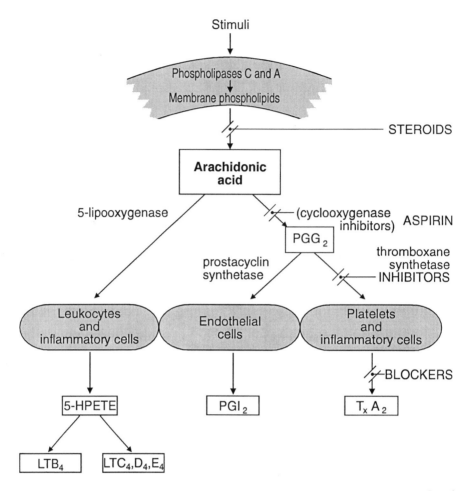

Fig. 1.4 Arachidonic acid (AA) pathways. The stimulation of phospholipases C and A leads to the production of AA (inhibited by steroids) from which different products can originate depending on the type of enzymes that prevail in different cells: AA is transformed into prostacyclin (PGI$_2$) in endothelial cells and into thromboxane A$_2$ (TxA$_2$) in platelets by cyclooxygenase (blocked by aspirin). AA is transformed into 5-hydroperoxyeicosatetraenoic acid (5-HPETE) and then into leukotrienes (LT) in both leukocytes and inflammatory cells by 5-lipooxygenase. When stimulated by adherent leukocytes, the endothelium can produce LT with vasoconstrictor and pro-inflammatory effects.

Endothelin. Under some conditions, endothelial cells can produce vasoconstrictor substances. The only one to be characterized is endothelin-1, a 21-amino acid peptide[23] derived from a longer peptide, "big" endothelin (which has only about 10% of the activity of endothelin), by the action of a converting enzyme. The conversion of "big" endothelin to endothelin-1 may occur in cells other than endothelial cells. It interacts with two types of receptors (ET$_A$ and ET$_B$) and activates phospholipase C. Although its half-life in plasma is only about 5 min, endothelin-1 has a very prolonged onset and duration of action.[24] Plasma levels in normal subjects are of the order of 1 pmol/l and much higher values have been reported in subjects with acute myocardial infarction (MI) and heart failure. It is not clear whether endothelin has a tonic physiologic function, but its release is reduced by NO and stimulated by thrombus and by interleukins.[25] Endothelial stimulation of smooth muscle contraction in response to hypoxia in some vascular beds does not seem to be caused by endothelin and could be due to superoxide production.[26]

Anticoagulant function

The surface of the endothelium is electronegative, thus repelling blood cells and platelets. Continuous production of NO prevents platelet adhesion and, together with PGI_2, reduces platelet aggregation. In addition, production and binding of anticoagulants by endothelial cells prevents the development of thrombosis at the normal blood/vessel-wall interface:[14]

1. Heparan sulfate is a locally produced endogenous heparin that remains bound to the cell surface and accelerates the inactivation of thrombin by plasma antithrombin III.
2. Thrombomodulin accelerates the activation of protein C by thrombin. Activated protein C inactivates factors V and VIII (with the interaction of protein S, also produced by endothelial cells). Thrombin bound to the complex protein C-thrombomodulin cannot activate platelets or cleave fibrinogen.
3. Normal endothelial cells secrete two plasminogen activators—a urokinase type (u-PA), which activates plasminogen in the fluid phase and a tissue type (t-PA), which is active only when bound to fibrin. They also produce an inhibitor of the plasminogen activators, plasminogen activator inhibitor-1 (PAI-1). Thrombin stimulates t-PA and u-PA secretion by endothelial cells, and activated protein C neutralizes PAI-1.

Thus, prevention of platelet adhesion, inactivation of thrombin, and lysis of fibrin prevent the formation and growth of thrombi on normal endothelium.

Activation of the endothelium

Interruption of the endothelial continuity not only removes all the anticoagulant and vasodilator functions of the endothelium but also exposes the subendothelium, which has several procoagulant functions such as adhesion of platelets to both von Willebrand's factor and collagen (with release of thromboxane A_2 and 5-HT leading to platelet aggregation) and exposure of tissue factor (TF), which activates factor VII. Thus, the physiologic response of the vessel wall to injury is local thrombus formation and vasoconstriction in order to prevent bleeding (see Figs 1.3A, B and 1.5A, B).

However, even without detectable histologic changes, the function of the endothelium can change from vasodilator to vasoconstrictor and from anticoagulant to procoagulant. Such changes can be induced by inflammatory or immune cytokines such as interleukin-1 (IL-1), tumor necrosis factor (TNF) and linfotoxin, and by granulocyte-released cathepsin G and elastase.[27,28]

Activation of the endothelium has several major effects:

1. It decreases the production of EDRFs and of PGI_2, hence reducing vasodilator, anti-adhesive and anti-aggregation platelet functions, and increases production of the powerful vasoconstrictor endothelin.
2. It increases the expression of adhesive receptors for leukocytes and platelets, and of receptors for platelet-activating factor (PAF).
3. It expresses TF on the luminal surface, thus activating factor VII.
4. It increases the production of PAI-1 and depresses that of plasminogen activators.
5. It may express Ia antigens; thus, endothelial cells can act as antigen-presenting cells.

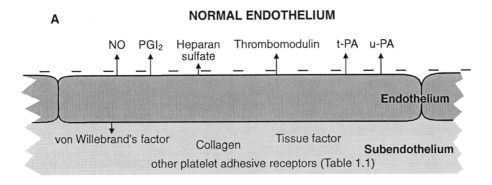

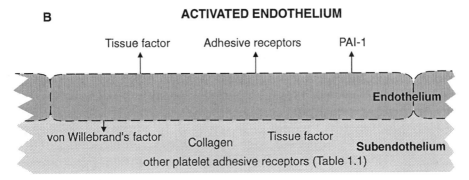

Fig. 1.5 Anticoagulant role of normal endothelium (A) and procoagulant role of activated endothelium (B). The anticoagulant properties are due to electronegative charges and to the production of nitric oxide (NO) (which antagonizes platelet adhesion), prostacyclin (PGI$_2$) (which antagonizes platelet aggregation), heparan sulfate (which catalyzes binding of antithrombin III to thrombin), thrombomodulin (which activates protein C), and tissue and urokinase plasminogen activators (t-PA and u-PA) (which activate plasminogen). Activation of the endothelium causes the loss of anticoagulant functions, the expression of adhesive receptors for leukocytes and platelets, the production of TF and endothelin, and a greatly enhanced production of PAI-1. The adhesion of leukocytes to activated endothelium results in the production of leukotrienes.

■ *Activation of the endothelium in epicardial coronary arteries sets the stage for local thrombosis and vasoconstriction.* ■

1.3.2. Smooth muscle coat

In muscular arteries and arterioles, the immediate physiologic adaptations of the vessel lumen to local and systemic hemodynamic needs are provided by physiologic changes in vasomotor tone, but adaptations to persistent hemodynamic changes or to pathologic stimuli involve substantial biologic changes in SMCs. The notion that the function of SMCs is not restricted to the mechanical regulation of vessel caliber is important because they comprise the most abundant cell type in the arterial wall. Proliferation and hyperplasia of the media take place in arterial hypertension; SMC migration into the intima, with proliferation and intercellular matrix production, is a major common response to physical, chemical and inflammatory stimuli.[9]

Smooth muscle cells produce and digest extracellular matrix and have the potential to produce angiotensin-II and growth factors such as PDGF, which can cause proliferation of dedifferentiated SMCs and contraction of mature cells. They also release inflammatory cytokines such as IL-1 and TNF.[28]

Extracellular matrix production and digestion

Smooth muscle cells are the main source of the extracellular matrix (collagens, elastin, glycoproteins [GP], and proteoglycans) into which SMCs are embedded. They can also produce enzymes involved in the fibrinolytic balance controlling extracellular matrix digestion and hence cell migration, multiplication, and vascular wall remodeling.[29]

Production of and response to mitogens and vasoconstrictors

Smooth muscle cells have paracrine and autocrine functions because they produce mediators that can cause contraction or growth of adjacent cells, as well as of the same cells.

Some mitogens and vasoconstrictors have a common signal transduction pathway by being coupled to diacylglycerol generation and protein kinase C activation. The vasoconstrictor or proliferative effect in response to growth factors such as PDGF and to constrictor factors such as angiotensin-II and 5-HT depends on the SMC phenotype: cells in the proliferative phenotype respond with increased protein synthesis and proliferation, and cells in the mature contractile phenotype respond with contraction.[30] There is suggestive evidence that, in atheroma, cell clones may acquire an independent proliferative capacity (as in benign tumors) (see Ch. 8).

Source and targets of inflammatory mediators

IL-1 and TNF produced by macrophages, SMCs, or endothelial cells are active on both endothelial cells and SMCs themselves: SMCs represent the potentially largest source and target because of their greater cellular mass in the vessel wall.[31]

■ *Alterations of SMCs resulting in an enhanced constrictor response to vasoactive stimuli and/or cytokine production may set the stage for coronary vasoconstriction, spasm, and thrombosis, and for a proliferative response when the cells are in a proliferative phenotype.* ■

1.3.3 Adventitia

The adventitia is the interface of the vessel wall with the perivascular fluid and its thickness is proportional to the size of the vessel. Thus, in larger vessels the adventitia is supplied with vasa vasorum and lymphatic channels. It is composed of loose connective tissue with sparse indwelling cells and abundant intercellular matrix providing a sheet supporting perivascular nerves, as well as vasa vasorum and lymphatics for arteries. The network of vasa vasorum increases very considerably at the site of atherosclerotic plaques, but no information is available on the role or the adaptive changes of lymphatic vessels. Indwelling inflammatory cells infiltrating the surrounding nerve structures are also abundant at the site of atherosclerotic lesions, but the cause and consequences of such infiltrates have not been investigated appropriately. Cells residing in the adventitia can release a variety of powerful substances: mast cells can release histamine, which has a powerful dilator effect on small vessels, but can have a constrictor effect on larger vessels; mast cells, eosinophils, monocytes, granulocytes and macrophages can synthesize and release leukotrienes (metabolites of AA, with powerful chemotactic [LTB_4], inflammatory and vasoconstrictor [LTD_4, LTC_4 and LTE_4] effects) as well as thromboxane A_2 and other prostaglandins and interleukins.

On the arterial side of the circulation, the main function of the adventitia is that of favoring the elimination of substances diffusing into the wall from the bloodstream or produced locally and, for larger arteries, of providing oxygen and nutrients to the media through vasa vasorum.

Banding of a proximal segment of epicardial coronary artery with a loose cellophane layer causes intense smooth muscle proliferation, matrix production, and intimal thickening, a response similar to that observed following endothelial denudation (see Ch. 8). This intense proliferative reaction can be caused only by impairment of the mechanisms by which substances are normally removed from the vessel wall and/or by ischemia of the wall. Although the actual mechanism has not yet been elucidated, this observation suggests that the adventitia may have a role in the development of focal proliferative lesions in the vessel wall see Ch. 8).

1.4 THE BLOOD/VESSEL-WALL INTERACTION IN THROMBOSIS

Arterial thrombosis is a common, ultimate cause of MI, stroke and peripheral vascular disease. Nevertheless, these ischemic events are not only very rare, even in patients with extensive atherosclerosis, but they also occur unexpectedly. Precisely why and how a thrombotic event happens at a particular time in the life of an individual is unknown. In order to develop rational forms of therapy and prevention it is important to understand why and how the physiologic hemostatic process, designed to initiate a repair process of acute vessel damage, can itself become a mechanism of disease. The vast majority of arterial thrombi are mostly rich in platelets (white thrombi), held together by a variable amount of fibrin mesh; those (red) thrombi that are rich in red cells and fibrin, and which are the most common on the venous side, are rare and are usually associated with blood flow stasis (see Ch. 9). In general, the size of an arterial thrombus depends on the following:

a. the thrombogenicity of the arterial lesion
b. the hemodynamic effects of flow
c. the reactivity of the hemostatic system.

■ *Thus, the mechanisms that determine the evolution of thrombosis from a physiologic repair process to a mechanism of disease may be multiple.* ■

This section presents a broad outline of the following:

a. local thrombogenicity and hemodynamic effects of flow
b. platelet adhesion and aggregation
c. generation of thrombin
d. formation, limitation and lysis of thrombi
e. prothrombotic states.

1.4.1 Local thrombogenicity and hemodynamic effects of flow

A single monolayer of platelets adheres to the subendothelium following gentle denudation of normal arterial endothelium, but multiple layers deposit over a deeper or a repeated injury. More intense thrombogenic stimuli, such as grafts of nonbiocompatible segments of artery, lead to rapid and complete thrombotic occlusion of the vessel.

The arterial flow pattern is characterized by displacement of platelets towards the wall; thus, substances released by activated species of platelets may be concentrated and retained in the vessel wall. Stenoses are thought to enhance platelet interaction with the vessel wall, but common clinical observations suggest that this may not necessarily be the case because, in many stable patients, flow-limiting atherosclerotic plaques remain stable and elicit no signs or symptoms of myocardial ischemia for months or even years (see Ch. 9). The absence of thrombogenic effects of chronic critical coronary stenoses may be due to the absence of local thrombogenic activation in chronic lesions and to the increased velocity of flow (which removes and dilutes activated platelets and coagulation activation products). Thus, in the absence of a marked local thrombogenicity, it is difficult for a mural thrombus to become occlusive until flow is interrupted or retarded, for the following reasons:

a. platelet clusters are broken and carried downstream
b. activated coagulation factors are continuously diluted
c. fibrinolytic factors are continuously supplied.

However, when the local thrombogenicity is intense or flow is ultimately arrested (because of the growth of the thrombus or because of local or distal vasoconstriction), blood distal and proximal to the occlusion becomes stagnant, giving rise to a red-cell-rich thrombus.

1.4.2 Platelet adhesion and aggregation

The composition of arterial thrombi, in which platelets predominate, indicates that these blood elements play a fundamental part in the initiation and progression of arterial mural thrombosis. The formation of platelet thrombi occurs in three steps—platelet adhesion, activation, and release reaction with amplification of the reaction. Coming into contact with subendothelial structures, macrophages, activated leukocytes, and endothelial cells activated by inflammatory cytokines, platelets adhere through the expression of membrane integrins, a family of GP that act as receptors on the platelet membrane. These receptors are specific for each component of the extracellular matrix (see Table 1.1). The main subendothelial adhesive protein is represented by von Willebrand factor.

Platelet adhesion is followed by platelet activation and degranulation through the release reaction that causes amplification of platelet activation (see Fig. 1.6). The release reaction products, 5-HT, thromboxane A_2, adenosine diphosphate (ADP) and PAF, are potent independent but interacting agonists in the activation of platelets. The most potent platelet activator is thrombin, followed by collagen, thromboxane A_2 and ADP. At physiologic concentrations, 5-HT, and epinephrine promote platelet aggregation in combination with the other agents.

Activated platelets aggregate through the attachment of GP IIb–IIIa receptors to fibrinogen strands. (The deficit of GP IIb-IIIa causes the syndrome of thromboasthenia, a severe bleeding disorder.) Activated platelets are stimulated to contract and release the content of dense granules (ADP, 5-HT), α-granules (platelet factor 4 [PF_4]) and β-thromboglobulin [βTG], both of which have antiheparin action, adhesive and coagulant proteins, as well as PDGF (which stimulates cellular growth or causes smooth muscle contraction) and transforming growth factor β (TGFβ) (which inhibits proliferation and migration of SMCs). The activation of phospholipase-C and phospholipase A_2 liberates AA from the membrane phospholipids, which metabolize to PGI_2 and thromboxane A_2 (see Fig. 1.4). Aggregated platelets provide a necessary membrane support for the initiation of coagulation, as

Table 1.1 Platelet membrane glycoproteins mediating adhesion and aggregation

Glycoprotein receptors	Ligands
Adhesion	
Ib–IX	von Willebrand factor*, thrombin
Ia–IIa	Collagen
Ic–IIa	Fibronectin
Vitronectin receptor	Vitronectin, von Willebrand factor, fibronectin, fibrinogen, thrombospondin
IV (GP IIIb)	Thrombospondin, collagen
Aggregation	
IIb–IIIa	Fibrinogen†, von Willebrand factor, fibronectin, thrombospondin, vitronectin

*von Willebrand factor is the main adhesive ligand for platelets: its absence causes von Willebrand disease. The other adhesive proteins have modulatory roles unless von Willebrand factor is absent or reduced
†Fibrinogen is the main aggregating ligand

described below. Platelets can also modulate fibrinolysis as they carry the inhibitor of fibrinolysis, PAI-1.

1.4.3 Generation of thrombin

The generation of thrombin is the final, critical step in the activation of coagulation because thrombin is responsible for the formation of insoluble fibrin from its soluble precursor fibrinogen. The source of thrombin is the activation of factor X within the prothrombinase complex via the intrinsic and extrinsic coagulation pathways. Selective limitation of thrombin generation at the site of vascular injury is determined by:

a. the factors that localize the reaction on a supporting surface
b. its rapid inactivation in flowing blood.

The formation of coagulation enzymes is regulated by the interaction of an inactive enzyme or zymogen (such as factors VII, X, IX, or prothrombin), an active converting enzyme or serine protease (such as activated factors VIIa, Xa, IXa, or thrombin) and a cofactor—required to localize the reaction on a supporting surface—(such as TF, and factors V or VIII), which must form a multimolecular complex on an appropriate natural surface (activated platelets, white blood cells, and activated endothelial cells).[32]

Thus schematically, the activation of coagulation proceeds in three main phases:

1. The conversion of prothrombin to thrombin results from the prothrombinase complex (factor Xa, factor Va, phospholipid surface, and Ca^{2+}) acting on prothrombin: the formation of factor Xa results from the intrinsic factor X-ase complex (factor IXa and factor VIII+Ca) or from the extrinsic factor X-ase complex (factor VIIa and TF) (see Fig. 1.7).
2. Thrombin formed from the prothrombinase complex interacts with fibrinogen to produce fibrin monomers, but can be neutralized by the antithrombin–heparin complex or by binding to thrombomodulin (see Fig. 1.8).
3. Fibrin monomers formed by the action of thrombin on fibrinogen polymerize to form soluble fibrillar strands of fibrin. Thrombin-activated factor XIII (factor XIIIa) stabilizes fibrin by cross-linking fibrin strands.

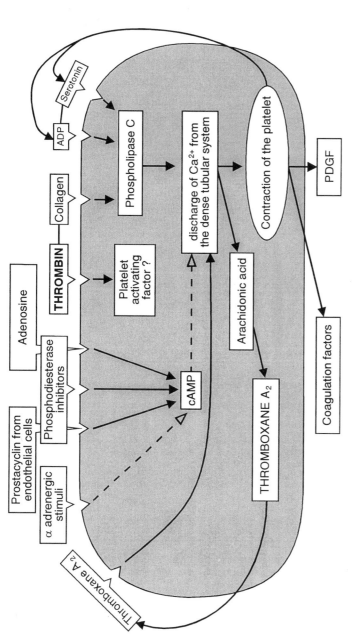

Fig. 1.6 Activation of platelets that leads to their contraction and aggregation. Thrombin is by far the most important physiologic activator, followed by collagen; ADP and serotonin have modulatory roles. The stimulation of $Ca^{2(+)}$ discharge from the dense tubular system leads to contraction of the platelet, with extrusion of secretory granules, and to production of thromboxane A_2 (which has a positive feedback on Ca^{2+} discharge), platelet-derived growth factor (PDGF), and coagulation factors. Platelet activation is inhibited by prostacyclin, adenosine, and phosphodiesterase inhibitors, which increase the levels of cyclic adenosine monophosphate (cAMP), and is favored by α-adrenergic stimulation, which lowers the levels of cAMP. Aggregated platelets represent one of the macromolecular surfaces that localizes coagulation factors. Thus, thrombin formation (due to a primary activation of the intrinsic or extrinsic coagulation pathways) and primary platelet activation can initiate the hemostatic and thrombotic chains of event.

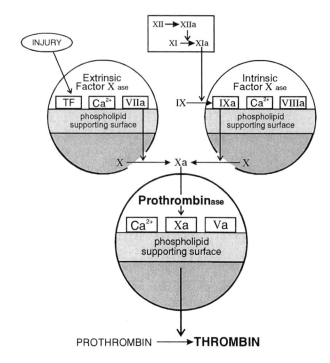

Fig. 1.7 Main steps in the coagulation cascade. The scheme illustrates the importance of the binding of the Xase and prothrombinase complexes to the same biologic phospholipid supporting surface, which is essential for both the localization and amplification of the reactions. TF, factor VIII, and factor V are responsible, respectively, for the binding of (a) the extrinsic factor X activation complex (extrinsic Xase), (b) the intrinsic factor X activation complex (intrinsic Xase), and (c) the prothrombinase complex. The principal positive and negative feedback mechanisms of these reactions are represented in Figures 1.8 and 1.9.

The binding of the multimolecular complexes to the natural surfaces, mediated by cofactors V and VIII, leads to:

a. a dramatic acceleration of the reaction (which becomes several orders of magnitude faster than in the fluid phase of blood)
b. the localization of thrombus formation.

It also protects critical activating factors, generated within the macromolecular complexes within the thrombus, from inactivation by potent plasma inhibitors that are active in flowing blood (i.e. antithrombin III, α_2-macroglobulin, α_1-antitrypsin).

These enzymatic reactions either are accelerated by positive feedback produced by activator factors on their own activation (both factor Xa and thrombin increase their own formation rates by catalyzing the activation of factors V and VII, respectively) (see Fig. 1.9), or are suppressed if:

a. the converting enzyme is inhibited (such as the inhibition of thrombin by antithrombin)
b. the cofactor is inactivated (such as the inactivation of factors Va and VIIIa by protein C)
c. the surface receptors essential for the assembly of the macromolecular complex are either sequestered or inhibited (such as the lack of expression of TF in non-activated endothelium) by the lipoprotein-associated coagulation inhibitor.[33]

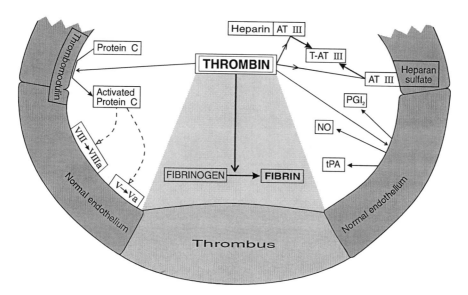

Fig. 1.8 Multiple effects of thrombin. In addition to its main effects of activating platelets and transforming fibrinogen to fibrin, thrombin has several effects that control the coagulation process: it stimulates production of prostacyclin (PGI_2), nitric oxide (NO), and tissue plasminogen activator (t-PA) by normal endothelium; it binds to antithrombin III (ATIII) through endothelium-bound heparan sulfate and through heparin in the fluid phase, and it activates protein C (through thrombomodulin) which inactivates factors Va and VIIIa on normal endothelium.

For example, on the one hand thrombin is inhibited by antithrombin III (which also inhibits factors IXa, Xa, XIa, and XIIa) and the thrombin–antithrombin reaction rate is accelerated several orders of magnitude when antithrombin III binds to heparin sulfates on the endothelial surface or to heparin in the fluid phase (see Fig. 1.10). On the other hand, thrombin exerts a negative feedback on the coagulation system of adjacent normal endothelium by:

a. binding to thrombomodulin (because thrombomodulin activates protein C, which in turn inactivates factors Va and VIIIa)
b. stimulating the release of NO and PGI_2 (see Fig. 1.8). Thrombin can be inhibited by hirudin, an anticoagulant produced by leeches (now being tested in clinical trials).

The rate of thrombin generation can be evaluated indirectly by measurement of the following:

a. the fragment cleaved during transformation of prothrombin to thrombin, prothrombin fragment 1 + 2 (F_{1+2})
b. the peptide cleaved by the action of thrombin on fibrinogen, fibrinopeptide A (FPA)
c. the binding of thrombin to antithrombin III, to form thrombin–antithrombin III complexes (T–AT).

Blood levels of these markers of thrombin formation provide information on the intensity of thrombin generation and also help in dating the time at which it occurs. For example, levels of FPA and T–AT, each with a half-life of 5 min, can remain elevated after a burst of thrombin generation occurring up to about 25 min earlier, whereas levels of F_{1+2}, with a half-life of about 90 min, can remain elevated up to 9 h after the burst of thrombin generation.

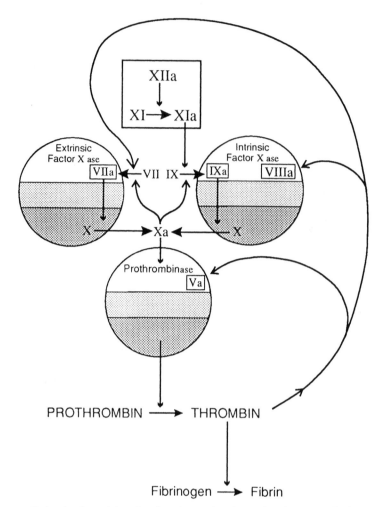

Fig. 1.9 Principal positive feedback mechanisms in the coagulation cascade.
Factor Xa activates factors VII and IX; thrombin activates factors V, VIIa, and VIII.

1.4.4 Formation of fibrin and localization, limitation and lysis of thrombus

Following the generation of fibrin monomers by the action of thrombin on fibrinogen, polymerization and cross-linking take place with formation of a fibrin mesh. Stabilization of the fibrin mesh by cross-linking occurs in the presence of factor XIIIa, derived from factor XIII and activated by thrombin (see Fig. 1.11). The formation of fibrin from fibrinogen is confined to the site of vessel wall injury by a number of mechanisms:

1. The binding to a biologic surface of the macromolecular complex that initiates the intrinsic and extrinsic pathways that activate factor X (intrinsic and extrinsic X-ase) and subsequently of the prothrombinase complex, leads to the localization of the thrombus. Locally formed thrombin activates platelets and generates fibrin.
2. Confinement of thrombus to the site of injury is also favored by the following:

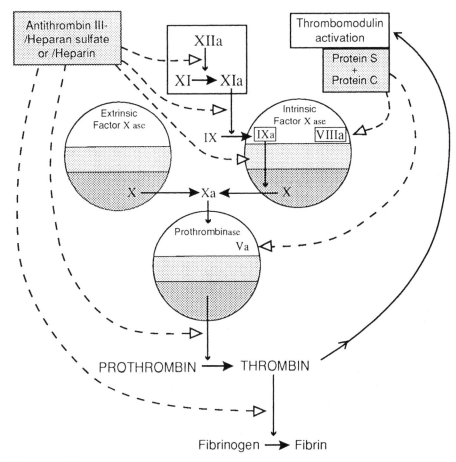

Fig. 1.10 Principal negative feedback mechanisms in the coagulation cascade.
Thrombin binding to thrombomodulin on normal endothelium activates the protein
C/protein S complex (which inactivates factors Va and VIIIa); heparin and heparan sulfate binding to antithrombin III inactivates factors XIIa, XIa, and IXa and also inactivates thrombin and fibrin formation.

   a.   stimulation on adjacent normal endothelium of NO and PGI_2 production
   b.   heparin sulfate
   c.   thrombin activation of thrombomodulin and of t-PA release.
3. The propagation of thrombus is limited by dilution of activated coagulation factors in
    flowing blood, by inactivators triggered by the thrombus, such as protein C (which
    inactivates factors Va and VIIIa), and by plasmin (which digests fibrin) (see Fig. 1.12).
4. Fibrin binds coagulation and fibrinolysis factors that facilitate both thrombus growth
    and thrombus lysis:
   a.   thrombin bound to fibrin is protected from inactivation by heparin–antithrombin
       III complexes; thus, thrombin bound to fibrin may continue to mediate platelet
       activation and fibrin formation in spite of heparin or thrombolytic therapy
   b.   binding to fibrin of plasminogen and of t-PA (normally produced by endothelial
       cells and stimulated by thrombin) greatly increases the activation of plasmino-
       gen.

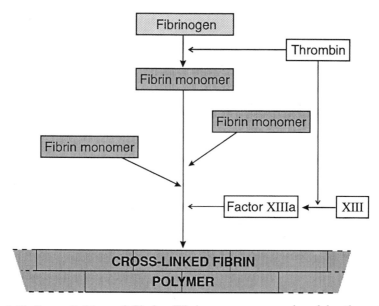

Fig. 1.11 Cross-linking of fibrin. Fibrin monomers produced by the action of thrombin on fibrinogen are cross-linked by factor XIII activated by thrombin.

The local formation of plasmin from plasminogen localizes the lysis of fibrin to the very site of the thrombus, thus modulating its growth and contributing to its limitation. Plasminogen can be activated by the circulating activator u-PA and by circulating t-PA; both u-PA and t-PA are inhibited by the circulating inhibitor PAI-1. Circulating PAI-1 production is increased by activation of the endothelium but PAI-1 is also contained in platelets in considerable amounts and is, therefore, present within thrombi. Because of the fibrin binding of t-PA, plasmin is formed locally and is confined to the vicinity of the thrombus without significant escape into the bloodstream. Thus, the localization of plasmin formation is insured by:

a. the enhanced release of t-PA from adjacent normal endothelium by thrombin
b. the fibrin specificity of t-PA
c. the inactivation of free circulating plasmin by α_2-antiplasmin
d. the inhibition of excess circulating t-PA by circulating PAI-1.

1.4.5 Prothrombotic states

The physiologic response to acute vascular injury culminates in two simultaneous and mutually amplifying processes:

a. adhesion, activation, and aggregation of platelets
b. the rapid generation of thrombin, resulting from the local activation of the intrinsic and extrinsic activation of factor X by the specific X-ase complexes.

The concept of a prothrombotic state implies that the physiologic response of the hemostatic system to local injury is enhanced and probably leads to the more rapid development of larger thrombi. Although hypercoagulant states associated with some specific defect in natural anticoagulant mechanisms are known,[34] the concept of a prothrombotic state as a common predisposing factor to arterial thrombosis is still ill-defined.[35]

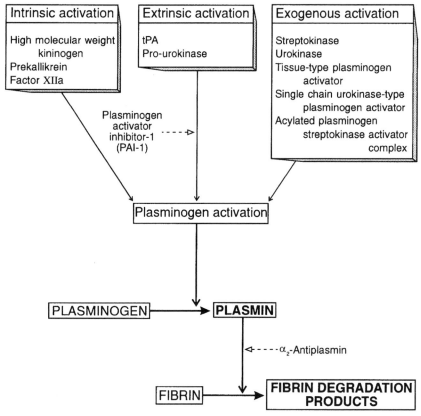

Fig. 1.12 Degradation of fibrin by plasmin. Plasminogen can be activated by intrinsic, extrinsic, and exogenous activators. The role of intrinsic activation is normally a minor one. Tissue plasminogen activator (t-PA) and pro-urokinase are inhibited by PAI-1. Plasmin is inhibited by antiplasmin.

Intense vascular injury can rapidly cause occlusive arterial thrombosis even in the presence of a perfectly normal hemostatic equilibrium (see Ch. 6). However, lesser injuries may lead to total occlusion only when the balance of the hemostatic system is tipped towards thrombosis (prothrombotic state). This tipping of the balance towards thrombosis may result from increased adhesiveness and aggregation of platelets and/or a defective modulation of the coagulation cascade.

Increased platelet adhesiveness and aggregation

Increased platelet aggregation ex vivo, decreased platelet survival, and increased plasma levels of platelet-released products have been reported in patients with arterial ischemic syndromes. However, the large variation in platelet responses ex vivo to aggregating agents in normal individuals, and the possibility that increased platelet activation in individuals with ischemic arterial disease represents a physiologic rather than a pathologic response to acute and chronic vessel-wall damage, prevent firm conclusions being made. The evidence that the presence of larger platelets is associated with an increased risk of ischemic heart disease (IHD) (see Ch. 12) is compatible with the hypothesis of a platelet-derived prothrombotic state, but the observed correlation could have been mediated through other unidentified variables such as subclinical inflammatory states or abnormal immunoreactivity.

■ *The study of the pathogenetic role of enhanced platelet reactivity in cardiac ischemic events is not easy because, when present, it may occur only before the event takes place (a few days or weeks) or it may involve only a minority of platelets—sufficient, however, to trigger the adhesion and activation of normal platelets at critical moments.* ■

Defective modulation of the coagulation cascade

The normal mechanisms that turn on the coagulation cascade are extremely powerful, and it is unlikely that they could be further enhanced. It would seem more likely that a prothrombotic state could result from defects in the equally powerful mechanisms that turn off thrombosis (a single molecule of activating factor may give rise to 1000 molecules of the next protease in the cascade, but 999 of them are immediately inactivated) and that activate fibrinolysis.

The negative feedback mechanisms of the coagulation cascade regulate three types of protein transformation:

a. generation of serine proteases (inhibition by antithrombin not only of factor Xa and of thrombin but also of factors IXa, XIa, and XIIa)
b. production of activated cofactors (inhibition by protein C of factors Va and VIIIa, following binding of thrombin to thrombomodulin)
c. degradation of fibrin (activation of plasminogen by plasminogen activators) (see Figs 1.10 and 1.12).

■ *Each of these three main mechanisms can be internally modulated at intermediate steps.* ■

The state of activation of thrombosis can not be assessed by measuring the plasma concentrations of inactive enzymes, converting enzymes, or cofactors as, under normal conditions, their levels do not influence the reaction rate. Conversely, the plasma concentration of their cleavage reaction products (each of which has a finite life in plasma) provides some indications of the rate at which the system is activated. Thus, for example (as discussed in 1.4.3), the rate of formation of thrombin from prothrombin can be assessed from the plasma levels of prothrombin fragment 1 + 2 (F_{1+2}), fibrinopeptide A, and thrombin–antithrombin (T–AT) complexes; the rate of activation of protein C can be assessed from the plasma levels of protein C activation peptide (PCP). According to the same principle, the activation of the fibrinolytic system can be assessed from fibrin degradation products and from the plasmin–antiplasmin (PAP) complex.

Deficiency of proteins C and S and antithrombin is often associated with persisting enhancement of the formation of thrombin (as assessed by cleavage reaction products) and with venous, rather than arterial, thrombosis, and has been found to be associated with enhanced activity of the hemostatic system. A similar increase in thrombin formation in vivo has been reported in normal elderly individuals, but this may be a reflection of increased concurrent vascular damage and repair processes.[36]

An increased PAI-1 activity in young patients after MI was found to be predictive of the occurrence of successive ischemic events, but this relation could be an indirect one as PAI-1 is one of the acute-phase reaction proteins. The significant value of high levels of fibrinogen and factor VII for predicting IHD events would seem to contradict the line of reasoning presented above, but the relationship with fibrinogen and factor VII levels could also be an indirect one as they may be correlated with other long-acting causal factors (see Ch. 12). The possible role of the TF pathway inhibitor[33] is under consideration.

■ *Study of the possible pathogenetic role of prothrombotic states in cardiac ischemic events is not easy for the following reasons:*

a.   *they may result from multiple mechanisms*
b.   *they may present only a few days or even hours before the event*
c.   *they may have a significant pathogenetic role in some patients, but not in others.* ■

REFERENCES

1. Corral-Debrinski M, Stepien G, Shoffner JM, Lott MT, Kanter K, Wallace DC. Hypoxemia is associated with mitochondrial DNA damage and gene induction: Implications for cardiac disease. J Am Med Ass 1991;*266:*1812.
2. Breitbart RE, Andreadis A, Nadal-Ginard B. Alternative splicing: A ubiquitous mechanism for the generation of multiple protein isoforms from single genes. Ann Rev Biochem 1987;*56:*467.
3. Hirzel HO, Tuckschmid CR, Schneider J et al. Relationship between myosin isoenzyme composition, hemodynamics, and myocardial structure in various forms of human cardiac hypertrophy. Circ Res 1985;*57:*729.
4. Schwartz K, Lecarpentier Y, Martin JL et al. Myosin isoenzymic distribution correlates with speed of myocardial contraction. J Mol Cell Cardiol 1981;*13:*1071.
5. Maisel AS, Motulsky HJ, Insel PA. Externalization of β-adrenergic receptors promoted by myocardial ischemia. Science 1985;*230:*183.
6. Heathers GP, Yamada KA, Kanter EM, Corr PB. Long-chain acylcarnitines mediate the hypoxia-induced increase in α-adrenergic receptors in adult canine cardiac myocytes. Circ Res 1987;*61:*735.
7. Currie RW, Karmazyn M, Kloc M, Mailer K. Heat-shock response is associated with enhanced postischemic ventricular recovery. Circ Res 1988;*63:*543.
8. Zhao M, Zhang H, Robinson TF, Factor SM, Sonnenblick EH, Eng C. Profound structural alterations of the extracellular collagen matrix in postischemic dysfunctional ("stunned") but viable myocardium. J Am Coll Cardiol 1987;*10:*1322.
9. Gordon D, Reidy MA, Benditt EP, Schwartz SM. Cell proliferation in human coronary arteries. Proc Natl Acad Sci USA 1990;*87:*4600.
10. Freissmuth M, Casey PJ, Gilman AG. G proteins control diverse pathways of transmembrane signaling. FASEB J 1989;*3:*2125.
11. Lefkowitz RJ, Caron MG. Adrenergic receptors: models for the study of receptors coupled to guanine nucleotide regulatory proteins. J Biol Chem 1988;*263:*4993.
12. Hadcock JR, Malbon CC. Down-regulation of β-adrenergic receptors: agonist-induced reduction in receptor mRNA levels. Proc Natl Acad Sci USA 1988;*85:*5021.
13. Churchill WC. Angiotensin II: Hemodynamic regulator or growth factor? J Mol Cell Cardiol 1990;*22:*739.
14. Jaffe EA. Cell biology of endothelial cells. Hum Pathol 1987;*18:*234.
15. Vane JR, Anggard EE, Botting RM. Regulatory functions of the vascular endothelium. New Engl J Med 1990;*323:*27.
16. Furchgott RF, Zawadski JV. The obligatory role of endothelial cells in the relaxation of arterial smooth muscle by acetylcholine. Nature 1980;*288:*373.
17. Palmer RM, Ashton DS, Moncada S. Vascular endothelial cells synthesize nitric oxide from L-arginine. Nature 1988;*333:*664.
18. Moncada S. The L-arginine-nitric oxide pathway. Acta Physiol Scand 1992;*145:*201.
19. Myers PR, Minor RL, Guerra R Jr, Bates JN, Harrison DG. Vasorelaxant properties of the endothelium-derived relaxing factor more closely resemble S-nitrosocysteine than nitric oxide. Nature 1990;*345:*161.
20. Rees DD, Palmer RM, Moncada S. Role of endothelium-derived nitric oxide in the regulation of blood pressure. Proc Natl Acad Sci USA 1989;*86:*3375.

21. Vallance P, Collier J, Moncada S. Effects of endothelium-derived nitric oxide on peripheral arteriolar tone in man. Lancet 1989;*2*:997.
22. Feletou M, Vanhoutte PM. Endothelium-dependent hyperpolarization of canine coronary smooth muscle. Br J Pharmacol 1988;*93*:515.
23. Yanagisawa M, Kurihara H, Kimura S et al. A novel potent vasoconstrictor peptide produced by vascular endothelial cells. Nature 1988;*332*:411.
24. Clarke JG, Benjamin N, Larkin SW et al. Endothelin is a potent long-lasting vasoconstrictor in man. Am J Physiol 1989;*257*:(Heart Circ Physiol *26*):H2033.
25. Miyauchi T, Yanagisawa M, Tomizawa T et al. Increased plasma concentrations of endothelin-1 and big endothelin-1 in acute myocardial infarction. Lancet 1989;*2*:53.
26. Vanhoutte PM, Shimokawa H. Endothelium-derived relaxing factor and coronary vasospasm. Circulation 1989;*80*:1.
27. Stern DM, Kaiser E, Nawroth P. Regulation of the coagulation system by vascular endothelial cells. Haemostasis 1988;*18*:202.
28. Bevilacqua MP, Gimbrone MA. Inducible endothelial functions in inflammation and coagulation. Seminars in Thrombosis and Hemostasis 1987;*13*:425.
29. Sperti G, Van Leeuwen R, Quax P, Maseri A, Kluft C. Cultured rat aortic vascular smooth muscle cells digest naturally produced extracellular matrix: involvement of plasminogen-dependent and plasminogen-independent pathways. Circ Res 1992;*71*:385.
30. Berk BC, Alexander RW, Brock TA, Gimbrone MA Jr, Webb RC. Vasoconstriction: A new activity for platelet-derived growth factor. Science 1986;*232*:87.
31. Libby P, Ordovas JM, Birynyi LK, Auger KR, Dinarello CA. Inducible interleukin 1 expression in human vascular smooth muscle cells. J Clin Invest 1986;*78*:1432.
32. Mann KG, Nesheim ME, Church WR, Haley P, Krishnaswamy S. Surface-dependent reactions of the vitamin K-dependent enzyme complexes. J Am Soc Hematol 1990;*76*:1.
33. Broze GJ Jr, Warren LA, Novotny WF, Higuchi DA, Girard JJ, Miletich JP. The lipoprotein-associated coagulation inhibitor which inhibits the factor VII-tissue factor complex also inhibits factor Xa: insight into its possible mechanisms of action. Blood 1988;*71*:335.
34. Bauer KA, Rosenberg RD. The pathophysiology of the prethrombotic state in humans: insights gained from studies using markers of hemostatic system activation. Blood 1987;*70*:343.
35. Hirsh J. Hypercoagulability. Semin Hematol 1977;*14*:409.
36. Bauer KA, Weiss LM, Sparrow D, Vokonas PS, Rosenberg RD. Aging associated changes in indices of thrombin generation and protein C activation in humans. J Clin Invest 1987;*80*:1527.

CHAPTER	# The pump function of the heart, as affected by IHD
2	

INTRODUCTION

The earliest and most obvious consequence of myocardial ischemia is a transient abolition of contractile function that becomes irreversible if ischemia persists and myocardial infarction (MI) develops.

Myocardial ischemia and MI are typically regional, involving only one part of the ventricular wall usually within the territory of distribution of a major epicardial coronary artery. The resulting impairment of the ventricular pump function is due not only to the loss of contractile elements, transiently or persistently effected by ischemia, but also to the disruption of the normal synergy of contraction. The lack of a synergic contraction produces regional alterations of the contractile function in the remaining normal myocardium that differ from those encountered in global ventricular pressure or volume overload and in diffuse myocardial diseases.

This chapter summarizes the basic features of the heart as a pump and of cardiac contractility, which are useful for the understanding and assessment of myocardial dysfunction in ischemic heart disease (IHD).

2.1 THE HEART AS A PUMP

For each cardiac cycle the pump function is conditioned by the functional anatomy of the ventricles and by the disruption caused by ischemia or MI. It is determined by the initial stretching of the sarcomeres due to the diastolic filling of the ventricles (preload), by the aortic pressure against which the blood is ejected (afterload) and by the inotropic and lusitropic state of the myocytes.[1] (Inotropic and lusitropic state are defined as the intrinsic contractile properties of myocytes, unrelated to preload or afterload, that are influenced by the rate of interaction between actin and myosin.) The energy cost of myocardial contraction depends on the external work of the ventricle and on the efficiency of the pump. The heart rate (i.e. the number of times the pump is actuated per minute) determines the cardiac output per minute and also influences preload, afterload, and inotropic state.

2.1.1 Functional anatomy of the ventricles

The shape of the two ventricles is quite different: the left resembles an elongated cone, the right is crescentric in cross-section and forms a shallow "U" between inflow and outflow.

The thickness of the left ventricular wall is about three times that of the right. These structural differences have a profound influence on the pump function: whereas the right ventricle is suited to operate as a *volume pump,* the left is suited to operate more as a *pressure pump* and generates systolic pressures about five times higher than the right. The contraction of the left ventricular myocardium contributes to right ventricular emptying, with bulging of the septum and traction of the right ventricular free wall. Distortion of the left ventricular shape by MI has a profound influence on its performance as a pump, particularly when aortic pressure is elevated. This notion provides the basis for the concept that the remodeling process postinfarction can be influenced by therapeutic interventions such as the chronic use of angiotensin-converting enzyme (ACE) inhibitors (see Chs. 7 and 21).

Myocytes represent about 60% of cardiac volume, the remaining 40% being represented by interstitial tissue with fluid, collagen, blood vessels, and blood (the latter comprising about 10% of cardiac volume). Myocytes account for only about 30% of cells in the heart, the remaining 70% being represented by endothelial cells, fibroblasts, and smooth muscle cells (SMCs). Given the considerable vascularity of the myocardium, it has been postulated that the intravascular pressure and the diastolic content of blood in coronary vessels may contribute to determine diastolic fiber length—the "garden hose effect."[2] This mechanism seems to play some physiologic role and may also contribute to reducing local myocardial work and oxygen consumption in areas of myocardium distal to a critical coronary obstruction with a low perfusion pressure, which would then result in shorter diastolic fiber length.

Myocardial cells, as well as being connected to each other in series through the intercalated discs, are connected sideways. They are arranged in *bundles* forming a series of overlapping layers oriented in different directions and joined by tightly interwoven strands of connective tissue. The bundles are fixed to the fibrous skeleton of the heart and surround the ventricles, crossing each other at different angles in different layers (see Fig. 2.1).[3-5] Ejection of blood results from shortening of the interwoven bundles of myocardial cells along their varied directions, with a resulting reduction in the minor diameter of the cavity by about 25% and shortening of its distance from apex to base by about 10%. Shortening of each sarcomere contributes to these volume changes in variable proportions according to its spatial orientation, to the pull from the adjacent sarcomeres in series, and to the friction against the other structures in parallel. The complex geometric arrangement of the fibers raises doubts about the possibility of applying the mechanics of skeletal muscle (with essentially parallel fibers) to the whole heart.

The sympathetic innervation of the ventricles is also segmental and stimulation of isolated branches of cardiac nerves causes localized changes of contractile function in the distal segment of the wall.[6]

It is still not clear whether some areas of myocardial wall are critical for coordinated contraction (acting like the hinges of a door) and if their destruction by myocardial necrosis or scarring is particularly disruptive to the synergy of ventricular contraction. It is also unknown whether interruption of branches of cardiac nerves can influence the development of asynergy of contraction and of arrhythmias.

In order to generate intraventricular pressure the myocardial wall must generate tension: the tension (T) required to generate pressure (P) increases with the radius (R) of the cavity and is inversely proportional to the thickness of the wall (h). This relationship is approximated by the law of Laplace which, when applied to a sphere as a first approximation, is: $T = (P \times R)/2h$. In order to generate a given intraventricular pressure, therefore, the tension required is higher when the radius is large and the wall thickness is small: $P = (T \times 2h)/R$.

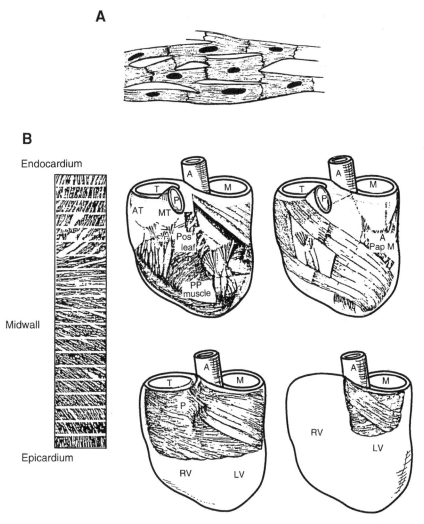

Fig. 2.1 Variable orientation of muscle bundles in the myocardium of left ventricular wall. A. Interconnections between muscle fibers. **B.** Reconstruction obtained by gradually peeling the external and mid-wall layers (right); and in a transverse section across the free wall of the left ventricle (left). The widely variable direction in which muscle bundles shorten prevents the straightforward application of the concepts of muscle mechanics derived from muscles in which fibers are parallel. Synchronous, coordinated contraction and relaxation of these differently oriented bundles are essential for efficient ventricular function. Disruption of coordination and synchrony may vary according to the sites of ischemia and infarction and can affect the efficiency of ventricular contraction also independent of the mass of myocardium lost to contraction. (Modified from refs 3 and 4.)

The right ventricle, with its crescentric form, larger radius and thinner wall, is less suited to the generation of pressure than the conical thicker-walled left ventricle. When the end-diastolic volume (EDV) becomes larger, the tension required to generate a given pressure increases; conversely, where the thickness of the wall is increased by hypertrophy, the tension that must be developed by an individual muscle fiber is reduced. During systole, wall tension decreases as the ventricle becomes smaller and the walls thicken.

2.1.2 Systolic–diastolic interaction and ventriculoarterial coupling

The definition of systole and diastole differs according to the point of view from which they are considered:

a. in *clinical terms* systole begins with the first heart sound and ends with the second sound
b. in *hemodynamic terms* different periods are recognized according to transvalvular gradients
c. in terms of the underlying *fundamental contractile process* it is useful to separate, conceptually, the period during which cross-bridges are interactive, from the period during which they are completely inactivated and when fibers are stretched passively by the filling pressure (see Fig. 2.2)

According to the Laplace law, the left ventricle unloads itself gradually during ejection as its volume decreases and the wall thickens. This unloading is conditioned by the compliance of the aorta and large arteries and by the resistance of systemic arterioles. During the last third of systole and the early part of diastole, *load-dependent relaxation* and *cross-bridge inactivation* occur together.[7] *Afterload* (i.e. a load not initially borne by the resting muscle) influences the stroke volume (SV) and ejection fraction (EF) (see 2.1.4) and has opposite effects on the duration of contraction, depending on the time at which it is applied: increased afterload prolongs contraction when applied during the initial two-thirds of systole but shortens it when applied later. Ischemia delays cross-bridge inactivation.

■ *These opposite effects of afterload may contribute to increased asynergy of contraction and relaxation by magnifying regional heterogeneity of duration and extent of contraction in adjacent myocardial fiber bundles: when regional ischemia, necrosis, and scarring delay local activation and alter the duration of contraction, the maximum pulling of some muscle bundles on others may occur in early systole and prolong contraction, or in late systole and shorten contraction.* ■

As the generation of tension in the ventricular wall increases ventricular pressure, the atrioventricular valves close and contraction remains *isovolumic*—although not isometric, as the shape of the cavity changes—until the semilunar valves open. Myocardial fibers then shorten rapidly and contraction remains practically *isotonic* during the ejection of the SV until the semilunar valves close. Relaxation is then isovolumic until the atrioventricular valves open and subsequently practically isotonic with rapid fiber lengthening.

The SV results from the difference between the EDV and the end-systolic volume (ESV). The ratio of SV to EDV represents the EF. In turn EDV depends on:

a. ESV
b. the diastolic filling (see above).

ESV depends on:

a. EDV
b. the force of contraction
c. afterload. The number of beats per minute determines the *cardiac output* (SV × heart rate).

Major links exist between abnormalities of contraction, relaxation preload, and afterload:

1. *Incomplete emptying* of the ventricle, as a result of contractile abnormality, increases ESV. This increased volume of blood in the ventricle reduces subsequent diastolic filling.

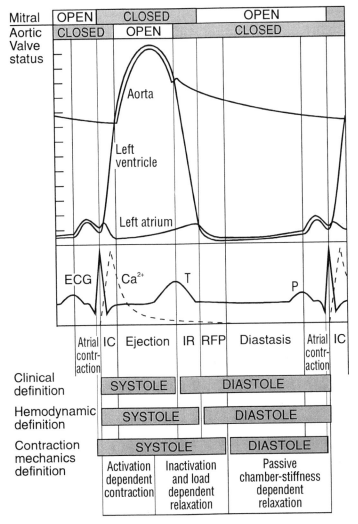

Fig. 2.2 Delimitations of systole and diastole. Systole and diastole can be delimited in several ways. For the *clinical* definition, systole begins with mitral valve closure (MC) and ends with aortic valve closure. For the *hemodynamic* definition, systole begins with MC, includes isovolumic contraction (IC) and relaxation (IR) and ends with mitral valve opening. For contraction mechanics, systole begins immediately after the onset of the QRS wave, but before MC and continues until all cross-bridges are inactivated after the rapid filling period (RFP) until the beginning of diastasis. The dashed line indicates the time course of cytosolic Ca^{2+} concentration. (Modified from ref. 7.)

2. *Incomplete filling* of the ventricle, as a result of relaxation abnormalities, reduces diastolic compliance and decreased atrial contribution reduces preload. The reduced amount of blood at the end of diastole reduces subsequent systolic emptying, i.e. SV.
3. Increased afterload due to hypertension and/or increased impedance to ejection increases systolic wall tension, reduces systolic emptying, and increases ESV; in normal ventricles, SV is maintained at the expense of an increased EDV: in ventricles with impaired systolic reserve, increased afterload and increased impedance reduce SV.

2.1.3 Diastolic priming of the pump

The EDV sets the initial *average* fiber length (preload), which conditions the *force* of contractions. The direction and position of the individual fibers within the wall condition the amount of their lengthening during diastole, in the same way as they condition their shortening during systole. Changes in EDV are brought about by changes in end-diastolic pressure. The relationship between changes in diastolic pressure and changes in volume defines the *chamber stiffness* of the ventricle, which increases progressively with the filling pressure so that, at low pressure, small variations in distending pressure cause large changes in volume, whereas at high pressures the variations in volume are small.

The stiffness of the myocardium is partly related to the interwoven course of the muscle bundles and to the resistance to stretch of the connective tissue that surrounds them in the different directions (parallel elastic component), but it is also evident in papillary muscles where fibers have a nearly parallel orientation with an elastic component predominantly in series. A certain degree of stiffness is also intrinsic to the myocardial fibers, since it decreases in skinned fibers, and some may also be intrinsic to the cross-bridge. The chamber stiffness is increased by myocardial hypertrophy and by interstitial myocardial fibrosis.

Arterial compliance decreases with age and, therefore, impedance to left ventricular ejection, systolic and pulse pressure and left ventricular load increase with age, leading to myocardial hypertrophy.[8,9]

End-diastolic volume depends on end-diastolic pressure and stiffness of the ventricle, but it is influenced by ESV, by the lusitropic state of myocardial fibers and by the synergy of relaxation, both of which condition early systolic filling, particularly during tachycardia.[10] ESV may increase considerably in MI with aneurysm formation, but this increased ESV is localized and does not contribute directly to the preloading of myocardial fibers. The average lusitropic state of myocardial fibers is determined by the rate of removal of calcium from troponin-C, independent of the other determinants of diastolic filling. For example, it can be greatly enhanced by β-adrenergic stimulation which becomes an essential adaptation during tachycardia caused by exercise. Myocardial ischemia and asynchronous regional relaxation of the ventricular wall reduce the global rate of ventricular relaxation.[11,12] The

Table 2.1 Determinants of diastolic function in IHD*

	Determinant
Rapid filling	Lusitropic state (i.e. inactivation of cross-bridges)
	Synergy of relaxation and hypertrophy
	End-systolic blood volume and ventricular suction
	Atrioventricular pressure gradient
Diastasis	Amount of blood in the ventricle at the beginning of diastasis
	Chamber stiffness** and duration of diastasis
Atrial filling	Amount of blood in the ventricle at the end of diastasis
	Atrial contraction, ventricular chamber stiffness**

  * Myocardial ischemia can reduce early diastolic filling by causing increased ESV and delayed asynergic relaxation. It can also impair diastasis and atrial pressure by incomplete relaxation or regional rigor. Myocardial infarction and fibrous scarring increase ESV and chamber stiffness

  ** Passive chamber stiffness is determined by fibrosis and hypertrophy

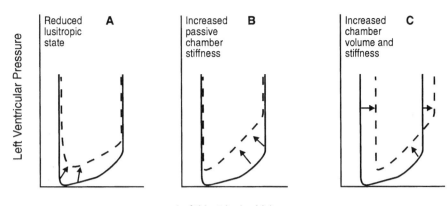

Fig. 2.3 Schematic relationship between diastolic ventricular volume and filling pressure. The continuous line indicates the normal pressure–volume relation: in the initial part of diastole, large changes in volume are associated with a small increase in pressure (low chamber stiffness); in the last part of diastole, small changes in volume are associated with a larger increase in pressure (high chamber stiffness). **A.** A reduced lusitropic state is associated with a reduced early relaxation of the ventricle because of slow inactivation of cross-bridges. **B.** An increased passive chamber stiffness is associated with a larger increase in pressure for the same increase in volume throughout diastole. **C.** An increased residual volume, due to infarction, for example, is associated with an increased chamber stiffness; thus the pressure–volume curve indicated by the dashed line in **B** is displaced to the right, and greater end-diastolic volume and pressure are required to accommodate the SV entering from the left atrium. (Modified from data in refs 10–12.)

consequent impairment of diastolic ventricular filling may become critical for systolic function during tachycardia.

Filling of the ventricle occurs in three phases: early filling (*rapid filling*), mid-filling (*diastasis*), and late-filling (*atrial priming*); the duration of diastole influences diastasis.

1. *Rapid filling* is conditioned by a number of factors:
    a. lusitropic state, i.e. the rate of active inactivation of cross-bridges—which is accelerated by β-adrenergic stimulation and reduced by ischemia
    b. ESV and elastic recoil of the ventricle—which is actively deformed during systole (particularly relevant when systolic shortening is great)
    c. synchrony of regional relaxation (particularly important at fast heart rates)
    d. atrioventricular pressure gradient.
    It also increases during exercise—in spite of tachycardia—because of the enhanced lusitropic state, and decreases during ischemia because of the delayed and asynchronous regional relaxation.
2. *Diastasis* is associated with *passive filling* related to the duration of diastole, the extent of rapid filling, the atrioventricular pressure gradient, and ventricular compliance (which depends both on the thickness and on the stiffness per unit volume of the ventricular wall but not on the myofibrillar deactivation process). (The compliance of the right ventricle is greater than that of the left only because its wall is thinner, not because its stiffness per unit volume is smaller.)

3. *Atrial priming* depends on the force and timing of atrial systole, on ventricular compliance and on the degree of filling during diastasis. Because it increases diastolic pressure only at the very end of diastole (when increased ventricular myocardial fiber length affects volume ejected), it enables atrial pressure and diastolic pressure to remain low (thus giving a low extracoronary flow resistance) throughout the remainder of diastole.

Thus, ventricular filling and the consequent priming of the pump may be decreased by reduced ventricular emptying, reduced rapid filling, increased chamber stiffness, and lack of atrial contraction. Reduced early filling decreases early peak transmitral blood flow and indirectly increases end-diastolic flow. Conversely, increased chamber stiffness and lack of atrial contraction decrease end-diastolic flow and indirectly increase early peak diastolic flow.

The *lusitropic state of the heart* can be defined by the varying rate of inactivation of cross-bridges; it is typically increased by β-adrenergic stimulation, which makes the heart relax more rapidly at the beginning of diastole, and is reduced by ischemia, which impairs early diastolic relaxation by delayed inactivation of cross-bridges.

In IHD the diastolic components of pump function (see Table 2.1) may be impaired because ischemia causes increased ESV, delayed and asynchronous relaxation, and rigor of ischemic segments, thus reducing filling.[12] Infarction also causes alterations to the ventricular wall structure by fibrosis and hypertrophy and geometric structural changes of the cavity with impaired late filling (see Fig. 2.3). Defective ventricular filling results in increased atrial and diastolic ventricular pressure (which is greater when the atrial contraction is lacking), with consequent retrograde blood stasis and impaired subendocardial perfusion in segments of the wall distal to critical stenoses (see Ch. 4).

2.1.4 Systolic function of the pump

The systolic function of the ventricle is influenced by the interaction of three somewhat independent variables—preload, afterload, and myocardial inotropic state—as well as by the synergy of contraction.

Preload

Preload is determined by the diastolic priming of the pump, which, together with chamber stiffness, determines myocardial fiber length. The relation between the diastolic priming and systolic function is described by the Starling curve, which, for a given inotropic state, describes how increased preload (EDV) increases force and velocity of contraction, SV and EF with unchanged ESV (see Fig. 2.4). The continuous beat-to-beat adjustment of right and left ventricular SV is mediated by changes in EDV in the two ventricles according to a Frank–Starling mechanism. A descending limb of the curve after its plateau has not been convincingly demonstrated in humans. Preload contractile reserve depends on resting EDV:[13] the lower the EDV, the greater the preload contractile reserve.

Afterload

Afterload is determined by the ventricular pressure during ejection and influences the quantity of blood ejected. Its effects vary in relation to wall thickness and to the radius of the ventricle. Moderately increased afterload mildly enhances contractile force—at least in animal models—by the *homeometric mechanism* (Anrep effect), but increased afterload at constant EDV reduces contraction velocity and SV and increases ESV (see Fig. 2.4).[14] Normal, but not failing, ventricles can restore SV as long as sufficient preload reserve (Starling effect)

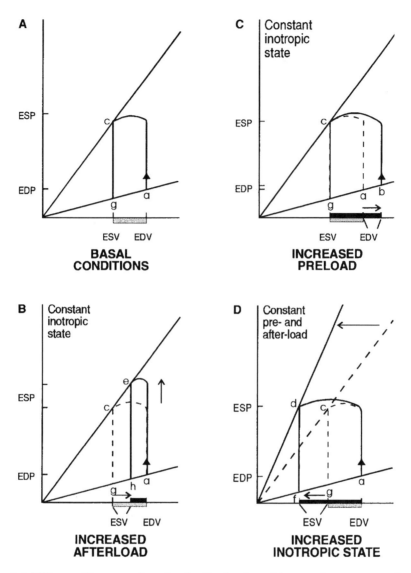

Fig. 2.4 Effects of increased preload, afterload, and inotropic state on a theoretical reference pressure–volume curve. A. The reference pressure–volume curve. **B.** When inotropic state and preload are kept constant, an increase in afterload reduces stroke volume (SV) and increases ESV; the new end-systolic pressure–volume point "e" remains on the same line. **C.** When inotropic state and afterload are kept constant, an increase in end-diastolic pressure (preload) from "a" to "b" increases EDV and SV, but ESV remains constant. The end-systolic pressure–volume point "c" remains unchanged. **D.** When preload and afterload are kept constant, an increased inotropic state increases SV as ESV is reduced; the end-systolic pressure–volume point "d" is displaced to the left on a different line. In practise, the interpretation of changes in the slope of the line on which end-systolic pressure–volume points lie (**D**) is made difficult by the uncertainty of the intercept of the line with the abscissa, as, when multiple end-systolic pressure-volume points are determined, it often does not pass through zero.

remains available. Afterload also conditions the duration of systole and the onset of relaxation (see 2.1.2). Increased afterload impairs ventricular systolic emptying more when the radius of the cavity is large and the thickness of the wall is small, because of the Laplace law (see 2.1.1).

■ *Thus, dilated ventricles are much less tolerant of high systolic blood pressure than are normal ventricles, particularly in the absence of hypertrophy, and acute left ventricular failure can develop in response to a sudden increase of systemic arterial blood pressure.* ■

2.1.4.3 Inotropic state

Inotropic state determines ventricular performance independent of both preload and afterload. Positive inotropic stimuli, at a given preload and afterload, increase the amount and rate of Ca^{2+} delivery to troponin-C (and/or its sensitivity to Ca^{2+}) and, hence, the force and velocity of contraction increase SV and reduce ESV (see Fig. 2.4). The inotropic state of myocardial fibers can be increased acutely by the following:

a. postextrasystolic potentiation[15] or paired electric stimulation,[16] which increase the release of Ca^{2+} from intracellular stores
b. β-adrenergic stimulation, which controls the levels of cyclic adenosine monophosphate (cAMP) and hence calcium availability for binding to troponin-C
c. tachycardia
d. exogenous inotropic agents such as cardiac glycosides, sympathomimetic agents, caffeine, theophylline, amrinone, and their derivatives
e. blood levels of calcium.

The inotropic state can also be changed tonically as Ca^{2+} sensitivity is modified by genetic programing. For example, velocity of contraction can vary according to the synthesis of myosin heavy chain (MHC) isoforms (α-MHC with a high ATPase activity and velocity of shortening and β-MHC with low ATPase activity and velocity of shortening).[17]

In IHD the systolic components of the pump function (see Table 2.2) may be impaired both by irreversible loss of myocytes (and by their replacement with fibrous tissue) and by

Table 2.2 Determinants of systolic function in IHD★

Determinant of systolic function are:
  • number of residual myocardial cells
  • inotropic and lusitropic state
  • preload (end-diastolic pressure and chamber stiffness)
  • afterload (impedance to ejection)
  • synergy of contraction and relaxation
  • fibroelastic hindrance to shortening.

Thus, impairment of systolic pump function can be caused by:
  • regional or patchy loss of fibers and fibrosis
  • asynergy of contraction and relaxation
  • decreased preload and increased afterload
  • reduced inotropic state.

★Permanent loss of myocardial fibers or transient dysfunction due to ischemia, stunning, hibernation, fibrosis, hypertrophy, geometric changes of the cavity, and asynergy of contraction may alter considerably the relative importance of the parameters that are known to control the contractile process under physiologic conditions

transient impairment of contraction due to ischemia, stunning, and hibernation (see Ch. 7). In the presence of cardiac failure, it is also impaired by a reduced inotropic state of remaining myocytes.[18]

2.1.5 Stroke work and efficiency of the pump

In order to appreciate the relation between myocardial *contraction* and the *ejection of blood* (i.e. SV), it is useful to consider in physical terms the external work performed by the heart during each beat.

The work of the ventricle per beat, i.e. the stroke work, is the product of systolic ventricular pressure, P, and SV, i.e. P × SV. (More correctly the work should be expressed as $\int PdV$, as both the pressure and the volume ejected vary in time, but the difference in the final calculation is small.) An additional 3–10% of useful work is performed by the ventricles in accelerating blood, i.e. increasing its kinetic energy, which is subsequently transformed into pressure at the periphery. Stroke work is determined by the following:

a.   fiber length, which in normal conditions, depends on EDV
b.   afterload (aortic pressure)
c.   the inotropic state of the fibers at each initial length.

For any given level of inotropic state the ventricle will perform more work (larger SV, greater pressure, or both) as end-diastolic pressure, hence volume, hence fiber length, increases (Frank–Starling mechanism). For any given EDV and afterload, work varies according to the changes of SV caused by variations of the inotropic state.

■ *The same external work can be performed by various combinations of SV and P: for the same EDV and inotropic state, SV is reduced when P increases.* ■

The efficiency of the pump depends on the amount of internal work that the ventricle must perform in order to overcome internal elasticity and sheer stress caused by internal friction and by the interwoven course of the muscle bundles. This internal work is mostly degraded to heat, but is also partly returned as useful work during diastole in the form of active suction of blood into the ventricle when the heart operates at short end-systolic sarcomere lengths. The ratio of useful work to total energy required to perform it defines the efficiency of the ventricle.

The efficiency of ventricular contraction ranges between 5 and 20% and is dependent on:

a.   type of work
b.   inotropic state
c.   EDV
d.   the heart rate.

For a given stroke work the efficiency is greatest when the SV is large, the generated pressure low, the EDV small, and the velocity of contraction low. (When systolic pressure is high, the cost of elevating pressure during the isovolumic phase is higher; when EDV is large, the tension required to generate pressure is higher [Laplace law]; when the speed of contraction is great, the energy expenditure is greater because of the rapid turnover of the cross-bridges and the greater amount of internal work.) The efficiency is greater when the SV is high and the heart rate is low (for a given EDV and a given systolic pressure) because the energy cost of switching on the contractile machinery more times per minute is greater than that of having a larger SV. (The relation between performance of the heart and myocardial oxygen consumption is discussed in Ch. 4.)

It follows that, in order to provide a given cardiac output, the ventricle operates more economically (i.e. requiring less oxygen and hence less coronary blood supply) with a rather large SV and low heart rate, a small EDV, and a low ESV, and with a low contraction velocity and systolic pressure. However, these working conditions, which result in optimal efficiency at rest and during moderate exercise, are not optimal when output has to be increased greatly: during severe physical exercise SV cannot increase much further without increasing EDV, so that the increase of heart rate is essential; contraction and relaxation velocity must also increase to allow time for diastolic filling. Accordingly, in pathologically dilated ventricles, an elevated heart rate and a small SV may be more economic than a larger SV associated with a further increase in EDV, particularly when systolic pressure is elevated.

2.2 CLINICAL ASSESSMENT OF LEFT VENTRICULAR CONTRACTILE FUNCTION

The possibility of quantifying the contractile function of the heart has interested physiologists and clinicians for over a century. This problem can be tackled by substantially different, although interrelated, complementary approaches:

a. assessment of the *average inotropic and lusitropic state of myocardial fibers* in conditions that involve the myocardium uniformly
b. assessment of the *performance of the ventricular pump as a whole* as an overall indication of its adequacy for the circulatory function
c. assessment of the *regional contractile function* and of the synergy of contraction and relaxation in diseases that affect the myocardium segmentally, such as IHD.

The acid test for the clinical usefulness of these approaches is their ability to achieve the following:

a. to separate normal from abnormal behavior in patients *without* obvious disease at rest or to assess residual contractile reserve during hemodynamic stress
b. to quantify the severity of the abnormality and follow its changes during the course of the disease or as a result of interventions
c. to provide clues to the underlying abnormality of cardiac function.

The choice of how to assess contractile function depends, therefore, on the questions that need to be answered.

2.2.1 Definition of the problem

In patients with IHD the myocardium is diseased, not uniformly but usually in discrete regions that are large in transmural MI, or are patchily distributed in small, diffuse areas of cell necrosis. Regional myocardial ischemia, necrosis, and scarring are often associated with variable degrees of hypertrophy and interstitial fibrosis. Episodes of cardiac failure are associated with a reduction of inotropic state that is potentially reversible. The loss of contractile elements and their transient dysfunction may be variably compensated for by hypertrophy and increased inotropic state of the myocardium not affected by necrosis or ischemia. Thus, impairment of pump function is the result not only of the average function of myocardial fibers, but also of the following:

a. their residual number
b. the degree of interstitial fibrosis of localized necrosis or scarring
c. the synergy of contraction and relaxation
d. ventricular chamber stiffness and preload
e. afterload, particularly when EDV is large
f. the average inotropic and lusitropic state of nonischemic myocardium.

For clinical purposes, therefore, it is as important to quantify cardiac contractile function as it is to establish the prevailing causes of the abnormality. In groups of patients, estimates of inotropic state are useful to study the effects of interventions and the mode of action of drugs. In individual patients, such estimates may be useful when they provide clues to the following:

1. The extent to which the impairment of pump function is caused by
    a. reduced inotropic state
    b. regional or patchy loss of fibers and fibrosis
    c. asynergy of contraction and relaxation
    d. impaired diastolic filling of the ventricle
    e. valvular or mechanical abnormalities that influence preload and afterload,
2. The extent to which the potential compensatory mechanisms of residual contractile reserve (dilation, hypertrophy, sympathetic stimulation) have been exhausted.

Clinicians would like very much to develop a single, possibly numeric, index that would separate patients from normal subjects and would provide a grading of the severity of myocardial involvement.

2.2.2 Average inotropic and lusitropic state of myocardial fibers

Assessment of the average inotropic and lusitropic state of myocardial fibers loses significance when the behavior of individual myocardial fibers is neither uniform nor synchronous. Such an assessment is valid in normal hearts as measurements of inotropic state have been shown to be sensitive indicators during interventions known to modify contractility. However, in the presence of large regional inhomogeneities, such as areas of myocardial ischemia or of necrosis or scarring, measurements of the average inotropic or lusitropic state of myocardial fibers and of their changes must be interpreted with caution.

The *assessment of the average inotropic state* of myocardial fibers is derived from the systolic parameters described below.

Measurements taken during the *systolic isovolumic* phase, as peak dP/dt, measured by a tip manometer catheter (if occurring before aortic valve opening), or $dP/dt/DP_{40}$ (value of dP/dt at a developed systolic pressure of 40 mmHg) are relatively insensitive to moderate changes in preload and to changes in afterload. Maximal velocity of shortening (V_{max}) calculated from dP/dt has no practical advantage over these less elaborate indices. The isovolumic phase indices are of little value in assessing basal level of contractility and in comparing inotropic state among patients, because of the very wide overlap with normal values.[19] They are heavily influenced by asynergy of contraction, by the loss of fibers, and by myocardial fibrosis, and are of no use in separating these various abnormalities. However, because they are relatively insensitive to preload and afterload they are useful in assessing acute changes in average inotropic state during heart catheterization.

Measurements taken during the *ejection* phase—such as velocity of contractile fiber shortening (V_{cf}), which relates the velocity of myocardial wall shortening (measured by angiography or echocardiography) to wall stress measured simultaneously—are fairly sensitive to changes in inotropic state and can separate groups of patients from normal subjects at rest better than can isovolumic phase indices, but they are considerably influenced by afterload. Their usefulness is, therefore, limited to conditions in which afterload remains constant and to the comparison of groups of patients. The effects of afterload could be taken into account by relating percentage fractional shortening to end-systolic stress.[20]

■ *Except where patients with valvular abnormalities are concerned, when it is desirable to separate the myocardial from the mechanical component of impairment of function, the characterization of the average inotropic state of myocardial fibers at rest is of rather limited practical use in assessing individual patients with IHD, but it may be useful for investigating the effects of interventions.* ■

The *assessment of the average lusitropic state* is derived from the rate of ventricular relaxation, assessed from the peak negative dP/dt (which is influenced by afterload) or from the half-time of the slope of the descending limb of the ventricular pressure curve ($t_{0.5}$),[21] which is independent of systolic and diastolic pressure and SV, and is only moderately influenced by wall stiffness. It is increased by asynchrony of relaxation, ischemia, reperfusion, β-blockade, and old age and is reduced by β-adrenergic stimulation. Measurement of ($t_{0.5}$) can be useful in assessing changes of lusitropic state in the same patient. Changes in late diastolic filling can result from reduced lusitropic state or from changes in passive chamber stiffness.

2.2.3 Global ventricular pump function

Ventricular pump function indicates directly the actual handling of the SV by the ventricle. It reflects not only the inotropic and lusitropic state of average myocardial fibers and regional contractile function but also the variable relationship between EDV, pressure, fiber length, afterload, and valvular or mechanical dysfunction. Global ventricular pump function cannot be assessed simply by measuring SV or end-diastolic ventricular pressure, but requires an evaluation based on the following:

a. construction of Starling curves
b. measurement of ventricular EF
c. assessment of ventricular diastolic filling
d. construction of ventricular pressure–volume curves.

Measurements of cardiac output and left ventricular end-diastolic pressure cannot be used on their own to assess ventricular function because they are markedly influenced by total blood volume, by venous return (see Ch. 3), and by acute changes in afterload.

The evaluation of global ventricular function from *Starling curves* was the first approach that allowed the separation of normal from obviously abnormal ventricular function, but it does not adequately separate normal subjects from patients with mild disease. In fact, in pathologic conditions the variable relation between EDV, pressure, and fiber length introduces a considerable spread of values along the abscissa of the Starling curves and the level of adrenergic stimulation causes a spread of values along the ordinate for any given initial fiber length, generating a family of Starling curves.[22] A ventricle that is enlarged because of MI, for example, with a high end-diastolic pressure but with well-functioning and normal remaining myocardium, will appear to be on a depressed function curve. Two ventricles, although on the same point on a Starling curve, may have different levels of adrenergic stimulation and of residual contractile reserve.

Among ejection phase indices, *EF* is currently the most fashionable for assessing individual patients in clinical practise. In normal ventricles it is sensitive to changes in myocardial inotropic state, but it is markedly influenced by afterload and by heart rate (when not associated with proportionate increases of β-adrenergic stimulation).[23]

In spite of these limitations, measuring EF using angiographic, nuclear, and cross-sectional echocardiographic techniques has gained great popularity as a means of indicating, with a single numeral, global ventricular function. The advantages of this index of ventricular function are its intuitive relation to the extent of ventricular emptying, its very wide range of values (from above 80% to below 10%), and its general relation to clinically judged heart function and prognosis. The shortcomings are twofold:

1. Being a ratio, it gives no information on the ventricular volume, so that a low value of EF can result from a normal EDV and a very small SV (for example during tachycardia at rest), as well as from an abnormally large EDV and a normal SV (i.e. a large ESV).
2. It does not provide information on the segmental or global nature of the myocardial abnormality.

Although values of EF below 50% should be considered abnormal, in borderline cases they should be related to SV or to ESV, which appears more closely correlated with ventricular function and with prognosis than EF.[24]

Left ventricular rate of filling[25] can be measured by the same techniques used to measure EF, provided that they have adequate temporal resolution; it is directly influenced by the parameters that control isovolumic relaxation and early filling. Peak diastolic rate of filling or mitral blood flow velocity also seems to provide an early sign of ventricular dysfunction; it is also indirectly influenced by changes in end-diastolic filling and, in healthy individuals, the rate of filling increases when they simply move from the supine to the standing position.[26]

The use of *pressure–volume loops* has been proposed because in animals the end-systolic pressure–volume relation seems to be (to a reasonable extent) independent of preload and afterload and influenced only by the inotropic state.[27] This approach is the most useful for assessing the global response of the myocardium to inotropic stimuli and its residual contractile reserve when challenged by an increased workload, as the end-systolic pressure–volume point is displaced in proportion to the inotropic changes.

In theory, pressure–volume loops constructed during hemodynamic stimulation allow the effects of preload, afterload, and inotropic and lusitropic state to be separated, according to the scheme presented in Figure 2.4.

- For a given EDV, when afterload increases, SV decreases, but the end-systolic pressure–volume point remains on the same slope.
- For a given afterload, SV and stroke work vary in proportion to EDV but the end-systolic pressure–volume point remains on the same slope.
- The diastolic part of the pressure–volume curve provides information on the lusitropic state.

> • For any value of afterload and EDV, changes in the inotropic state cause proportionate changes in SV and the end-systolic pressure–volume point moves to a different slope.

The independence of the slope of end-systolic pressure–volume points from EDV and afterload allows its noninvasive definition; end-systolic pressure–volume points can be measured by echocardiography or by angioscintigraphy, and end-systolic pressure by measurements of arterial blood pressure.[28]

The practical difficulty in separating normal from abnormal ventricular function by this approach is related to the fact that the intercept of the slope joining the end-systolic points, obtained at the same inotropic state, does not pass through zero[29] and often varies, intercepting either the ordinate or the abscissa of the pressure–volume graph.

■ *The assessment of global ventricular function, like that of the average inotropic state of the myocardial fibers, does not allow the precise interpretation of the contribution made by either loss of contractile elements or reduced inotropic state to impaired pump function.* ■

2.2.4 Regional contractile function

In patients with IHD, a comprehensive assessment of ventricular pump function requires definition of the following:

a.   the size of the segment of the ventricular wall with impaired contractility
b.   its potential reversibility upon relief of ischemia, stunning, or hibernation (see Chs 7 and 24)
c.   the extent to which enhanced function of normal regions compensates for reduced function of abnormal regions and their contractile reserve
d.   the contribution made by asynergy of contraction and relaxation among different regions to impaired pump function.

Thus, in addition to the assessment of global ventricular function by pressure–volume curves, information on regional contractile function is also required. The rate of segmental wall thickening and thinning provides more accurate information than local inward and outward movements of the wall, which may also be caused by passive movements of the wall (see Ch. 24).

This comprehensive set of data will eventually be obtained in three dimensions using the most advanced technology, such as ultra-fast computerized tomographic angiography and magnetic resonance imaging, but it has already been obtained experimentally by echocardiography.[30]

■ *However, even when characterized by this comprehensive set of parameters* obtained at rest, *interpreting the abnormalities found in contractile function is complicated by the uncertainty about not only their possible reversibility but also the extent to which compensatory hypertrophy and sympathetic activity are present or are already exhausted at the time of the measurements.* ■

For patients in whom ischemia, stunning, or hibernation (see Chs 7 and 24) do not contribute to pump dysfunction, a most relevant clinical question is "What is the extent of the heart's contractile reserve when it faces increased workload?" An exercise test would be by far the most informative way of assessing cardiac response (although other tests may be easier to apply) because it reproduces the physiologic stimulation and can be directly related to the level of physical activity that a patient performs during daily life. However, exercise tolerance is conditioned by other factors besides ventricular pump function. Thus, ideally, it would be desirable to evaluate regional ventricular contractile function during a stress test by one of the methods mentioned above.

2.2.5 Practical conclusions

After assessing the potentially reversible regional defects in contractile function, physicians are often called upon to make an assessment of left residual ventricular contractile function at a particular point in time in the course of a patient's disease, in order either to choose the appropriate treatment or to assess prognosis. The amount of detailed information that it is desirable to have should be weighed against not only the inconvenience, risk, and cost of the investigations, but also the possibility that, during a careful follow-up, sequential, although less comprehensive, assessment, may help to characterize the evolution of the disease state better than even the most sophisticated measurements at a single point in time.

REFERENCES

1. Katz AM. Influence of altered inotropy and lusitropy on ventricular pressure–volume loops. J Am Coll Cardiol 1988;*11:*438.
2. Watanabe J, Levine MJ, Bellotto F et al. Effects of coronary venous pressure on left ventricular diastolic distensibility. Circ Res 1990;*67:*923.
3. Robb JS, Robb RC. The normal heart: anatomy and physiology of the structural units. Am Heart J 1942;*23:*455.
4. Streeter DD, Spotnitz HM, Patel DP, Ross J, Sonnenblick EH. Fiber orientation in the canine left ventricle during diastole and systole. Circ Res 1969;*24:*339.
5. Sommer JR, Scherer B. The geometry of cell and bundle appositions in cardiac muscle: Light microscopy. Am J Physiol 1985;*248* (Heart Circ Physiol 17):H792.
6. Randall WC, Wechsler JS, Pace JB, Szentivanyi M. Alterations in myocardial contractility during stimulation of the cardiac nerves. Am J Physiol 1968;*214:*1205.
7. Brutsaert DL, Sys SU. Relaxation and diastole in the heart. Physiol Rev 1989;*69;*1228.
8. Nichols WW, O'Rourke MF, Avolio AP et al. Effects of age on ventricular–vascular coupling. Am J Cardiol 1985;*55:*1179,
9. Avolio AP, Chen SG, Wang RP, Zhang CL, Li MF, O'Rourke MF. Effects of aging on changing arterial compliance and left ventricular load in a northern Chinese urban community. Circulation 1983;*68:*50.
10. Zile MR. Diastolic dysfunction: detection, consequences, and treatment. Part 2: Diagnosis and treatment of diastolic function. Mod Concepts Cardiovasc Dis 1990;*59:*1.
11. Lima JAC, Weiss JL, Guzman PA, Weisfeldt ML, Reid PR, Trail TA. Incomplete filling and incoordinate contraction as mechanisms of hypotension during ventricular tachycardia in man. Circulation 1983;*68:*928.
12. Miyazaki S, Guth BD, Miura T, Indolfi C, Schulz R, Ross J Jr. Changes of left ventricular diastolic function in exercising dogs without and with ischemia. Circulation 1989;*81:*1058.
13. Lee JD, Tajimi T, Patritta J, Ross J Jr. Preload reserve and mechanisms of afterload mismatch in the normal conscious dog. Am J Physiol 1986;*19:*H464.
14. Ross J Jr, Covell JW, Sonnenblick EH, Braunwald E. Contractile state of heart characterized by force–velocity relations in variably afterloaded and isovolumic beats. Circ Res 1966;*18:*149.
15. Yue DT, Burkhoff D, Franz MR et al. Postextrasystolic potential of the isolated canine left ventricle: relationship to mechanical restitution. Circ Res 1985;*56:*340.
16. Frommer PL, Robinson BF, Braunwald E. Paired electrical stimulation. A comparison of the effects on performance of the failing and nonfailing heart. Am J Cardiol 1966;*18:*738.

17. Mahdavi V, Chambers AP, Nadal-Ginard B. Cardiac α and β myosin heavy chain genes are organized in tandem. Proc Natl Acad Sci USA 1984;*81*:2626.

18. Morgan JP. Mechanisms of disease: abnormal intracellular modulation of calcium as a major cause of cardiac contractile dysfunction. New Engl J Med 1991;*325*:625.

19. Petersen KL, Skloven D, Ludbrook P, Uther JB, Ross J Jr. Comparison of isovolumic and ejection phase indices of myocardial performance in man. Circulation 1974;*49*:1088.

20. Borow KM, Green LH, Grossman W, Braunwald E. Left ventricular end-systolic stress–shortening and stress–length relations in humans. Normal values and sensitivity to inotropic state. Am J Cardiol 1982;*50*:1301.

21. Gilbert JC, Glantz SA. Determinants of left ventricular filling and of the diastolic pressure-volume relation. Circ Res 1989;*64*:827.

22. Sarnoff SJ, Berglund E. Starling's law of the heart studied by means of simultaneous right and left ventricular function curves in the dog. Circulation 1954;*9*:706.

23. Ross J Jr. Afterload mismatch and preload reserve: a conceptual framework for the analysis of ventricular function. Prog Cardiovasc Dis 1976;*18*:255.

24. White HD, Norris RM, Brown MA, Brandt PWT, Whitlock RML, Wild CJ. Left ventricular end-systolic volume as the major determinant of survival after recovery from myocardial infarction. Circulation 1987;*76*:44.

25. Zoghbi WA, Bolli R. Editorial. The increasing complexity of assessing diastolic function from ventricular filling dynamics. J Am Coll Cardiol 1991;*17*:237.

26. Plotnick GD. Changes in diastolic function—difficult to measure, harder to interpret. Am Heart J 1989;*118*:637.

27. Spratt JA, Tyson GS, Glower DD et al. The end-systolic pressure–volume relationship in conscious dogs. Circulation 1987;*75*:1295.

28. Feldman T, Borow KM, Lang RM et al. Differentiation of simultaneous changes in preload, afterload, peripheral resistance and left ventricular performance: clinical assessment of myocardial mechanics. Am J Noninvasive Cardiol 1987;*1*:30.

29. Kass DA. Evaluation of left ventricular systolic function. Heart Failure 1988;*4*:198.

30. Rein AJJT, Lewis N, Sapoznikov D, Gotsman MS, Lewis BS. Quantitation of regional ventricular asynergy using real-time two-dimensional echocardiography. Int J Med Sci 1982;*18*:457.

CHAPTER 3

General principles of the circulation of the blood

INTRODUCTION

The function of the circulation of the blood is to transport substrates and waste products to and from organs and tissues in proportion to their respective and changing needs. Proper control of the circulation insures that the composition of the interstitial fluid surrounding the cells is optimal for their metabolic function at any given moment. The distribution of blood flow to the different organs in proportion to their needs is accomplished by two closely integrated control mechanisms:

a. the *central autoregulation* of the systemic arterial pressure, which is designed to maintain constant pressure when cardiac output varies over the short term
b. the *local autoregulation* of flow to each organ and tissue, which is largely under local metabolic control and which is designed to adjust local vascular resistance so that the supply of blood to each organ is constantly proportional to the local level of cellular metabolism, independent of the level of systemic arterial pressure over a wide range (see Fig. 3.1A).

The systemic circulation can thus be seen as a distribution system that provides the same pressure at the inflow to each organ and tissue, largely independent of the variations of cardiac output. From this distribution system, each organ and tissue takes as much blood flow as is required by its current needs (see Table 3.1), largely independent of the value of arterial pressure (autoregulation of flow) (see Fig. 3.1B).

The integrated central neurohumoral control of total peripheral vascular resistance and of cardiac output normally maintains systemic arterial pressure within a fairly narrow range. In so doing, it exerts a finer modulation on the redistribution of peripheral blood flow, which is superimposed on local organ and tissue metabolic control.

This chapter summarizes very briefly some general information that is useful for a better understanding of the pathophysiology of ischemic heart disease (IHD).

3.1 BASIC ARCHITECTURE AND FUNCTION OF THE VASCULAR SYSTEM

The structure of each section of the vascular system is designed to serve a special function to optimal effect. Although the vascular bed presents particular adaptations in the different

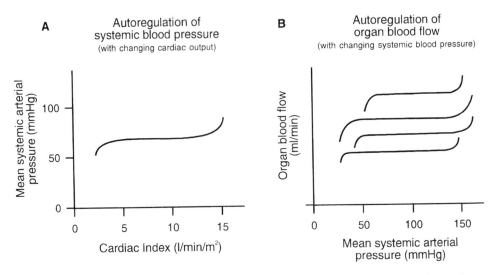

A Autoregulation of systemic blood pressure (with changing cardiac output)

B Autoregulation of organ blood flow (with changing systemic blood pressure)

Fig. 3.1 Schematic illustration of the regulation of the circulation. A. Systemic autoregulation of the circulation is designed to maintain blood pressure constant when cardiac output varies. This phasic function is controlled by the baroreceptor reflex. Thus, in young healthy adults, when cardiac output varies over a wide range during isotonic exercise the mean arterial pressure remains constant. The magnitude of the autoregulation can be grasped by considering that, in the presence of fixed resistance, a fivefold increase in cardiac output from 3 to 15 l/min/m² would be associated with a fivefold increase in mean arterial pressure. The efficiency of the reflex control decreases slightly with age and in hypertensive patients. The magnitude of the deviation from perfect autoregulation is indicated by the deviation from the horizontal. **B.** Circulation through the organs is designed either to maintain flow proportional to local metabolic needs when systemic pressure varies, or to vary flow independently of systemic pressure, according to local metabolic needs. Thus, for each organ, flow remains constant over a certain range of systemic blood pressure: at the extremes of the range, flow begins to decrease when the pressure drop is too great and to increase when the pressure rise is too great. Nervous and humoral controls are superimposed on local organ autoregulation in order to coordinate perfusion among different organs of the body while maintaining a constant level of arterial blood pressure. This neurohumoral modulation influences the tissue oxygen extraction, which increases when flow is reduced by vasoconstrictor stimuli and vice versa. In the resting state, the extent of the neural modulation varies among different organs.

organs in parallel with the aorta, the structure of each of the successive segments considered in series (arteries, arterioles, capillaries, venules, veins) is similar in different organs.

3.1.1 Aorta and proximal large arteries

The walls of these vessels are largely composed of elastic tissue designed to allow distension during systole and to accommodate part of the kinetic energy of the stroke volume (SV) and return it during diastole. Thus, this proximal section of the systemic arterial system functions as a dynamic systolic reservoir, modulating the sudden changes in pressure that would occur if the SV were to be ejected into a system of rigid tubes. During diastole, it returns the preload volume and part of the pressure stored as elastic energy during systole. The pressure waveform is thus progressively delayed and modified by wave reflection in peripheral arteries. The reduction of elasticity with age decreases the dynamic systolic reservoir func-

Table 3.1. Peripheral distribution of cardiac output and oxygen consumption.

Organ or tissue	Resting O_2 consumption as percentage of total body	Resting flow as percentage of cardiac output	Maximal increase of local flow above resting flow	Predominant mechanism of control of flow
Heart	11	4	6-fold	Local
Brain	20	13	3-fold	Local
Skeletal muscle	30	21	25-fold	Local
Splanchnic	25	24	7-fold	Neural
Kidney	7	19	2-fold	Neural
Skin	2	9	20-fold	Neural
Other	5	10	—	—

tion and pulse pressure increases, even for comparable values of SV. This increase of systolic pressure increases ventricular afterload. The velocity of propagation of the pressure wave increases when the elasticity of the vessel decreases.

3.1.2 Muscular arteries

Organs and tissues are connected to the large distensible elastic arteries by arteries provided with a thick tunica media containing smooth muscle, which allows them to maintain vessel-wall shear stress within narrow limits when flow varies by flow-mediated local dilation, and also to maintain the caliber of the lumen constant when the distending pressure changes, as well as to dilate and constrict in response to neurohumoral stimuli. The caliber of the muscular arteries is controlled by tonic flow-mediated release of endothelial-derived relaxing factors (EDRFs) (see Ch. 1). The intrinsic regulation of vessel caliber, in response to pressure changes, is controlled by myogenic tone. These intrinsic regulations can be modulated by neurohumoral controls. Prearteriolar vessels contribute to resistance and hence determine perfusion pressure at the origin of arterioles. Their caliber (and hence their flow resistance) is also under the control of locally generated autacoids (such as EDRFs) and neural and humoral substances directly acting on vascular smooth muscle tone (see Ch. 1).

3.1.3 Arterioles

These vessels, provided with a thick muscular media (with a high wall-to-lumen ratio), are influenced by local metabolites diffusing into the interstitial fluid. *They represent the major site of resistance to flow and hence are the site of the largest pressure drop.* They are thus eminently suited to control the amount of flow to each organ and tissue at any time and the pressure at the arterial end of the capillaries, even when the nerve supply to the organ is interrupted. They are the major site of local autoregulation of flow by the metabolic control of vascular tone, but they are also influenced by neurohumoral stimuli and local autacoids.

3.1.4 Capillaries

Capillary walls are very thin (and fenestrated in some organs) but sufficient to sustain transmural pressure because of their small caliber (Laplace law for a cylinder [see 3.3.2]). They have a considerable resistance to flow and hence there is a large pressure drop between the arteriolar end (about 30 mmHg) and the venous end (about 15 mmHg), which creates the pressure gradients necessary for proximal filtration and distal resorption of solutes. Not all capillaries are perfused at all times: their recruitment and derecruitment alternates under the control of precapillary sphincters and is influenced by local oxygen consumption, by inflow and outflow pressure, and by neurohumoral stimuli. The density of capillaries perfused has a major influence on the process of exchange.

Capillaries represent the site at which the fundamental function of the circulation is accomplished—the exchanges between blood and tissue that maintain the homeostasis of the interstitial fluid.

Exchanges occur by diffusion along concentration gradients through endothelial cells for gases and lipid-soluble substances (which pass freely through capillary membranes), or through pores for water-soluble substances. Fluid movement between blood and interstitial fluid occurs along pressure gradients as a result of the differences between transcapillary hydrostatic and colloid osmotic pressures; the difference favors filtration near the arterial end and resorption near the venous end of the capillary. Fluid not resorbed is returned to the systemic circulation by the lymphatics; total lymphatic flow is approximately 4–5 l per 24 h and carries an equivalent of one-half to one-quarter of the total plasma albumin.

Increased filtration can occur because of the following:

a.   increased surface area available for exchange (recruitment of capillaries not previously perfused)
b.   increasing precapillary or postcapillary pressure
c.   increasing surface permeability per unit surface area (increasing the diameter of the pores).

Precapillary pressure increases when arterioles dilate; postcapillary pressure increases when venous pressure rises or veins constrict. Permeability is determined by the level of transmural capillary pressure and to a major extent by humoral substances.

Intercapillary distance conditions the uniformity and velocity of diffusion in the tissues: the shorter the distance between capillaries, the faster the equilibration within the tissue. Thus, when, under resting conditions, there is plenty of time available to reach concentration equilibrium, few capillaries are perfused and they continually alternate during low metabolic activity. During maximal metabolic activity, however, all are recruited but the transit time is shortened.

3.1.5 Venules and veins

The vessels of the venous system that collect the blood from the site of exchange are characterized by thin, highly distensible walls with a well-developed smooth muscle coat. In the supine position, pressure at the venous end of capillaries is about 15 mmHg; this represents the driving pressure for the return of blood to the heart. Both the deep and superficial veins of the legs have thicker muscular coats and also sets of regularly spaced one-way valves that interrupt and subdivide the hydrostatic pressure during orthostatism (see 3.3.4). The venous return to the heart is also favored by compression of surrounding tissues. Besides the transport of blood back to the heart, the venous system serves a major function as a blood reservoir, thus modulating the return of the blood to the heart (see 3.2.2), and can also influence capillary pressure and hence the process of exchange (see 3.1.4).

3.2 REGULATION OF CARDIAC OUTPUT

When individual organs vary their flow, the fractional distribution of cardiac output must change accordingly. The control of cardiac output at any given moment is the integrated result of two components—the amount of blood that the heart is set to pump (pump function) and the amount of blood with which the heart is presented (venous return). The following examples illustrate this dual form of control:

1. In resting supine healthy subjects, when the heart rate is increased by atropine or by electric stimulation, cardiac output remains practically unchanged; as the rate is increased the SV decreases and atrial pressure decreases slightly[1] (as venous return is not stimulated at the same time).
2. In supine healthy subjects, when venous return is increased by expansion of blood volume or by compression of the lower half of the body by a positive-pressure suit, right atrial pressure increases by 10 mmHg or more but cardiac output increases by only 10–20% because the activity of the heart is not increased simultaneously.[2]
3. When the heart rate is increased following an artificial increase in venous return, as described in (2) above, cardiac output increases proportionally, as SV remains unchanged.[3]
4. Adrenergic stimulation and exercise increase both venous return and cardiac pump function (heart rate, diastolic filling, and contractility). Thus, cardiac output can increase maximally.
5. When cardiac pump function is impaired because of extremely reduced heart rate or right heart dysfunction, the right atrial pressure rises and the venous return to the heart becomes impaired (acute and chronic neurohumoral influences profoundly affect this condition).

3.2.1 Regulation of pump function

For any given level of cardiac function (heart rate and inotropic state), venous return influences cardiac output according to the Frank–Starling mechanism by modifying the filling pressure. In healthy, *supine* individuals the heart normally operates *near the plateau* of the Starling curve—this explains the small increase in cardiac output when venous return is increased artificially, and its reduction with decreased blood volume or increased venous pooling. In the healthy, *upright* subject, the heart normally operates *on the ascending limb of the curve;* thus an increased venous return and filling pressure (reduced venous pooling or increased blood volume) can increase SV (Frank–Starling mechanism) and cardiac output (see Fig. 3.2).

When the venous return is in the low or normal range, an increase in cardiac pump function (higher heart rate or contractility) does not increase cardiac output as the heart cannot pump out more blood than it receives, but a decrease in cardiac function will reduce output.

3.2.2 Regulation of venous return

The separation of venous return from cardiac output is a rather abstract concept but it may help in the understanding of the principles that regulate the circulation of the blood. At any given time the venous return of the heart is controlled by:

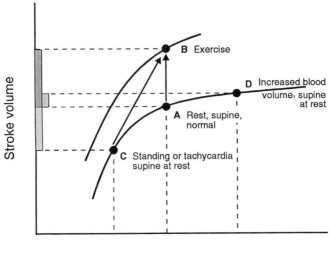

End-diastolic pressure

Fig. 3.2 Schematic relation between ventricular end-diastolic pressure and stroke volume (SV). In individuals at rest in a supine position, the ventricle operates near the plateau of the Starling curve (point A): a larger increase in filling pressure causes only a small increase in SV, but a small reduction in filling pressure causes a large decrease in SV. In individuals resting in the upright position, and also when they are resting in the supine position during tachycardia, the ventricle operates on the lower, steeper part of the curve (point C). During exercise, the heart moves on a steeper Starling curve and SV increases more in the standing than in the supine position.

a.   right atrial pressure
b.   capacitance of the venous bed
c.   distribution of flow through low- and high-capacitance vascular beds.[4]

A decrease of *right atrial pressure* increases the driving pressure and hence facilitates the venous return; the opposite occurs when right atrial pressure is increased. Increased cardiac pump function and decreased intrapleural pressure increase venous return by decreasing right atrial pressure.

When the *capacitance of the vascular bed* relative to total blood volume increases because of diffuse venodilation or because of reduced total blood volume, venous return is reduced; the opposite occurs in the presence of venoconstriction or increased blood volume.

These mechanisms involving right atrial pressure and capacitance of the venous bed often operate in opposition. For example, elevated atrial pressure increases the distending pressure in the veins and hence their volume, but reduces the driving pressure towards the right atrium.

The greater the compliance of a given venous bed relative to its resistance to flow, the greater the changes in volume that accompany changes of flow through it.

The distribution of blood volume in the different sections of the vascular bed differs completely from the distribution of the resistance to flow: arterioles and capillaries, which account for about 85% of resistance, contain a minimal fraction of the total blood volume, whereas the largest fraction of total blood volume (65%) is contained in venules and veins, which account for only 15% of the resistance to flow; hence, veins comprise the major area of capacitance in the vascular bed. Of the remaining 35% of total blood volume, approximately 10% is contained in the heart, 10% in the lungs, 10% in the arterial system, and 5% in the capillaries.

The venous system conditions the return of blood to the heart, not only because it is the largest reservoir but also because it is the most sensitive to influences of distending pressure (small wall-to-lumen ratio and large distensibility) and to changes in smooth muscle tone (low distending pressure).

Total blood volume is normally 70 ml/kg or 2850 ml/m^2 body surface area; the plasma volume is about 40 ml/kg and the ratio of the volume of red cells to the volume of plasma (body hematocrit) is about 0.45. The hematocrit is about 10% higher in large vessels because the small vessels contain more plasma than red cells. When total blood volume decreases, the venous reservoir is less distended and venous pressure decreases (unless full neurohumoral compensation occurs); conversely, when total blood volume is expanded, venous pressure increases.

Variations of flow through muscles, heart, brain, and kidneys will not be accompanied by appreciable changes in the venous blood volume of these organs because the compliance of their venous beds is low relative to their resistance. Conversely, an increase in flow through the skin and through the splanchnic bed is associated with a considerable increase in blood content in the venous bed because its compliance is high relative to its resistance. Thus, when a large fraction of the cardiac output is distributed through splanchnic or cutaneous beds, venous return is hampered; conversely, when a large fraction of cardiac output is distributed through muscles, the venous return is facilitated. The local and neurohumoral control of the distribution of flow between venous beds with high or low compliance, and the control of the capacitance of the venous system, have key roles in the determination of venous return. It is important to note that, in contrast to vascular resistance, which is mainly controlled by local metabolic factors, control of the capacitance bed is largely neurohumoral.

3.3 CIRCULATORY REGULATION

Resistance is distributed unevenly along the successive segments of the systemic circulation connecting the aorta with the right atrium: on average, approximately 5% is provided by the arteries and 60% by the arterioles—a relatively short segment of the vascular bed—and the remainder is divided between about 20% along the capillaries and about 15% along the venules and veins. Accordingly, the major drop in pressure occurs rather abruptly at the arteriolar level, where the local metabolic vascular control takes place. A second drop occurs gradually between the arteriolar and venous ends of the capillaries. The last drop also occurs gradually, along venules and veins.

The average vascular resistance results from the integrated values of resistance of the various organs and tissues connected in parallel to the aorta. Among these parallel circuits, with the exception of the skin and kidneys, vascular resistance and tissue perfusion depend on the degree of local metabolic activity. In each organ and tissue, under resting conditions, arterioles have a variable, inherent basal tone even after denervation; from this level they dilate in proportion to the metabolic activity of the tissue, varying flow in proportion to the fourth power of the radius (see 3.3.2) (in muscles, during maximal exercise, flow can increase 25-fold; see Table 3.1). Metabolites released into the interstitial fluid (adenosine, hydrogen and potassium ions, CO_2), as well as reduced oxygen tension and increased osmolarity, directly cause relaxation of smooth muscle and also indirectly inhibit the vasoconstrictor response to adrenergic stimulation.

■ *This means that metabolically active tissue tends to become functionally disconnected from nervous vasoconstrictor control during increased demand, to insure adequate local blood supply.* ■

A major function of blood flow is the delivery of oxygen in proportion to its utilization. Oxygen delivery results from oxygen transport and from extraction. However, venous oxygen saturation at rest varies markedly in the various organs, being minimal in the heart and maximal in the kidneys and skin. The capacity for extracting oxygen increases with tissue metabolic activity and when flow becomes inadequate.

3.3.1 Control of systemic arterial pressure

Systemic arterial pressure is under *tonic control,* which maintains its level approximately constant over the long term (days, months), and *phasic control,* which maintains blood pressure constant from instant to instant when cardiac output varies (see Fig. 3.1A). The mechanisms of tonic control are multiple and incompletely understood. They include control by the kidneys of fluid and electrolyte balance, tonic production of EDRFs, stretch receptor (baroreceptor) changes, and architectural changes in vascular smooth muscle and the arteriolar wall, as well as resetting of the central control mechanism. The mechanisms of phasic control are largely mediated by the baroreceptor reflex arc. The efficiency of this phasic control is quite remarkable considering that, for example, a fivefold increase of cardiac output during exercise would result in a fivefold increase of arterial pressure if there were no phasic control mechanisms capable of producing a fivefold decrease in total peripheral resistance.

Total systemic vascular resistance thus varies inversely with cardiac output according to an equilateral parabola. Alternatively, conductance (the inverse of resistance) varies linearly with cardiac output (see Fig. 3.3). Hence, the state of the resistive vessels cannot be characterized only by the calculated values of systemic arterial resistance or conductance. For example, similarly high values of resistance can be encountered with normal arterial pressure and low cardiac output or with high arterial pressure and normal cardiac output. Changes of resistance can be interpreted directly only when cardiac output does not change; otherwise, they must be interpreted according to the diagram in Figure 3.3. Conversely, the extent of change in resistance or conductance is immediately defined by the value of mean arterial pressure for each level of cardiac output.

■ *According to these diagrams, the tonic central control of systemic arterial pressure sets the isopressure line along which the phasic control makes resistance or conductance vary when cardiac output changes. The phasic control becomes slightly less perfect with age, so that mean systemic arterial pressure tends to increase slightly when cardiac output increases. In hypertensive subjects the tonic central control of arterial pressure is reset at a higher level, and, during exercise, the phasic control does not succeed in maintaining the mean pressure, at a constant level.* ■

3.3.2 Vasomotor regulation of vessel caliber

The vasomotor control of vessel caliber influences resistance, wall tension, and wall shear stress.

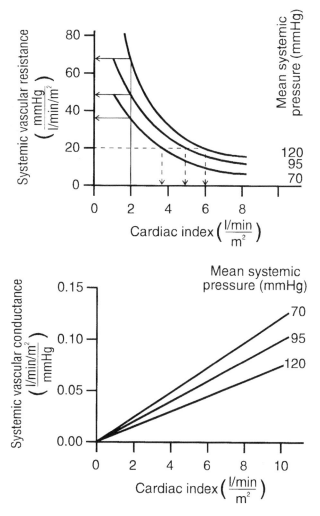

Fig. 3.3 Schematic relation between cardiac output and systemic vascular resistance (SVR) and systemic vascular conductance (SVC) as a function of mean systemic arterial pressure (MSP). SVR is calculated as the ratio of MSP to cardiac output/m² body surface area (cardiac index): the relation is described by a series of parabolic curves. SVC is calculated as the ratio of cardiac index to MSP: the relation is described by a series of straight lines passing through zero. It should be noted that each curve for SVR and each line for SVC is defined by the value of MSP. The same value of SVR (20 in the example) can be obtained with variable values of cardiac index and MSP (from 120 to 70). Conversely, the same value of cardiac index (2 in the example) can be associated with variable values of SVR from less than 40 to more than 60, depending on the value of MSP. Therefore, values of SVR or SVC have no precise meaning for the identification of abnormal systemic vasoconstriction or vadodilation, unless referred to the corresponding values of MSP or of cardiac index. Conductance presents the advantage of a linear relation to cardiac output for each value of MSP.

Resistance to flow

Flow (F) between two points in a vessel is determined by the driving pressure $(P_1 - P_2)$ between the two points and by the resistance to flow (R), i.e. $F = (P_1 + P_2)/R$.

In a tube, the resistance to flow (R) is described by the formula of Poiseuille, $R = (1 \times 8h/\eta r^4$. This relationship indicates that the radius of the tube (r) has the major role in the control of resistance relative to its length (1), the thickness of the wall (h) and to the viscosity of the blood (η) (as it enters the formula with the fourth power). This formula is only an approximation of the situation in vivo because flow is pulsatile, blood is corpusculated, and, in particular, because blood vessels are not rigid tubes and driving pressure represents also the distending pressure that controls their caliber. However, the formula serves the purpose of indicating that a 10% reduction in radius may cause an increase in resistance of nearly 50%. Variations in vessel caliber influence resistance in proportion to its basal value; changes in the caliber of vessels with negligible resistance to flow, such as muscular arteries, have negligible effects on flow compared with changes in the caliber of arterioles.

Wall tension

The radius of a distensible vessel (r) is determined by the equilibrium between the distending pressure (P) (intravascular $-$ tissue pressure), the tension of the wall (T) and its thickness (h) (Laplace law for a cylinder): $T = (P \times r)/h$. The tension of the wall is largely dependent on the distending pressure, on the radius of the vessel, and on the thickness of the smooth muscle coat. The radius of the vessel is influenced by vasomotor tone. Maintenance of constant tension is the basis of the myogenic control of vascular smooth muscle tone (see Ch. 5): when pressure increases, the radius must decrease in order to maintain constant tension; when pressure decreases, the radius must increase to keep tension constant.

Wall shear stress

The frictional forces between flowing blood and endothelial surface, for a given blood viscosity, depend on the flow velocity. Within arteries, flow velocity is highest at the center of the vessel and decreases as a parabolic function towards the wall. Flow-mediated vasodilation limits the increase of wall shear stress when blood flow increases.

3.3.3 Pulmonary circulation

The function of the pulmonary circulation is that of distributing blood to the site of gas exchange, matching local perfusion to ventilation with the least resistance to flow. The vascular components of this function are summarized below.

Resistance to flow

The pulmonary circulation has a very low resistance to flow (about one-fifth of the systemic). Normally, the calculated pulmonary vascular resistance decreases with increasing flow at constant left atrial pressure and with increasing left atrial pressure at constant flow, because of recruitment of vessels previously not perfused and vessel distensibility. Pulmonary artery pressure increases proportionately when left atrial pressure and pulmonary vascular resistance increase. In healthy individuals, pulmonary artery pressure increases by only a few millimeters of mercury during maximal exercise. Furthermore, the right or left branch of the pulmonary artery can be totally occluded by inflating a balloon catheter, without a measurable increase in pulmonary artery pressure at rest or during exercise for comparable levels of cardiac output. These findings give a measure of the degree of reduction of the pulmonary vascular cross-section necessary to cause pulmonary hypertension.

Blood volume

The volume of blood in the pulmonary circulation is about 10% of total blood volume and increases only to a small extent (up to 12–15% of total blood volume) when left atrial pressure is elevated in the early stages of mitral stenosis or in acute left ventricular failure. Thus, the pulmonary circulation cannot serve as a reservoir of blood for sudden increases of cardiac output, as generally thought.[3]

Blood flow

The distribution of blood flow is normally influenced by gravity: it is highest at the bases and lowest at the apex in the upright position; it is higher in the dorsal than in the frontal regions in the supine position. The distribution of blood flow is similar to that of blood volume. In chronic left atrial hypertension, the distribution of blood flow can become balanced in the early stages and inverted in the advanced stages (greater at the apex than at the base) because of increased vascular resistance in the more dependent zones, due to organic and functional factors. In pulmonary hypertension, the distribution of flow is normal or balanced.

Capillary exchange

Normal capillary permeability to fluid is low, and efficient lymphatic drainage into the systemic veins of the chest insures a normal interstitial fluid volume in the lungs. Acute transudation of fluid caused by an excessive increase in capillary pressure and/or capillary permeability causes a large accumulation of interstitial fluid (interstitial edema)—up to several hundred milliliters—before producing intra-alveolar edema. When chronic interstitial fluid accumulation is caused by elevated left atrial pressure its distribution is largely gravity dependent, but this is not so when it is caused by primary capillary damage.

The endothelial cells of the lung capillaries also play an important metabolic part through uptake and release of various bioactive materials: they are the site of transformation of angiotensin-1 to angiotensin-2 and of inactivation of bradykinin; they remove and inactivate nonepinephrine, 5-hydroxytryptamine, histamine, and certain prostaglandins and they produce prostacyclin. This handling of bioactive materials by the lungs is important because they continuously "filter" the entire cardiac output in an amount equal to the total blood volume each minute.

3.3.4 Effect of posture on intravascular pressure

Because of gravity, intravascular pressures at any given level within the body are the algebraic sum of the pressures generated by the heart and of hydrostatic pressure (1 cmH_2O/cm vertical height). Obviously, the effect of hydrostatic pressure is minimal in the supine position (where the effect is limited to the dorsoventral thickness of the body) and maximal in the erect position when measured at the level of the feet; in resting subjects of average height, arterial and venous pressures are about 90 mmHg higher here than at the level of the heart (1 cmH$_2$O corresponds to 1.36 mmHg). Conversely, arterial pressure measured in the hands when held above the head is about 60 mmHg lower than at the level of the heart. Because posture affects pressure to the same extent in arteries and veins, it does not influence arteriovenous pressure gradients, but does proportionately affect transmural and filtration pressure (when extravascular tissue pressure does not increase also with gravity, as in the brain, spinal cord, and splanchnic bed).

When the subject is erect and at rest, the volume of blood in the legs increases by several hundred milliliters and capillary filtration is much greater; thus, fluid resorption must increase proportionately. The volume of blood in the heart and lungs decreases by about 20% and the SV is also about 20% lower. Normally, reflex tachycardia tends to reduce the drop in cardiac output and reflex vasoconstriction maintains systemic arterial pressure.

3.3.5 Effects of physical exercise

The effects of isometric and isotonic exercise on blood flow through muscles and on the circulation differ considerably.

Isometric exercise reduces blood flow through the working muscles because blood vessels are squeezed by contraction, but it causes a large increase in systemic arterial pressure that is of reflex origin and largely independent of the size of the muscle mass involved. It cannot be sustained for more than a few minutes because it is largely anaerobic.

Isotonic rhythmic exercise can increase muscle blood flow over 25 times as the vasodilation in working muscles is compensated for by reflex constriction in other beds (predominantly splanchnic and kidney). Cardiac output increases in proportion to the increased body oxygen consumption (up to five or six times the resting level) and total vascular resistance is reduced proportionately, so that mean arterial pressure increases only slightly in young subjects, moderately in middle-aged subjects, and slightly more in hypertensive subjects. In normotensive individuals this increase is mainly related to an increased systolic pressure. Cardiac output increases because of:

a.   increased venous return from low-capacitance beds, reduced flow through high-capacitance beds (splanchnic), and generalized venous constriction
b.   increased tachycardia and increased inotropic and lusitropic state.

From the very beginning of even moderate exercise (such as taking a few steps), the massaging action of the muscles squeezes the blood out of the leg veins. The venous valves, which were incompetent during resting erect posture because of the excessive dilation, become competent and venous pressure in the feet decreases by about 60 mmHg. This increases venous return to the heart and brings filling pressure and end-diastolic SV closer to the resting supine level (see Fig. 3.2).[4] Oxygen transport increases, not only because of the increased cardiac output, but also because of increased tissue extraction, with considerable widening of the average arteriovenous difference in oxygen content. Prolonged exercise is associated with a reflex increase of blood flow through the skin—which is caused by the increased temperature of the blood, and which contributes to the dispersion of the heat generated by muscular work—and with some hemodynamic adaptations.

For every steady state of physical exercise there is a carefully controlled level of cardiac output, systemic pressure, pulmonary ventilation, and deep body temperature. The levels are maintained as precisely as at the resting level and the controlling feedback systems are the same in exercise as during rest—only the setting point has been changed. These changes and the new setting of the control mechanism are not determined by a single factor but by a combination of several.

The increase in cardiac output is approximately linear with work load and total body oxygen consumption. Initially, the increase is larger in the supine than in the sitting position. Mean arteriovenous oxygen difference increases progressively up to about 10–13 volumes, being wider in the sitting than in the supine position. SV and end-diastolic volume (EDV) are initially about 25% lower in the sitting or standing than in the supine position, but during heavy exercise they become similar. A transient reduction in end-diastolic ventricular volume occurs at the beginning of mild exercise because of the increased heart rate and inotropic state, but at higher work loads the end-diastolic left ventricular volume and the SV increase considerably. Thus, in the supine position and at submaximal work loads, heart rate is the main determinant of cardiac output. In sitting and standing positions, SV (which is lower than in the supine position at rest) contributes much more significantly to the increase in cardiac output. At maximal work loads, SV increases in all conditions.[5] The SV also increases when the heart rate response is reduced, for instance by conduction disturbances or following β-blocking drugs and with age.[6] This can occur only at the expense of a larger EDV.

In normal conditions, the rate-limiting factor needed to attain the maximal level of oxygen consumption possible for an individual is represented by the circulatory function.[7] The form of stress presented by exercise is, therefore, the most suitable for assessing the adequacy of the heart's function.

REFERENCES

1. Weissler AM, Leonard JJ, Warren JV. Effects of posture and atropine on the cardiac output. J Clin Invest 1957;*36*:1656.
2. Frye RL, Braunwald E. Studies on Starling's law of the heart. I. The circulatory response to acute hypervolemia and its modification by ganglionic blockade. J Clin Invest 1960;*39*:1043.
3. Giuntini C, Maseri A, Bianchi R. Pulmonary vascular distensibility and lung compliance as modified by dextran infusion and subsequent atropine injection in normal subjects. J Clin Invest 1966;*45*:1770.
4. Rothe CF. Physiology of venous return: An unappreciated boost to the heart. Arch Intern Med 1986;*146*:977.
5. Upton MT, Rerych SK, Roeback JR Jr et al. Effect of brief and prolonged exercise on left ventricular function. Am J Cardiol 1980;*45*:1154.
6. Rodeheffer RJ, Gerstenblith G, Becker LC, Fleg JL, Weisfeldt ML, Lakatta EG. Exercise cardiac output is maintained with advancing age in healthy human subjects: cardiac dilation and increased SV compensate for a diminished heart rate. Circulation 1984;*69*:203.
7. Astrand PO. Quantification of exercise capability and evaluation of physical capacity in man. Prog Cardiovasc Dis 1976;*19*:51.

4 | The coronary circulation

INTRODUCTION

The coronary circulation is designed to supply the myocardium with blood for its widely and rapidly changing needs. It supplies oxygen in amounts varying over a six- to eightfold range, carries substrates, and removes metabolic waste products, all in order to insure optimal working conditions for myocardial cells. This demanding function takes place in an organ that generates its own perfusion pressure. Thus, in the ventricular wall, extravascular tissue pressure during systole exceeds intravascular pressure—with consequent vessel collapse—so that blood flow exhibits a 180-degree phase shift, in that it enters the wall during diastole and leaves it during systole.

When myocardial metabolic requirements remain constant, the autoregulation of coronary blood flow (CBF) maintains flow nearly constant over a wide range of aortic pressure by reducing vasomotor tone when aortic pressure decreases, and vice versa.

In basal resting conditions the tone of coronary resistive vessels is high and CBF is at its lowest level. This intrinsically high resting basal tone provides the coronary circulation with the ability to increase flow by reducing vasomotor tone when myocardial oxygen consumption increases.

The metabolic control of CBF, which reduces the vasomotor tone of resistive vessels in order that myocardial perfusion can increase to match requirements, is very precise. In a given individual, myocardial extraction of oxygen does not increase during increased heart work up to submaximal levels (except under extreme circumstances such as ischemia or cardiac failure). Resting myocardial oxygen extraction varies between different individuals depending on the level of neurohumoral modulation of CBF (see 4.3.4).

The physiologic ability of CBF to increase above resting levels and to match any augmentation of myocardial oxygen consumption is defined as *coronary flow reserve*.

When coronary arterioles are maximally dilated, flow depends on two factors:

1. The first factor is prearteriolar coronary perfusion pressure (i.e. the pressure at the origin of the arterioles, which are the site of metabolic control of flow), which is determined by aortic pressure and resistance of arterial segments interposed between the aorta and the origin of the arterioles (i.e. the epicardial coronary arteries and prearteriolar vessels).

2. The second factor is the tissue compressive forces in the left ventricular wall; these prevent flow during systole and may also impair flow during early diastole in the subendocardial layers of the myocardium when coronary perfusion pressure at the origin of arterioles is significantly lower than left ventricular pressure, particularly during tachycardia, which shortens the duration of diastole. (Coronary perfusion pressure at the origin of arterioles may become much lower than intraventricular systolic pressure in the presence of aortic stenosis, epicardial coronary artery stenoses, and prearteriolar vessel constriction.)

The intrinsic mechanisms that control the autoregulation of CBF in isolated hearts can be modulated by the autonomic nervous system and by a variety of humoral substances carried by the bloodstream or produced by the endothelium. Under physiologic conditions, when myocardial oxygen consumption remains constant this neurohumoral modulation of flow is associated with proportional opposite changes of myocardial oxygen extraction, so that coronary sinus oxygen saturation decreases with vasoconstriction and increases with dilation of coronary resistive vessels.

This chapter discusses the following:

a. the functional anatomy of the coronary circulation
b. the distribution of coronary vascular resistance
c. the regulation of oxygen transport and CBF
d. myocardial oxygen consumption.

4.1 FUNCTIONAL ANATOMY

A review of the functional anatomy of the coronary circulation is useful in order to understand better the basis of its regulation. The coronary circulation is composed of three vascular systems arranged in series:

a. an arterial system that brings blood to the site of tissue exchange and controls most of the resistance to blood flow
b. a meta-arteriolar and capillary system that controls the local microdistribution of blood flow and hence blood–tissue exchanges
c. a venous segment that collects capillary blood, influences capillary recruitment and controls the intramyocardial volume of blood at the end of diastole and hence influences the end-diastolic myocardial fiber length.

4.1.1 The arterial system

Traditionally, two compartments in series have been considered in the coronary arterial system—conductive vessels and resistive vessels. However, the physiologic functions of the coronary arterial system can be better understood by considering it as being composed of three, rather than two, compartments arranged in series (see Fig. 4.1).[1] The physiologic role of these three *functional* compartments are distinctly different, although their borders cannot be clearly defined anatomically or histologically:

1. The proximal compartment is represented by the large epicardial coronary arteries, which have a conductive and capacitance function, and a negligible pressure drop along their length.
2. The intermediate compartment is represented by prearteriolar vessels, interposed between large epicardial arteries and arteriolar vessels. These vessels have a

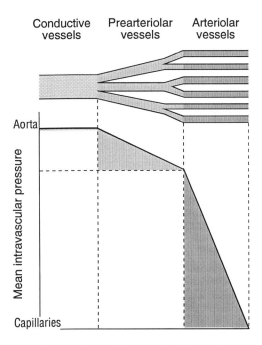

Fig. 4.1 Schematic illustration of the subdivision of coronary arterial vessels into conductive, prearteriolar and arteriolar vessels. The pressure drop along conductive vessels is negligible; that through prearteriolar vessels is appreciable, and that through arteriolar vessels is the largest. Prearteriolar vessels, by definition, are not exposed to myocardial dilator metabolites because of either their extramyocardial position or their size.

measurable pressure drop along their length as they offer some resistance to flow but are *not under direct vasomotor control by diffusable myocardial metabolites* because of their extramyocardial position or size. Their specific function is to maintain pressure at the origin of arterioles within a narrow range when aortic pressure and coronary flow vary.

3. The distal segment is represented by the arterioles, the site at which interstitial fluid composition and myocardial metabolites *directly and continuously* influence coronary vascular resistance.

Epicardial conductive coronary arteries

These arteries offer a negligible resistance to flow *until* they are 1 mm or less in diameter. At their distal end, the profile of the pressure drop as a function of caliber has not been established; the anatomic border with prearteriolar vessels is therefore ill-defined. A functional definition, therefore, could state that conductive arteries extend up to the point where the pressure at the end of diastole in resting conditions is measurable, i.e. only about 1–2 mmHg lower than in the aorta. The site where the pressure drop exceeds this level may occur before or after the arteries enter the ventricular wall. Conductive arteries have both distribution and capacitance functions.

Distribution function. The pattern of branching and tapering of epicardial coronary arteries minimizes blood kinetic energy losses and wall shear stress, but, in normal adults, both left and right coronary arteries exhibit a diameter range that can vary by as much as threefold among different individuals. This complicates the angiographic assessment of "normal" caliber in patients with coronary atherosclerosis.

Capacitance function. During systole, epicardial coronary arteries accumulate elastic energy as they increase their blood content up to about 25% because of anterograde flow from the aorta and retrograde flow from intramyocardial vessels. This elastic energy is transformed into blood kinetic energy at the beginning of diastole and contributes to the prompt reopening of intramyocardial vessels that had been squeezed closed by systole (see 4.2.2). This systolic storage of blood is increased by β-adrenergic stimulation and reduced distal to critical coronary stenoses in proportion to the decrease in poststenotic pressure.

Adaptation to increased flow. The basal lumen diameter and systolic capacitance of coronary arteries are likely to be optimal for resting flow. The smooth muscle structure of the arterial wall allows for increases of lumen and capacitance above resting levels when release of endothelial-derived relaxing factors (EDRFs) increases with flow (see Chs 1 and 5). Such an adjustment can help to minimize the increase in shear stress and to accommodate a larger fraction of blood in a shorter systole when blood flow is increased during effort-induced tachycardia.

Adaptation to changes in aortic pressure. When aortic pressure varies, the *myogenic regulation of coronary tone* (see Ch. 5) tends to maintain the vessel lumen constant by minimizing passive changes, as it responds with an increase of smooth muscle tone to a pressure rise and with a decrease of tone to a pressure drop. The intrinsic regulation of myogenic tone is modulated by humoral and neural stimuli (see Ch. 5).

Histologic structure of epicardial coronary arteries. As previously stated, the muscular structure of epicardial coronary arteries enables them to undergo major changes in caliber and capacitance. The endothelial lining of the intima provides the sensorieffector mechanisms that respond to increased shear stress by releasing nitric oxide (NO) and possibly other dilators towards the media, relaxing the smooth muscle and thus increasing the vessel diameter. The rather sparse nerve endings in the adventitia of these vessels, compared with prearteriolar and arteriolar vessels, suggests that the caliber of large epicardial arteries is not under intensive nerve control.

The wall-to-lumen ratio of epicardial coronary arteries is about 1:4 and about 60% of the wall thickness is represented by the media, which is composed of several layers of smooth muscle cells (SMCs). This allows powerful phasic and tonic adjustments to be made in response to changes in intravascular pressure and myogenic tone, as well as to changes caused by neurohumoral stimuli. At the border with the adventitia, the media is perfused by vasa vasorum, which can greatly increase in number in the presence of atherosclerotic plaques.

In the *adventitia* there are sparse synaptic connections between nerves and SMCs at the border with the media. In pathologic conditions, inflammatory cell infiltrates and neoformation of vasa vasorum may occur. The *intima* is lined with a layer of endothelial cells supported by connective tissue and is separated from the media by a continuous elastic membrane. The intima is the site where molecules and small particles such as immune complexes carried by the bloodstream are deposited and where SMCs migrate and proliferate. It also incorporates mural thrombi when they became covered by endothelial cells.

Interarterial connections. There is some overlap at the border between territories perfused by major arteries; anastomotic connections exist in normal hearts between branches of the same coronary artery as well as between different coronary arteries. Such anastomotic branches are of considerable importance as they are the channels from which collaterals arise when a pressure gradient develops as a result of critical stenoses of one of the parent arter-

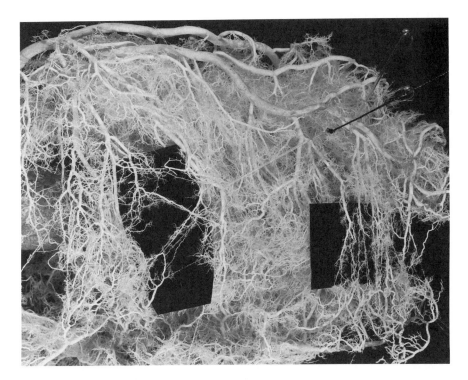

Fig. 4.2 Anastomotic interarterial communications in the interventricular septum of a normal heart. Some anastomotic branches course in a slightly downward direction across the septum, joining the anterior descending artery on the right to the posterior descending artery on the left. Some run nearly at right angles and lie on the left side of the septum. These vessels may be large in number but are usually small in size. (From ref. 2.)

ies. These anastomotic arterial vessels differ markedly in number, size, and distribution between animal species and between individuals of the same species: for example they are prominent in guinea pigs and dogs, less so in pigs and rats, and practically absent in sheep. In normal human hearts, interarterial anastomoses 50–200 μm in caliber are abundant (see Fig. 4.2) particularly in the subendocardium and septum (similar to the distribution most commonly found in pigs), whereas epicardial anastomoses, usually found in dogs, are less common.[2–4] *Blood can flow through these anastomotic branches only in the presence of a pressure gradient* between their origin and their termination: thus, in order to maintain patency across these anastomoses and avoid stagnant flow, a pressure gradient must develop intermittently or during some phases of the cardiac cycle between the parent branches, under normal conditions.

Prearteriolar vessels

These vessels, although contributing to coronary flow resistance, are not *directly* involved in the process of metabolic autoregulation of flow because of their extramyocardial position and/or size. The extramyocardial portion of these vessels accounts for a sizable pressure drop (see 4.2.4) but their proximal and distal ends cannot be precisely defined anatomically.

As the resistance to flow of these vessels determines the pressure drop at the origin of the arterioles, their function is to maintain pressure at the origin of arterioles within a range optimal to ensure a reasonably constant forward driving pressure (see Fig. 4.1).

Adaptation to increased flow. If prearteriolar resistance (R) remained constant, the pressure drop at the origin of arterioles relative to aortic pressure (ΔP) would increase linearly with flow (Q) (as $Q = \Delta P/R$), meaning that the pressure drop would double when flow doubled. However, prearteriolar vessels dilate progressively and minimize the pressure drop through them, as flow causes release of EDRFs, mediated by wall shear stress.

Adaptation to changes in aortic pressure. Prearteriolar vessels constrict when aortic pressure increases and dilate when aortic pressure falls as a result of changes in myogenic tone; thus, as previously stated, they maintain the pressure at the origin of arterioles within a narrow range. When aortic pressure falls and full dilation of prearteriolar vessels is insufficient to maintain pressure constant at the origin of arterioles, metabolically mediated arteriolar dilation (see 4.3.3) contributes to maintain flow constant.

Architecture of intramural prearteriolar vessels. Along their course and with their distal branches, epicardial coronary arteries provide branches that enter the left ventricular myocardium at right angles and course directly through the walls towards the endocardium. These penetrating branches divide in a tree-like pattern and give off small branches with gradually diminishing caliber (see Fig. 4.3A), the terminal branches often anastomosing with adjacent ones in the subendocardial zones.

The histology of prearteriolar vessels is similar to that of epicardial coronary arteries but their adventitia is more densely innervated.

Arteriolar vessels

Arterioles are responsible for the metabolic control of CBF. They are the site of a substantial fraction of coronary flow resistance and dilate progressively in response to increased release of metabolites by surrounding myocardial cells into the interstitial fluid. They are also responsible for maintaining flow constant when pressure falls at their origin. For arterioles, as for the other segments, the histologic definition of the proximal and distal borders is blurred. As the resting diameter of the vessels that exhibit the most obvious increase in caliber during metabolic vasodilation is of the order of 100 μm, these may represent the most critical section of arteriolar vessels.

Over their length, the vasomotor response to interstitial fluid composition varies gradually with vessel size because the diffusion distance necessary for interstitial fluid equilibration with the vessel wall increases progressively with the thickness of the vessel wall. At the distal end, the relative contribution of precapillary sphincters and meta-arterioles to the overall resistance to flow and the metabolic control of flow is not precisely known.

Adaptation to flow changes. These vessels continuously adapt their caliber in response to changes in the surrounding interstitial fluid composition brought about by changes in myocardial metabolic state. This function can be modulated by neural and humoral stimuli acting on the arterioles themselves and/or on prearteriolar vessels.

Adaptation to pressure changes. These vessels are relatively spared from increases of aortic pressure, but dilate when their inflow pressure decreases, in response to an increased concentration of vasodilator metabolites in the interstitial fluid, and tend to maintain flow constant.

Histologic structure. Their remarkable capacity to control flow resistance is provided by their very thick muscular wall. Their wall-to-lumen ratio is 2:3, compared with 1:4 in conductive arteries. Some arterioles have intimal cushions at branching sites and these may provide arterioles with the possibility of regional, temporal, and spatial variability of flow (see ahead); they are very richly innervated.

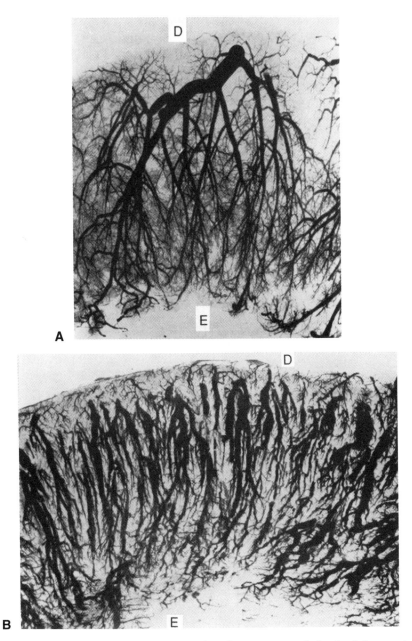

Fig. 4.3 Transmural course of arterial and venous vessels in the left ventricular free wall. A. The arterial blood supply is provided by branches running nearly perpendicularly from the epicardium to the endocardium, often giving off side branches at right angles. **B.** The venous drainage is provided by veins that run nearly perpendicularly from the endocardium (E) to the epicardium (D). (Modified from ref. 4.)

4.1.2 The meta-arteriolar and capillary segment

As arterioles subdivide and taper they terminate in precapillary sphincters (30–15 μm in diameter) composed of SMCs, which in turn lead into meta-arterioles (20–10 μm in diameter) that have very few SMCs.

Within the territory of distribution of each arteriole, intimal cushions and precapillary sphincters control the *regional* microdistribution of flow, which may alternate in adjacent regions (see ahead). The recruitment of the capillaries, one for each myocardial fiber, also originates here: there are about 3000 capillaries/mm^2 cross-sectional area of the myocardium, but their density is about 20% higher in inner than in outer layers.

4.1.3 Venules and veins

Venules (15–100 μm) have only isolated and poorly developed SMCs in their walls. The course of the veins in the free wall of the left ventricle differs from that of the arteries. The small veins in the subendocardial zone continue into large-caliber veins which course straight out to the epicardial surface (see Fig. 4.3B). There are numerous interconnections between venules and also between large veins. As blood in the venous system is at a very low pressure compared with that in the arterial system, smaller changes of distending pressure or of smooth muscle contraction are sufficient to influence the caliber, flow resistance, and upstream pressure of these vessels. Although the venous system contributes a detectable fraction of the total coronary flow resistance, and venous pressure can influence capillary recruitment and the blood volume content in the ventricular wall, the venous side of the coronary circulation has so far received scant attention.[5]

4.2 DISTRIBUTION OF CORONARY VASCULAR RESISTANCE

The vascular resistance is distributed in series along the coronary vascular bed, but it also varies in the parallel vascular segments in different layers of the ventricular wall and even within the same layer. Not only are coronary vessels distensible, undergoing passive and active changes in caliber, but also flow is pulsatile and extravascular compression in the ventricular wall is phasic, causing phasic changes in the caliber of different sections of the coronary vascular bed. During each cardiac beat, the cyclic changes in volume, resistance, and flow in successive vascular sections in series, are *out of phase*. The time taken by the successive sections of the vascular bed to fill after being squeezed during systole (indicated by their time constant, $t_{0.5}$, in analogy to the electric circuit of a condenser) is also variable in relation to their capacitance and their downstream vascular and extravascular resistance.

During systole the main site of cyclical storage of blood—"capacitance"—is in the section of the arterial tree that is outside the ventricular wall, i.e. the extramural arteries: blood enters epicardial arteries from the aorta and is also squeezed backward from intramural arteries. The elastic energy accumulated during systole helps to propel the blood through collapsed intramural vessels at the beginning of diastole. The time constant of this compartment is short (about 0.2 s).

During diastole the main site of capacitance is in intramyocardial vessels, as blood accumulates in the capillaries and intramyocardial venules and veins from which it was squeezed during systole. The vascular cross-section and myocardial compressive forces are large and the time constant of vessel filling during early diastole is long (about 1.5 s), and longer in subendocardial than subepicardial layers.

According to the Poiseuille formula (see Ch. 3.3.2), resistance generally varies inversely with the fourth power of the vessel radius; thus, small changes in coronary vessel caliber produce large changes in flow resistance of resistive vessels. For example, a 10% change in diameter involving uniformly all resistive vessels would produce approximately a 50% change in flow at constant coronary perfusion pressure. However, the evaluation of changes of coronary vasomotor tone according to conventional hemodynamic principles is complicated by the distribution of resistance and capacitance among the different segments of vascular bed, by variations in intramyocardial pressure in the different myocardial layers, and by the effect of heart rate. Comparative assessment of the behavior of vasomotor tone in the individual segments of the coronary bed is therefore valid only under carefully defined conditions, as changes in resistance in one segment can be compensated for by opposite changes in other segments in series (see 4.2.5).

The interaction of intramyocardial compressive forces and vascular cross-section of resistive segments with coronary perfusion pressure varies in the parallel circuits that connect large arteries to large veins in inner and outer layers of the ventricular wall, and, at the microvascular level, it also varies within each layer; this is defined as *in-parallel* distribution of resistance. The distribution of resistance along parallel vessels in inner and outer layers is best described by a series of pressure/flow curves (see 4.2.3). The understanding of the in-parallel distribution of resistance requires some knowledge of intramyocardial tissue pressure, vascular cross-section, and capacitance. (For details see the review by Hoffman in reference 6.)

In each parallel circuit, the distribution of resistance varies along the successive segments connecting arteries to veins: this is defined as the *in-series* distribution of resistance. The integrated in-parallel and in-series distribution of resistance determines total CBF for each level of aortic pressure.

4.2.1 Transmural distribution of intramyocardial tissue pressure

Accurate measurements of interstitial tissue pressure across the left ventricular wall are beset with technical problems, not only because of the mechanical distortions introduced by the measuring devices but also because of the local effects of solid tissue pressure around the vessels. However, there is reasonable agreement that intramyocardial pressure during systole is close to intraventricular pressure in subendocardial layers and to intrathoracic pressure in subepicardial layers, decreasing in a linear fashion from endocardium to epicardium.[7]

Interstitial pressure in the right ventricular wall during systole is proportionally lower than in the left ventricular wall, as systolic pressure in the right ventricle is about one-fifth of that in the left. *During systole*, intramyocardial pressure appears to be sufficiently high to prevent systolic flow across the whole wall (perhaps with the exception of the outermost layers) and to squeeze intramyocardial blood *forward* out of the capillaries, venules and veins towards the coronary sinus and *backward* from subendocardial and midwall layers towards epicardial arteries. However, as pressure is higher in subendocardial layers, subendocardial vessels are compressed more than subepicardial vessels.

During diastole, intramyocardial pressure is low across the different layers and is only slightly higher in the subendocardial layer than in the subepicardial layer.[7] However, when left ventricular diastolic pressure is elevated, the subendocardial intramyocardial pressure increases because of the resulting left ventricular distension and the increased tissue pressure.

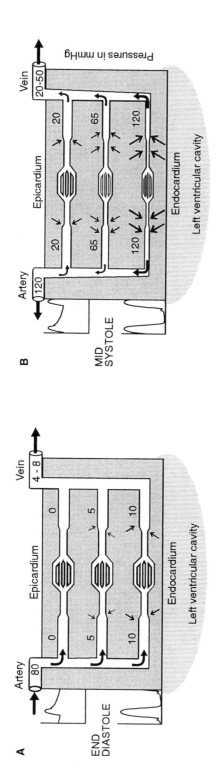

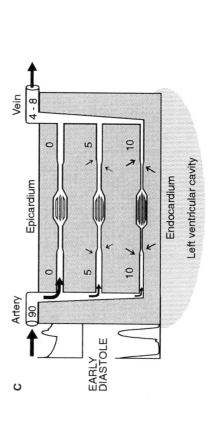

80

4.2.2 Distribution of capacitance

The volume of blood contained in the coronary circulation is about 15–20% of myocardial mass, depending on the vascular tone, and most of this volume is contained in intramyocardial vessels, particularly capillaries, venules, and veins. The vascularity of subendocardial layers is 10–20% greater than that of subepicardial layers.[8] The distribution of blood also varies during the cardiac cycle—during systole, epicardial coronary arteries accumulate blood. However, the volume of blood in epicardial arteries is small compared with the intramyocardial blood volume; thus, the time constant of filling and emptying is of the order of 0.2 s for large epicardial arteries and 1.5 s for intramyocardial vessels.[9]

During systole, most of the blood entering the left coronary artery (10–25% of flow per beat) is stored in the epicardial arteries (more so during adrenergic stimulation).[10] Moreover, particularly during isovolumic ventricular contraction, blood is also squeezed retrogradely into the epicardial arteries from the arterial intramyocardial vessels.[11] At the same time, intramyocardial blood is squeezed out into the venous side of the heart.

During diastole, the blood stored in epicardial arteries in systole is very rapidly propelled into intramyocardial vessels, which have emptied to a variable extent during systole. The magnitude of these cyclical blood volume variations is greater and their time course longer in subendocardial layers because, as previously indicated, their vascular volume is greater than that of subepicardial layers and because they are exposed to higher extravascular pressures during systole. Thus, the time needed for them to refill and resume their maximal caliber is much longer for subendocardial than subepicardial vessels; this contributes to the impairment in subendocardial perfusion that occurs during tachycardia (see Fig. 4.4).

4.2.3 Distribution of resistance in parallel

The in-parallel distribution of resistance among different layers across the ventricular wall can be studied by pressure/flow curves, which provide information on the differences in vascular and extravascular resistance *between* subendocardial and subepicardial layers of the ventricular wall. However, also *within* the same layer, the vascular resistance of parallel vascular segments branching from conductive arteries and connecting to conductive veins varies and causes a spatial and temporal heterogeneity of blood flow.

Effects of tissue pressure on transmural pressure/flow relationships during maximal coronary vasodilation

The interaction between perfusion pressure, intramyocardial pressure, and vascularity (i.e. between extravascular and vascular resistance and the effects of heart rate) across the thickness of the left ventricular wall are best assessed by considering pressure/flow relations in

Fig. 4.4 Schematic illustration of the changes in interstitial and intravascular pressures and vessel caliber across the left ventricular free wall during the cardiac cycle. A. In end-diastole, the vascular cross-section of the resistance beds is mainly determined by metabolic demands, when coronary flow is not exhausted, and by the difference between interstitial and intravascular pressures, when the vessels are maximally dilated. **B.** During systole, interstitial tissue pressure is greater in endocardial than in mid- or epicardial layers (120, 65, 20 mmHg); blood is squeezed out of the myocardium into the arterial and venous sides, more in the inner than in the outer layers of the wall. **C.** In early diastole, interstitial pressure decreases rapidly, but inner vessels that have been more intensely squeezed during systole take longer to reach their full diastolic dimensions. (Modified from ref. 7.)

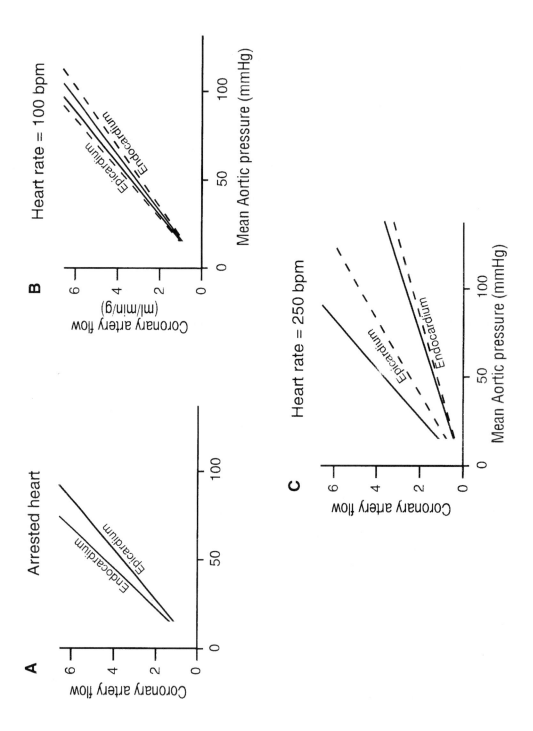

82

arrested and beating hearts, following maximal vasodilation, and in inner and outer layers of the ventricular wall.

In the *complete absence* of coronary tone, flow is linearly related to pressure (except in the lowest part of the curve where changes in pressure cause important changes in vessel lumen). The slope of the linear portion of this pressure/flow curve defines the maximal coronary conductance, i.e. the minimal coronary resistance. When expressed in terms of flow per unit volume of tissue, the slope of the curve defines the specific coronary conductance and is determined by the cross-sectional area of the resistive vascular bed per unit volume of myocardium. The slope is less when vasomotor tone is not completely abolished or when the vascular cross-sectional area is reduced, either because of a reduced number or reduced cross-section of vessels, or because of increased tissue mass in myocardial hypertrophy. Pressure/flow relations reflect only the transmural distribution of vascular resistance in arrested, fully vasodilated hearts, whereas in working hearts they also reflect the effect of the systolic–diastolic interaction caused by cyclic myocardial extravascular compression.

In nonbeating hearts, maximal conductance is higher in subendocardial than in subepicardial layers. In beating hearts, conductance is lower in subendocardial layers and decreases progressively with tachycardia, particularly in the presence of left ventricular hypertrophy (see Fig. 4.5).[12,13] In the intermediate layers of the wall the behavior of conductance varies gradually between these two extremes. The difference between coronary perfusion pressure of intramyocardial arterial branches and extravascular tissue compression (which is related to systolic ventricular pressure) is a major determinant of overall subendocardial flow resistance, particularly during tachycardia; this becomes relevant in the presence of aortic stenosis or epicardial coronary obstruction, and also of prearteriolar constriction.

During ventricular contraction, subendocardial and midwall arteries and arterioles become more narrowed relative to those in the subepicardium (as more blood is squeezed backward) and hence *at the onset of diastole they present a higher resistance to flow and take longer to resume their full diastolic caliber.* Under normal conditions, early diastolic pressure and the systolic expansion of conductive arteries (which transforms kinetic energy of blood flow into potential elastic energy during systole) during diastole contribute to the propulsion of blood into the partially or totally collapsed intramural vessels, reducing the time required for their return to full diastolic caliber. This effect is more critical for subendocardial vessels, which, as described, have a longer time constant for filling as they are more intensely squeezed during systole. Tachycardia impairs subendocardial blood flow because the time constant of diastolic filling of intramyocardial vessels does not shorten with heart

---

Fig. 4.5 Difference in transmural coronary flow resistance assessed from pressure/flow relation in maximally vasodilated dog hearts. The relation between perfusion pressure and flow is linear except at very low distending pressure (not shown on the graph). The larger the increase in flow for a given increase in perfusion pressure, the lower the resistance to flow. In the arrested heart, resistance is lower in subendocardial than in subepicardial layers **(A),** indicating a greater subendocardial vascular cross-section of resistive vessels. In the beating heart (——) **(B)** at a heart rate of 100 beats/min, resistance becomes slightly lower in subepicardial than in subendocardial layers, indicating that, in the presence of maximal coronary vasodilation, systolic compression reduces flow more in subendocardial than in subepicardial layers. The effect of systolic compression on flow resistance becomes dramatic at a heart rate of 250 beats/min **(C)**. This effect is accentuated markedly by the presence of myocardial hypertrophy (---). (From data reported in refs 12 and 13.)

rate and becomes a limiting factor for the perfusion of subendocardial layers if arteriolar pressure is low relative to intraventricular pressure.

Given a sufficiently high perfusion pressure, a sufficiently long diastole, and adequate systolic expansion of conductive arteries or an adequate subendocardial coronary flow reserve, the subendocardium can be adequately perfused. However, when perfusion pressure at the origin of arteriolar vessels is significantly lower than systolic ventricular pressure, and with smaller systolic expansion of conductive arteries (as in the presence of aortic stenosis, coronary obstructions, or prearteriolar coronary vasoconstriction), perfusion becomes jeopardized earlier in inner than in outer layers of the ventricular wall. Inner layers then become even more susceptible to ischemia if diastolic time is short and if myocardial oxygen consumption increases. Selective dilation or constriction of subepicardial resistive vessels can influence perfusion pressure of subendocardial arteriolar vessels and hence subendocardial flow (see Ch. 6).

Heterogeneity of regional microperfusion within the same myocardial layer

The pattern of branching and the level of tone in individual prearterioles, arterioles, and capillary sphincters determine differences in regional CBF, which is not abolished by vasodilation induced by adenosine infusion. In addition, cyclic variations in local tone every 30–90 s[14] contribute to a temporal heterogeneity of perfusion in the same region.

This conclusion can be inferred from a large body of studies that show convincingly considerable regional differences in myocardial blood flow (assessed by the microsphere technique) within the same myocardial layer, as well as temporal variations within the same region. This temporal and spatial heterogeneity is considerable—from 40 to 160% of the mean in the same region and up to threefold larger in adjacent regions.[15,16] The smaller the volume of myocardium examined, the greater the variability.[14] In addition to the heterogeneity of perfusion detectable by the microsphere technique, there is considerable heterogeneity at the capillary level.

Regional temporal heterogeneity of microvascular flow seems to be a generalized phenomenon common to other vascular beds and would serve the purpose of optimizing blood–tissue exchanges. It is consistent with observations of regional variability of myocardial oxygen tension, venous oxygen saturation, and concentration of metabolites in adjacent areas of ventricular myocardium.[17,18] The control mechanisms responsible for this spatial cyclical variation of microvascular perfusion are unknown.

The intermittent changes in tone that occur with either changes in resistance or with the opening and closing of vessels enable *recruitment* and *derecruitment* of parallel vascular units (which contribute to local microheterogeneity of perfusion and can modulate total coronary resistance) to take place. This additional modulatory mechanism of total vascular resistance has received little consideration and is difficult to assess.

4.2.4 Distribution of resistance in series

Pressure/flow curves provide information on the total flow resistance across the parallel vascular beds interposed between large epicardial coronary arteries and large epicardial veins, but provide no information on the in-series distribution of resistance along the successive vascular segments. The individual contribution of successive coronary vascular segments to total resistance can be inferred from the progressive drop in mean pressure from the aorta to the coronary sinus. Although such an inference is an approximation because the vascular cross-section, intravascular pressure gradients, and flow vary considerably during the cardiac cycle and are out of phase, the magnitude of the drop roughly reflects the distribution of resistance, which seems to be as follows: about 10% of total resistance occurs in vessels larger than 500 µm in diameter; 30% occurs in vessels between 500 and 100 µm; 40% occurs in vessels between 100 µm and capillaries, and 20% occurs between capillaries and large veins.

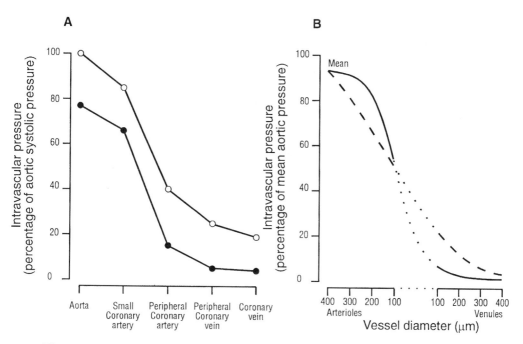

Fig. 4.6 Pressure gradients along the coronary vascular bed. A. In anesthetized dogs, systolic (○) and diastolic (●) pressures are expressed as percentages of systolic aortic pressure in a small epicardial coronary artery (resected and cannulated retrogradely), in a peripheral coronary artery (resected and cannulated anterogradely), in a peripheral coronary vein (resected and cannulated retrogradely), and in a coronary vein (cannulated anterogradely). The greatest drop in pressure occurs between epicardial coronary branches (small coronary artery cannulated retrogradely) and precapillary segments (small coronary artery cannulated anterogradely), where the major fraction of flow resistance occurs, but a measurable pressure drop occurs between the aorta and small epicardial coronary artery branches (thus obviously part of prearteriolar vessels). (From data presented in ref. 19.) **B.** Mean coronary pressure drop from the aorta to small epicardial coronary arteries and veins in a rabbit heart measured by the servo-nul technique on the surface of the epicardium. The greatest pressure drop occurs at the level of arterial vessels 100 µm in diameters. The profile of the pressure drop may change in different conditions. During infusion of dipyridamole (dashed curve) the pressure drop increases across large vessels (prearteriolar), indicating that they failed to dilate in proportion to the increased blood flow. (From data presented in ref. 20.)

Measurements of intravascular pressure have been obtained using fluid-filled tubes:

a.   in small tertiary myocardial coronary artery branches
b.   at the "precapillary" level
c.   at the "postcapillary" level
d.   in epicardial coronary veins (see Fig. 4.6A).

The pressure gradients between these points were shown to vary considerably during neural stimulation and pharmacologic intervention, but the interpretation of the relative changes is complicated by the failure to maintain heart rate and aortic pressure constant and by the lack of simultaneous measurement of flow changes.[19] Studies performed by a servo-nul technique on epicardial vessels confirm the existence of a continuous distribution of pressure drop, with a 20 mmHg pressure gradient between the aorta and vessels 0.2 mm in diameter and a 35 mmHg pressure gradient in arterioles up to 0.1 mm in diameter. About 55% of estimated total vascular resistance is distal to arterioles 0.1 mm in diameter, the remaining 45% being proximal, thus suggesting that the metabolic autoregulation of vascular resistance takes place mainly in those arteriolar vessels of about 100 mm (see Fig. 4.6B).[20] However, when these vessels dilate, resistance across the other prearteriolar segments (which also contribute a significant pressure drop, but are not directly influenced by the composition of the interstitial fluid) must also decrease to allow flow to increase maximally. A direct positive feedback mechanism leading to prearteriolar vessel vasodilation in response to an increased flow is represented by the flow-mediated local release of EDRFs by endothelial cells.

The in-series distribution of coronary resistance is modulated by neural and humoral vasomotor stimuli that may have widely different, and even opposite, effects on successive segments of the coronary vascular bed and in subendocardial and subepicardial resistive vessels (see Ch. 5).

4.2.5 Integration of flow resistance in series and in parallel

Considering the segmental, in-parallel, and in-series distribution of coronary vascular resistance, CBF is determined by the ratio of aortic pressure (AOP) minus right atrial pressure (RAP) and the sum of segmental coronary resistance: $CBF = (AOP - RAP)/(r_0 + r_1 + r_2 + r_3)$, where r_0 is the resistance across conductive arteries, normally negligible, r_1 is the average resistance across prearterioles in the parallel vascular beds, r_2 is the average resistance across arterioles, the main site of regulation of flow, and r_3 is the average resistance interposed between arterioles and the right atrium. Metabolic autoregulation at the arteriolar level is the main compensatory mechanism for increased resistance in the other segments. Increased resistance in a large artery influences all downstream vessels, but increased resistance of prearteriolar vessels may be patchily distributed among parallel vessels and hence patchily affects downstream vessels. The values of r_1, r_2, and r_3 differ along parallel vascular beds, in particular in subendocardial and subepicardial vessels. Thus, even when total coronary vascular resistance and hence total blood flow remain the same, the transmural distribution of resistance and hence of blood flow may vary.

The pressure drop at the end of each segment depends on the flow resistance through all preceding segments, as well as on flow. Pressure in the right atrium is somewhat lower than pressure at zero flow along the preceding vascular segments. The zero flow pressure is higher in subendocardial layers than in subepicardial layers, but the interpretation of pressure at zero flow (critical closing pressure) is made difficult by the changes in caliber of the vessels with decreasing distending pressure.[6]

4.3 REGULATION OF OXYGEN TRANSPORT AND CORONARY BLOOD FLOW

In normal resting humans and in unanesthetized dogs, mean left CBF exhibits considerable individual variations. These variations are largely dependent on heart rate, but, when expressed per beat, flow corresponds to about 1 ml/g myocardium. Right ventricular flow per unit volume of tissue is about 75% of that in the left ventricular myocardium.[6] In normal resting conditions, the individual variability of flow values not accounted for by heart rate values is a result of differences in resting myocardial oxygen consumption (MVO_2) for the same heart rate and a variable degree of myocardial oxygen extraction.[21]

During submaximal exercise in both humans and dogs, CBF increases in line with MVO_2 (see Fig, 4.7).[22] In unanesthetized dogs, subendocardial flow is about 15% greater than subepicardial flow and is related to a greater shortening of subendocardial fibers[23] and to a higher oxygen consumption.[18] The ratio of endocardial to epicardial blood flow (endo–epi ratio) decreases with tachycardia during maximal vasodilation (see Fig. 4.8).

At any level of CBF, oxygen delivery to the myocardium is determined by two factors— the rate of oxygen transfer from capillaries to myocardial cells and the supply of oxygen to the capillaries. The rate of oxygen transfer is affected by the PO_2 gradient between cells and

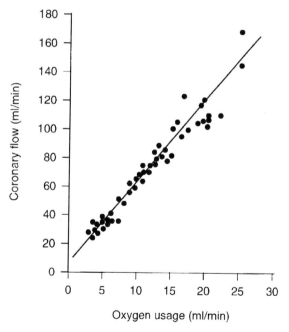

Fig. 4.7 Relation between myocardial oxygen uptake and coronary blood flow. The relation between myocardial oxygen uptake and CBF is linear over a sevenfold range during exercise in dogs. The coronary sinus oxygen saturation remains practically constant over this wide range, indicating the heart's remarkable ability to match myocardial oxygen supply with demand without changing oxygen extraction. (From data presented in ref. 22.)

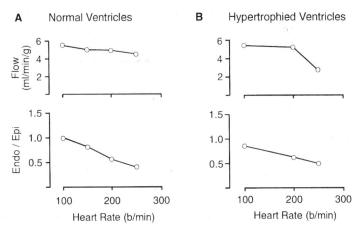

Fig. 4.8 Effect of tachycardia on mean and transmural blood flow (endo/epi ratio) in fully dilated normal and hypertrophied ventricles (the latter being 100% heavier). As the heart rate increases from 100 to 250 beats/min during maximal adenosine-induced coronary dilation of resistive vessels, mean flow decreases slightly in normal ventricles **(A)** and markedly in hypertrophied ventricles **(B)** (in which subepicardial flow also decreases). The endo/epi ratio decreases equally in normal and hypertrophied hearts, but the absolute drop in subendocardial flow is greatest in hypertrophied hearts because of the larger decrease in mean flow. (From data presented in ref. 13.)

capillaries, the intercapillary distance, and the oxygen/hemoglobin dissociation curve. The oxygen supply to myocardial tissue is determined by the arterial oxygen content, by the blood flow, and by the PO_2 gradient, which determines average myocardial oxygen extraction. The metabolic regulation of CBF is subject to *neurohumoral modulation* by vasomotor stimuli that cause reciprocal changes in myocardial oxygen extraction when MVO_2 remains constant. The possibility of CBF increasing above resting levels and matching increased MVO_2 without changes in myocardial oxygen extraction is defined as *coronary flow reserve*.

4.3.1 Rate of oxygen tissue transfer

The rate at which oxygen is transferred from blood to tissues depends on the gradient of PO_2. The value of PO_2 is about 90 mmHg in arterial blood and about 20–25 mmHg in the coronary sinus blood under basal conditions, whereas tissue PO_2 values as low as 1–5 mmHg have been recorded in the myocardium.[17] As arteriovenous shunting (assessed by microsphere recovery in the coronary sinus) is negligible, nonuniform oxygen extraction at the capillary level could be explained by the regional, temporal, and spatial heterogeneity of myocardial blood flow.[14–16] Capillaries with very high flow may act as "functional" shunts for oxygen, increasing *mean* oxygen saturation of the coronary sinus.

Recruitment of capillaries during increased metabolic activity could considerably reduce the effective intercapillary distance. However, as coronary flow increases, the *average* time spent by blood in the capillaries becomes shorter (from about 5 s at rest to about 1 s during peak exercise).

Even for the same end-capillary PO_2/tissue gradient, the oxygen extraction can increase considerably when the hemoglobin/oxygen dissociation curve becomes shifted to the right,

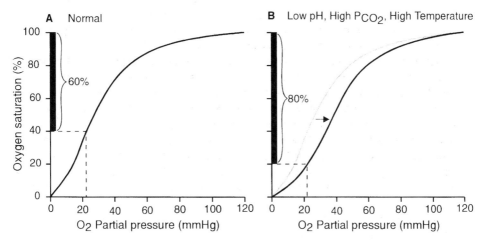

Fig. 4.9 Effect of the shape of the oxygen–hemoglobin dissociation curve on myocardial oxygen extraction. At low pH, high PCO_2 and high temperature (such as during increased cardiac work), the oxygen–hemoglobin dissociation curve is displaced to the right so that, for example, at the same PO_2 of 22, oxygen saturation may decrease from 40 to 20% and oxygen extraction may increase from 60 to 80%. In the range of PO_2 values observed in the coronary sinus, the oxygen–hemoglobin dissociation curve is steepest: small changes in PO_2 are associated with large changes in venous oxygen saturation. During coronary vasodilator stimuli that increase blood flow without increasing oxygen consumption, coronary sinus oxygen saturation is high and small changes are associated with large changes of PO_2. Therefore, in the absence of changes in MVO_2, the effects of coronary constrictor stimuli are best assessed by measuring oxygen saturation in the coronary sinus, and the effects of dilator stimuli are best assessed by measuring coronary sinus PO_2.

because pH decreases or PCO_2 and local temperatures rise. At the low levels of PO_2 present in coronary sinus blood, the oxygen dissociation curve is at its steepest and, therefore, not only are small changes in PO_2 associated with large changes in both myocardial oxygen extraction and coronary blood oxygen saturation but also small shifts of this curve have a considerable effect on oxygen dissociation from hemoglobin (see Fig. 4.9).

The physiologic role of myoglobin, which can store oxygen for only a few beats, is still unclear.[24]

4.3.2 Determinants of oxygen supply

For any given *rate* of oxygen transfer set by the factors discussed in the previous section, the *total amount* of oxygen taken up by the myocardium or MVO_2 (expressed as ml O_2/min/100 g myocardium) depends on CBF (expressed as ml/min/100 g myocardium) and arteriovenous difference in oxygen concentration $[A-V]O_2$ (expressed as volume O_2/100 ml blood): $MVO_2 = CBF \times [A-V]O_2$.

At constant blood flow, oxygen delivery to the myocardium can only increase by 20–30% as basal oxygen extraction is about 60%.

The following examples illustrate the effects of changing CBF (at constant MVO_2) on $[A-V]O_2$, myocardial oxygen extraction, coronary sinus oxygen saturation and PO_2:

1. Assuming a 100% saturation and an O_2 content of 1.35 volumes per g hemoglobin, for a normal value of 15 g hemoglobin arterial blood carries 20.25 volumes O_2 per 100 ml blood to which 0.3 volumes of dissolved O_2 are to be added.

   Assuming a 40% coronary sinus O_2 saturation, which normally corresponds to a PO_2 of 25 mmHg, the venous O_2 content is 8.10 volumes O_2 per 100 ml blood. Thus, the coronary $[A-V]O_2$ is 12.15 volumes per 100 ml blood, which corresponds to a myocardial O_2 extraction of 60%. (With this level of myocardial extraction and a resting MVO_2 of 8 ml O_2/100 g myocardium, CBF must be 65.8 ml/min/100 g.)

2. A 25% reduction of CBF (from 65.80 to 49.35) at constant MVO_2 requires $[A-V]O_2$ to increase from 12.15 to 16.21 volumes and myocardial O_2 extraction to increase from 60 to 80%, coronary sinus O_2 saturation to decrease from 40 to 20%, and PO_2 to decrease from about 25 to about 19 mmHg (assuming no changes occur in pH, PCO_2 or temperature).

3. Halving CBF at a constant MVO_2 would be impossible because myocardial O_2 extraction cannot double (as it is already 60%).

4. Doubling CBF from 65.8 to 131.6 ml/min/100 g, at constant MVO_2, would cause $[A-V]O_2$ to decrease from 12.15 to 6.1, myocardial O_2 extraction to decrease from 60 to 30%, coronary sinus O_2 saturation to increase from 40 to 70%, and PO_2 to increase from 25 to 43 mmHg.

5. Reducing hemoglobin content to one-half 7.50% at constant MVO_2 would require a doubling of resting CBF (and a fourfold increase when MVO_2 doubles).

6. Doubling of ventricular mass by myocardial hypertrophy would not affect MVO_2/g and hence flow/g, but it would require doubling of resting flow through main coronary arteries (the combination of doubling ventricular mass and halving hemoglobin concentration would require doubling of resting flow/g, but a fourfold increase in resting flow through main coronary arteries).

Whenever a decrease in coronary flow is compensated for by increased oxygen extraction, the supply of substrates and removal of metabolic waste products is decreased. When percentage oxygen saturation falls in the arterial blood, not only is the arterial oxygen content reduced, but the PO_2 at the arterial origin of the capillary is also reduced, and with it the PO_2 blood/tissue gradient.

4.3.3 Metabolic regulation of coronary blood flow

During exercise, coronary flow increases in proportion to myocardial oxygen requirements (see Fig. 4.7) without changes occurring in myocardial oxygen extraction; this behavior can also be observed in isolated denervated hearts, indicating a direct, close feedback loop between myocardial metabolic activity and coronary flow resistance, which is responsible for the autoregulation of CBF.[21,22]

Autoregulation of coronary blood flow

When metabolic requirements do not vary, the heart, like other organs, exhibits an intrinsic tendency to maintain blood flow constant despite changes in arterial perfusion pressure, as long as the intrinsic capacity to autoregulate flow is retained. Variation of coronary perfusion pressure in the beating heart, in the presence of unaltered myocardial metabolic requirements, can be achieved only by perfusing the coronary arteries separately from the aorta, so that aortic pressure remains constant when coronary arterial pressure is varied. Pressure/flow curves in such an artificial model of a working heart with intact vascular tone show that, when perfusion pressure is varied, flow remains nearly constant over a mean perfusion pressure range of about 60–120 mmHg. The level at which flow remains constant is determined by the level of myocardial oxygen consumption:[25] when this is low, the plateau of flow is low; when oxygen consumption is high, the plateau is high (see Fig. 4.10). Over this range, a *slight* increase of flow may result from a coronary perfusion pressure effect on myocardial oxygen consumption or from imperfect autoregulation; in the latter case, the slope of the plateau defines the deviation from perfect autoregulation. Autoregulation becomes less perfect in the presence of myocardial hypertrophy, particularly in subendocardial layers.

In the presence of intact vascular tone, the plateau of the pressure/flow relationship varies across the thickness of the left ventricular wall: in subepicardial layers it extends down to about 35 mmHg in anesthetized dogs and to about 25 mmHg in conscious dogs, which have lower heart rates; in subendocardial layers the plateau extends only to about 70 mmHg in anesthetized dogs and to about 40 mmHg in conscious dogs (see Fig. 4.11).[26,27] Thus, in the beating heart, subendocardial layers compensate for the reduction of perfusion pressure much less well than subepicardial layers, in spite of their larger vascular cross-section. In contrast, at the opposite end of the plateau, when coronary artery pressure is elevated beyond the range of autoregulation, flow increases less in subepicardial than in subendocardial layers because the latter have a larger cross-section of resistive vessels.[6]

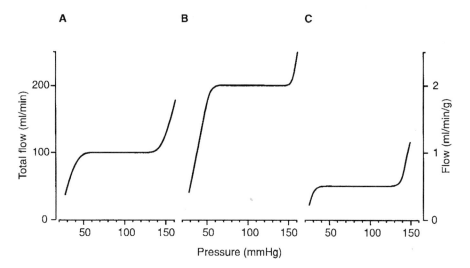

Fig. 4.10 Autoregulation of coronary blood flow in anesthetized dogs: A, normal myocardial oxygen consumption; **B,** high myocardial oxygen consumption or low arterial oxygen content; **C,** low myocardial oxygen consumption. In the presence of coronary autoregulation, flow is determined by the level of MVO_2, by the oxygen content of the arterial blood, and by the neurohumoral modulation of coronary vasomotor tone. When cardiac work remains constant, flow also remains practically constant over a wide range of values of coronary perfusion pressure. The deviation of the pressure/flow curve from a horizontal line indicates the deviation from perfect autoregulation: the relation applies equally to measurements of flow per gram or for the total left ventricle (assuming a weight of 100 g). Autoregulation fails when pressure either decreases or increases beyond its range. The level of the plateau depends on both MVO_2 and arterial oxygen content. Halving of arterial oxygen content is approximately equivalent to the doubling of MVO_2. (From data presented in ref. 28.)

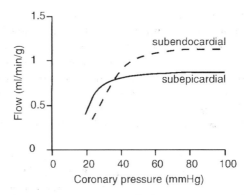

Fig. 4.11 Relation between coronary perfusion pressure and flow in subendo-cardial and subepicardial layers in the presence of coronary autoregulation in conscious dogs. Perfusion is slightly higher in subendocardial layers where flow begins to decrease when coronary perfusion pressure falls below about 40 mmHg. In subepicardial layers flow begins to decrease only when perfusion pressure falls below about 25 mmHg. In conscious dogs, the plateau of the pressure/flow curve extends to much lower values than in anesthetized animals because of their lower resting heart rate and MVO_2. (From data presented in ref. 28.)

The time taken to autoregulate when pressure is changed is of the order of several seconds because, when pressure is suddenly elevated, flow increases promptly and takes over 10 s to return to the plateau level.

The mechanisms responsible for maintaining a constant flow when pressure increases, are not necessarily exactly the same as those involved in maintaining flow when pressure decreases. The myogenic mechanism is likely to be predominantly involved in autoregulation when pressure is increased, but is likely to interact, during the initial seconds of the change, with metabolic autoregulation. Metabolic autoregulation has a dominant role when aortic pressure falls below resting levels.

When MVO_2 increases, the effector arm of the control system is represented by increased leakage of vasodilator metabolites from myocardial cells into the interstitial space and possibly by reduced tissue PO_2 and increased PCO_2 levels (see Ch. 5.2.1). Metabolites diffusing into the arteriolar walls cause concentration-dependent smooth muscle relaxation, and upon entering the bloodstream they are promptly washed away and/or degraded and do not produce systemic effects. The resulting arteriolar dilation causes flow to increase and closes the feedback loop by reducing the metabolite concentration in the interstitial space and vessel wall and by increasing tissue PO_2; thus, a new dynamic equilibrium is reached and flow is reset at a higher level. Conversely, when heart activity is reduced, extracellular diffusion of metabolites decreases, tissue PO_2 increases, and PCO_2 decreases; thus vasodilation is reduced and flow is reset to a lower level.

When prearteriolar pressure decreases below resting values, because of increased resistance in conductive or prearteriolar vessels, the initial decrease in flow causes reduced washout of metabolites, decreased tissue PO_2, and increased PCO_2, and hence greater arteriolar dilation with restoration of flow and a new dynamic equilibrium.

■ *In normal conditions the tuning of metabolic regulation is so fine that, in a given individual, when myocardial oxygen consumption increases, flow is adjusted over a very wide range of oxygen consumption* without appreciable changes in myocardial O_2 extraction, *as long as sufficient coronary flow reserve is available, but changes in myocardial oxygen extraction can be produced by both neurohumoral modulation and pharmacologic stimuli.* ■

4.3.4 Neurohumoral modulation of coronary flow

For any level of MVO_2, average coronary vascular resistance, and hence flow, can be modulated by a wide variety of neurotransmitters, by vessel wall autacoids, and by drugs acting on different segments of resistive vessels. Neurotransmitters are released at nerve endings; some autacoids are generated locally (EDRFs, prostaglandins) or produced by cells in the adventitia (histamine, kinins, leukotrienes); and others may be released locally by platelets (thromboxane A_2, serotonin), formed during blood clotting (thrombin) or carried in the bloodstream (see Chs 1 and 5). The physiologic role of neurohumoral modulation above that of metabolic coronary autoregulation is not clear, but its effect is easily appreciated when it is not associated with changes in myocardial metabolism and hence in oxygen uptake.

When myocardial oxygen uptake remains constant, any change in flow caused by neurohumoral modulation must be mirrored by a proportional change in oxygen extraction, so that vasodilation or constriction are associated, respectively, with a proportional increase or decrease in coronary sinus PO_2 and oxygen saturation. As myocardial high-energy phosphate stores are sufficient only for a few beats, changes in coronary sinus oxygen saturation reflect, practically instantaneously, the variations in coronary vasomotor tone of resistive vessels (which determine flow) when myocardial oxygen consumption remains constant. For example, vasodilation resulting in the doubling of flow above the level set by the metabolic control must be accompanied by a halving of myocardial oxygen extraction (and hence by an increase in coronary sinus oxygen saturation). Vasoconstrictor stimuli that reduce flow, increase oxygen extraction, thus causing a reduction in oxygen saturation and in PO_2 in the coronary sinus blood. Conversely, vasodilator stimuli that produce vasodilation in excess of that required by metabolic needs, reduce oxygen extraction and hence increase oxygen and PO_2 saturation in the coronary sinus. In resting humans, abolition of α-adrenergic tone causes an approximately 10% increase in CBF and a proportional increase in coronary sinus oxygen saturation, indicating the presence of a tonic basal, nervous coronary vasoconstrictor tone (see Ch. 5.4.1). Subepicardial vessel constriction can prevent transmural blood flow "steal." Conversely, subepicardial vasodilation with luxury perfusion can exacerbate subendocardial ischemia distal to flow-limiting stenoses (see Ch. 6).

Because of the shape of the oxygen dissociation curve, measurement of coronary sinus PO_2 levels provides a more sensitive index of changes in oxygen extraction at high blood flow, and measurement of oxygen saturation provides a better index of changes in oxygen extraction at low blood flow (see Fig. 4.9).

If neurohumoral or pharmacologic stimulation of subendocardial and subepicardial vessels are not the same, average coronary sinus values will tend to reflect the most prominent and diffuse effect. The extent of neurohumoral modulation of coronary flow becomes more difficult to evaluate when stimuli also influence myocardial contractile activity, so that the end result with regard to coronary vascular resistance is the algebraic sum of the myocardial metabolic effect and the vasomotor neurohumoral modulation.

4.3.5 Coronary flow reserve

The maximal coronary flow above resting levels that can be achieved by maximal vasodilation depends on:

a. the perfusion pressure at the origin of the arteriolar vessels relative to interstitial tissue pressure
b. the total vascular cross-section per unit volume of tissue (which implies the complete recruitment of parallel vessels)
c. the level of heart rate.

When the coronary vascular bed is maximally dilated (so that resistance remains fixed at its minimum level), there is an approximate linear relationship between pressure and flow

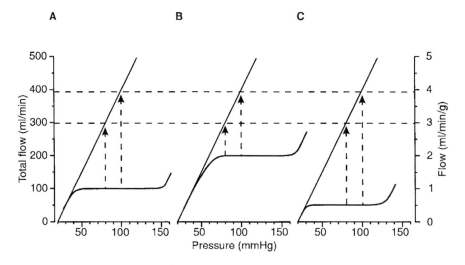

Fig. 4.12 Coronary flow reserve as a function of coronary perfusion pressure and resting flow in a normal ventricle. Conditions in **A, B,** and **C** are as in Figure 4.10. Under maximal coronary vasodilation, the pressure/flow relation is linear over a wide range of pressures. This relationship is independent of the level of resting flow (the position and slope of the straight line are the same in A, B, and C and represent the maximal level of flow attainable at any value of coronary perfusion pressure). In the presence of normal coronary autoregulation, resting flow (which is mainly determined by the level of MVO_2 and of arterial oxygen content), remains constant over a large intermediate range of values of coronary perfusion pressure (thick lines in A, B, and C). For each pressure value, the difference between the thick line (resting coronary flow) and the oblique straight line represents the coronary flow reserve. Therefore, in the normal range of perfusion pressures, coronary flow reserve decreases with coronary perfusion pressure and is lowest when resting flow is highest (dashed lines and arrows correspond to perfusion pressures of 80 and 100 mmHg in A, B, and C). The maximal absolute flow attainable at any given perfusion pressure is the same in A, B, and C, independent of the value of resting flow. However, when expressed as multiples of resting flow in A, B, and C, coronary flow reserve at a perfusion pressure of 80 mmHg is three, one-half, and six times the resting values, respectively; at a pressure of 100 mgHg it is four, two, and nine times resting values. In nonhypertrophied ventricles, the values of coronary flow reserve are the same when expressed as flow per gram or as total flow for the whole left ventricle (assuming a weight of 100 g in the dog) or through a main coronary branch. (Modified from ref. 28.)

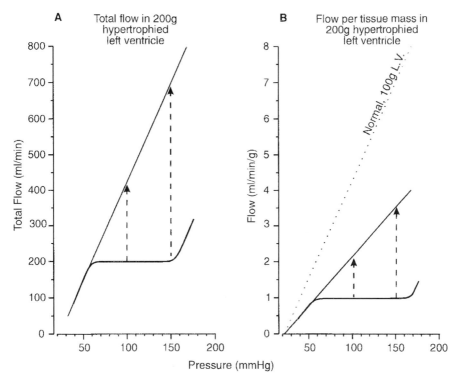

Fig. 4.13 Coronary flow reserve in hypertrophied ventricles. Assuming a doubling of ventricular mass, resting flow per gram of myocardium remains the same but total flow through any large coronary branch doubles. The slope of the pressure/flow curve remains the same when expressed in terms of total flow (**A**), but decreases when flow is expressed in terms of flow per gram of tissue (**B**), as the number of resistive vessels per unit volume of tissue approximately halves. Coronary flow reserve at pressures of 100 and 150 mmHg is the same—double, and 3.5 times the basal flow, respectively, independent of the way that flow is expressed, i.e. per gram or total. (Modified from ref. 28.)

so that perfusion pressure determines the possible increase in flow above resting levels. Resting flow per gram of tissue is in turn determined by the level of myocardial oxygen consumption and by its neurohumoral modulation. Therefore, *coronary flow reserve* must be thought of as *relative* rather than an *absolute* value that depends on four variables:[28]

a.   resting level of flow
b.   cross-sectional area of resistive vessels per unit volume of myocardium and myocardial mass
c.   extracoronary flow resistance
d.   perfusion pressure.

   The *perfusion pressure* that determines flow for any given level of vascular resistance is the pressure at the origin of arteriolar vessels. During maximal coronary dilation, the slope of the pressure/flow curve is very steep; the increase of coronary flow reserve with increasing pressure is, therefore, very substantial (see Fig. 4.12). Under physiologic conditions the coronary perfusion pressure that determines myocardial blood flow corresponds closely to aortic pressure. Aortic pressure is not the determinant of flow in the presence of epicardial

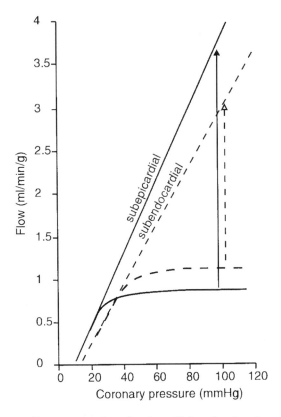

Fig. 4.14 Coronary flow reserve in subepicardial and subendocardial layers of the myocardium. In physiologic conditions, coronary flow reserve is lower in subendocardial layers, where there is a higher basal flow and a lower pressure/flow curve: this difference increases progressively with tachycardia and with elevation of diastolic pressure. (From data reported in ref. 27.)

coronary artery stenoses because the perfusion pressure that determines CBF is then the poststenotic coronary pressure and poststenotic pressure varies with transstenotic blood flow (see Ch. 6). In the presence of aortic stenosis, coronary perfusion pressure is similar to aortic pressure but lower than systolic ventricular pressure, which is the determinant of intramyocardial tissue pressure. For this reason, aortic stenosis can cause an impairment of coronary flow reserve similar to that caused by proximal coronary artery stenosis. The impairment of coronary flow reserve increases during exercise as the transstenotic aortic pressure gradient increases.

The *resting level of flow* determines the possible *further* increase for any given level of perfusion pressure and vascular resistance. The higher the resting level, the lower the absolute and percentage increase that remains available above that level as a reserve (see Figs. 4.12 and 4.13).

The *cross-sectional area of resistive vessels per unit volume of myocardium* influences coronary flow conductance and hence the slope of the pressure/flow curve in inner and outer layers of the ventricular wall (see Fig. 4.14). The greater the vascular cross-sectional area (i.e. the greater the conductance), the steeper the slope of the pressure/flow curve (the greater the increase in flow per unit increase in pressure). In the presence of maximal vasodilation the vascular conductance per unit volume of myocardium can be reduced because:

a. the total number of resistive vessels per unit volume is decreased,
b. the lumen of individual vessels is reduced, or
c. hypertrophy of myocardial cells indirectly decreases the vascular cross-section per unit of myocardial volume.

Extravascular compressive forces reduce coronary flow reserve in subendocardial layers during tachycardia (see Fig. 4.15) and when diastolic ventricular pressure becomes elevated.

Thus, for a given perfusion pressure and vascular conductance, coronary flow reserve is less when resting flow is high, for example during high resting heart work, anemia, hypoxia, or inappropriate coronary vasodilation. For the same resting level of flow and conductance, coronary flow reserve is less when prearteriolar coronary perfusion pressure is low relative to ventricular systolic pressure because of aortic stenosis or significant coronary artery stenosis (epicardial or prearteriolar), and when complete vasodilation is not achieved. For the same level of resting flow and arterial pressure at the origin of arteriolar vessels, coronary flow reserve is less when the vascular cross-section is reduced in either absolute or relative terms (i.e. because of myocardial hypertrophy) and (in subendocardial layers) also during tachycardia.

General principles for the assessment of coronary flow reserve

Coronary flow reserve is often reported in terms of total flow through a coronary artery branch measured with a flowmeter in animals or with a Doppler catheter in man, rather than flow per gram of tissue. In normal hearts this corresponds to a correction factor for the total weight of myocardium perfused by the branch, but, in the presence of myocardial hypertrophy, the increase of myocardial mass leads to a relative reduction in the vascular cross-section of resistive vessels per gram of tissue, although it does not influence resting flow per gram.

In the presence of myocardial hypertrophy, when total flow is measured, the pressure/flow curve maintains the same slope (as the cross-sectional area of resistive vessels remains the same), but resting flow is increased in proportion to the increase in myocardial mass. When flow per gram is measured, resting flow remains the same, but the slope decreases in proportion to the increase in tissue mass (as this indirectly reduces the cross-sectional area of resistive vessels) (see Figs 4.13 and 4.15).

In *animal models*, coronary flow reserve is commonly assessed from the peak level of coronary reactive hyperemia: when CBF through a large epicardial artery is suddenly interrupted for a period of a few seconds and then released, there is a transient, large increase in blood flow above resting values. This increase in flow can also be observed following a very short diastolic single-beat occlusion but is maximal following an occlusion of 15–20 s (showing no further increase thereafter). The peak increase of flow above preocclusion levels is considered to be indicative of the maximal coronary flow achievable in that arterial branch. This is true only as a first approximation because, at constant myocardial work load and coronary perfusion pressure, flow values nearly twice those of peak reactive hyperemia have been observed by prolonged infusion of adenosine (i.e. for more than 20 min) (see Fig. 4.16);[29,30] this could be attributable to further gradual vasodilation or to gradual recruitment of parallel vessels.

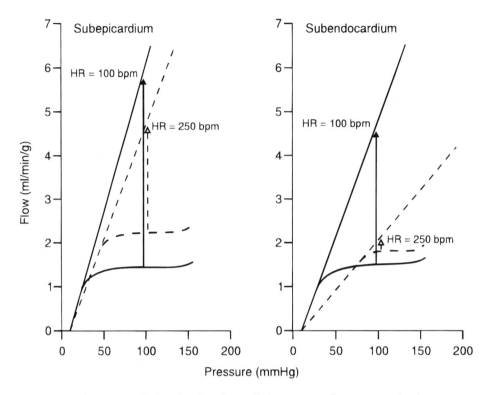

Fig. 4.15 Subepicardial and subendocardial coronary flow reserve in the presence of ventricular hypertrophy. Coronary flow reserve decreases dramatically during tachycardia in subendocardial layers (right panel) and, to a lesser extent, in subepicardial layers (left panel) also. This decrease is due to a combination of the effects of tachycardia on the pressure/flow relation during maximal dilation (dashed line) and the increase of MVO_2 caused by tachycardia. (From data presented in ref. 13.)

Peak reactive hyperemia is commonly expressed as multiples of resting flow and must be thought of as a relative rather than an absolute index, in the same manner as coronary flow reserve. The practise of expressing peak reactive hyperemia as a percentage increase above preocclusion levels is necessitated by the fact that the occluded branch varies in size, and there is no information on the mass of myocardium it perfuses, i.e. flow per gram. In fact, the absolute value of peak reactive hyperemia through an artery is mainly determined by resting flow, perfusion pressure, and conductance. In turn, the resting flow through the arterial branch is influenced, not only by all the factors that determine flow per unit volume of myocardium, but also by the presence of myocardial hypertrophy (which increases resting flow through the branch in proportion to the increase of ventricular mass), as flow per unit volume is largely independent of the presence of hypertrophy. In the presence of hypertrophy that doubles myocardial mass, resting flow through the artery doubles and peak reactive hyperemia is reduced by 50%, although the absolute peak flow remains the same.

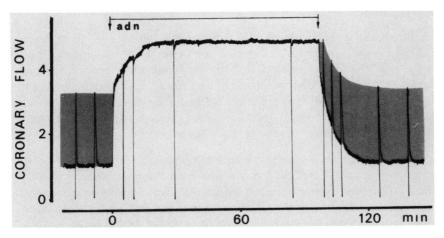

Fig. 4.16 Variability of coronary flow reserve as estimated by peak reactive hyperemia. Continuous recording of circumflex coronary artery blood flow played back at low speed. Resting flow is about 1 ml/min/g, following two 15 s interruptions of coronary flow in control conditions (before time zero), peak reactive hyperemia reaches 3.5 ml/min/g. During adenosine infusion (adn), peak flow becomes higher than in control conditions, reaching a maximum of 4.7 ml/min/g. In control conditions, therefore, peak reactive hyperemia is much lower than observed 20 min after the onset of adenosine infusion. During adenosine infusion, interruption of coronary flow is not followed by any detectable reactive hyperemia as adenosine-induced dilation is already maximal. (Modified from ref. 30.)

An accurate assessment of coronary flow reserve would require measurement of flow per gram of myocardium at rest and during *maximal* coronary vasodilation to be related to perfusion pressure. Measurements of absolute flow through coronary artery branches or through the coronary sinus allow only estimates of percentage increase above the resting level, which cannot be related to flow per gram; hence, it becomes impossible to establish whether a reduced flow reserve is due to an increased resting flow. However, a crucial aspect is the achievement of maximal vasodilation: the response to standard doses of a vasodilator drug may not induce the same degree of coronary vasodilation in all patients under all circumstances.

Although the concept of coronary reserve is useful in understanding the intrinsic physiologic regulation of coronary blood flow, recent evidence indicates that, during ischemia, flow can be increased by vasodilator drugs.[31,32] Thus, some coronary flow reserve can still be present during ischemia. It is not clear whether, during ischemia, the further drug-induced dilation occurs at the level of arteriolar or prearteriolar vessels or is patchily distributed in the "ischemic" territory.

4.4 MYOCARDIAL OXYGEN CONSUMPTION

The rate of myocardial oxygen consumption (MVO_2) has the key role in determining CBF. It therefore becomes important to establish:

a. what are the main factors that set the level of myocardial metabolic activity and hence oxygen consumption
b. how MVO_2 can be assessed in clinical conditions.

MVO_2 is about 15% higher in the subendocardium than in the subepicardium.

4.4.1 Determinants of MVO$_2$

The most important determinant of MVO$_2$ is cardiac contraction, as in the nonbeating heart MVO$_2$ decreases to only 15–20% of that in normal resting conditions. (It is also influenced by the type of substrate utilized: it is slightly higher when using predominantly fatty acids than when using carbohydrates. Catecholamines do not appear to have a direct oxygen-wasting effect.)[33] Most of the time, particularly during exercise, the factors that control metabolic activity *vary concurrently.* However, when they are artificially separated in experimental conditions they appear to rank in the following order:

1. *Heart rate.* The number of times per minute that contraction is activated is *by far* the main determinant of MVO$_2$ in dogs and humans. When heart rate is increased above resting levels by electric pacing, myocardial oxygen uptake approximately doubles when heart rate is doubled.[33,34] However, this is probably an underestimate of the total physiologic effects of heart rate during exercise,[28] as during pacing (but not during exercise) the stroke volume (SV) decreases proportionally (see Ch. 3), causing ventricular volume and wall tension to decrease, and no adrenergic stimulation to occur (see Fig. 4.17).

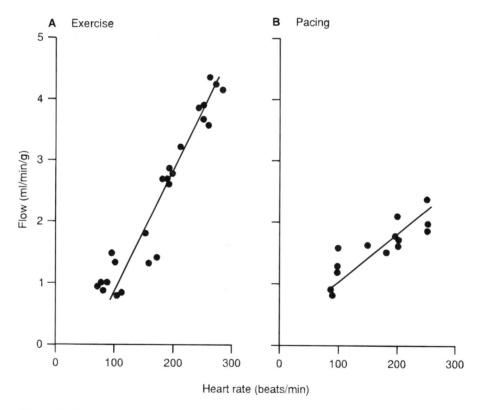

Fig. 4.17 Increase in average transmural myocardial blood flow during exercise (A) and pacing-induced tachycardia (B). During exercise, flow increases approximately threefold when heart rate doubles; during pacing, flow approximately doubles when heart rate doubles. (Modified from ref. 28.)

2. *Myocardial inotropic state.* In dogs, MVO_2 increases by about 30% when dP/dt is doubled by extrasystolic potentiation or by norepinephrine at constant heart rate, aortic pressure, and cardiac output.[35]

3. *Aortic pressure.* In dogs, myocardial oxygen uptake approximately doubles as mean aortic pressure is increased from 75 to 175 mmHg at constant heart rate and SV.[36]

4. *Stroke volume.* In dogs, myocardial oxygen uptake increases by only about 20% when SV is increased by 60% at constant heart rate/systolic blood pressure product.[33]

In some conditions encountered in clinical practise the determinants of MVO_2 do *not* vary concurrently: for example, ventricular volume, SV, and wall tension decrease during paroxysmal or pacing-induced tachycardia; conversely, in the failing heart, inotropic drugs that increase oxygen consumption reduce ventricular volume and wall tension.

During physical exercise the relationship between total body oxygen consumption and MVO_2 can vary. The same total body oxygen consumption during effort can be attained with a lower cardiac work load and hence a lower MVO_2 and blood flow when

a. the peripheral organ blood flow is distributed more efficiently so that a lower cardiac output is required

b. the heart works more economically (i.e. produces the same cardiac output with a lower heart rate, blood pressure, and contractility).

4.4.2 Clinical assessment of MVO_2

Measurement of MVO_2 requires the determination of mean CBF and of the coronary arteriovenous difference in oxygen content. As coronary sinus sampling is required, and as the measurement of coronary flow presents considerable methodologic problems, a number of indirect indices, obtainable noninvasively, have been proposed. Of these, the heart rate/systolic blood pressure product ($HR \times SBP$) is the simplest and yet appears to be the one that correlates most closely with measured changes in MVO_2 in a variety of physiologic and experimental conditions.

In dogs, during changes of preload, afterload, and contractility, either separate or combined, the heart rate/systolic blood pressure product was found to be the noninvasive index that most accurately predicted relative changes in myocardial oxygen consumption (with a 10% error when preload and afterload were changed and with a 13% error when inotropic state was changed). In addition, during submaximal bicycle exercise, the product of heart rate and systolic blood pressure in humans gives the closest correlation with measured CBF and MVO_2 compared with the other indices currently used, including the tension/time index and the triple product.[37]

In normal volunteers exercising at about 10 times the resting total body oxygen consumption (i.e. 10 METs, where 1 MET is one metabolic equivalent of basal, resting oxygen consumption), coronary blood flows of the order of 250 ml/min/100 g were measured, i.e. about three times the average resting values.[37] This increase is of the same order of magnitude as that obtained by the microsphere technique in exercising dogs (see Fig. 4.17).

■ *It can, therefore, be estimated that, on average, the doubling of heart rate/systolic blood pressure product is associated with a twofold increase in myocardial blood flow, and doubling of heart rate with a threefold increase.* ■

REFERENCES

1. Maseri A, Crea F, Cianflone D. Myocardial ischemia caused by distal coronary vasoconstriction. Am J Cardiol 1992;*70:*1602.
2. Baroldi G, Mantero O, Scomazzoni G. The collaterals of the coronary arteries in normal and pathologic hearts. Circ Res 1956;*4:*223.
3. Fulton WFM. Arterial anastomoses in the coronary circulation: II Distribution, enumeration and measurement of coronary arterial anastomoses in health and disease. Scot Med J 1963;*8:*466.
4. Farrer-Brown G. Patterns of the microvasculature in normal and diseased hearts. Acta Cardiol Brux 1974;*19:*119.
5. Wong AYK, Armour JA, Klassen GA et al. The dynamics of the coronary venous system in the dog. J Biomech 1984;*17:*173.
6. Hoffman JIE, Spaan JAE. Pressure-flow relations in coronary circulation. Physiol Rev 1990;*70:*331.
7. Hoffman JIE, Baer RW, Hanley FL et al. Regulation of transmural myocardial blood flow. J Biochem Eng 1985;*107:*2.
8. Crystal GJ, Downey HF, Bashour FA. Small vessel and total coronary blood volume during intracoronary adenosine. Am J Physiol 1981;*241:*H194.
9. Douglas JE, Greenfield JC Jr. Epicardial coronary artery compliance in the dog. Circ Res 1970;*27:*921.
10. Vatner SF, Hintze TH, Macke P. Regulation of large coronary arteries by beta-adrenergic mechanisms in the conscious dog. Circ Res 1982;*51:*56.
11. Chilian WM, Marcus ML. Phasic coronary blood flow velocity in intramural and epicardial coronary arteries. Circ Res 1982;*50:*775.
12. Bache RJ, Cobb FR. Effect of maximal coronary vasodilation on transmural myocardial perfusion during tachycardia in the awake dog. Circ Res 1977;*41:*648.
13. Bache RJ, Vrobel TR, Arentzen CE, Ring WS. Effect of maximal coronary vasodilation on transmural myocardial perfusion during tachycardia in dogs with left ventricular hypertrophy. Circ Res 1981;*49:*742.
14. King RB, Bassingthwaighte JB. Temporal fluctuations in regional myocardial flows. Eur J Physiol 1989;*413:*336.
15. Marcus ML, Kerber RE, Ehrhardt JC et al. Spatial and temporal heterogeneity of left ventricular perfusion in awake dogs. Am Heart J 1977;*94:*748.
16. Sestier FJ, Mildenberger RR, Klassen GA. Role of autoregulation in spatial and temporal perfusion heterogeneity of canine myocardium. Am J Physiol 1978;*235:*H64.
17. Skolasinska K, Harbig K, Lubbers DW et al. PO_2 and microflow histograms of the beating heart in response to changes in arterial PO_2. Basic Res Cardiol 1978;*73:*307.
18. Franzen D, Conway RS, Zhang H, Sonnenblick EH, Eng C. Spatial heterogeneity of local blood flow and metabolite content in dog hearts. Am J Physiol 1988;*254* (Heart Circ Physiol *23*):H344.
19. Klassen GA, Armour JA, Garner JB. Coronary circulatory pressure gradients. Can J Physiol Pharmacol 1987;*65:*520.
20. Chilian WM, Layne SM, Klausner EC, Eastham CL, Marcus ML. Redistribution of coronary microvascular resistance produced by dipyridamole. Am J Physiol 1989;*256* (Heart Circ Physiol *25*):H383.
21. Feigl E. Coronary physiology. Physiol Rev:1983;*1.*
22. Khouri EM, Gregg DE, Rayford CR. Effect of exercise on cardiac output, left coronary flow and myocardial metabolism in the unanesthetized dog. Circ Res 1965;*17:*427.
23. Bell JR, Fox AC. Pathogenesis of subendocardial ischemia. Am J Med Sci 1974;*268:*2.

24. Wittenberg JB. Myoglobin-facilitated oxygen diffusion: role of myoglobin in oxygen entry into muscle. Physiol Rev 1970;*50:*559.

25. Bache RJ, Cobb FR, Greenfield JC Jr. Effect of increased myocardial oxygen consumption on coronary reactive hyperemia in the awake dog. Circ Res 1973;*33:*588.

26. Guyton RA, McClenathan JE, Newman GE, Michaels LL. Significance of subendocardial S–T segment elevation caused by coronary stenosis in the dog. Am J Cardiol 1977;*40:*373.

27. Canty JM Jr. Coronary pressure–function and steady-state pressure–flow relations during autoregulation in the unanesthetized dog. Circ Res 1988;*63:*821.

28. Hoffman JIE. A critical view of coronary reserve. Circulation 1987;*75(suppl I):*1.

29. L'Abbate A, Camici P, Trivella MG et al. Time dependent response of coronary flow to prolonged adenosine infusion: doubling of peak reactive hyperaemic flow. Cardiovasc Res 1981;*15:*282.

30. Dalle Vacche M, Trivella MG, Pelosi G et al. Modello della doppia risposta vasodilatatrice coronarica all'adenosina. Cardiologia 1987;*32:*1009.

31. Aversano T, Becker LC. Persistence of coronary vasodilator reserve despite functionally significant flow reduction. Am J Physiol 1985;*248* (Heart Circ Physiol *17*):H403.

32. Ball RM, Bache RJ. Distribution of myocardial blood flow in the exercising dog with restricted coronary artery inflow. Circ Res 1976;*38:*60.

33. Rooke GA, Feigl EO. Work as a correlate of canine left ventricular oxygen consumption, and the problem of catecholamine oxygen wasting. Circ Res 1982;*50:*273.

34. Baller D, Bretschneider HJ, Hellige G. A critical look at currently used indirect indices of myocardial oxygen consumption. Basic Res Cardiol 1981;*76:*163.

35. Braunwald E. Control of myocardial oxygen consumption: physiologic and clinical considerations. Am J Cardiol 1971;*27:*416.

36. Ross J Jr, Sonnenblick EH, Kaiser GA et al. Electroaugmentation of ventricular performance and oxygen consumption by repetitive application of paired electrical stimuli. Circ Res 1982;*50:*273.

37. Kitamura K, Jorgensen CR, Gobel FL, Taylor HL, Wang Y. Hemodynamic correlates of myocardial oxygen consumption during upright exercise. J Appl Physiol 1972;*32:*516.

Regulation of coronary vasomotor tone

INTRODUCTION

Our present understanding of the control of coronary vasomotor tone is only approximate as the mechanisms of contraction and relaxation of smooth muscle are more complex, varied, and less well explored than those of skeletal and cardiac muscle. The dominant feature of smooth muscle appears to be an extreme variability in its response to stimuli. This variability can be observed not only in the smooth muscle of different vascular beds but also in different segments of the same vascular bed, such as arteries, arterioles, and veins, as well as in the same segment of vascular bed in different species or under different experimental conditions.

The complexities are increased in the coronary circulation because arterioles, prearterioles, and large arteries are subjected to distinct intrinsic mechanisms of vasomotor control, mediated by oxygen consumption (metabolically mediated arteriolar dilation), flow (flow-mediated prearteriolar and arterial vasodilation), and pressure (myogenic control of tone).

On the one hand, assessing precisely the specific effects of a given vasoactive stimulus requires carefully controlled experimental conditions in which as many variables as possible are controlled. In experimental conditions, vascular segments are isolated, pressure, flow and oxygen consumption are kept constant, afferent nerves and receptors are blocked, nerve branches are electrically stimulated, and neurotransmitters are infused into the vessel.

On the other hand, the findings obtained in carefully controlled artificial conditions cannot easily be extrapolated to intact organisms in which the resting vasomotor tone may be different and variably influenced by local and systemic feedback control mechanisms. In intact organisms also, the results obtained with specific agonists and blockers should be interpreted with caution because not only is the effect of stimulation or blockade of one mechanism in one vascular segment influenced by its basal tone but also the vasomotor changes induced in one segment can elicit reactive changes in proximal or distal segments. The part played by any mechanism identified in acute experimental conditions is even less certain in chronic pathologic conditions, where some abnormal or defective mechanisms of control may be compensated for by others.

The aims of this chapter are as follows:

a. to summarize the information currently available regarding the major distinctive features of smooth muscle structure and function
b. to present the general relationship between constrictor stimuli and constrictor response in coronary vessels and
c. to review:
    • the experimental findings on the control of tone by locally released autacoids
    • the neural regulation of tone
    • the effects of the intracoronary infusion of neurotransmitters in man.

5.1 MAJOR DISTINCTIVE FEATURES OF SMOOTH MUSCLE STRUCTURE AND FUNCTION

In order to analyze the regulation of coronary vasomotor tone, some basic information is required on the major histologic and functional distinctive features of vascular smooth muscle, as well as on its mechanisms of contraction and relaxation.[1,2]

5.1.1 Histologic and physiologic features

The tunica media of coronary arteries is composed of vascular smooth muscle cells (SMCs) (about 3 μm in diameter and 30–130 μm long), arranged circularly or spirally with a small angle around the lumen, mechanically interconnected by collagen fibrils and often also electrically connected through gap junctions. These SMCs, like those in other vascular beds, differ greatly from skeletal and cardiac muscle.

Specific features of smooth muscle

In SMCs, surface open vesicles (or caveolae) increase the membrane surface by about 75%. Actin and myosin filaments are much less regularly arranged (thus smooth muscle shows no cross-striations), and their relative numbers vary largely among different types of muscle. They appear to be attached to dense bodies scattered in the cytoplasm and connected by filaments of intermediate size (10 μm) representing the equivalent of the Z lines in striated muscles. Tropomyosin is a component of the actin filament; troponin is absent. The sarcoplasmic reticulum is less well developed than in striated muscle and has a variable role in the control of cytoplasmic Ca^{2+} levels in vessels of different sizes (more so in conductive arteries than in arterioles).

Resting membrane potential ranges between −40 and −60mV. The relation between resting membrane potential, action potential, and contraction varies in different vascular segments and possibly even in the same segment in different species, as well as with time and with the nature of the stimulus. Contraction may also develop independently of membrane depolarization. The same stimulus may produce contraction or relaxation, or have no effect, in different vascular segments—and even in the same segment in different species. Vascular SMCs can trigger their own contraction because the membrane tends to depolarize spontaneously and thus generates rhythmic changes in wall tension or, more often, a sustained contraction (myogenic tone).

Compared with skeletal and cardiac muscle, vascular smooth muscle contracts much more slowly, because it takes several seconds to reach peak tension as actomyosin ATPase rates are 20–30 times slower than in striated muscle. The response of an SMC to a single stimulus is often a sustained contraction, which can generate considerable force and is usually maximal when the cell is stretched to about 150% of resting length.

Although the tension cost is 30- to 500-fold less for smooth than for skeletal muscle, high-energy phosphate stores are sufficient for only a few contractions. Carbohydrates play a substantial part as an energy source (more than 30%) and vascular smooth muscle can function anaerobically for relatively long periods.

Vascular smooth muscle is generally organized in functional units of variable numbers of cells connected by gap junctions through which an action potential can spread rapidly, so that their contraction becomes synchronized. For example, mechanical injury produced by the tip of a needle to a segment of artery produces a localized ring contraction due to electrotonic propagation of the mechanically induced local depolarization.[3]

■ *Thus, vascular tone may be determined not only by the various mechanisms that control contraction and relaxation of individual cells, but also by the intercellular connections and, hence, by the number of cells recruited into the contraction.* ■

5.1.2 Smooth muscle contraction and relaxation

In smooth muscle, as in other types of muscle, excitation–contraction coupling is triggered by an increase of cytosolic Ca^{2+} concentration from about 10^{-7} to 10^{-5}.[2,4] However, the relationship between increased cytosolic Ca^{2+} concentration and contraction appears to be quite variable and depends on the nature of the stimulus. In the process of excitation–contraction coupling, the action of Ca^{2+} on regulatory proteins in smooth muscle is distinctly different from that in striated and skeletal muscle, in which the increase of cytosolic Ca^{2+} removes the inhibition of the regulatory proteins so that the cross-bridges can interact. In smooth muscle, actin and myosin have little tendency to form cross-bridges or to split adenosine triphosphate (ATP), and the role of Ca^{2+} is to turn on the activation process.

The triggering rise in cytosolic Ca^{2+} can be produced by electromechanical coupling (spontaneous or induced by external stimuli) following an action potential and/or a graded depolarization, and/or pharmacomechanical coupling independent of changes in membrane potential. These mechanisms may operate separately or together. The increased cytosolic Ca^{2+} can derive either from the sarcoplasmic reticulum (as contraction can occur in the absence of extracellular Ca^{2+} and be blocked by ryanodine, which prevents Ca^{2+} release from the sarcoplasmic reticulum) or from the extracellular space entering through *voltage-operated channels* (which are open upon depolarization of the membrane and blocked by calcium-antagonist drugs) and/or *receptor-operated channels* (which are opened upon activation of receptors for various stimulant substances and are not blocked by calcium-antagonist drugs) (see Fig. 5.1). Effects not mediated by changes in membrane potential require receptor activation on each individual cell by the transmitter diffusing through the interstitial space; conversely, effects mediated by changes in membrane potential can be transmitted rapidly by the depolarization process through gap junctions to all the cells connected in functional units.

The molecular mechanism through which cytoplasmic free Ca^{2+} regulates contraction is complex. It is thought to be through phosphorylation of myosin light chains by a light-chain kinase (MLCK) that is activated upon the binding of Ca^{2+} to calmodulin. Phosphorylated myosin light chains combine with the actin and split ATP, thus initiating cross-bridge cycling, which continues as long as cytoplasmic Ca^{2+} remains high. When Ca^{2+} falls below the threshold level, the

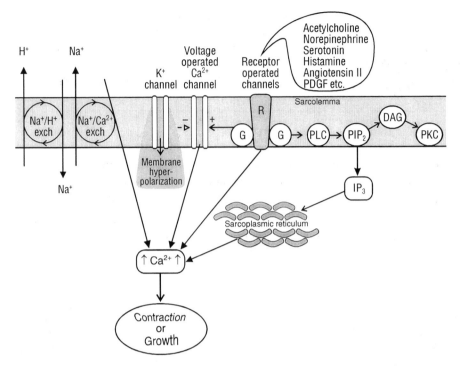

Fig. 5.1 The various mechanisms of cytosolic Ca²⁺ increase in smooth muscle cells. Ca^{2+} enters the cell by exchange with Na (which enters via Na^+/H^+ exchange), and via voltage- and receptor-operated channels. Activation of receptor-operated channels also causes release of inositol triphosphate (IP_3) and triggers the release of Ca^{2+} from the sarcoplasmic reticulum. Potassium-channel openers increase the polarization of the sarcolemma and reduce Ca^{2+} entry through voltage-operated channels. (G, G protein; PLC, phospholipase C; PIP_2, phosphoinositol diphosphate; DAG, diacylglycerol; PKC = phosphokinase C.)

concentration of the calcium–calmodulin complex falls, the active form of MLCK decreases, and relaxation tends to prevail. Relaxation can be produced by a second enzyme, myosin light-chain phosphatase, which dephosphorylates the myosin light chains. Unlike skeletal and cardiac muscle, the cross-bridge cycle can stop in conditions that involve a variety of actin–myosin interactions, including a "latch" state of cross-bridges in which they remain attached and maintain force, but cycle very slowly with minimal energy expenditure.[5] A state of "rigor," similar to that observed in striated muscle, can occur also in smooth muscle when ATP concentration is reduced to very low levels during prolonged contraction.

This phosphorylation/dephosphorylation mechanism appears to be responsible for rapid contractions, whereas sustained contractions seem to be mediated by a different mechanism as, over time, cytosolic Ca^{2+} concentration and phosphorylated myosin may decrease towards control values, whereas contraction persists. Under these conditions it appears that a specific Ca^{2+}-sensitive enzyme, protein kinase C, becomes associated with the plasma membrane and is responsive to Ca^{2+} influx rather than to changes in Ca^{2+} concentration (see Fig. 5.2).

The process of pharmacomechanical coupling seems to operate through the activation of membrane phosphotidylinositides with the formation of inositol triphosphate (IP_3) and diacyl-glycerol.[6] IP_3 seems to be responsible for liberating Ca^{2+} from the sarcoplasmic reticulum and diacylglycerol for the activation of protein kinase C, which increases Ca^{2+} sensitivity. Thus, the intensity of contraction is influenced by intracellular Ca^{2+} stores and, in turn, the size of intracellular Ca^{2+} stores is influenced by extracellular Ca^{2+} concentration and Ca^{2+} currents.

The role and importance of these mechanisms in the control of contractile response varies with the types of stimulus and muscle to which it is applied. The complexities in this field are epitomized by the observation that acetylcholine may produce contraction of coronary arteries in pigs, either with no change in membrane polarization or with hyperpolarization of the membrane.

The *process of relaxation* is also complex and incompletely understood. The major extra-

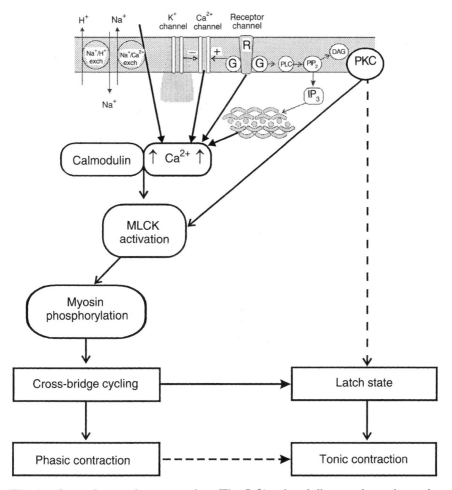

Fig. 5.2 Smooth muscle contraction. The Ca^{2+}–calmodulin complex activates the myocardial light-chain kinase (MLCK), which phosphorylates myosin. Phosphokinase C (PKC) (activated by diacylglyceride; DAG) contributes to the activation of MLCK. Cross-bridge cycling, initiated by activation of MLCK, causes phasic contraction. Cross-bridges can stop in the latch state and cause tonic contractions; PKC can also cause the latch state. Repeated phasic contractions can result in tonic contraction when their duration overlaps. Thus, the mechanisms of increased smooth muscle tone can be multiple.

cellular efflux of Ca^{2+} seems to occur through the calmodulin-stimulated Ca^{2+} transport ATPase and only partly through the Na/Ca^{2+} pump, but Ca^{2+} accumulation by the sarcoplasmic reticulum is likely to have a dominant role in the decrease of cytosolic Ca^{2+} (see Fig. 5.3).[7] As well as a reduction in cytosolic Ca^{2+}, relaxation requires dephosphorylation of the myosin molecule by a phosphatase activated by cyclic guanosine monophosphate (cGMP). The processes that control cGMP production are multiple and summarized in Fig. 5.4. cGMP is degraded by phosphodiesterases. Cyclic adenosine monophosphate (cAMP) also causes smooth muscle relaxation by phosphorylation of MLCK (which reduces its affinity with the calcium calmodulin complex) and by enhancing Ca^{2+} uptake into the sarcoplasmic reticulum.[2,4,8]

The main mechanisms that are responsible for reducing smooth muscle tone can be summarized as follows:

1. Blockers of the L (see below) calcium channel (calcium antagonists) reduce Ca^{2+} entry into the cell.
2. Nitric oxide (NO), exogenous NO donors and atrial natriuretic factor increase cGMP

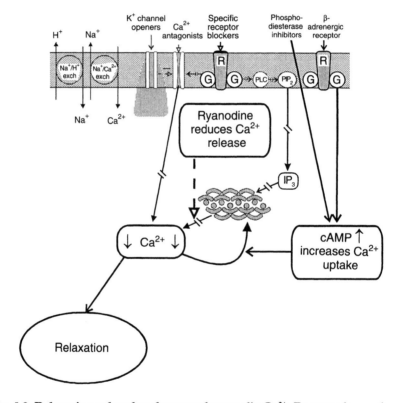

Fig. 5.3 Relaxation related to decreased cytosolic Ca^{2+}. Decreased smooth muscle tone can result from reduced Ca^{2+} entry through voltage- and receptor-operated channels (Ca^{2+} antagonists, K^+-channel openers), specific receptor blockers, reduced Na^+ entry, reduced Ca^{2+} release from the sarcoplasmic reticulum (ryanodine), or from increased uptake into the sarcoplasmic reticulum caused by cAMP (β-adrenergic stimulation or phosphodiesterase inhibitors). (G, G protein; PLC, phospholipase C; PIP_2, phosphoinositol diphosphate; cAMP, cyclic adenosine monophosphate.)

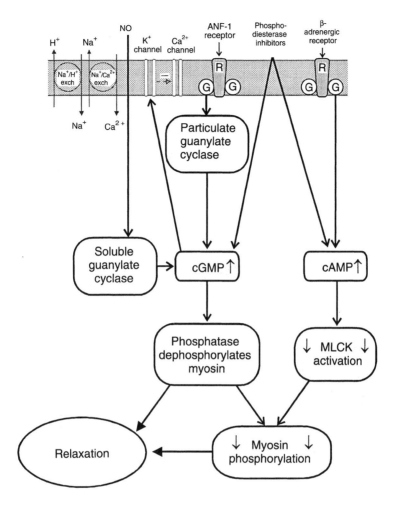

Fig. 5.4 Additional mechanisms of smooth muscle relaxation. Nitric oxide (NO) and atrial natriuretic factor-1 (ANF-1) increase cyclic guanosine monophosphate (cGMP), which activates the phosphatase that causes dephosphorylation of myosin; cGMP also favors K^+-channel opening, increasing membrane polarization. Cyclic adenosine monophosphate (cAMP) inhibits myosin light-chain kinase (MLCK) activation, thus reducing myosin phosphorylation. Smooth muscle tone can, therefore, also be reduced through mechanisms unrelated to cytosolic Ca^{2+} concentration. (G, G protein.)

(which activates the phosphatase involved in the dephosphorylation of myosin light chains and activates potassium channels).
3. β-Adrenergic stimulation increases cAMP (which enhances Ca^{2+} uptake into the sarcoplasmic reticulum and reduces MLCK activation).
4. Potassium-channel openers which increase membrane potential.
5. Phosphodiesterase inhibitors reduce cAMP and cGMP degradation.
6. Ryanodine-like agonists reduce Ca^{2+} release from the sarcoplasmic reticulum.
7. Specific receptor blockers for vasoconstrictor agonists.

The importance of these mechanisms for producing vasodilation varies in different types of vessels and according to the actual cause of constriction: for example, the effect of calcium antagonists will be greatest when the mechanism responsible for increased tone is an increase in intracellular Ca^{2+}; the effect of nitrates will be greatest when the mechanism of increased tone is a reduced level of cGMP, and the effect of potassium-channel openers will be greatest when membrane polarization is reduced.

■ *The multiple modes of stimulation of contraction, the variable intracellular transduction of the signals into phasic and sustained "latch" contraction, and the multiple processes that determine SMC relaxation, suggest that abnormalities of coronary vasomotor tone may result from a wide variety of cellular and subcellular mechanisms, each of which would be best treated by a specific vasodilator.* ■

5.1.3 Control of coronary vasomotor tone by calcium and potassium channels

Interest in the mechanisms of control of coronary vasomotor tone by calcium and potassium channels on the plasmalemma of SMCs derives from the availability of a number of compounds that can block calcium channels, thus reducing intracellular calcium, and open potassium channels, thus raising membrane potential and making the cell less excitable. Two types of voltage-operated calcium channels have been identified in smooth muscle—the L type, with a long activation time, and a T type, with a short activation time.

Calcium-channel blockers began to be used for the treatment of angina pectoris, myocardial ischemia and hypertension in the late 1970s, when the importance of calcium in the control of smooth muscle tone in coronary and systemic arterial beds became accepted. Since then, the mechanisms by which calcium channels control coronary smooth muscle tone have received considerable attention. Their main mechanism of action is the blocking of the L type, voltage-operated channel. The notion of "calcium antagonists" was proposed by Fleckenstein[9] and Godfraind,[10] and the calcium antagonist drugs now in use belong to three types of compounds developed from the original drugs verapamil, nifedipine, and diltiazem. Their diverse molecular structures explain their differing modes and sites of action on both cardiac function and vascular beds.[11] These differences may depend on the prevalence of binding sites for the individual compounds, on the open or closed state of the channel (as nifedipine does not require entry of the cell through the channel), and on additional intracellular actions of the various compounds.

The activation that allows calcium channels to open when the membrane becomes depolarized depends on the phosphorylation of the channel, which is influenced by intracellular cAMP (and hence by adrenergic tone); in smooth muscle it is also influenced by α-adrenergic stimulation. By changing the polarization of the membrane, the function of potassium channels also influences that of voltage-operated calcium channels.[12]

Potassium-channel openers are a new and heterogeneous class of compounds that, in addition to opening potassium channels on the plasmalemma and causing hyperpolarization of the cells, may exert other effects in different cells.[13] The effect of hyperpolarization on vascular smooth muscle is reduction of vasomotor tone.[14] Endogenous potassium-channel openers have been identified and a number of drugs with similar effects are already in an advanced phase of pharmacologic and clinical characterization (see Fig. 5.5).[15] Various subtypes of potassium-channel openers have been identified: these include voltage-gated, ion-gated, ligand-gated, and second-messenger-gated (IP_3, cAMP, ATP) channels. Endogenous and synthetic potassium-channel openers have also been identified. Endothelium-dependent hyperpolarizing factor (EDHF) is one of the endogenous openers of ligand-gated potassium channels that can be stimulated by shear stress and pulsatility, by acetylcholine, by substance P, and by calcitonin gene-related peptide (CGRP). Synthetic

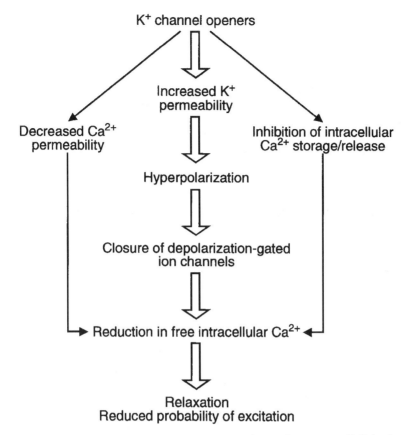

Fig. 5.5 Mechanisms of action of potassium-channel openers. Cellular hyper-polarization is unlikely to be the only mechanism of action of potassium-channel openers and reduction of intracellular Ca^{2+} contributes to their relaxant effect on smooth muscle. (Modified from ref. 15.)

potassium-channel openers include several classes of compounds: the most widely studied are related to cromokalim, pinacidil, nicorandil, and thioformamide derivatives.

Neither the segmental distribution of calcium and potassium channels in conductive, prearteriolar, and arteriolar vessels nor their role on the modulation of local vasomotor tone has been investigated.

■ *Calcium antagonists and potassium-channel openers should be expected to have the greatest therapeutic efficacy when the abnormal coronary constriction is related to excessive cytosolic Ca^{2+} or to resting depolarization of the cell membrane, respectively. They are also likely to be efficacious when the abnormal constriction occurs in vessels in which vasomotor tone is strongly influenced by calcium or potassium channels.* ■

5.2 SEGMENTAL CORONARY VASOMOTOR CONTROL AND RESPONSE

The intrinsic mechanisms of vasomotor control are not the same in conductive arteries, prearterioles, and arterioles: arterioles are mainly under metabolic control, but prearterioles and conductive arteries are under only neural, humoral, and myogenic control. These three arterial components of the arterial system may not have the same levels of resting vasomotor tone, and exhibit different responses to neurohumoral vasoactive stimuli.

The effects of constrictor and dilator stimuli on the various segments of the coronary circulation are influenced by the following:

a. the segmental basal tone and local mechanisms of control of tone
b. the type and density of receptors on the endothelium and smooth muscle,
c. the distribution of terminal nervous branches
d. the reactivity of the vessel to constrictor stimuli, related to the specific intracellular signal transduction mechanisms of contraction and relaxation (such as the development of the sarcoplasmic reticulum) of the smooth muscle cells.[8]

The constriction observed in normal segments of epicardial conductive arteries can be magnified geometrically at the site of subintimal plaques that occupy the lumen of pliable arteries with preserved tunica media (see Ch. 9).

■ *Only knowledge of the specific mechanisms of segmental control of coronary vasomotor tone will allow the design of specific drugs capable of dilating selectively those segments in which abnormal coronary constriction develops.* ■

5.2.1 Myogenic and metabolic control

Coronary vessels undergo changes in caliber when transmural distending pressure varies. Passive changes of caliber are opposed by the myogenic autoregulation of tone, which tends to maintain the tension of the vessel wall (and hence the lumen) within a narrow range when distending pressure varies (i.e. the tone increases when pressure increases, and vice versa). In epicardial coronary arteries, transmural distending pressure is determined only by aortic pressure, but, in intramyocardial vessels, transmural pressure is also influenced by cyclical extravascular myocardial compressive forces; their distending pressure is therefore, the difference between intraluminal and extraluminal pressure.

The myogenic control of vasomotor tone differs in arterial, arteriolar, and venous beds and is incompletely understood. In some types of smooth muscle, stretching can elicit increased spontaneous contraction.[16] Cell stretching in response to pulsatile changes in pressure can influence SMC membrane permeability and hence tension and/or the frequency of spontaneous tonic contractions, thus contributing to the maintenance of basal intrinsic vasomotor tone. The spontaneous rhythmic contractions observed in rings of excised epicardial coronary arteries[17] are consistent with the possibility that myogenic tone and contractions can develop independently of external cellular stimulation. The role of myogenic control of vasomotor tone in resistive vessels is difficult to assess, as it cannot be easily separated from the effects of simultaneous release of endothelial-derived relaxing factors (EDRFs), induced by stretching, and from metabolic autoregulation.[18]

The metabolic control of vasomotor tone involves only those vessels exposed to the effects of interstitial concentrations of catabolites and PO_2, i.e. the arterioles in the definition given in Chapter 4.

Adenosine was proposed as the major component of myocardial metabolic regulation of flow, but it is not the only one. A "micro-hypoxia" model proposes that adenosine production reflects ATP degradation, resulting from a local myocardial imbalance between oxygen supply and demand, and is compatible with evidence of temporal and spatial heterogeneity of myocardial perfusion. An alternative "normoxia" model explains adenosine production in terms of the cytosolic ratio of ATP to adenosine diphosphate. Adenosine, diffusing into the interstitial space and arteriolar wall, can activate smooth muscle A_2 adenosine receptors which initiate smooth muscle relaxation by activation of cGMP cyclase, with consequent activation of the phosphatase that induces dephosphorylation of myosin. Adenosine can also produce vasodilation by its effect on the vascular endothelium. It is also produced by endothelial cells and could represent another endothelial regulator of vasomotor tone, but the control of its luminal or abluminal release has yet to be elucidated. Not all experimental data are consistent with adenosine being the only mediator of metabolic control: decreased PO_2, increased extracellular PCO_2, K^+ and osmotic pressure are thought to be possible additional contributors to the metabolic control of coronary vasomotor tone.[19] Neither adenosine nor tissue acidosis can account for the chronic dilation of resistive vessels in response to critical coronary stenosis.[20,21]

In arterioles the metabolic regulation of flow directly opposes the local effects of constrictor stimuli and compensates for increased resistance in proximal segments.

5.2.2 Influence of basal tone on vasomotor response

Vascular segments, with low vasomotor tone, dilate less in response to dilator stimuli than do consticted segments. In pharmacologic experiments the dilator effect of agonists is usually studied on preconstricted vessels, but the dilator effects observed in such models may be less relevant to physiologic conditions and may apply to a different extent to arteriolar, prearteriolar, and arterial vessels in relation to their basal tone.

In arteriolar vessels, vasomotor tone is highest or near maximal in resting conditions because myocardial metabolism at rest is low; it decreases when myocardial demand increases above basal conditions or when perfusion pressure decreases below basal conditions. In prearteriolar vessels the intrinsic resting tone is influenced by both the level of aortic pressure and flow.

In epicardial conductive arteries, resting tone appears to be set at an intermediate level of tone, as on average they exhibit an approximately similar percentage dilation and constriction, respectively, in response to a variety of dilator and constrictor stimuli,[22,23] and those vessels that respond more strongly to vasodilator stimuli respond less to constrictor stimuli, and vice versa (see Fig. 5.6).[23] Dilator and constrictor responses are greater in distal coro-

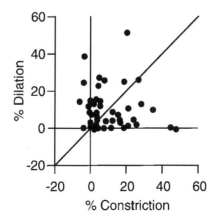

Fig. 5.6 Dilator versus constrictor response of angiographically normal coronary artery segments. The segments that dilate more following isosorbide dinitrate, constrict less in response to ergonovine, and vice versa, suggesting that the vasomotor response is influenced by basal tone. The 45 degree diagonal line represents the response to be expected if the vessels had the same basal tone and the same degree of dilator and constrictor response. (Modified from ref. 23.)

nary arteries with diameters less than 1.5 mm than in larger proximal arteries.[24]

The intrinsic tone is modulated by neurohumoral stimuli: for example, the tone of resistive vessels at rest is decreased by sympathectomy or α-blockade. The "basal" tone of conductive epicardial arteries is, on average, higher in the early morning than in the afternoon (see Chs 9 and 19).

■ *The effect of a dilator or constrictor stimulus should, therefore, be related to the level of pre-existing vasomotor tone.* ■

5.2.3 Variability of segmental vasomotor response to vasoactive stimuli

In the coronary circulation, the vasomotor response of conductive arteries, prearterioles, and arterioles to the same vasoactive drugs can be markedly different and dose dependent,[25-27] and can cause secondary vasomotor changes in other vascular segments connected in series.

For example, dipyridamole exerts its dilator effect by reducing the degradation rate of adenosine and, therefore, dilates directly only those vessels that are *tonically* exposed to endogenous adenosine; the increase of coronary flow caused by arteriolar dilation can, however, elicit secondary *flow-mediated* dilation of the upstream segments (i.e. prearterioles and arteries). In contrast, low doses of nitrates cause maximal dilation of epicardial conductive arteries with minimal increase of coronary blood flow. This very selective dilation cannot be attributed to differences in basal tone, which in arterioles is high. Furthermore, some agonists that stimulate EDRF production can maximally dilate conductive arteries, at the same time causing either a mild increase in flow (e.g. substance P) or no change at all (e.g. CGRP); others may dilate conductive arteries at low doses, but constrict them at higher doses (e.g. acetylcholine and serotonin [5-HT]), and some may constrict conductive arteries while further dilating distal resistive vessels (e.g. acetylcholine at high doses) (see 5.5.1).

Ergonovine and high doses of 5-HT and acetylcholine cause a dose-dependent mild degree of constriction of normal epicardial coronary arteries; in contrast, neuropeptide Y (NPY) and endothelin do not cause detectable constriction of epicardial coronary arteries at doses that cause intense constriction in distal coronary vessels (see Chs. 6 and 9).

Major variability of the vasomotor response has also been observed at the level of epicardial microvessels of different sizes.[28] For example, sympathetic nerve stimulation, infusion of norepinephrine, and infusion of 5-HT were found to constrict vessels more than 0.1 mm in diameter and to dilate smaller vessels. The dilation of smaller vessels could be caused by metabolically mediated dilation of arteriolar vessels in order to provide compensation for constriction of more proximal vessels. Differences in vasomotor response to vasoactive stimuli were also reported for subepicardial and subendocardial vessels.[29]

■ *Thus, the definition of vasoactive drugs merely as either coronary dilators or coronary constrictors, without specifying the coronary segment on which they act and their dose, is no longer acceptable.* ■

5.2.4 Response to constrictor stimuli in normal and abnormal vessels

The response of the coronary arteries to constrictor stimuli should be considered in terms of the effect such stimuli have on normal arteries and the response of abnormal arteries to vasoactive stimuli (see Fig. 5.7).[30]

In *normal arteries*, the effects of constrictor agents can be defined in pharmacologic terms according to their potency and efficacy. *Potency* is defined by the position of the dose–response curve with respect to concentrations of the agonist: the lower the dose

Normal Vessels: Response to different stimuli

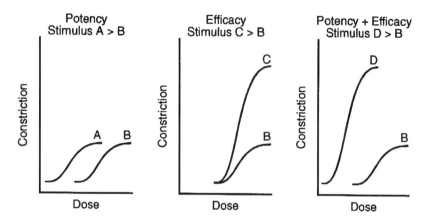

Abnormal vessels: Response to the same stimulus

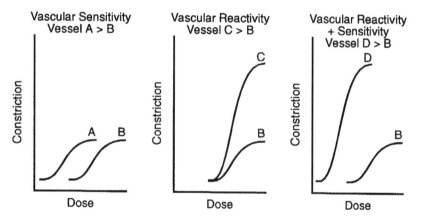

Fig. 5.7 Vasoconstrictor stimuli and constrictor response. The vasoconstriction in response to stimuli of different potency and efficacy in normal arteries is illustrated in the top panels; the response of abnormal arteries having different sensitivity and reactivity to the same stimulus is illustrated in the bottom panels. Top left: stimulus A is more potent than stimulus B; the same constriction is caused by a lower dose of the agonist. The maximal lumen reduction achieved is the same; therefore, the efficacy of the two stimuli is similar. Top center: stimulus C is more efficacious than B and elicits a greater maximum constriction. Top right: stimulus D is more potent and efficacious than stimulus B; it causes greater constriction at a lower dose. Bottom left: the sensitivity of vessel A is greater than that of vessel B as vessel A develops the same constriction as vessel B at lower doses of the same agonist. Bottom center: the reactivity of vessel C is greater than that of vessel B as vessel C develops a greater constriction than vessel B at the same dose of agonist. Bottom right: both the reactivity and sensitivity of vessel D are greater than those of vessel B as it develops greater constriction at lower doses of agonist. (Modified from ref. 30.)

required to generate a response, the greater the potency; this term makes no statement about the maximal response. *Efficacy* is defined by the range of the response, irrespective of the dose, and can, therefore, describe the maximal response that can be obtained with the agonist.

In terms of constriction, a *potent* agonist will produce its effect at very low molar concentrations. However, the effect may well be slight and within the physiologic range of constriction. Conversely, an *efficacious* agonist produces a response that, when maximal, may be well beyond the physiologic range for the vessel. The vasomotor response is more complex for agonists that act on different components of the vessel wall—endothelium, smooth muscle, and nerve endings. The overall effect on the vessel lumen is the algebraic sum of the dilator or constrictor effects of each individual component, which is usually dose dependent. In these cases, only the constrictor response can be defined in terms of potency and efficacy.

In *vessels reacting abnormally,* the vasoconstrictor response should be defined in terms of the sensitivity and reactivity of the vessel to constrictor stimuli, compared with that of normal vessels: for example, the abnormal vessels may exhibit hypersensitivity, resulting in a degree of constriction similar to that of normal vessels but occurring in response to a lower dose of constrictor agent; alternatively, it may exhibit hyperreactivity, resulting in a contraction greater than that of normal vessels in response to the same dose of constrictor agent.

Thus, according to the above considerations, in arteries without significant subintimal plaques, occlusive epicardial coronary artery spasm could, in theory, result either from extremely efficacious stimuli capable of inducing vessel occlusion, even in the absence of any abnormality of coronary arteries, or from hyperreactivity of a segment of the artery that causes complete occlusion in response to stimuli that produce constriction only within the physiologic range in adjacent coronary segments (see below).

Vasoconstrictor response of normal coronary arteries

Normal epicardial coronary arteries in experimental animals and humans respond to a variety of constrictor stimuli with a mild, uniform reduction in diameter (10–20%). The identification of an abnormal vasomotor response is straightforward when a normally dilator stimulus causes constriction, but is difficult to establish when the response to constrictor stimuli varies with the dose of the agonist and/or seems only slightly greater than normal, as the constrictor response is also influenced by resting vasomotor tone.

Several constrictor substances have been identified recently that can cause myocardial ischemia at very low doses in the normal coronary circulation, but such constrictor stimuli exert their action predominantly on small vessels rather than on epicardial coronary arteries (see Ch. 6). It seems, therefore, that no constrictor stimuli so far identified are sufficiently efficacious to cause segmental occlusive spasm in normal epicardial coronary artery branches.

Hypersensitivity to constrictor stimuli

A typical example of hypersensitivity to constrictor stimuli is illustrated by observations on aortic strips taken from cholesterol-fed rabbits:[31] the dose–response curve of these strips to low doses of ergonovine and 5-HT was shifted to the left by three orders of magnitude, whereas maximal constriction increased only by about 30%. These findings indicate the development of remarkable hypersensitivity, but only very mild hyperreactivity, to these constrictor agents. The increased sensitivity to constrictor stimuli can be due to defective production of EDRFs or to enhanced sensitivity of SMCs to constrictor stimuli. Whatever its cause, increased sensitivity to constrictor agents alone cannot cause occlusive spasm. Indeed, large doses of ergonovine failed to produce occlusive coronary artery spasm in hypercholesterolemic rabbits, despite severe reduction of the coronary artery lumen by cholesterol deposits.[32] This may not be surprising, because patients with variant angina have plasma cholesterol values similar to those in patients with the common syndrome of chronic stable angina, and variant angina has not been reported in patients with familial hypercholesterolemia (see also 6.2.4 and Chs 9 and 19).

Hyperreactivity to constrictor stimuli

A typical example of segmental coronary hyperreactivity is provided by the experimental model of coronary artery spasm developed in miniature swine 3 months after endothelial denudation (see Ch. 6).[33] In this model, the reduction in luminal diameter at the level of the spastic segment after administration of histamine or 5-HT was several-fold greater than that in adjacent branches. A similar local coronary hyperreactivity has also been documented during provoked and spontaneous coronary artery spasm in patients with variant angina (see Fig. 5.8).[34] The data available from both the miniature swine model and patients with variant angina indicate that local coronary hyperactivity is more prevalent than hypersensitivity, because the doses of constrictor agents that cause segmental occlusive spasm are not distinctly lower than those that cause constriction in nonspastic vessels and in other segments of the spastic vessels. This type of analysis can also apply to prearteriolar and arteriolar vessels.

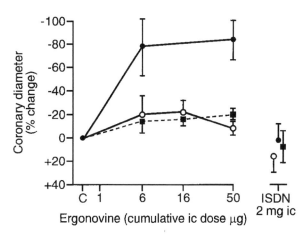

Fig. 5.8 Plot of the dose–response relation of the change in coronary diameter after intracoronary ergonovine (mean ± 1 SD): ● segments of vessels with coronary spasm in patients with variant angina; ○, segments of other vessels without coronary spasm in the same patients after the same injection; ■, segments of vessels in patients without variant angina. The percentage narrowing in spastic segments is several-fold that in the nonspastic arteries in the same patients and controls, but the segmental reduction in caliber occurs over the same range of doses, indicating a local hypercontractile response. The dilator effect of a 2 mg intracoronary bolus of isosorbide dinitrate (ISDN) in spastic and reference segments does not differ significantly. (Modified from ref. 34.)

The effect of vasoactive stimuli with multiple sites of action, i.e. endothelium and SMCs, must be interpreted with caution, because in chronic disease processes it can be influenced not only by the function of the endothelium but also by the response of the smooth muscle and its basal tone.

■ *Rational prevention of the effects of constrictor ischemic stimuli on coronary vessels must be based on the combined assessment of the stimulus (physiologic or abnormal), and the vasomotor response (physiologic or abnormal). Specific prevention of coronary constriction caused by abnormal stimuli or by an abnormal local response would require different approaches.* ■

5.3 LOCAL CONTROL OF CORONARY VASOMOTOR TONE BY AUTACOIDS

Isolated organs and vessels have an intrinsic regulation of vasomotor tone that is variably modulated by locally released autacoids with paracrine and autocrine functions. The endothelium, being the interface between blood and the vessel wall, represents a key sensory-effector transducer of vasoactive stimuli carried by the bloodstream or produced by flow for the control of smooth muscle tone.[35] The intrinsic mechanism of control that has received the greatest attention is the endothelial-derived production of dilator factors (one or more EDRFs). However, the endothelium also produces prostacyclin and endothelin, and SMCs and other resident cells in the vessel wall produce vasoactive autacoids that can contribute to the local modulation of vasomotor tone (see Ch. 1).

5.3.1 Endothelial-mediated vasomotor control

As indicated in Chapter 1, there appear to be at least two EDRFs. NO was identified as a mediator that can mimic most of the physiologic effects of EDRF in biologic assays, and has been referred to as the endogenous nitrate: it could be released from a compound (S-nitrosocysteine) stored in lysosome-like organelles, the effects of which mimic those of EDRF more closely than NO. Within the SMC, NO exerts its dilator effect by activating soluble guanylate cyclase and increasing cGMP. Although NO has been shown convincingly to exert important biologic functions, it does not appear to be the only EDRF, as it cannot account for all the vasodilator effects produced by stimulation of endothelial cells, and an EDHF that opens potassium channels has been identified.

The role of EDRFs on vascular tone has been studied by observing the effects of agonists on isolated normal blood vessels with the endothelium either intact or removed. This approach allows only speculation about the possible physiologic functions of EDRFs. A much more rational approach has been the use of inhibitors of the synthesis of NO, as representative of the EDRFs.

The inhibition of NO synthesis by systemic administration of L-*N*-monomethyl-L-arginine (LNMMA) in intact animals results in a prompt increase in systemic arterial pressure, which persists until the administration of arginine (the natural substrate for NO synthesis) competitively removes the inhibition. This observation demonstrates that tonic NO production exerts an evident physiologic role as a tonic vasodilator of resistive vessels. This effect has also been observed in the human forearm (see Ch. 1).

In basal conditions the local tonic release of EDRF may not be equally important in arterial, prearteriolar, and arteriolar segments of the coronary circulation, and NO and EDHF distribution and predominant effects may not be similar in the three compartments. The role of NO has been explored in humans by intracoronary infusion of LNMMA; the caliber of conductive arteries was found to decrease very slightly, flow failed to change, and the effect of intracoronary acetylcholine was abolished in conductive arteries but not in resistive vessels.[36] This lack of complete inhibition may be explained not only by an inadequate dose of LNMMA but also by the presence of a non-NO-dependent effect of acetylcholine, such as stimulation of EDHF release (see 5.5.2).

In the coronary circulation, the segmental distribution of different EDRFs and their receptor coupling, are poorly elucidated; however, one of their major hemodynamic roles is the continuous adaptation of coronary lumen to blood flow, in order to reduce both blood shear stress on the wall of conductive arteries and prearteriolar resistance when flow increases (see Ch. 4). Flow not only stimulates production of NO but also activates an endothelial potassium channel to release endogenous vasodilators.[37] Endothelial cells produce angiotensin-converting enzyme that inactivates bradykinin, a powerful stimulus for EDRF release. Different types of endothelium can release EDRFs at widely different rates according to the agonist.[38] Porcine aortic endothelial cells exhibit a tonic release of endothelin.[39] No information is available on the release of endothelin in coronary arteries, but threshold concentrations of endothelin can potentiate the constrictor response to norepinephrine and 5-HT in excised human coronary arteries.[40]

5.3.2 Effects of substances released by vascular resident cells

Smooth muscle cells can produce angiotensin II, which, together with cellular growth factors also produced by endothelial cells (platelet-derived growth factor, fibroblast-derived growth factor, epidermal growth factor, transforming growth factor β), stimulate proliferation of SMCs when they are in the proliferative phenotype, but cause constriction when they are in the contractile phenotype. Cellular growth is inhibited by heparan sulfate, prostacyclin and NO (for details see the review by Dzau et al in reference 41).

Whether prostacyclin has a tonic dilator role in coronary resistance is not clear but, in humans, indomethacin causes a reduction of coronary blood flow (CBF) and increased myocardial oxygen extraction, which could be mediated by inhibition of prostacyclin synthesis.[42]

In pathologic conditions, inflammatory cells (such as mast cells), present in the wall, may produce histamine and leukotriene D_4, which cause coronary vasoconstriction.[43,44] Activated macrophages and SMCs produce cytokines that can activate the endothelium, prevent its production of prostacyclin and EDRFs, and express adhesive receptors to leukocytes (see Ch. 1). Polymorphonuclear granulocytes, which adhere to activated endothelium, can produce leukotrienes.[45]

These substances can cause coronary constriction in unstable angina at sites of activated endothelium.

5.4 NEURAL INFLUENCES ON CORONARY VASOMOTOR TONE

Coronary vessels are densely innervated by both sympathetic and parasympathetic efferent divisions of the autonomic nervous system, which form a lattice-like tubular sheet at the border between adventitia and media.[46]

The spatial association between nerve fibers and smooth muscle is not clear because fluorescent techniques and light microscopy lack the resolution necessary to draw precise conclusions concerning functional blood vessel innervation, whereas electron microscopy, which does provide the necessary detail, does not lend itself easily to a comprehensive three-dimensional view of sufficiently large segments of vessel wall. The information available suggests that nerve endings are much sparser in epicardial coronary arteries than in arterioles. The distribution of nerve endings is denser at the adventitial–medial border than at the intimal–medial border and the inner layers of the media are more sensitive to circulating than to neurally released transmitters.[3]

Neurotransmitters are synthesized both in the cell body (whence they are transported down the terminal axon to the branches, where they are stored in varicosities) and in the terminal varicosities. From the varicosities they are released on nerve stimulation by a process of exocytosis.

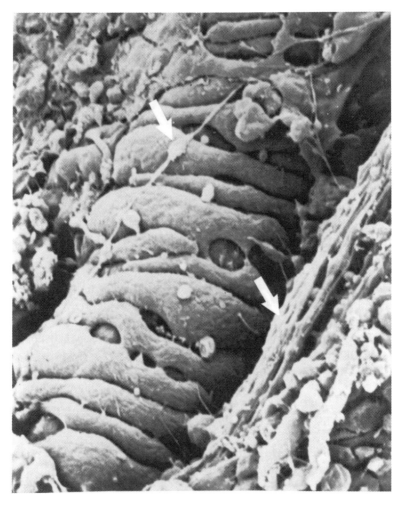

Fig. 5.9 Scanning electron micrograph of the adventitial surface of the smooth muscle cells of an arteriole. The nerve fibers are indicated by the white arrows. The varicosities are in contact with some of the smooth muscle cells that run perpendicularly surrounding the vessel. (Modified from ref. 47.)

Table 5.1 Putative nonadrenergic noncholinergic transmitters. *

Transmitter	Abbreviation
Adenosine triphosphate	ATP
5-Hydroxytryptamine	5-HT
γ-Aminobutyric acid	GABA
Dopamine	DA
Peptides	
Neuropeptide Y/pancreatic polypeptide	NPY/PP
Calcitonin gene-related peptide	CGRP
Substance P	SP
Vasoactive intestinal polypeptide/peptide HI	VIP/PHI
Angiotensin	A II
Enkephalin/endorphin	Enk/End
Somatostatin	ST
Neurotensin	NT

    * Modified from ref. 49

The separation between varicosities and SMCs varies between about 0.05 and 0.5 µm, being smaller in arterioles than in large arteries. As neurotransmitters reach their specific receptors on SMCs by molecular diffusion through the interstitial space, their concentration decreases progressively with the distance from the varicosities toward the vessel lumen. In general, therefore, the neuromuscular relationship in smaller vessels is more intimate than that in the larger. The action of the transmitter is diffuse in the outer part of the tunica media in larger arteries, but becomes more localized to the proximity of the synaptic cleft in smaller ones (see Fig. 5.9).[47]

The neurotransmitters released by the varicosities can bind to receptors, can be variably taken up by the varicosity, or can be inactivated and degraded or diffuse towards the vessel lumen, where they may either interact with endothelial receptors or be transported in the bloodstream. The process of neurotransmitter diffusion across the vessel wall depends on wall thickness and local degradation. Thus, the assessment of nerve function from estimates of the neurotransmitter concentration within the bloodstream is very indirect.

The traditional concept of sympathetic and parasympathetic innervation begins to appear rather simplistic, because nonadrenergic, noncholinergic neurotransmission has been convincingly demonstrated in various vascular beds[48] and the number of putative transmitters that have been identified is growing rapidly (see Table 5.1).[49] Peripheral transmission of nervous stimuli in adrenergic and cholinergic nerves can also be modulated by substances that modify the neurotransmission process, either by prejunctional modulation of the transmitter release from the terminal neurons, or by postjunctional modulation of the time course or of the extent of action of the transmitter (see Fig. 5.10).

Several transmitter substances have been shown to coexist in the same varicosity. They can be secreted together as cotransmitters in variable proportions (influenced by the rate of nerve stimulation) and one can modulate the release or the peripheral action of the other. For example, norepinephrine can be released upon nerve stimulation by exocytosis together with ATP and possibly with NPY.

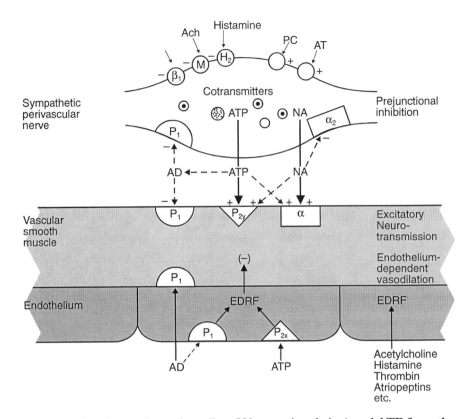

Fig. 5.10 Corelease of noradrenaline (NA norepinephrine) and ATP from the terminal varicosities of a sympathetic perivascular nerve. Neuronal release may be modulated both by feedback mechanisms (respectively on P_1 and α_2 neuronal receptors; AD, adenosine and from other mediators. Acetylcholine (Ach) acting on M receptors, histamine acting on H_2 receptors, β-receptor (β_1) stimulation and hyperosmolarity have inhibitory actions; prostacyclin (PC) and angiotensin (AT) appear to have facilitatory actions on release of neurotransmitters. In some sympathetic nerves neuropeptide Y can also be released, depending on the frequency of stimulation. Thus, the effects of sympathetic nerve stimulation can vary considerably (EDRF, endothelial-derived relaxing factors). (Modified from ref. 48.)

The effects produced by binding of the transmitter to the receptor (excitatory or inhibitory) vary depending on the type of receptor and the site at which it is situated—nerve ending, SMC, or endothelial cell. At present, our knowledge of the physiologic role of nonadrenergic, noncholinergic neurotransmission is still rather scanty.

5.4.1 Adrenergic influences

The release of norepinephrine is modulated by a number of substances, among which norepinephrine itself exerts a negative feedback effect (see Fig. 5.10). Following its release, norepinephrine binds to adrenergic receptors and/or is removed from the tissue by degradation inside the affected cells by the enzymes catechol-*o*-methyl transferase and monoamine oxidase and by reuptake into the nerve terminals. Only a small, variable fraction is removed by the bloodstream. For this reason, measurement of norepinephrine levels in the effluent blood from a vascular bed, as an index of neuroadrenergic stimulation, provides useful information only if the other major pathways of tissue removal are constant.

Both α_1- and α_2- and both β_1- and β_2- adrenergic receptors have been identified through their affinity for norepinephrine, epinephrine, isoproterenol, and phenylephrine and through their response to antagonist drugs. All can be found in vascular smooth muscle, but their proportion varies both among different vessels and in proximal and distal segments. β_1 Receptors are also present in myocardial cells and are responsible for the positive chronotropic, dromotropic, and inotropic effects of catecholamines. α_2 Receptors are also present in adrenergic nerve terminals and are responsible for the negative feedback of norepinephrine on its release. Both α_1 and α_2-receptor stimulation cause coronary constriction, whereas both β_1- and β_2-receptor stimulation cause vasodilation.[50]

Norepinephrine is the most powerful endogenous agonist for α- and β_1 receptors, but has practically no effect on β_2 receptors at physiologic concentrations. Epinephrine, produced and released by the adrenal glands and reaching the vascular smooth muscle via the bloodstream, is a very weak agonist for β_1 receptors and a weak agonist for α receptors, but is a powerful agonist for β_2 receptors. (β_2 Receptors are much more numerous in skeletal muscle than in myocardial arterioles and epinephrine produces a very much greater dilation in skeletal muscles than in the myocardium.) The synthetic compound isoproterenol is as powerful as norepinephrine for β_1 receptors and as powerful as epinephrine for β_2 receptors, but has practically no effect on α receptors. Conversely, phenylephrine, also a synthetic compound, is a very powerful agonist for α receptors, but has no effect on β_1 or β_2 receptors.

Electric stimulation of sympathetic nerves causes moderate coronary constriction mediated by α-receptor stimulation (it is not clear yet whether these receptors are α_1 or α_2, or both) and indirect dilation of resistive vessels mediated by increased myocardial metabolic activity. The increase in coronary flow resistance caused by maximal nerve stimulation is only about one-quarter of that produced by intravenous or intracoronary infusion of norepinephrine. In fact, nerve stimulation is rather crude in that it stimulates all fibers. Naturally occurring nerve stimulation may cause different vasomotor effects by selectively stimulating specific fibers at specific rates, thus determining the release of mediators in different combinations and at different sites. Pharmacologic stimulation of coronary β_1 and β_2 receptors causes a modest reduction of coronary flow resistance (20–30%). Epicardial coronary arteries show changes in caliber similar in direction to, but even smaller in magnitude than, those of resistive vessels in response to nervous and pharmacologic α- and β-receptor stimulation. α-Adrenergic blockade reduces coronary vascular resistance at rest and also during heavy exercise, but may exacerbate ischemia distal to critical stenoses (see Ch. 6).

Electric stimulation of adrenergic nerves causes initial modest vasoconstriction with increased coronary flow resistance, which is followed by sustained major vasodilation secondary to increases in heart rate, in blood pressure, and in inotropism and, hence, in myocardial metabolic activity. Following β_1 adrenergic blockade with atenolol, maximal adrenergic nerve stimulation causes only a 20–30% increase in coronary resistance, which is prevented by phentolamine. The degree of constriction caused by adrenergic nerve stimulation in the coronary circulation is many times smaller than that in skeletal muscle and skin.[50]

The physiologic neurotransmitter norepinephrine, released at the varicosities in the border between adventitia and media, exerts its most profound action on the media before ultimately reaching the endothelium. In contrast, epinephrine released into the bloodstream from the adrenal glands, first meets endothelial receptors and then smooth muscle receptors in the media.

The effect of dopaminergic nerves on the coronary vasculature is still unknown. Intravenous infusion of dopamine causes coronary dilation, partly mediated by increased myocardial metabolic activity but also directly (occurring also in the presence of β_1 blockade). This direct vasodilator effect is mild, mediated in part by inhibition of norepinephrine release from sympathetic nerves and in part by stimulation of dopaminergic receptors (as it can be prevented by haloperidol, a specific dopaminergic-receptor blocker).

■ *The effect of adrenergic vasoactive stimuli on coronary vasomotor tone can be quite variable because it is the integrated result of their direct effect on the smooth muscle, their endothelium-mediated effects, the basal level of vasomotor tone, and the effect on myocardial oxygen consumption. The direct and indirect effects both depend on the type, number, and function of adrenergic receptors and on their coupling with the intracellular mechanisms that control contraction and relaxation.* ■

5.4.2 Cholinergic control

Acetylcholine is the classic cholinergic neurotransmitter, which under some circumstances, may be coreleased with ATP, with vasoactive intestinal polypeptide, or with CGRP.[48] It acts on nicotinic receptors in nervous ganglia and on muscarinic receptors in the cardiovascular system. The cardiovascular effect of parasympathetic nerves, mediated by muscarinic receptors, is selectively blocked by atropine. In the tissues and bloodstream, acetylcholine is almost immediately degraded by acetylcholinesterase. In coronary vessels, muscarinic receptors are located:

a. on the endothelium, where the activation causes release of EDRF and hence vasodilation
b. on SMCs, where their activation causes contraction
c. on sympathetic nerve varicosities, where their activation inhibits norepinephrine release.

The vasomotor effects of vagal stimulation depend not only on the direct effect on smooth muscle but also on the indirect effect attributable to endothelial stimulation, as well as on basal vasomotor tone and on the reflex changes induced by the stimulation. The transmitter released by the nerve varicosities first reaches adrenergic varicosities and SMCs in the media and progressively diffuses towards the endothelium and the lumen. The results of experimental studies on the effects of vagal stimulation are species dependent and controversial.[50]

In dogs, but not in pigs, when heart rate is maintained constant by pacing, electrical vagal stimulation produces a 20–30% reduction in coronary flow resistance, which is quite modest compared with the near-maximal coronary dilation caused by intracoronary infusion of acetylcholine in the presence of normal endothelial function. The effect on large epicardial arteries has not been studied. The overall effect of cholinergic nerve stimulation is determined by the ratio of receptor density in smooth muscle, in the endothelium, and in adrenergic nerve varicosities, and by the rate of acetylcholinesterase degradation of acetylcholine in the vessel wall.

5.4.3 Purinergic and peptidergic control

The information available suggests that there may be a role for nonadrenergic, noncholinergic nervous control of the coronary circulation. The main candidate for neurotransmission in purinergic nerves is ATP. Two types of purinergic receptors have been identified on the basis of their agonist potency order:[49] P_1, which is most sensitive to adenosine and least sensitive to ATP, is present on endothelial cells (stimulates release of EDRF), on SMCs (mediates relaxation) and on sympathetic nerve varicosities (inhibits norepinephrine release); P_2, which is most sensitive to ATP and least sensitive to adenosine, is present on endothelial cells (stimulates EDRF release) and on SMCs (mediates constriction). As adenosine infusion causes maximal dilation of resistive vessels, but only a small increase in the caliber of epicardial coronary arteries compared with that produced by nitrates, it is possible that the density of P_1 receptors is much greater in resistive vessels than in extramyocardial coronary arteries. ATP can be released from nerve terminals, endothelial cells, and platelets and from myocardial cells during ischemia. Adenosine is produced from degradation of ATP and can be released from myocardial cells and platelets; it is also produced by endothelial cells. In coronary vessels, peptidergic nerves have been identified by immunohistochemistry, but so far their possible role has been investigated only very indirectly by intravenous or intracoronary administration of peptidergic transmitters (see 5.5.1 and Ch. 6).

■ *Nonadrenergic, noncholinergic neurotransmission appears to have only a modulatory role on adrenergic and cholinergic physiologic control of the cardiovascular functions so far explored, but it may be more important in pathologic conditions.* ■

5.4.4 Reflex control

Coronary vasomotor tone is also under the influence of cardiac reflexes, both indirectly, through changes in myocardial contractile (and hence metabolic) activity, and directly, by nervous regulation of vessel caliber. Afferent stimuli, arising outside the heart (from chemoreceptors in the carotid bodies, and from mechanoreceptors in the carotid sinus, aortic arch, and lungs), may produce efferent stimuli that influence coronary flow resistance. When myocardial contractile activity is maintained constant, reduction of pressure in the carotid sinus increases coronary flow resistance and, conversely, an increase in pressure reduces coronary resistance; stimulation of chemoreceptors and inflation of the lungs also reduces coronary flow resistance.[51,52] Reflex effects on the coronary circulation from other visceral organs, such as the gallbladder, esophagus, and stomach, suggested by anecdotal clinical observations, have so far not been satisfactorily explored. Reflexes also originate from chemoreceptors and mechanoreceptors, which form a diffuse network of fibers throughout all chambers of the heart.[53] These receptors are connected to the central nervous system via unmyelinated fibers traveling with the vagi, and also by means of both myelinated and unmyelinated fibers traveling with the sympathetic nerves.[54] Their effect on coronary vasomotor tone is unknown. Cardiac afferent fibers stimulated by substance P also appear capable of generating axon reflexes, which may be important in the phasic and tonic autoregulation of local vascular perfusion, but their role has not been clearly established.[55]

5.5 EFFECTS OF INTRACORONARY INFUSION OF VASOACTIVE SUBSTANCES

Differences between species, organs, and vascular segments, with regard to their vasomotor response to the same agonists, may be very considerable.[38,50] Studies are, therefore, required in order to assess the segmental vasomotor response of the human coronary circulation, and one of the ways in which this can be achieved is by direct intracoronary infusion of vasoactive substances. This rather crude approach has the advantage of eliminating the systemic reflex vasomotor changes that could be induced by systemic administration of these substances, but the disadvantage that this route of administration may reflect conditions in vivo for only some agonists (such as 5-HT, which can be released by platelets) and not for others, such as acetylcholine and the various neuropeptides, that exert their physiologic effects on the vessel wall from the adventitial side of the wall rather than from the bloodstream.

Studies have been performed in patients with "angiographically normal" coronary arteries, catheterized because of "atypical" chest pain, and in patients with angiographically detectable coronary atherosclerosis. Within the limitations mentioned above, the studies summarized below have confirmed the existence of considerable variations in the segmental response of the coronary circulation, and have allowed the detection of abnormalities in the vasomotor response of different groups of patients.

5.5.1 Studies on the coronary endothelial function of epicardial coronary arteries

The data available indicate that, in atherosclerotic coronary segments, the vasomotor response to acetylcholine and other vasoactive stimuli that cause vasodilation in normal vessels is characterized by failure to dilate, or even by constriction. This abnormal response,

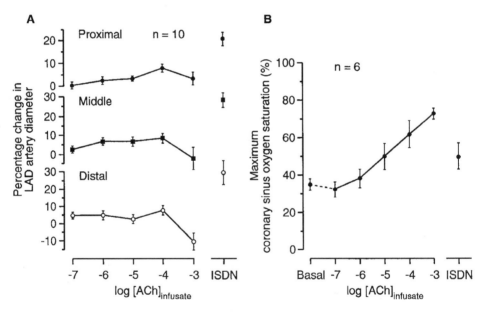

Fig. 5.11 Different and dose-dependent effects of acetylcholine on conductive and resistive coronary arteries. In patients with angiographically normal coronary arteries, plots of percentage change in luminal diameter of the proximal (●), middle (■), and distal (○) segments of the left anterior descending coronary artery (**A**), and in coronary sinus oxygen saturation (**B**) associated with 2 min intracoronary infusions of increasing concentrations of acetylcholine (log [ACh]$_{infusate}$). Mild dilation of conductive arteries at low doses is followed by constriction at high doses. However, the resistive vessels continue to dilate further at high doses (as indicated by the further large increase in coronary sinus oxygen saturation in the absence of any change in the determinants of myocardial oxygen consumption). Dilation following intracoronary injection of 2 mg isosorbide dinitrate (ISDN) is also reported. The increase in coronary sinus oxygen saturation observed after ISDN is much smaller than that observed after acetylcholine, suggesting that at least part of the large increase in flow caused by acetylcholine is not nitric oxide-dependent. (Modified from ref. 59.)

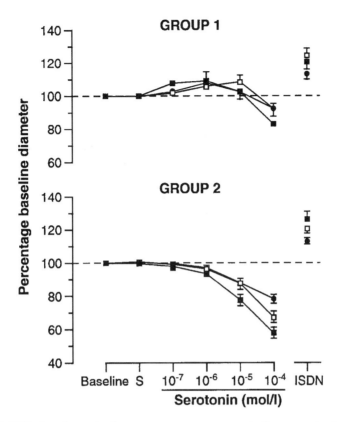

Fig. 5.12 Effects of serotonin on coronary segments from control subjects and patients with stable angina. The mean ($\pm$SEM) change from base line in the luminal diameter of proximal (●), middle (□), and distal (■) arterial segments is shown after a 2 min infusion of saline (S), increasing concentrations of serotonin and an intracoronary injection of isosorbide dinitrate (ISDN). The coronary segments from the controls (Group 1) show a small progressive dilation at lower concentrations of serotonin, but constriction (more marked in the distal segments) at the highest concentration. The segments from the patients with coronary atherosclerosis (Group 2) fail to dilate and develop greater constriction than controls. Distal segments constrict more than proximal segments. (Modified from ref. 60.)

observed not only in epicardial segments but also in resistive vessels, is commonly attributed to defective production of EDRF, by analogy with the results obtained in endothelial denuded *previously normal* vessels, but its mechanisms are likely to be more complex.

The potential interest of a defective dilator response derives from the possibility that it could favor the development of myocardial ischemic episodes by constrictor stimuli and may reflect a local endothelial dysfunction, including a thrombotic tendency. A review of available information reveals that the physiologic endothelial control of coronary vasomotor tone and its alterations are still incompletely understood.

The dilator effect of acetylcholine in angiographically normal epicardial coronary arteries is considerably smaller than that produced by nitrates; it decreases with age and with the presence of coronary risk factors. It also has a constrictor effect on atherosclerotic segments and each of these different effects occurs in the presence of a preserved dilator response to nitrates.[56–59]

The effect of acetylcholine on angiographically normal coronary arteries is dose dependent.[59] The same segments that dilate mildly at lower doses constrict at higher doses, indicating that endothelium-mediated dilator effects prevail at low doses whereas direct smooth muscle constrictor effects prevail at high doses. The effect of acetylcholine on resistive vessels is markedly different from that observed in proximal conductive arteries: a very large increase in CBF occurs at doses that produce constriction of angiographically visible epicardial coronary arteries (see Fig. 5.11). The very large increase in flow caused by acetylcholine (compared with that caused by intracoronary nitrates) suggests that it may possibly stimulate the production of EDHF, as well as of NO. Even higher doses cause ischemia, but without a reduction in coronary sinus oxygen saturation below resting values, which is compatible with inhomogeneous dilation and constriction of parallel coronary vessels (see Ch. 6).

5-HT also produces dose-dependent effects on angiographically normal epicardial arteries: at low doses it has a mildly dilator effect and at high doses a constrictor effect. On atherosclerotic arteries it has a mildly constrictor effect (see Fig. 5.12 and Ch. 6).[60,61]

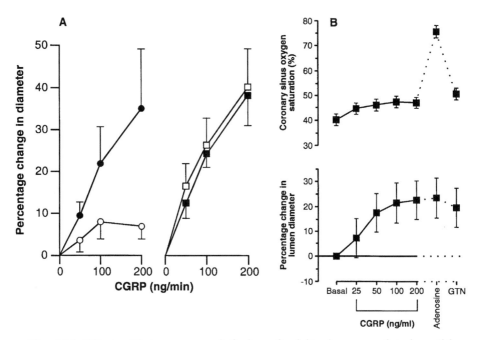

Fig. 5.13 Effects of intracoronary infusion of calcitonin gene-related peptide (CGRP) in patients with normal coronary arteries and in those with atherosclerotic coronary arteries. A. In patients with angiographically normal coronary arteries significant increases in diameter occur with increasing doses of CGRP in all segments, but the increase is greater in segments of smaller diameter (1.5–2.7 mm circumflex artery [●], mid-left anterior descending artery [LAD] [■], and distal LAD [□]) than in those of larger diameter (3.1 mm proximal LAD [O]). B. The increase in diameter of atherosclerotic mid-LAD segments is not significantly different from that observed in normal arteries. There is only a small increase in coronary sinus oxygen saturation, which increases markedly following intracoronary infusion of adenosine and only mildly following glyceryl trinitrate (GTN). As the changes in coronary sinus oxygen saturation are not associated with changes in the determinants of myocardial oxygen consumption, they indicate that CGRP and GTN cause a much smaller degree of dilation of resistive vessels than adenosine. (Modified from refs 62 and 64.)

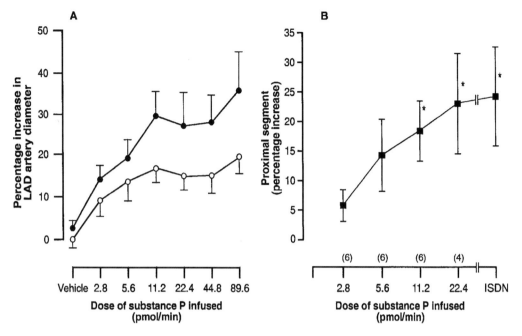

Fig. 5.14 **Effect of substance P on epicardial coronary artery diameter in patients with normal coronary arteries and in those with atherosclerotic coronary arteries. A.** In patients with angiographically normal coronary arteries the increase in left anterior descending (LAD) coronary artery diameter in response to substance P is dose dependent and is greater in distal (●) than in proximal (○) vessels. The maximal dilation of epicardial branches was associated with only a 50% increase in flow. **B.** Proximal, smooth segments of stenotic vessels show a preserved dilator response to substance P not significantly different from that observed in **A.** Thus, in patients with detectable coronary atherosclerosis, the dilator response to substance P may be preserved. As substance P does not have a direct constrictor effect, it should be a more specific indicator of endothelial dysfunction than acetylcholine which, also having a constrictor effect, may reflect an hyperreactivity of coronary smooth muscle. (Modified from refs 63 and 65.)

The findings with agonists that are known to stimulate release of EDRF, but which have no direct constrictor effects on the smooth muscle, are quite different from those of acetylcholine. CGRP and substance P cause dose-dependent dilation of epicardial coronary arteries with a maximum effect similar to that produced by nitrates. The maximal epicardial artery dilation was found to be associated with only minimal increase of flow with CGRP and an average 50% increase with substance P. In most atherosclerotic segments, substance P and CGRP produced a maximal degree of dilation comparable to that observed in angiographically normal segments and to that obtained with nitrates (see Figs 5.13 and 5.14).[62–65] In contrast, bradykinin had a significantly lower dilator effect on atherosclerotic segments than on normal coronary segments.[66] The segmental coronary constrictor effects of NPY and endothelin on small coronary vessels, rather than on conductive coronary arteries, are described in Chapter 6.

These observations show that agonists that exert their dilator effect by a mechanism mediated by the endothelium, can have markedly different, and even opposite, vasomotor effects on the caliber of epicardial coronary arteries and on flow. These differences can be related to differences in the distribution of receptors in endothelial and smooth muscle cells, or to their intracellular coupling in different vascular segments.

5.5.2 Mechanisms of the variability of segmental endothelium-dependent coronary dilation

The lack of effect of CGRP on flow,[64] and the minor effect of substance P,[63] are in sharp contrast to the marked increase in flow caused by acetylcholine[59] (in spite of its direct constrictor effect on smooth muscle). In humans, as the increase in flow caused by acetylcholine is much greater than that caused by intracoronary injection of nitrates, it cannot be attributable only to NO. This conclusion is consistent with the effects of intracoronary LNMMA reported above.[36] The major dilator effect of both CGRP and substance P on epicardial coronary arteries, and their much smaller effect on flow compared with that of acetylcholine, may be due to a different density or type of receptors for these agonists in the two types of vessels, and/or to a different coupling of the receptors with NO and EDHF production mechanisms.[14]

5.5.3 Implications of defective endothelial function

Both endothelial denudation and blockade of NO synthesis are associated with an enhanced dilator response to exogenous NO donors such as nitrates, but it is not clear to what extent this enhanced dilator response is due to increased basal tone.[67,68] Defective EDRF production has also been observed in vessels with regenerated endothelium following its denudation. In endothelium-denuded vessels, a paradoxical response can be attributable only to deficient EDRF production, but in chronic conditions a paradoxical constrictor response could also be attributable to an enhanced constrictor response of the smooth muscle. Independent of its actual mechanisms, there is convincing evidence that the response of human epicardial coronary arteries to a variety of vasoactive stimuli tends to shift toward coronary constriction with advancing age, with increasing levels of risk factors, and with angiographically detectable coronary atherosclerosis:[56–58] this constrictor response can also be detected in resistive vessels (see Ch. 9).[69]

■ *The clinical significance of the abnormal coronary vasomotor response caused by endothelial dysfunction in experimental animals is uncertain because in humans compensatory mechanisms are likely to intervene. The extensive coronary atheroma detectable in the majority of middle-aged individuals who died of noncardiac causes, without any evidence of IHD (see Ch. 8), indicates that even obvious coronary atherosclerosis per se may not necessarily be associated with signs of IHD.* ■

REFERENCES

1. Somlyo AP. Excitation–contraction coupling and the ultrastructure of smooth muscle. Circ Res 1985;*57*:497.
2. Hathaway DR, March KL, Lash JA, Adam LP, Wilensky RL. Vascular smooth muscle: a review of the molecular basis of contractility. Circulation 1991;*83*:382.
3. Keatinge WR. Blood-vessels. British Med Bull 1979;*35*:249.
4. Morgan JP, Perreault CL, Morgan KG. The cellular basis of contraction and relaxation in cardiac and vascular smooth muscle. Am Heart J 1991;*121*:961.

5. Murphy RA, Aksoy MO, Dillon PF, Gerthoffer WT, Kamm KE. The role of myosin light chain phosphorylation in regulation of the cross-bridge cycle. Fed Proc 1983;*42:*51.

6. Berridge MJ, Irvine RF. Inositol triphosphate, a novel second messenger in cellular signal transduction. Nature 1984;*312:*315.

7. Murad F. Cyclic guanosine monophosphate as a mediator of vasodilation. J Clin Invest 1986;*78:*1.

8. Ashida T, Schaeffer J, Goldman WF et al. Role of sarcoplasmic reticulum in arterial contraction: comparison of ryanodine's effect in a conduit and a muscular artery. Circ Res 1988;*62:*854.

9. Fleckenstein A. Calcium antagonism in heart and smooth muscle. J Wiley, New York, 1983.

10. Godraind T, Kaba A. Blockade or reversal of contraction induced by calcium and adrenaline in depolarized arterial smooth muscle. Br J Pharmacol 1969;*36:*549.

11. Reuter H. Ion channels in cardiac cell membrane. Ann Rev Physiol 1984;*46:*473.

12. Nelson M, Patlak J, Worley J, Standen N. Calcium channels, potassium channels and the voltage dependence of arterial smooth muscle tone. Am J Physiol 1990;*259:*C3.

13. Latorre R, Oberhauser A, Labarca P, Alvarez O. Varieties of calcium-activated potassium channels. Ann Rev Physiol 1989;*51:*385.

14. Standen NB, Quayle JM, Davies NW et al. Hyperpolarizing vasodilators activate ATP-sensitive K$^+$ channels in arterial smooth muscle. Science 1989;*245:*177.

15. Edwards G, Weston AH. Potassium channel openers and vascular smooth muscle relaxation. Pharmacol Ther 1990;*48:*237.

16. Kalsner S. Coronary artery reactivity in human vessels: some questions and some answers. Fed Proc 1985;*44:*321.

17. Godfraind T, Miller RC. Pharmacology of coronary arteries. In: De Bakey ME, Gotto AM Jr (eds). Factors influencing the course of myocardial ischaemia. Elsevier, Amsterdam, 1983, p.101.

18. McHale PA, Dubé GP, Greenfield JC Jr. Evidence for myogenic vasomotor activity in the coronary circulation. Prog Cardiovasc Dis 1987;*30:*139.

19. Olsson RA, Bünger R. Metabolic control of coronary blood flow. Prog Cardiovasc Dis 1987;*29:*369.

20. Gewirtz H, Brautigan DL, Olsson RA, Brown P, Most S. Role of adenosine in the maintenance of coronary vasodilation distal to a severe coronary artery stenosis. Observations in conscious domestic swine. Circ Res 1983;*53:*42.

21. Gewirtz H, Weeks G, Nathanson M, Sharaf B, Fedele F, Most AS. Tissue acidosis. Role in sustained arteriolar dilatation distal to a coronary stenosis. Circulation 1989;*79:*890.

22. Lablanche JM, Didier B, Delforge M et al. La vasomotricité coronaire chez l'homme. Description d'une méthode de quantification et valeurs normales. Arch Mal Coeur 1986;*79:*13.

23. Maseri A, Bertrand M, El Tamimi H. Study of the vasomotor response of human stable coronary artery stenoses. 1995; in preparation.

24. Tousoulis D, Kaski JC, Bogaty P et al. Reactivity of proximal and distal angiographically normal and stenotic coronary segments in chronic stable angina. Am J Cardiol 1991;*67:*1195.

25. Winbury MM, Howe BB, Hefner MA. Effect of nitrates and other coronary dilators on large and small coronary vessels: hypothesis for the mechanism of action of nitrates. J Pharmacol Exp Ther 1969;*168:*70.

26. Cohen MV, Kirk E. Differential response of large and small coronary arteries to nitroglycerin and angiotensin. Circ Res 1973;*33:*445.

27. Young MA, Vatner S. Regulation of large coronary arteries. Circ Res 1986;*59:*579.

28. Marcus ML, Chilian WM, Kanatsuka H, Dellsperger KC, Eastham CL, Lamping KG. Understanding the coronary circulation through studies at the microvascular level. Circulation 1990;*82:*1.

29. Domenech RJ, MacLellon PR. Transmural ventricular distribution of coronary blood flow during coronary beta$_2$ adrenergic receptor activation in dogs. Circ Res 1980;*46:*29.

30. Maseri A, Davies G, Hackett D, Kaski JC. Coronary artery spasm and coronary vasoconstriction: the case for a distinction. Circulation 1990;*81:*1983.

31. Henry PD, Yokoyama M. Supersensitivity of atherosclerotic rabbit aorta to ergonovine: mediation by a serotonergic mechanism. J Clin Invest 1980;*66:*306.

32. Crea F, Von Arnim T, Allwork SP, Jadhav A, Thompson GR, Maseri A. Failure of experimental atherosclerosis to sensitize coronary arteries to spasm in hypercholesterolemic rabbits. Am Heart J 1985;*109:*491.

33. Shimokawa H, Tomoike H, Nabeyama S, Yamamoto H, Araki H, Nakamura M. Coronary artery spasm induced in atherosclerotic miniature swine. Science 1983;*221:*560.

34. Hackett D, Larkin S, Chierchia S, Davies G, Kaski JC, Maseri A. Induction of coronary artery spasm by a direct local action of ergonovine. Circulation 1987;*75:*577.

35. Bassenge E, Busse R. Endothelial modulation of coronary tone. Prog Cardiovasc Dis 1988;*30:*349.

36. Lefroy DC, Crake T, Uren NG, Davies GJ, Maseri A. Effect of inhibition of nitric oxide on epicardial coronary artery caliber and coronary blood flow in man. Circulation 1993;*88:*43.

37. Cooke JP, Rossitch E Jr, Andon NA, Loscalzo J, Dzau VJ. Flow activates an endothelial potassium channel to release an endogenous nitrovasodilator. J Clin Invest 1991;*88:*1663.

38. Christie MI, Griffith TM, Lewis MJ. A comparison of basal and agonist-stimulated release of endothelium-derived relaxing factor from different arteries. Br J Pharmacol 1989;*98:*397.

39. Boulanger C, Lüscher TF. Release of endothelin from the porcine aorta. Inhibition by endothelium-derived nitric oxide. J Clin Invest 1990;*85:*587.

40. Yang ZH, Richard V, von Segesser L et al. Threshold concentrations of endothelin-1 potentiate contractions to norepinephrine and serotonin in human arteries. A new mechanism of vasospasm? Circulation 1990;*82:*188.

41. Dzau VJ, Gibbons GH, Cooke JP, Omoigui N. Vascular biology and medicine in the 1990s: scope, concepts, potentials, and perspectives. Circulation 1993;*87:*705.

42. Friedman PL, Brown, EJ, Gunther S et al. Coronary vasoconstrictor effect of indomethacin in patients with coronary-artery disease. New Engl J Med 1981;*305:*1171.

43. Godfraind T, Miller RC. Effects of histamine and the histamine antagonists mepyramine and cimetidine on human coronary arteries in vitro. Br J Pharmacol 1983;*79:*979.

44. Letts LG, Newman DL, Greenwald SE, Piper PJ. Effects of intra-coronary administration of leucotriene D$_4$ in the anaesthetized dog. Prostaglandins 1983;*26:*563.

45. Tippins JR, Antoniw JW, Alison MR, Garvey B, Maseri A. A platelet-activating factor antagonist, WEB 2086, inhibits neutrophil-dependent increase in coronary resistance in the rabbit isolated, blood-perfused heart. Cardiovasc Res 1992;*26:*162.

46. Shepherd JT. The heart as a sensory organ. J Am Coll Cardiol 1985;*6:*83B.

47. Uehara Y, Suyama K. Visualization of the adventitial aspect of the vascular smooth muscle cells under the scanning electron microscope. J Electron Microsc 1978;*27:*157.

48. Burnstock G, Kennedy C. A dual function for adenosine 5′-triphosphate in the regulation of vascular tone. Circ Res 1985;*58:*319.

49. Burnstock G, Kennedy C. Is there a basis for distinguishing two types of P$_2$-purinoceptor? Gen Pharmac 1985;*16:*433.

50. Young MA, Knight DR, Vatner S. Autonomic control of large coronary arteries and resistance vessels. Prog Cardiovasc Dis 1987;*30:*211.

51. Ito BR, Feigl EO. Carotid baroreceptor reflex coronary vasodilation in the dog. Circ Res 1985;*56:*486.

52. Ito BR, Feigl EO. Carotid chemoreceptor reflex parasympathetic coronary vasodilation in the dog. Am J Physiol 1985;*249:*H1167.

53. Armour JA. Intrinsic cardiac neurons. J Cardiovasc Electrophysiol 1991;*2:*331.

54. Malliani A. Cardiovascular sympathetic afferent fibers. Rev Physiol Biochem Pharmacol 1982;*94:*11.

55. Armour JA. Instant to instant reflex cardiac regulation. Cardiology 1976;*61:*309.

56. Ludmer PL, Selwyn AP, Shook TL et al. Paradoxical vasoconstriction induced by acetylcholine in atherosclerotic coronary arteries. N Engl J Med 1986;*315:*1046.

57. Yasue H, Matsuyama K, Matsuyama K, Okumura K, Morikami Y, Ogawa H. Responses of angiographically normal human coronary arteries to intracoronary injection of acetylcholine by age and segment. Possible role of early coronary atherosclerosis. Circulation 1990;*81:*482.

58. Zeiher AM, Drexler H, Wollschläger, Just H. Modulation of coronary vasomotor tone in humans.

Progressive endothelial dysfunction with different early stages of coronary atherosclerosis. Circulation 1991;*83:*391.

59. Newman CM, Maseri A, Hackett DR, El-Tamimi HM, Davies GJ. Response of angiographically normal and atherosclerotic left anterior descending coronary arteries to acetylcholine. Am J Cardiol 1990;*66:*1070.

60. McFadden EP, Clarke JG, Davies GJ, Haider AW, Kaski JC, Maseri A. Effect of intracoronary serotonin on coronary vessels in patients with stable and variant angina. New Engl J Med 1991;*324:*648.

61. Golino P, Piscione F, Willerson JT et al. Divergent effects of serotonin on coronary-artery dimensions and blood flow in patients with coronary atherosclerosis and control patients. New Engl J Med 1991;*324:*641.

62. McEwan J, Larkin S, Davies G et al. Calcitonin gene related peptide is a potent dilator of human epicardial coronary arteries. Circulation 1986;*74:*1243.

63. Crossman DC, Larkin SW, Fuller RW, Davies GJ, Maseri A. Substance P dilates epicardial coronary arteries and increases coronary blood flow in humans. Circulation 1989;*80:*475.

64. Ludman PF, Maseri A, Davies GJ. Effects of calcitonin gene-related peptide on normal and atheromatous vessels and on resistance vessels in the coronary circulation in humans. Circulation 1991;*84:*1993.

65. Crossman DC, Larkin SW, Dashwood MR, Davies GJ, Yacoub M, Maseri A. Responses of atherosclerotic human coronary arteries in-vivo to the endothelium-dependent vasodilator Substance P. Circulation 1991;*84:*2001.

66. Rafflenbeul W, Bassenge E, Lichtlen P. Konkurrenz zwischen endothelabhängiger und nitroglycerin-induzierter koronarer vasodilation. Z Kardiol 1989;*78:*45.

67. Bassenge E, Stewart DJ. Interdependence of pharmacologically-induced and endothelium-mediated coronary vasodilation in antianginal therapy. Cardiovasc Drugs Ther 1988;*2:*27.

68. Moncada S, Rees DD, Schulz R, Palmer RMJ. Development and mechanism of a specific supersensitivity to nitrovasodilators after inhibition of vascular nitric oxide synthesis in vivo. Proc Natl Acad Sci USA 1991;*88:*2166.

69. Zeiher AM, Drexler H, Wollschläger H, Just H. Endothelial dysfunction of the coronary microvasculature is associated with impaired coronary blood flow regulation in patients with early atherosclerosis. Circulation 1991;*84:*1984.

Pathophysiologic principles

Experimental models of acute myocardial ischemia

INTRODUCTION

Experimental models are better suited for studying the consequences and pathogenetic mechanisms of ischemia than for investigating its etiology. Current experimental models of ischemia have been developed in accordance with prevailing views on the actual causes of ischemia in patients with IHD. Thus, their development has focused on the consequences of epicardial coronary stenosis, on the development of collaterals, and, more recently, on dynamic modulation of coronary stenosis. The possible role of distal coronary vessel constriction has received very little attention and models of coronary thrombosis have been developed more to study the consequences of infarction than to speculate on its causes. However, studies in anesthetized and conscious animals have provided useful details of some known pathogenetic mechanisms of ischemia and important information on the effects of ischemia on myocardial cells and cardiac function (see Ch. 7). They have elucidated the hemodynamic consequences of coronary stenoses and their effects on the development of collateral circulation, and have provided examples of patterns of intraluminal plugging and epicardial and distal coronary constriction. The most important information provided by experimental models can be summarized as follows.

Fixed stenoses begin to interfere appreciably with coronary flow reserve only when the diameter of the artery is reduced by more than 50%, corresponding to a 75% reduction of the lumen (see Ch. 8), but further reduction of diameter increases transtenotic resistance progressively and dramatically. In acute experiments, the increase in transtenotic resistance at rest can be compensated for by proportional dilation of resistive vessels until the diameter of the stenosis is reduced by about 90%, but this compensation requires the use of a significant fraction of coronary flow reserve, just for basic resting needs.

Decreased poststenotic coronary pressure, resulting from the buildup of the transtenotic pressure gradient, jeopardizes perfusion much more in subendocardial than in subepicardial layers. Poststenotic pressure decreases with increasing severity of the stenosis and, for the same severity of stenosis, it increases more than linearly with increasing flow. Distal to chronic stenoses, perfusion pressure is increased by collateral flow, which thus tends to restore coronary flow reserve in poststenotic areas.

Collaterals begin to develop by dilating preexisting anastomotic connections within hours of the establishment of a poststenotic pressure gradient and from newly formed connections between arterial systems. Collateral development reaches a maximum within a few months.

The extent of collateral development is variable from species to species and between individuals of the same species; it is largely genetically determined.

Dynamic stenoses—transient changes in epicardial coronary artery caliber—have a much greater effect on flow when occurring at the site of severe preexisting stenoses that already encroach upon the lumen than when occurring at the site of mild stenoses. Dynamic stenoses of epicardial coronary arteries can be caused by physiologic increase of coronary vasomotor tone, by occlusive spasm, by intravascular thrombosis, and by a combination of these causes; passive changes in caliber that are only secondary to a reduction in intravascular distending pressure do not seem to have significant pathogenetic roles.

Constriction of distal, small coronary vessels can impair flow also, in the absence of critical coronary artery stenoses.

Acute coronary thrombosis can cause persistent coronary artery occlusion.

6.1 EFFECTS OF FIXED EPICARDIAL CORONARY ARTERY STENOSIS

An epicardial coronary artery stenosis causes resistance to flow, so that the same flow across the stenotic segment can be maintained only if a transstenotic pressure gradient develops. As aortic pressure is obviously unaffected by the production of a coronary stenosis, the necessary transstenotic pressure gradient can become established only by a decrease in poststenotic pressure.

The initial tendency to impair flow, caused by the production of an epicardial coronary artery stenosis, is counteracted by the metabolic autoregulation of flow, which maintains flow constant when pressure at the origin of arterioles falls (see Ch. 4). In these conditions, the same flow is maintained in the presence of a lower poststenotic peripheral perfusion pressure at the expense of a reduction in the basal tone of arterioles. In this process of compensation a fraction of the coronary flow reserve is used merely to maintain resting flow. Thus, when myocardial demand increases, the maximal possible increase in flow above basal becomes less in the poststenotic area than in the rest of the ventricular wall perfused by normal vessels.

A readily comprehensible, although approximate, expression of the compensation for the presence of an epicardial coronary stenosis by resistive vessels is offered by the equation given in 4.2.5, where coronary blood flow (CBF) is determined by the ratio of the driving pressure, aortic pressure minus right atrial pressure (AOP − RAP) to resistance, which is the sum of epicardial coronary artery resistance (r_0), and preateriolar prearteriolar (r_1), arteriolar (r_2) and postarteriolar (r_3) resistance. Normally r_0 is negligible; r_1 and r_3 are small, and r_2 is the major determinant of flow. When a stenosis in an epicardial coronary artery causes r_0 to increase, flow will not fall as long as the sum of $r_1 + r_2 + r_3$ decreases, so that the denominator of the equation can remain constant.

The more severe the stenosis, the greater are transstenotic flow resistance, the poststenotic pressure drop, and the dilation of distal coronary vessels required to maintain an adequate flow. In turn, when myocardial demand increases, flow across the stenosis can increase only if the transstenotic pressure gradient increases, i.e. poststenotic pressure decreases further.

These adjustments have an inherent adverse effect. As resistive vessels dilate in order to maintain resting flow, the available coronary flow reserve is reduced in proportion to the drop in poststenotic pressure relative to aortic pressure. In turn, the drop in poststenotic perfusion pressure jeopardizes subendocardial perfusion when myocardial oxygen consumption (MVO_2) increases, diastole shortens, intraventricular pressure increases, and aortic pressure decreases below a critical level (see 6.1.1, 6.1.2 and 4.3.5).

In chronic conditions, the reduced poststenotic pressure favors the development of a collateral circulation, which in turn increases poststenotic pressure and thus tends to restore residual coronary flow reserve (see 6.1.3).

6.1.1 Pressure/flow relations across an epicardial coronary stenosis

Theoretical calculations indicate that the relation between transstenotic resistance and the degree of stenosis is highly nonlinear.[1] Resistance begins to increase appreciably only when stenoses exceed 50% internal diameter reduction (75% luminal stenosis), but then rises progressively more and more steeply: for example, it almost triples as the stenosis increases from 80 to 90%.

The resistance to flow is mainly determined by the minimal residual artery lumen relative to control conditions and, to a smaller extent, by the length of the stenosis (according to the Poiseuille formula; see 3.3.2). It is also influenced by the presence of another stenosis in series and by flow, because of the energy loss created by turbulence, especially in the presence of irregularities of the lumen. Such calculations are an oversimplification, not only because stenoses are often irregular and flow is pulsatile, so that the caliber of the stenosis may change in systole and diastole, but also because systolic capacitance is modified distal

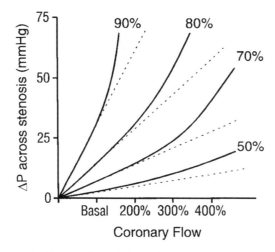

Fig. 6.1 Schematic illustration of the relation between transstenotic pressure gradient and blood flow. When the resistance (R) caused by the stenosis is fixed, in an ideal system, transstenotic pressure (ΔP) is linearly related to flow (F), F = ΔP/R and when flow doubles ΔP also doubles (dashed lines). The slope of the line depends on the severity of the stenosis. However, energy losses caused by turbulence at the site of the stenosis create a progressive flow-dependent increase in transstenotic pressure and the pressure/flow curves thus become curvilinear. At a constant aortic pressure, an appreciable transstenotic pressure gradient develops for a stenosis that reduces the diameter by more than 50% and increases progressively with its severity. For any given stenosis severity, transstenotic pressure increases more than linearly with flow. Thus, poststenotic pressure decreases progressively with increasing stenosis severity and, for a given severity of stenosis, it increases markedly with flow. The reduced poststenotic pressure may become insufficient to drive blood through maximally dilated arterioles, particularly in the subendocardium. In the absence of collateral flow, a 90% stenosis causes a drop in poststenotic pressure of more than 40 mmHg, which would barely be sufficient to maintain resting subendocardial flow; doubling of flow would require a drop in poststenotic pressure of more than 80 mmHg, which would cause transmural ischemia. (Modified from ref. 1.)

to the stenosis as a result of the decreased distending pressure and pulsatility. Nevertheless, such calculations give some idea of the order of magnitude of the effects of stenoses and imply that the transstenotic pressure gradient increases markedly with the severity of the stenosis and with the increase in flow (see Fig. 6.1). Measurements obtained in animals[2-4] confirm that a very large reduction in vessel lumen is needed to reduce resting coronary flow, even considering the inaccuracies that develop when estimating the degree of stenosis. When a stenosis is produced acutely, i.e. in the absence of a detectable collateral circulation, only reductions of 50–70% of internal diameter begin to reduce peak reactive hyperemia, and only reductions of 80–90% reduce resting flow (see Fig. 6.2).

As coronary flow reserve and peak reactive hyperemia are usually expressed in terms of percentage increases above basal flow, alterations in cardiac function can drastically change the relationship between coronary flow reserve and luminal dimensions of the stenosis. In the unanesthetized resting dog, for a given severity of stenosis and for comparable absolute values of maximal coronary flow (which depend on the level of aortic pressure [see 4.3.5]), resting coronary flow is low, so that both reactive hyperemia and coronary flow reserve above resting flow are substantially greater than in the anesthetized animal, in which resting coronary flow is high.

In unanesthetized resting dogs, peak reactive hyperemia (which may be taken as a gross indication of coronary flow reserve) starts to decline when the transstenotic pressure gradient at the end of diastole is about 5 mmHg (corresponding to an approximate 50% reduction in diameter); it then decreases rapidly, in proportion to the poststenotic pressure drop, disappearing completely when the transstenotic gradient is about 40 mmHg (a 60% gradient) and end-diastolic poststenotic pressure is about 20 mmHg (see Fig. 6.3).[2] In anesthetized animals (which have higher levels of resting MVO_2 and flow), reactive hyperemia starts to decline at minimal pressure gradients and disappears at about 30 mmHg transstenotic pressure gradient.[3-5]

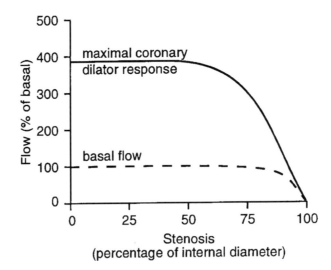

Fig. 6.2 Effect of stenosis severity on coronary flow reserve. In open chest dogs, only an acute reduction of coronary diameter to below 50% (a 75% reduction in lumen) begins to limit coronary flow reserve, but a stenosis reducing diameter to 50% still allows flow to increase about fourfold over resting values. Increases in the stenosis beyond 75% (a 94% reduction in lumen) dramatically reduce coronary flow reserve. Resting flow remains normal until the stenosis is about 90% (a 99% reduction in lumen). (Modified from ref. 4.)

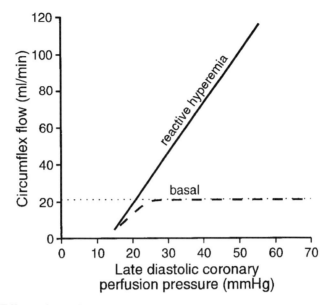

Fig. 6.3 Effect of a reduction in poststenotic pressure on reactive hyperemia and resting flow. In unanesthetized dogs, at constant aortic pressure, resting flow remains normal until late diastolic poststenotic pressure is reduced to about 25 mmHg (caused by a 90% stenosis in Fig. 6.2); however, peak reactive hyperemia decreases linearly fourfold as late diastolic perfusion pressure is reduced from 50 to 25 mmHg (caused by increasing the severity of the stenosis from 50 to 90% in Fig. 6.2). (From data presented in ref. 5.)

Although the disappearance of reactive hyperemia is commonly regarded as equivalent to a total loss of coronary bed dilatability, there is evidence that reserve dilatability is still available. In the presence of a stenosis that abolishes reactive hyperemia and causes a 20–30% decrease in basal coronary flow, the residual flow is almost doubled by the administration of nitroglycerin.[6] The dilatability of the ischemic bed has been confirmed by subsequent studies.[7,8] Whether this effect is related to dilation of prearteriolar or of arteriolar vessels is not yet known.

6.1.2 Transmural blood flow "steal"

When coronary flow reserve is reduced in subendocardial layers, the vasodilator reserve of subepicardial layers during increased myocardial work is still preserved. When subepicardial flow (and hence total flow) increases, therefore, poststenotic pressure falls; subendocardial flow then falls in proportion to the reduction in poststenotic perfusion pressure, and subendocardial ischemia develops because of the increase in subepicardial flow. Transmural "steal" can develop independently or together with intercoronary (lateral) "steal." This transmural redistribution—"steal"—of flow in favor of the subepicardium is more likely to produce ischemia when diastole is short, diastolic aortic pressure low, and MVO_2 high (see 4.3.5 and Table 6.1). In dogs, when the increase in CBF during exercise was reduced by one-third (using an hydraulic occluder on the circumflex artery),[9] only subendocardial flow was reduced (see Fig. 6.4).

Teleologically, therefore, a tonic constriction of subepicardial vessels distal to a critical stenosis would contribute to the maintenance of poststenotic perfusion pressure, thus pro-

Table 6.1 Mechanisms of subendocardial myocardial ischemia

In the presence of a coronary stenosis (or aortic stenosis), subendocardial ischemia may develop when poststenotic pressure decreases as a result of:

1. Increased stenosis severity (dynamic stenosis).
2. Increased transstenotic flow due to:
   a. increased MVO_2
   b. excessive vasodilation of subepicardial vessels caused by neurohumoral stimuli or drugs (even in the absence of increased cardiac work)
   c. a combination of (a) and (b).

Subendocardial ischemia is aggravated by:

1. Tachycardia, which increases oxygen consumption and reduces the duration of diastole.
2. Increased ventricular diastolic pressure, which increases the extravascular resistance in subendocardial layers.

tecting the subendocardium from ischemia; α-receptor-mediated tonic vasoconstriction may serve this purpose.[10] However, neural control may prove to be more complex, as a low poststenotic pressure has been reported to unmask sympathetic vasoconstriction in subendocardial layers: α_2-mediated coronary constriction, produced by electric stimulation of sympathetic nerves, was found to increase poststenotic resistance and even to cause ischemia in the presence of a critical stenosis, but not in its absence.[11] In conscious dogs, ischemia during exercise[12] can be attenuated by intracoronary α_2-adrenergic receptor blockade; in anesthetized dogs, subendocardial ischemia can be reduced by epidural anesthesia.[13] Epicardial blood flow steal may be reduced by theophylline[14] and subendocardial ischemia

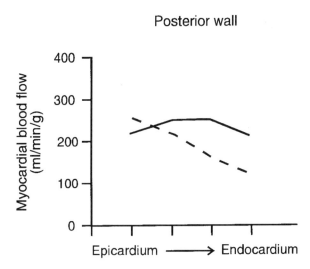

Fig. 6.4 Effect of a reduction in coronary flow during exercise on the transmural distribution of flow. A 30% reduction in left circumflex coronary blood flow during exercise in dogs (dashed line) is associated with a normal flow in subepicardial layers and a reduced flow in subendocardial layers compared with exercise under basal conditions (continuous line). Thus, a 30% reduction in total coronary blood flow during exercise may cause only mild subendocardial ischemia (as increased myocardial oxygen extraction partially compensates for the decreased blood flow). (Modified from ref. 9.)

may be increased by serotonin (5-HT).[15] Transmural blood flow steal may be increased by nitrates and calcium antagonists, but the overall effect of these drugs is complex as it also involves dilation of dynamic stenoses and prearterioles (see Ch. 10).

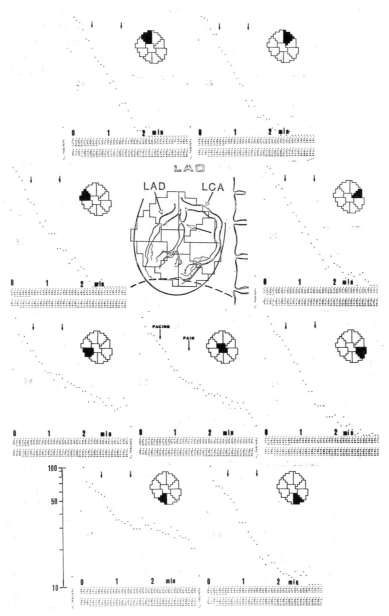

Fig. 6.5 Reduction of coronary blood flow during pacing-induced myocardial ischemia in patients. Precordial washout of ^{133}Xe, injected into the left coronary artery, was dramatically reduced by pacing-induced myocardial ischemia (arrows) in the myocardial regions perfused by the stenosed obtuse marginal coronary artery, but not in those perfused by the normal circumflex coronary artery. Small black arrow, onset of pacing; long arrow, slowing of the washout curve; thick arrow, stenosis. The reduction probably resulted from the elevation of pulmonary wedge pressure (from 5 to 20 mmHg) and, possibly, from ischemia-induced vasoconstriction. (Modified from ref. 16.)

6.1.3 Effect of elevated left ventricular diastolic pressure on poststenotic flow

Increased diastolic ventricular pressure is transmitted through the myocardial wall, decreasing linearly from the subendocardium to the subepicardium, and causing an increase in extravascular diastolic resistance to flow in subendocardial layers.

In the presence of normal coronary flow reserve, an even transmural distribution of flow is maintained (even when diastolic ventricular pressure is increased), by compensatory dilation of subendocardial resistive vessels. However, in the presence of a stenosis, subendocardial perfusion becomes impaired when poststenotic pressure is reduced relative to subendocardial extravascular pressure.

This mechanism of reduction of subendocardial flow by increased diastolic ventricular pressure represents a positive feedback mechanism by which the impairment of contractile function caused by ischemia further impairs subendocardial perfusion in the same area; it may also impair flow through subendocardial collaterals and may cause ischemia in other areas distal to critical stenoses.

For the same increase in diastolic ventricular pressure, the impairment of flow distal to a stenosis is greater when diastole is short, myocardial demand high, and diastolic aortic pressure low. A marked reduction in perfusion to ischemic myocardium can be demonstrated in patients with flow-limiting stenosis during pacing-induced ischemia (see Fig. 6.5).[16] The ischemia-induced impairment of perfusion is attributable to increased end-diastolic pressure, but a vasoconstrictor component can not be ruled out.

6.1.4 Chronic effects of stenoses: development of collateral circulation

Collaterals develop from preexisting anastomotic channels, as a result both of the establishment of a pressure gradient between their origin and termination and of chemical mediators; they also develop from newly formed microvessels, which establish new communications between adjacent vascular beds as a result of tissue ischemia.

Intercoronary arterial anastomoses are present in variable numbers in different mammals: they are so numerous in guinea pigs that they can prevent infarction even during sudden proximal coronary occlusion of a major coronary branch; they are more numerous in dogs than in pigs and rats and are virtually absent in rabbits (see Fig. 6.6).[17] Their presence and number in different species, and possibly in different individuals, are likely to be genetically determined. The patency of such anastomoses requires blood flow through them, which can occur only as a result of a pressure gradient developing from intermittent alternating constriction of parent branches. When a continuous pressure gradient develops, anastomoses gradually enlarge as blood flow through them increases.

A pressure gradient of about 10 mmHg in the resting unanesthetized dog, caused by a reduction in lumen of 70–80%, has been shown to elicit the development of collateral flow.[5,18] It seems, therefore, that the blood flow shear stress provided by the pressure gradient is a sufficient stimulus to elicit enlargement of interarterial anastomoses, when present[17–19] (as ischemia is unlikely to be present with such a small pressure gradient). Ischemia is also unlikely to contribute to the enlargement of collaterals that run on the epicardial surface or through nonischemic myocardium, but it can favor the formation and development of collaterals running within the ischemic zone.

The available data do not support convincingly the possibility that, in the presence of stenoses, further development of collaterals can be produced in the long term by bursts of exercise or by vasodilator drugs. It is possible that the pressure gradient in itself is a maximal stimulus for enlargement of existing anastomoses, but ischemia is required for the formation and development of new anastomotic connections. In animals with no coronary

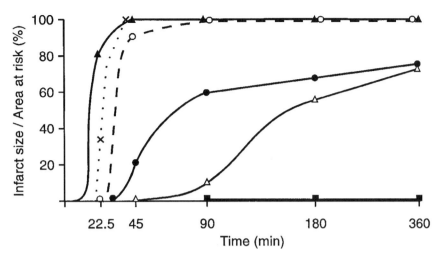

Fig. 6.6 Variable effects of sudden coronary occlusion on infarct size as a fraction of the anatomically perfused area at risk in different animal species. At one extreme, in guinea pigs (■) no infarction develops because of the presence of well developed intercoronary anastomoses. At the other extreme, in rabbits (▲), rats (×), and pigs (○), the whole area at risk becomes rapidly infarcted because of the lack of sufficiently developed interarterial anastomoses. In dogs (●) and cats (△), only a fraction of the area at risk becomes infarcted over a period of about 6 h because intercoronary anastomoses provide partial protection and cause a more gradual development of infarction. (Modified from ref. 17.)

stenoses, sustained exercise, prolonged for weeks, failed to produce detectable changes in anastomotic connections.

Newly formed interarterial connections can also develop in the *absence* of preexisting anastomoses. This was clearly demonstrated following mammary artery implants in the myocardium of dogs with gradual total occlusion of a major coronary artery.[20] The collateral blood supply provided by such newly formed vessels varied between different animals, but was always rather small compared with that provided by interarterial anastomoses. Microvascular occlusion was also shown to promote coronary collateral growth[21] as a result of ischemia or of pressure gradients at the coronary microvascular level. Following long-term embolization, however, collateral resistance was reduced only by about 50–75%, which represents a small change compared with the 10–30-fold reduction caused by chronic occlusion of a major coronary branch. The formation of vessels that establish new communications between adjacent arterial territories and their development is likely to be determined and influenced by vascular growth factors[17,22] and by heparin.[23]

The relative roles of enlargement and formation of new anastomotic channels are likely to vary in different species and in different experimental conditions; the results of experimental studies must, therefore, be applied to humans with caution.

Collateral vessels enlarge by division of cells in preexisting arteriolar vascular connections, associated with migration of monocytes into the wall and subsequently with proliferation of smooth muscle cells (SMCs). Incorporation of radiolabeled thymidine into DNA and the appearance of mitotic spindles in SMCs can be detected within 24 h of the establishment of a critical stenosis. The initial tissue mass of the collateral vessel can increase by a factor of

10–20 and collateral function develops progressively over a period of weeks, continuing for 3–6 months following coronary occlusion.

Vessel growth needs not only cell proliferation, which would result in a reduction of lumen diameter, but also a process of remodeling, which facilitates vascular enlargement by controlled and graded destruction of the existing structure.

Anastomoses can provide a very considerable amount of blood flow; in dogs, they are maximal 3–6 months after a gradual coronary occlusion developing over a few days.[18]

■ *The very variable ability to provide collateral compensatory blood flow in different species depends primarily on the number, size, and location of preexisting intercoronary arterial anastomoses, and only minimally on the formation of new connections between previously separated arterial territories.* ■

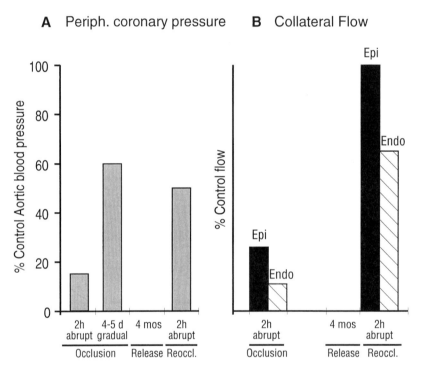

Fig. 6.7 Effect of sudden coronary occlusion on postocclusion coronary pressure and blood flow in unanesthetized dogs. Two hours after acute coronary occlusion, peripheral coronary pressure is still only 20% of aortic pressure, but with gradual occlusion developing over 4–5 days, peripheral coronary perfusion pressure is 60% of control aortic pressure. If the occlusion is then released and the artery reoccluded after 4 months, peripheral coronary perfusion pressure is 50% of control aortic pressure and only subendocardial flow is moderately reduced compared with control. In sharp contrast, when the artery is occluded suddenly before the development of collaterals, both epicardial (■) and endocardial (▨) blood flow are markedly reduced. Subsequently, once collaterals have developed, they are maintained for at least 4 months after the occlusion is released and provide near-complete protection during sudden coronary reocclusion, although the intercoronary pressure gradient between the origin and termination of collaterals had been abolished over this very long period. Collaterals remained patent most likely because of alternating constriction of parent branches.(Modified from ref. 18.)

6.1.5 Degree of functional compensation provided by collaterals in animals

The functional role of collaterals is to provide blood flow that protects against necrosis and gradually increases poststenotic pressure in the collateralized coronary arterial bed, eventually providing some coronary flow reserve. The protection provided by developing collaterals is a race against time. In both normal dogs and pigs, sudden coronary occlusion invariably causes myocardial infarction (MI), indicating that the function of normally available collaterals is totally inadequate to protect the myocardium from a sudden interruption of CBF in a major coronary artery. Conversely, a total occlusion produced gradually over a period of 3–7 days does not usually produce detectable myocardial necrosis in dogs or, over a longer period, in pigs.[17,18]

Experiments in isolated dog hearts, studied acutely following gradual total occlusion of a major coronary artery, indicate that collateral function, studied under maximal vasodilation, increases gradually up to 4 weeks, but then plateaus. In this model, collateral blood vessels replace only about 30% of the maximal conductance of the occluded artery, even at this late stage; this allows average flow rates under maximal vasodilation of the order of 300 ml/min/100 g compared with values of 750 ml/min/100 g distal to normal arteries,[17] with flow values of about 400 ml/min/100 g in the subepicardium and of 250 ml/min/100 g in the subendocardium. However, maximal vasodilation induced pharmacologically does not reproduce the mechanical features of myocardial contraction associated with vasodilation caused by increased work load. Enhanced systolic contraction may cause greater flow because of the massaging action of myocardial contraction on blood vessels, resulting in the greater systolic and diastolic interaction of flow (see Ch. 4). Six months after circumflex coronary artery occlusion in exercising unanesthetized dogs, myocardial blood flow, measured by the microsphere technique, can increase to the same extent (about 300%) in the posterior and the anterior papillary muscles.[24]

In dogs, collaterals often reach their full development and remain available for at least 4 months after the obstruction has been relieved; these vessels may adequately protect the myocardium in the event of subsequent reocclusion (see Fig. 6.7).[18] These results may apply to patients developing restenosis following angioplasty, or occlusion of aortocoronary bypass conduits in previously collateralized coronary arteries.

6.1.6 Determinants of collateral blood flow

The caliber and length of a collateral vessel determine its resistance and, at any given time, if collateral smooth muscle tone does not vary, flow through the vessel depends on the driving pressure between its site of origin in the parent vessel and its site of termination in the collateralized bed.

In the absence of a proximal stenosis in the parent vessel, pressure at the origin of angiographically visible collaterals is only a few millimeters of mercury lower than aortic pressure, even at high flow rates.

In dogs, after the administration of intracoronary adenosine, which brings about a large increase in flow to the normal myocardium, the reduction in retrograde blood flow from the cannulated distal end of the occluded artery is small, and is probably attributable to the dilator effect on the postocclusion vascular bed by the drug carried by collaterals.[25] Thus, in the absence of a pressure drop between the aorta and the origin of collaterals, collateral driving pressure and flow are determined largely by the pressure in the collateralized arterial territory. When the stenosis becomes more severe and when resistive vessels in the collateralized vascular bed dilate, poststenotic pressure decreases; thus, driving pressure (and, hence, flow through collaterals) increases. Conversely, when the stenosis becomes less severe and when resistive vessels in the collateralized bed constrict, poststenotic pressure increases; thus, driving pressure (and, hence, flow through collaterals) decreases. Dilation of collaterals does not increase collateral flow unless the collateralized bed is maximally dilated, but it does increase poststenotic pressure in the collateralized bed, thus increasing its coronary flow reserve; constriction of collaterals reduces poststenotic perfusion pressure and collateral flow to the collateralized bed.

When a critical stenosis is present in the parent vessel proximal to the origin of the collaterals, the pressure at the origin of the collaterals can be significantly lower than aortic pressure (but obviously higher than that in the collateralized territory), and decreases further when transstenotic flow increases. Thus, changes in flow across the stenosis in the parent vessel may influence the driving pressure across the collaterals when the pressure in the collateralized vessels does not decrease by exactly the same amount. As resistive vessels in the collateralized territory are already more dilated because poststenotic pressure is lower, they can undergo a lesser degree of further dilation. Thus, the presence of a stenosis in the parent vessel proximal to the origin of collaterals sets the scene for a possible reduction in driving pressure through collaterals and hence in collateral flow (interarterial collateral blood flow "steal").

In the presence of a pressure gradient between the aorta and the origin of collaterals, collateral blood flow can decrease when, with increasing flow, pressure at the origin of collaterals falls more than at their termination in the collateralized territory (where the decrease in pressure is limited because resistive vessels are already dilated in the basal condition). The conditions that predispose to intercoronary "steal" also produce transmural blood flow "steal" when they result in a reduction of poststenotic pressure in the collateralized territory (see Ch. 10).

Collateral flow can be increased by nitroglycerin and reduced by angiotensin and vasopressin but not by α-adrenergic stimulation.[26] Changes in collateral flow can be caused by variations in vasomotor tone in the collaterals themselves (when they are provided with a smooth muscle coat), in vessels proximal to the origin of collaterals, and in resistive vessels in the collateralized bed. Flow through collaterals running in the subendocardium can be reduced by increased ventricular diastolic pressure.

6.2 DYNAMIC CHANGES IN CORONARY STENOSES

As a growing body of clinical evidence indicates that epicardial stenoses can undergo transient changes in caliber, animal models have provided insight into the mechanisms that can modulate the caliber of the residual coronary lumen. When the stenosis is critical, even a minor dynamic modulation of the residual coronary lumen can have very important hemodynamic effects on poststenotic coronary pressure because of the exponential shape of the pressure/flow curve across a stenosis.

6.2.1 Passive changes in caliber

In dogs with an acute coronary stenosis, produced with a ligature to the point where reactive hyperemia is prevented, a decrease in flow has been noted following arteriolar dilation.[27,28] However, studies on isolated human coronary arteries with severe eccentric intraintimal stenosis show an increase in resistance of only 30% when inflow pressure is reduced from 100 to 50 mmHg, and flow remains constant when outflow pressure is reduced to zero, although the pressure gradient (and, hence, calculated resistance) increases.[29] Thus, isolated stenotic vessels tend to exhibit a "waterfall" phenomenon whereby flow is influenced only by inflow pressure, not by outflow pressure. This occurs when the main site of resistance is at the level of the stenosis and the stenosis is compliant, acting as a Starling resistor. It seems, therefore, that the reduction in flow observed in the studies cited above[27,28] depends on the chosen model of stenosis (external ligature) or on the secondary effects of reduced pressure on small distal vessels.

The behavior of flow was totally different in isolated arteries when the same degree of luminal reduction was created by an internal balloon rather than by external constriction (ligature). With external constriction, the flow rate decreased when outflow pressure was reduced, whereas with an internal balloon (mimicking more closely human coronary stenosis), the flow rate increased when outflow pressure was reduced. This difference in behavior could be explained by the wrinkling and crumpling effect of the ligature on the arterial wall, if the intraluminal protrusion of the wall is dynamically opposed by distending pressure.[30] Furthermore, an external coronary constrictor prevents myogenic autoregulation of tone, which tends to maintain caliber constant when distending pressure falls. In an unanesthetized dog, complete proximal occlusion of an epicardial coronary artery by a snare is associated with a reduction in distal diameter of less than 10% (see Fig. 6.8).[31]

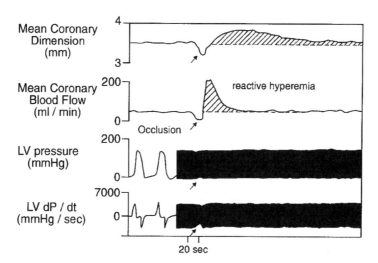

Fig. 6.8 Effect of sudden decrease of coronary artery pressure on distal caliber. Occlusion of the circumflex coronary artery causes only a 0.3 mm reduction of the diameter of the coronary artery beyond the site of occlusion (arrow), although distending pressure is reduced by about 80%. Release of the occlusion is followed by a transient increase of coronary blood flow due to reactive hyperemia and by dilation of the distal artery due to flow-dependent release of EDRF. Systolic left ventricular (LV) pressure remains constant; left ventricular peak relaxation and contraction (dP/dt) fall during occlusion. (Modified from ref. 31.)

It appears rather unlikely that passive changes in caliber of epicardial coronary arteries have any significant pathogenetic role in the genesis of myocardial ischemia in patients, for three reasons:

a. when distal pressure drops, myogenic autoregulation tends to maintain the lumen constant
b. when proximal perfusion pressure falls, the consequent decrease in lumen is small
c. when distal pressure falls, the passive reduction of caliber may act as a Starling resistor.

6.2.2 Intravascular plugging

An interesting model of acute intermittent coronary occlusion[32-34] can be produced in dogs by fitting a tight plastic ring around an epicardial coronary artery; this considerably reduces or abolishes reactive hyperemia. In this model, flow tends to exhibit cyclic fluctuations, with a gradual decrease towards zero and a brisk return to control values (see Fig. 6.9). These fluctuations have been shown convincingly to be caused by gradual accumulation and subsequent sudden fragmentation of platelet thrombi. Inhibition of cyclo-oxygenase, thromboxane A_2 synthetase and blockade of 5-HT or α-adrenergic receptors, but not administration of nitroglycerin or heparin, were shown to reduce or abolish the cyclical flow interruptions. The combination of thromboxane A_2-receptor blockers and serotoninergic antagonists has been reported to be more effective than the thromboxane A_2-receptor blockers alone.

In this acute model, the local accumulation of platelets is caused by the combination of endothelial disruption, with severe stenosis and wrinkling of the intima which cause local turbulence and increased wall shear stress. Platelet adhesion to the vessel wall remains weak and platelet aggregates can be broken loose and dislodged by the increasing pressure gradient and mechanical movements of the vessel. This model does not leave much room for vasoconstriction at the site of the stenosis, as the wall is constricted from the outside, causing medial SMC geometry to be profoundly disrupted. In other models of vessel wall injury with no concomitant stenosis, platelet deposition at the site of endothelial denudation is associated with vasoconstriction but not with total occlusion.[35]

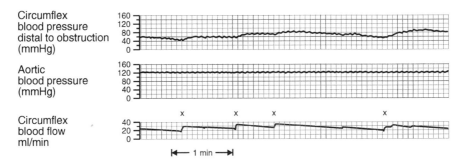

Fig. 6.9 Intermittent cyclic reduction of coronary blood flow caused by transient platelet aggregation. At the site of an acutely induced coronary stenosis in open chest dogs, gradual accumulation of platelets causes cyclic gradual reductions of transstenotic flow, with a brisk return to normal when the platelet thrombus is suddenly fragmented and carried downstream. (Modified from ref. 32.)

6.2.3 "Physiologic" coronary constriction

In unanesthetized dogs, changes in caliber of epicardial coronary arteries in response to a variety of constrictor stimuli are fairly minor. They do not exceed a 10–20% reduction in diameter (corresponding to a 19–36% reduction in cross-sectional area), even following massive neural electric stimulation; or pharmacologic stimulation with norepinephrine, 5-HT, angiotensin, ergonovine, or thromboxane A_2; or after endothelial denudation. Denudation of the endothelial lining and dysfunction of the endothelium can alter its response to several vasoactive stimuli from dilation to constriction (see 5.2 and Ch. 9). Because this degree of response is consistently observed in normal animals following such diverse stimuli, it would seem reasonable to define it as within the "physiologic" range—the quotation marks being intended to allow consideration of the possibility that such minor vasomotor changes could also be caused by pathologic mechanisms.

In normal epicardial coronary arteries, constriction within this "physiologic" range does not obstruct flow and is easily compensated for by minimal dilation of resistive vessels because of the highly nonlinear relation between the degree of stenosis and resistance up to about 50% reduction in diameter.

In the presence of a subintimal plaque that encroaches significantly upon the lumen without increasing the rigidity of the wall, in theory even a degree of constriction within this "physiologic" range may impair flow. Indeed, a subintimal plaque could act as a lever, magnifying the effects of constriction if the vessel wall remains sufficiently pliable. This concept can be grasped intuitively if one imagines that when, say, 80% of the lumen is occupied by a plaque, even a small degree of contraction of the smooth muscle can obliterate the remaining 20% of the lumen. However, this geometric magnification of the response is attenuated by rigidity of the wall, and atrophy of the smooth muscle surrounding the plaque (see Ch. 9).

6.2.4 Occlusive coronary artery spasm

In the absence of a subintimal plaque that encroaches to a significant extent on the coronary lumen, only an exceptional degree of constriction, intense enough to cause reduction of the lumen by 90%, can reduce resting CBF. Until the control of epicardial coronary tone is better understood, only a degree of segmental constriction that occludes or almost occludes the artery should be defined as "spasm" if this term is to retain its literal meaning.

Attempts to develop experimental models of occlusive coronary artery spasm began only after observation of its clinical role. As discussed in 5.2.4, this rare, extreme, degree of coronary constriction, often local, could result from two distinct types of mechanism, as follows:

1. The first mechanism could involve an alteration of the vessel wall that makes it hyperreactive so that it responds with a much more intense contraction to "ordinary" constrictor stimuli, that would otherwise produce only a degree of vasoconstriction within the "physiologic" range.
2. The second mechanism could involve stimuli that are so powerful that they cause total or subtotal occlusion, even in the absence of any hyperreactivity of the vessel wall.

As in variant angina, spasm usually (although not invariably) occurs at the site of an angiographically detectable atherosclerotic plaque; hypercholesterolemia has been induced in several animal species with the aim of making the coronary arteries hyperresponsive to constrictor stimuli. As already reported in 5.2.3, in hypercholesterolemic rabbits aortic rings exhibit a much greater sensitivity to constrictor agents[36] that is, they begin to contract at doses that are one to three orders of magnitude smaller (shift of the dose–response curve to the left; see 5.2.4). The development of experimental hypercholesterolemic models of spasm neglected the clinical observation that hypercholesterolemia is not a feature of variant angina. Cholesterol-fed rabbits with very severe narrowing of coronary arteries caused by cholesterol deposits have failed to develop ischemia in response to very high doses of constrictor agents, suggesting that the intensity of coronary constriction was not sufficient to impair flow, even in the presence of very significant subintimal plaques;[37] this is consistent with the lack of reports of variant angina in patients with familial hypercholesterolemia. Therefore, this very large displacement to the left of the dose–response curve, caused by hypercholesterolemia, does not appear to be associated with increased intensity of contraction (which is an essential feature of coronary spasm), as seen in variant angina.

So far, the only model capable of mimicking some of the features of variant angina has involved miniature pigs.[38] Segmental coronary artery endothelial denudation by a balloon catheter, with and without induction of hypercholesterolemia, was found to be associated with complete coronary occlusion in response to histamine and 5-HT in the presence of only minimal subintimal plaques. The authors inferred that the repair processes in the months following intimal injury made the arterial wall locally hyperreactive to constrictor stimuli that produced only a "physiologic" degree of coronary constriction in the unaffected coronary artery branches. Such a model fails to respond to ergonovine (thus mimicking only in part those patients with variant angina) and the mechanism of increased coronary reactivity to histamine leading to occlusive spasm remains unknown (see Ch. 9).

No pharmacologic stimuli that are consistently capable of causing coronary artery spasm in normal animals have been identified; however, occasionally, local occlusive coronary spasm may be observed during dissection of epicardial coronary arteries for the implantation of flowmeters in anesthetized pigs and occasionally also in dogs.

6.2.5   Combination of intravascular plugging and vasoconstriction

Vascular endothelial and intimal damage promptly bring about adhesion of a monolayer of platelets when the injury is minimal, and aggregation of platelets in multiple layers when the injury is more severe. Thromboxane A_2, 5-HT, platelet-aggregating factor (PAF), and platelet-derived growth factor, all released by platelets and thrombin, are powerful vasoconstrictors and, in carotid arteries with internal denudation, constriction proximal and distal to the site of balloon denudation was found to be proportional to the number of platelets deposited.[35] The degree of constriction was only a 10% reduction in diameter at the site of small injuries with limited platelet deposition and 20% at the site of large injuries with major platelet deposition; this degree of constriction is within the limits of the "physiologic" response to constrictor stimuli. It appears, therefore, that in previously normal arteries not even a combination of endothelial denudation and platelet deposition can produce a constrictor stimulus strong enough to result in occlusive spasm. As stated above, theoretically, it would be possible for such a degree of constriction to impair flow by geometric magnification of the stenosis, in segments with fresh or recent thrombus resulting in a pliable stenosis (see Ch. 9); however, such a possibility has not been explored experimentally.

6.3 SMALL CORONARY VESSEL CONSTRICTION

There is increasing evidence, from experimental observations and clinical studies, that myocardial ischemia can also be caused by constriction of small coronary vessels. However, the possibility that distal coronary vessel constriction may cause myocardial ischemia cannot be easily demonstrated in experimental studies, as it can be inferred only indirectly from the lack of angiographic evidence of epicardial coronary artery spasm during the infusion of the constrictor agents that produce ischemia. The existence of mechanisms capable of producing myocardial ischemia by constriction of distal coronary vessels is convincing, but the site of such constriction in response to different pharmacologic stimuli may vary.

Studies on coronary embolization involving intracoronary injection of increasing numbers of microspheres provide the background for interpreting the effects of blockade of the coronary microcirculation on the development of myocardial ischemia.

6.3.1 Microembolization by microspheres

Coronary microembolization with microspheres of known caliber produces more areas of ischemia in the subepicardium than in the subendocardium.[39] This occurs because of both the greater arterial vascularity of the subendocardium and its extensive plexiform arrangement with anastomoses, compared with the lesser degree of vascularity of the subepicardium and its more frequent terminal arteriolar distribution. Areas of ischemia are found distal to occluded arterioles with no distal anastomoses and are interspersed among areas of increased flow.[39] (Mean flow actually increases following mild and moderate degrees of embolization.)[40]

The most comprehensive of these studies,[40] with microspheres 26 μm in diameter, showed that, in dogs, it was necessary to inject a total of about 60 000 microspheres/g myocardium in order to abolish reactive hyperemia totally. At this point, although the number of embolizing microspheres was 50% higher in subendocardial than subepicardial layers, flow was about 50% lower in the subepicardium. Moreover, in spite of the abolition of reactive hyperemia, infusion of adenosine increased subepicardial flow by 90% and subendocardial flow by 160%, indicating that nonembolized arterioles could dilate further and confirming the observation that peak reactive hyperemia does not indicate the maximum vasodilation possible (see 4.3.5). Elevation of the ST-segment appeared when about 70 000 microspheres/g myocardium had been injected; this was not abolished when flow was increased by adenosine, and developed when subendocardial blood flow was still normal. The extent of necrosis produced by intracoronary injection of microspheres in dogs is reduced by α-adrenergic blockade, suggesting that α-adrenergic-mediated vasoconstriction contributes to the development of ischemia.[39]

6.3.2 Ischemia caused by pharmacologic stimuli

Infusion of endothelin into the left anterior descending coronary artery (LAD) of anesthetized dogs caused a dose-dependent reduction in flow and severe myocardial ischemia (see Figs. 6.10 and 6.11) in the absence of angiographically detectable constriction of visible coronary arteries, but in association with doubling of the filling time of the distal LAD territory.[41] The reduction in flow was similar in subendocardial and subepicardial layers (see Fig. 6.12). In rabbits, intracoronary injection of N-formyl-L-methiomyl-L-leucyl-L-phenylamine caused shutdown of peripheral coronary secondary and tertiary branches with severe

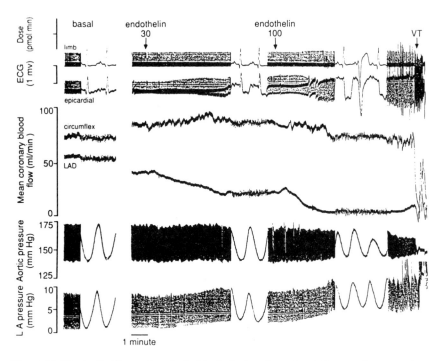

Fig. 6.10 Typical effect of endothelin infusion into the left anterior coronary artery (LAD) in anesthetized dogs. Basal and continuous recording, played back at low and high speeds, of left atrial (LA) and aortic pressure, LAD and circumflex blood flow (mean values) and ECG. Infusion of 3 pmol endothelin was started after the basal recordings (not shown). Progressive decrease of LAD flow associated with T–Q depression and ST-segment elevation on the epicardial ECG, and increase in LA pressure, develop at infusion rates of 30 and 100 pmol/min without detectable constriction of angiographically visible coronary branches. (Modified from ref. 41.)

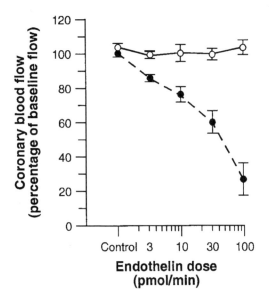

Fig. 6.11 Average dose-dependent reduction of myocardial blood flow caused by endothelin. Infusion of endothelin into the left anterior descending coronary artery (•– – –•) causes a dose-dependent reduction of flow; flow in the circumflex coronary artery (•——•]) remains constant. (Modified from ref. 41.)

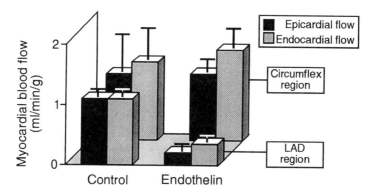

Fig. 6.12 Transmural reduction of myocardial blood flow across the left ventricular free wall caused by endothelin. Infusion of endothelin into the left anterior descending coronary artery (LAD) causes a similar reduction of flow in subendocardial (□) and subepicardial (■) LAD regions, compared with basal and circumflex regions. This is in sharp contrast to epicardial coronary stenoses, which cause predominantly subendocardial ischemia, and with microsphere embolization, which causes predominantly subepicardial ischemia. (From data presented in ref. 41.)

myocardial ischemia.[42] This tripeptide causes release of leukotrienes by polymorphonuclear granulocytes adhering to the coronary endothelium, and release of PAF.[43] These findings are of particular interest because granulocyte adherence to the activated endothelium could be a powerful constrictor stimulus to small coronary vessels in unstable angina.

Following adenosine-induced maximal dilation, intravenous infusion of angiotensin and phenylephrine in anesthetized dogs caused a marked reduction in flow.[44] It is not clear whether the constriction induced by these drugs involves prearteriolar or arteriolar coronary vessels. Regardless of the site of distal coronary vessel constriction, the reduction in flow was approximately similar in subepicardial and subendocardial layers, in accordance with the findings depicted in Figure 6.12. The uniform reduction of transmural blood flow caused by constriction of distal coronary vessels, contrasts with the predominantly subendocardial reduction of blood flow caused by epicardial coronary stenoses and with the predominantly subepicardial ischemia caused by microsphere embolization.

A review of angiographic pictures obtained following injection of neuropeptide Y in patients and of endothelin in dogs suggests that these substances can cause severe myocardial ischemia by diffuse constriction of small vessels. In fact, compared with control basal conditions, the caliber of larger epicardial branches appears unchanged following administration of the drugs; myocardial ischemia, therefore, can be attributable only to predominantly distal coronary artery constriction (see Ch. 9).

■ *Thus, a variety of neural and humoral stimuli, as well as local autacoids, can cause ischemia in normal experimental animals by constricting small coronary vessels rather than proximal epicardial coronary arteries. Such constriction seems to involve subepicardial and subendocardial microvessels equally.* ■

6.3.3 Ischemia caused by neural stimuli

Studies in animals with chronically implanted flowmeters and pressure transducers indicate that vasomotor tone of coronary resistive vessels is influenced markedly by stimuli that originate in the central nervous system, independent of myocardial oxygen demand. Coronary blood flow was found to vary more than twofold during sleep (in the absence of changes in heart rate and blood pressure in baboons) and to decrease markedly during surges of heart rate during REM sleep.[45,46] The nervous stimuli responsible for coronary constriction are conducted by sympathetic vessels, as constriction can be prevented by sympathectomy.

In normal dogs, transient coronary vasoconstriction was found to occur in response to presentation of classically conditioned aversion stimuli,[47] and myocardial ischemia developed in instrumented dogs 1–2 min after an attack of anger induced by watching other dogs eating their food.[48]

Vasoconstrictor centers appear to be located in the hypothalamus, as stimulation of some hypothalamic nuclei can cause a decrease in CBF[49] and coronary constriction.[50,51] The importance of the central regulation of CBF in myocardial ischemia is also suggested by the improvement of subendocardial perfusion by epidural anesthesia in experimental MI in dogs, independent of systemic hemodynamic changes.[13] Extensive β-adrenergic stimulation can cause direct myocardial damage characterized by necrosis with contraction bands, rather than by coronary vasoconstriction.[52]

6.4 ACUTE OCCLUSIVE EPICARDIAL CORONARY ARTERY THROMBOSIS

The most widely used method of occluding a coronary artery is by an external ligature, which causes a sudden total cessation of flow. In most animals this method of occlusion produces infarction unless the occlusion occurs very gradually. A gradual occlusion that does not cause infarction can be achieved by placing a cylinder with hygroscopic material (ameroid constrictor) around the artery, thereby reducing the lumen to complete occlusion over a period of days.[6] In dogs this allows time for the development of sufficient collaterals to provide full protection, so that no infarction, or only minor foci of necrosis, can be detected.

The formation of an occlusive coronary thrombus can result from three different basic mechanisms that can operate in isolation or in various combinations. First, thrombus formation may be proportional to the severity of mechanical injury caused to a previously normal vessel wall. This occlusive thrombosis would represent just the physiologic response of the hemostatic system to a severe mechanical injury in a normal vessel. Second, thrombus formation may be proportional to the intensity and duration of the local thrombogenic stimulus, independent of an anatomic injury. Finally, thrombus formation exceeds the severity of the mechanical vessel wall injury and the intensity and duration of local thrombogenic stimuli because of an abnormally increased thrombotic tendency or reduced fibrinolysis.

In animal models without flow-limiting stenoses, only intense local thrombogenic stimuli were shown to be capable of causing occlusive thrombosis. Acute thrombotic coronary occlusion can be produced by introducing a copper coil into an epicardial segment of artery, or by continuous electric stimulation via the tip of an intracoronary catheter but, in arteries without stenosis, coronary occlusion cannot be caused by even a deep injury to a normal arterial wall. Only when intimal damage is associated with the presence of flow-limiting stenoses (see 6.2.2), can intermittent and permanent vessel occlusion occur, as in the model of Folts et al.[33]

6.4.1 Formation of a red thrombus

In dogs, the insertion of a 3 mm copper coil into the main left coronary artery is followed within about 5 min (range 0–15 min) by complete occlusion caused by a red thrombus, rich in red cells and fibrin.[53] This experiment demonstrates not only that, even in a previously healthy animal (and one not easily susceptible to thrombosis like the dog), an occlusive thrombus can develop very rapidly in response to a strong thrombogenic stimulus, but also that such rapidly developing thrombi are predominantly composed of red cells and fibrin, with few platelets (which do not have sufficient time to accumulate).

6.4.2 Formation of a white thrombus

The application of an anodal current to the coronary lumen via a stainless steel electrode[54,55] causes a local occlusive coronary thrombosis. The rate at which the thrombus develops depends on the intensity of the electric current and is of the order of about 1 h. Such thrombi are white and rich in platelets. When a low-intensity current is applied, thrombus formation may take several hours and may be inhibited by antiplatelet agents.[56] Thus, thrombi forming slowly in response to weak thrombogenic stimuli are predominantly composed of platelets, do not become occlusive if the thrombogenic stimulus is interrupted, and can be partially prevented by antiplatelet agents. As indicated above, a white, platelet-rich, occlusive thrombus can form at the site of a severe coronary stenosis associated with acute endothelial damage, as in Folts' model,[32,33] owing to the combination of endothelial denudation and/or activation and a high shear stress effect on platelets.

6.4.3 Animal models of unstable angina and myocardial infarction

In postmortem studies, unstable angina is often characterized by the presence of mural platelet fibrin thrombi, in which multiple layers, all of different ages, can be recognized: these findings are consistent with the frequently reported evolution of the disease, with anginal attacks alternating with asymptomatic periods lasting days or weeks. So far, it has been impossible to develop an animal model of unstable angina in which to test specific preventive therapies; this is because it is not clear why mural thrombosis, rather than representing a repair process, often recurs (in patients) at the same site after intervals of days or weeks, possibly in response to recurring, local thrombogenic stimuli. In previously healthy animals, the severity of local damage to previously normal vessels was found to be the main determinant of thrombus size;[35] however, in patients, some thrombi are not associated with histologically detectable fissure of atherosclerotic plaques (see Ch. 9). Although in animals a very severe acute stenosis can produce occlusive platelet thrombi due to endothelial damage and increased shear stress,[32–34] in patients with chronic effort-induced angina many critical stenoses remain stable for years and in some patients with unstable angina culprit lesions may not be severe. Repeated episodes of mural thrombosis in unstable angina may, therefore, result from thrombogenic stimuli differing from those responsible for the thrombus that forms in previously healthy animals as an acute repair mechanism, which is necessarily proportional to the severity of the injury.

■ *Within these limitations, animal models provide useful evidence that red thrombi (fibrin and red cell rich) result from very intense thrombogenic stimuli and irreversibly occlude the vessel in a few minutes. Conversely, white thrombi (platelet rich) develop in response to weaker thrombogenic stimuli and can occlude the vessel only if the stimulus is either very persistent or occurs at the site of a severe flow-limiting stenosis.* ■

REFERENCES

1. Klocke FJ. Measurements of coronary blood flow and degree of stenosis: Current clinical implications and continuing uncertainties. J Am Coll Cardiol 1983;*1*:31.
2. Canty JM Jr. Coronary pressure–function and steady-state pressure–flow relations during autoregulation in the unanesthetized dog. Circ Res 1988;*63*:821.

3. Folts JD, Gallagher K, Rowe GG. Hemodynamic effects of controlled degrees of coronary artery stenosis in short-term and long-term studies in dogs. J Thorac Cardiovasc Surg 1977;73:722
4. Gould KL. Pressure-flow characteristics of coronary stenoses in un-sedated dogs at rest and during coronary vasodilation. Circ Res 1978;43:242.
5. Gregg DE, Bedynek JL Jr. Compensatory changes in the heart during progressive coronary artery stenosis. In: Maseri A, Lesch M, Klassen GA (eds) Primary and Secondary Angina Pectoris. Grune & Stratton, New York, 1978.
6. Elliot EC, Khouri EM, Snow JA, Gregg DE. Direct measurement of coronary collateral blood flow in conscious dogs by an electromagnetic flow meter. Circ Res 1974;34:374.
7. Aversano T, Becker LC. Persistence of coronary vasodilator reserve despite functionally significant flow reduction. Am J Physiol 1985;248:H403.
8. Laxson DD, Dai XZ, Homans DC, Bache RJ. Coronary vasodilator reserve in ischemic myocardium of the exercising dog. Circulation 1992;85:313.
9. Ball RM, Bache RJ. Distribution of myocardial blood flow in the exercising dog with restricted coronary artery inflow. Circ Res 1976;38:60.
10. Feigl EO. The paradox of adrenergic coronary vasoconstriction. Circulation 1987;76:737.
11. Heush G, Deussen A. The effects of cardiac sympathetic nerve stimulation on perfusion of stenotic coronary arteries in the dog. Circ Res 1983;53:8.
12. Seitelberger R, Guth BD, Heusch G, Lee JD, Katayama K, Ross J Jr. Intracoronary α_2-adrenergic receptor blockade attenuates ischemia in conscious dogs during exercise. Circ Res 1988;62:436
13. Klassen GA, Bramwell RS, Bromage PR, Zborowska-Sluis DT. Effect of acute sympathectomy by epidural anesthesia on the canine coronary circulation. Anesthesiology 1980;52:8.
14. Crea F, Pupita G, Galassi AR et al. Effect of theophylline on exercise induced myocardial ischaemia. Lancet 1989;1:683.
15. Bache RJ, Stark RP, Duncker DJ. Serotonin selectively aggravates subendocardial ischemia distal to a coronary artery stenosis during exercise. Circulation 1992;86:1559.
16. Maseri A, L'Abbate A, Pesola A, Michelassi C, Marzilli M, De Nes M. Regional myocardial perfusion in patients with atherosclerotic coronary artery disease, at rest and during angina pectoris induced by tachycardia. Circulation 1977;55:423.
17. Schaper W, Görge G, Winkler B, Schaper J. The collateral circulation of the heart. Prog Cardiov Dis 1988;31:57.
18. Khouri EM, Gregg DE, McGranahan GM. Regression and reappearance of coronary collaterals. Am J Physiol 1971;220:655.
19. Schwarz F, Wagner HO, Sesto M, Hofmann M, Schaper W, Kübler W. Native collaterals in the development of collateral circulation after chronic coronary stenosis in mongrel dogs. Circulation 1982;66:303.
20. Unger EF, Sheffield CD, Epstein SE. Creation of anastomoses between an extracardiac artery and the coronary circulation: Proof that myocardial angiogenesis occurs and can provide nutritional blood flow to the myocardium. Circulation 1990;82:1449.
21. Chilian WM, Mass HJ, Williams SE, Layne SM, Smith E, Scheel KW. Microvascular occlusions promote coronary collateral growth. Am J Physiol 1990;258 (Heart Circ Physiol 27):H1103.
22. Kass RW, Kotler MN, Yazdanfar S. Stimulation of coronary collateral growth: current developments in angiogenesis and future clinical applications. Am Heart J 1992;123:486.
23. Sasayama S, Fujita M. Recent insights into coronary collateral circulation. Circulation 1992;85:1197.
24. Lambert PR, Hess DS, Bache RJ. Effect of exercise on perfusion of collateral-dependent myocardium in dogs with chronic coronary artery occlusion. J Clin Invest 1977;59:1.
25. Patterson RE, Kirk ES. Coronary steal mechanisms in dogs with one-vessel occlusion and other arteries normal. Circulation 1983;67:1009.
26. Hautamaa PV, Dai XZ, Homans DC, Bache RJ. Vasomotor activity of moderately well-developed canine coronary collateral circulation. Am J Physiol 1989;256 (Heart Circ Physiol 25):H890.
27. Walinsky P, Santamore WP, Wiener L et al. Dynamic changes in the hemodynamic severity of coronary artery stenosis in a canine model. Cardiovasc Res 1979;13:113.

28. Swartz J, Carlyle P, Cohn JW. Effect of dilatation of the distal coronary bed on flow and resistance in severely stenotic coronary arteries in the dog. Am J Cardiol 1979;*43:*219.

29. Logen S. On the mechanisms of human coronary artery stenosis. IEEE Transactions on biomedical engineering. Biomed Eng 1975;*22:*327.

30. von Arnim T, Crea F, Chierchia S, Maseri A. Influence of the chosen model of stenosis on pressure–flow relationships in isolated perfused arteries. Int J Cardiol 1985;*9:*81.

31. Vatner SF. Regulation of coronary resistance vessels and large coronary arteries. Am J Cardiol 1985;*56:*16E.

32. Folts JD. Experimental arterial platelet thrombosis, platelet inhibitors, and their possible clinical relevance. Cardiovasc Reviews & Reports 1982;*3:*370.

33. Folts JD, Crowell EB, Rowe GG. Platelet aggregation in partially obstructed vessels and its elimination with aspirin. Circulation 1976;*54:*365.

34. Willerson JT, Yao S-K, McNatt J et al. Frequency and severity of cyclic flow alternations and platelet aggregation predict the severity of neointimal proliferation following experimental coronary stenosis and endothelial injury. Proc Natl Acad Sci USA 1991;*88:*10624.

35. Lam JYT, Chesebro JH, Fuster V. Platelets, vasoconstriction, and nitroglycerin during arterial wall injury: a new antithrombotic role for an old drug. Circulation 1988;*78:*712.

36. Henry PD, Yokoyama M. Supersensitivity of atherosclerotic rabbit aorta to ergonovine: Mediation by a serotonergic mechanism. J Clin Invest 1980;*66:*306.

37. Crea F, von Arnim T, Allwork SP, Jadhav A, Thompson GR, Maseri A. Failure of experimental atherosclerosis to sensitize coronary arteries to spasm in hypercholesterolemic rabbits. Am Heart J 1985;*109:*491.

38. Shimokawa H, Tomoike H, Nabeyama S, Yamamoto H, Araki H, Nakamura M. Coronary artery spasm induced in atherosclerotic miniature swine. Science 1983;*221:*560.

39. Eng C, Cho S, Factor SM, Sonnenblick EH, Kirk ES. Myocardial micronecrosis produced by microsphere embolization: Role of an α-adrenergic tonic influence on the coronary microcirculation. Circ Res 1984;*54:*74.

40. Pelosi G, L'Abbate A, Trivella MG et al. Persistence of subendocardial perfusion after subtotal coronary embolisation. Cardiovasc Res 1988;*22:*113.

41. Larkin SW, Clarke JG, Keogh BE et al. Intracoronary endothelin induces myocardial ischemia by small vessel constriction in the dog. Am J Cardiol 1989;*64:*956.

42. Gillespie MN, Booth DC, Friedman BJ, Cunningham MR, Jay M, DeMaria A. fMLP provokes coronary vasoconstriction and myocardial ischemia in rabbits. Am J Physiol 1988;*254* (Heart Circ Physiol 23):H481.

43. Tippins JR, Antoniw JW, Alison MR, Garvey B, Maseri A. A platelet-activating factor antagonist, WEB 2086, inhibits neutrophil-dependent increase in coronary resistance in the rabbit isolated, blood-perfused heart. Cardiovasc Res 1992;*26:*162.

44. Johannsen UJ, Mark AL, Marcus ML. Responsiveness to cardiac sympathetic nerve stimulation during maximal coronary dilation produced by adenosine. Circ Res 1982;*50:*510.

45. Vatner SF, Franklin D, Higgins CB, Patrick T, White S, Van Citters RL. Coronary dynamics in unrestrained conscious baboons. Am J Physiol 1971;*221:*1396.

46. Kirby DA, Verrier RL. Differential effects of sleep stage on coronary hemodynamic function. Am J Physiol 1989;*256* (Heart Circ Physiol 25):H1378.

47. Billman GE, Randall DC. Mechanisms mediating the coronary vascular response to behavioral stress in the dog. Circ Res 1981;*48:*214.

48. Verrier RL, Hagestad EL, Lown B. Delayed myocardial ischemia induced by anger. Circulation 1987;*75:*249.

49. Bonham AC, Gutterman DD, Arthur JM, Marcus ML, Gebhart GF, Brody MJ. Electrical stimulation in perifornical lateral hypothalamus decreases coronary blood flow in cats. Am J Physiol 1987;*252:*474.

50. Weckman N. Local constriction and spasm of large arteries elicited by hypothalamic stimulation. Experientia 1960;*16:*34.

51. Gutstein WH, Anversa P, Beghi C, Kiu G, Pacanovsky D. Coronary artery spasm in the rat induced by hypothalamic stimulation. Atherosclerosis 1984;*135:*51.

52. Eliot RS, Todd GL, Clayton FC, Pieper GM. Experimental catecholamine-induced acute myo-cardial necrosis. Adv Cardiol 1978;*25:*107.

53. Van de Werf F, Bergmann SR, Fox KAA et al. Coronary thrombolysis with intravenously admin-istered human tissue-type plasminogen activator produced by recombinant DNA techology. Circulation 1984;*69:*605.

54. Salazar AE. Experimental myocardial infarction, induction of coronary thrombosis in the intact closed-chest dog. Circ Res 1961;*9:*1351.

55. Kodenat RK, Kezdi P, Stanles EL. A new catheter technique for producing experimental coro-nary thrombosis and selective coronary visualization. Am Heart J 1972;*83:*360.

56. Romson JL, Haack DW, Lucchesi BR. Electrical induction of coronary artery thrombosis in the ambulatory canine: a model for in vivo evaluation of anti-thrombotic agents. Thromb Res 1980;*17:*841.

7 | Consequences of myocardial ischemia

INTRODUCTION

Myocardial ischemia develops when coronary blood flow (CBF) becomes inadequate for the supply of oxygen and removal of carbon dioxide that are required for maintenance of the local oxidative metabolism. Coronary blood flow may become inadequate because of chronic or acute intraluminal obstructions or because of vasoconstriction.

Sudden impairment of myocardial oxidative metabolism does not alter all cardiac functions simultaneously. Repetitive and prolonged ischemic episodes cause transient adaptations (preconditioning) and prolonged contractile dysfunction (stunning and hibernation). Persistent ischemia causes irreversible myocardial cell injury and tissue necrosis. Ischemia, necrosis, and myocardial scarring can favor the development of fatal arrhythmias.

The metabolic and cellular consequences of myocardial ischemia have been studied by the sudden interruption of blood flow, by hypoxic perfusion from the perfusate of isolated hearts, and in isolated cardiac myocytes. Each approach has its advantages and disadvantages: the closer the model to the clinical situation, the less controlled the variables; the more carefully controlled the experimental condition, the more remote is the model from clinical pathophysiologic situations. Thus, isolated cardiac myocytes are subjected neither to the effects of stretching by adjacent cells, nor to the effects of interstitial fluid, nerve endings, and blood components; hypoxic isolated hearts are denervated and not subjected to the normal interactions with blood components. Even the consequences of coronary flow reduction in otherwise normal animals (often anesthetized) may not be exactly the same as those encountered in patients with preexisting dysfunction of coronary vessels, hemostatic system, or myocardium. However, animal studies have provided useful information regarding the basic response of the normal heart to ischemic insults, which is summarized in the following sections.

7.1 METABOLIC AND CELLULAR CONSEQUENCES OF MYOCARDIAL ISCHEMIA

Myocardial ischemia inhibits oxidative metabolism and causes depletion of high-energy phosphate stores. Thus, cellular functions are very rapidly altered.

7.1.1 Inhibition of oxidative metabolism

Inadequate oxygen supply prevents the formation of adenosine triphosphate (ATP) by oxidative phosphorylation. Concomitantly, glycogenolysis and anaerobic metabolism are accelerated but, as ischemia becomes more severe, anaerobic glycolysis slows markedly because of the inhibitory effects of acidosis and the accumulation of metabolites such as phosphate and potassium ions. Indeed, glycolysis and lactate production are much greater during high-flow hypoxia, which removes metabolites and supplies glucose, than during ischemia. Anaerobic glycolysis leads to phosphorylation to ATP of two molecules of adenosine diphosphate (ADP) per molecule of glucose converted to lactate, compared with 38 molecules of ATP created by complete oxidation of one molecule of glucose.[1,2]

7.1.2 Consequences of inhibition of oxidative metabolism

The inadequate oxygen supply and the consequent marked reduction in ATP production very rapidly cause depletion of high-energy stores, accumulation of catabolites, alterations of protein and lipid metabolism, and the formation of free radicals; in addition, when ischemia is reversible but prolonged or repetitive, it leads to alterations taking place in receptors and gene expression.

Depletion of high-energy phosphates and adenosine nucleotides

Creatine phosphate is almost completely depleted within 3 min of coronary occlusion and ATP is reduced to one-third within 10 min. ATP is degraded to adenosine via ADP and adenosine monophosphate. Adenosine can escape from the myocyte and is degraded to xanthine via inosine and hypoxanthine. Thus, the total adenosine nucleotide pool is also reduced to one-half within 10–15 min of the onset of ischemia, but the reduction may differ among various intracellular compartments. The complete reconstitution of the adenosine nucleotide pool takes days.[2]

Accumulation of catabolites

Metabolic end products accumulate as a result of the activation of glycolysis, lipolysis and ATP breakdown, with a rapid increase in tissue acidosis largely due to accumulation of lactate. Myocardial cell acidosis may contribute to the decline in contractile function. The accumulation of catabolites and of Na^+ causes a progressive increase in osmotic pressure within ischemic myocytes, which causes water influx and cell swelling.[2]

Protein metabolism

Both protein synthesis and protein degradation are energy-requiring processes and are, therefore, impaired during ischemia. Ischemia activates cellular proteases that may contribute to the degradation of enzymes and structural proteins in the cells; it also activates heat-shock proteins, which have a protective effect against potentially harmful substances. Thus, the effects of short episodes or mild degrees of ischemia depend on the balance between these two effects. Proteolytic degradation, together with osmotic-induced cell swelling, contribute to sarcolemmal disruption.

Lipid metabolism

Triglyceride fuel stores are much greater than glycogen stores; moreover, ischemia increases lipolysis through a catecholamine-dependent mechanism. During severe ischemia, free fatty acids and acylcarnitine accumulate because they cannot be oxidized in the absence of oxygen. When blood flow is not completely abolished, fatty acids accumulate in the myocardium and may have detrimental effects. Phospholipids, the major structural components of membranes, are degraded and, as a result, arachidonic acid accumulates and its metabolic pathways are enhanced.

Free radicals

Ischemia, and reperfusion following ischemia, cause the production of free radicals such as superoxide and hydroxyl radicals. Free radicals can be derived from a variety of processes, including the metabolism of thiols, flavins, and catecholamines, the autoxidation of xanthine, the oxidase-mediated conversion of hypoxanthine to xanthine from mitochondrial electron transport, and cyclooxygenase-mediated oxidation of arachidonate. The high reactivity of free radicals causes detrimental alterations in proteins, nucleic acids, and lipids that result in ischemic and postischemic dysfunction.[3]

Cellular and myocardial functional alterations

Changes in intracellular and extracellular electrolytes are very early consequences of ischemia. Major changes involve K^+ and Ca^{2+} ions. Loss of intracellular K^+ begins within seconds of the onset of myocardial ischemia and extracellular K^+ increases threefold (from 5 to 15 mM) during the first few minutes. The mechanism of this loss, which begins before substantial decrease of ATP, is incompletely understood and may be related to a variable decrease of ATP in different intracellular compartments. The decrease of the transmembrane K^+ gradient causes diastolic depolarization (with T–Q depression). At a later stage, the decrease of the action potential causes elevation of the ST segment in the ischemic zone. The early increase in cytosolic Ca^{2+} results from increased Ca^{2+} influx (partly related to the depolarization of the membrane) and decreased sequestration in the sarcoplasmic reticulum, whereas subsequent Ca^{2+} influx is due to sarcolemmal disruption. Intracellular accumulation of Ca^{2+} is thought to be one of the mechanisms of irreversible cell death.[4] Ischemia causes intense release of norepinephrine from nerve terminals and, in some experiments, increases the number of exposed β- and α-adrenergic receptors. Myocardial ischemia also causes microvascular damage through lack of oxygen and the effects of acidosis, ischemic catabolites, free radicals, and fibrin-derived peptides. Endothelial activation leads to adhesion and activation of leukocytes, with platelet adhesion and activation of thrombin, which extend endothelial damage.[5,6]

■ *Thus, the extent of microvascular injury may be influenced by the biologic response of the heart and blood vessels to the ischemic insult. In turn, the biologic response is determined by the individual conditions that precede and accompany the development of myocardial ischemia.* ■

7.2 SEQUENCE OF CARDIAC ALTERATIONS AT THE ONSET OF ISCHEMIA

The average adult human heart contracts about 100 000 times every 24 h and in so doing pumps 8000 l of blood. Yet myocardial energy stores are sufficient for less than 1 min and cellular functions are inhibited within a few seconds by ischemia; for this reason, a contin-

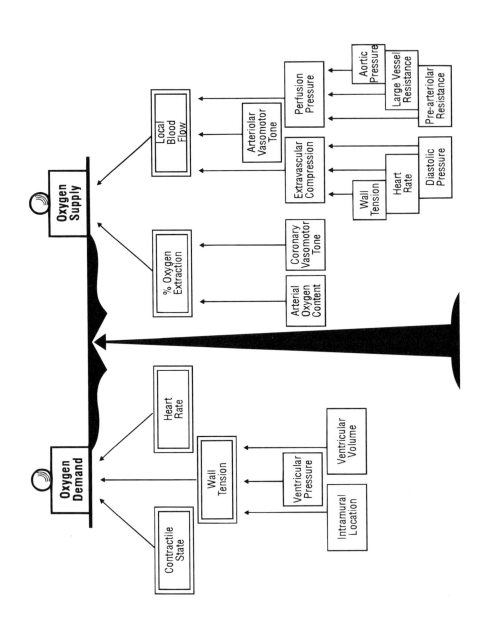

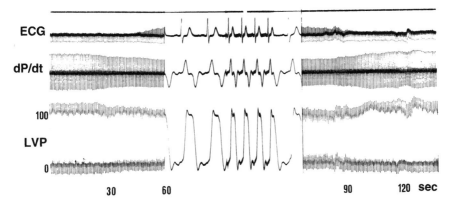

Fig. 7.2 Sequence of alterations during an ischemic episode caused by left anterior descending coronary artery spasm. The playback, at low and high speeds, of a spontaneous episode of silent ischemia recorded in the coronary care unit, shows a decrease in left ventricular peak relaxation and contraction dP/dt, and in systolic pressure and an increase in proto- and end-diastolic pressure clearly precedes the onset of peaking of T waves on the ECG, which is followed by slight ST-segment elevation. The episode resolved spontaneously. The sequence of events is similar to that observed during coronary angioplasty and in the dog following sudden coronary artery ligation. LVP: left ventricular pressure. dP/dt: left ventricular dP/dt. ECG: electrocardiographic tracing.

uous oxygen supply in proportion to metabolic requirements is essential. The importance of oxidative metabolism is also indicated by the very large cellular volume occupied by mitochondria (about 35%). When myocardial blood perfusion is impaired, the degree of imbalance between myocardial oxygen requirements and supply may vary considerably, depending on a large number of factors that influence the two sides of the equation (see Fig. 7.1). Contractile work accounts for about 80% of resting myocardial oxygen consumption, the remaining 20% being represented by that of the electrically arrested, noncontracting heart. The fraction of oxygen consumption associated with contractile work increases proportionately when heart activity increases above resting levels. During recovery from ischemic episodes, about 20% of myocardial oxygen consumption is used in the repair process. Hypoxia is used in some experimental models to produce ischemia, but the findings thus obtained may not be applicable to ischemia because, during hypoxia, the removal of catabolites is not impaired as flow is normal or even higher than normal.

The vulnerability of various cardiac functions to the development of myocardial ischemia can be assessed in experimental animal models as follows:

a. by following the temporal sequence of the abnormalities that develop upon sudden occlusion of a major coronary artery branch

Fig. 7.1 Determinants of the balance between myocardial oxygen consumption (demand) and coronary blood flow (supply). Demand is mainly determined by heart rate, wall tension and contractile state; supply is determined by oxygen extraction and blood flow. Oxygen extraction is mainly determined by the setting of coronary vasomotor tone (see Ch. 4) and by arterial oxygen content. Blood flow is determined by perfusion pressure at the origin of the arterioles, by arteriolar tone and by extravascular compressive forces.

b.   by reducing myocardial blood flow very gradually

c.   by increasing myocardial work gradually in the presence of a flow-limiting stenosis.

7.2.1 Effects of sudden coronary artery occlusion

Ligature of a major conductive artery is followed within 3–5 s by reduction in the velocity of ventricular relaxation and contraction, and, a few seconds later, by ST-segment elevation, increased end-diastolic pressure and decreased systolic arterial blood pressure. The sequence of hemodynamic and electrocardiographic events observed in experimental animals[7] and also during angioplasty[8] is similar to that observed in patients during episodes of occlusive epicardial coronary artery spasm (see Fig. 7.2),[9] i.e. a decrease in peak relaxation

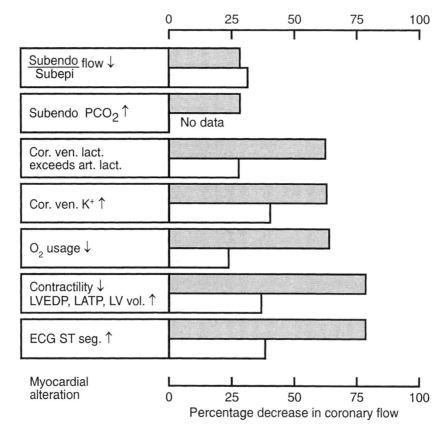

Fig. 7.3 Effect of graded flow reduction on myocardial metabolism and function. A 25% reduction of blood flow in the left anterior descending coronary artery of conscious dogs (■) causes a decrease in the subendo/subepicardial flow ratio and an increase in subendocardial PCO_2. A 50% reduction in flow causes a reduction in oxygen usage and detectable myocardial lactate and K^+ release. Only a 75% reduction of flow causes detectable reduction of contractility, and an increase in left ventricular end-diastolic and atrial pressures (LVEDP and LATP) and volume (LV), and ST-segment elevation. The reductions of flow sufficient to cause the same changes are smaller when flow is reduced in the left main coronary artery (□), possibly because this eliminates collateral flow from the circumflex artery. (Modified from ref. 10.)

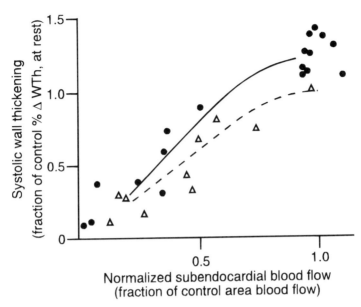

Fig. 7.4 Effect of graded reduction of total coronary blood flow on systolic thickening. In conscious dogs at rest ($\triangle$--$\triangle$) the extent of systolic thickening (WTh) decreases only slightly until flow is reduced by about 25%. During exercise (●—●) the systolic thickening is greater than at rest and a 25% reduction of blood flow causes only a barely detectable reduction of contraction. (Modified from ref. 11.)

dP/dt, followed by a decrease in peak contraction dP/dt, by an increase in early and end-diastolic pressure, and by a fall in systolic and pulse pressure.

Thus, when ischemia develops in the territory of a large coronary conductive artery, the development of ST-segment changes follows that of global left ventricular contractile abnormalities by a few seconds. Pain, when present, usually occurs only minutes later (see Ch. 14). The development of myocardial necrosis following persistent occlusion is described in 7.3.1.

7.2.2 Effects of graded reduction of coronary flow at rest in dogs

Graded reduction of CBF in anesthetized dogs allows assessment of the adaptive changes to mild inadequacy of perfusion, and of the degree of flow reduction required in order to produce the various abnormalities (see Fig. 7.3).[10] A 25% reduction of flow in the left anterior descending (LAD) coronary artery is associated with increased myocardial extraction of oxygen and with decreased oxygen consumption. Further reductions of flow are followed by decreases in the speed of left ventricular relaxation and contraction, then by ST-segment depression, elevation of end-diastolic pressure, decreased stroke volume, and finally by elevation of the ST segment, which develops when flow reduction is about 70%, so that myocardial ischemia becomes transmural. When flow is reduced in the main left stem coronary artery, lesser degrees of flow reduction are required to produce the same sequence of dysfunction, suggesting a contribution of collateral perfusion when flow is reduced only in the LAD or circumflex arteries.

In unanesthetized dogs, the relation between the reduction of myocardial blood flow and the impairment of contractile function is exponential: initially, the impairment of function

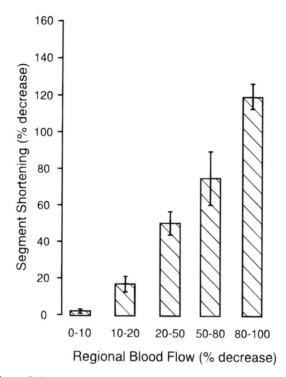

Fig. 7.5 Effect of decrease of subendocardial blood flow on systolic segment shortening. In conscious dogs the percentage decrease of subendocardial segment shortening is small until blood flow is reduced by 20%. Systolic bulging (segment lengthening) develops only when flow is reduced by more than 80%. (Modified from ref. 12.)

is small for a large decrease of flow; subsequently, further small reductions of flow cause greater impairment of contractile function (see Fig. 7.4).[11,12] An approximate 50% decrease of mean transmural blood flow in the territory of the left circumflex coronary artery is required in order to cause global left ventricular contractile dysfunction. Lesser degrees of flow reduction reduce the extent and peak velocity of thickening in the ischemic subendo-cardial layers. Local contractile function in subendocardial layers begins to fall slightly when regional subendocardial flow is reduced by 10–20% and becomes marked as flow decreas-es by 50–80%. Only segments with a flow reduction greater than 80% show paradoxical movement, with bulging of the ventricular wall (see Fig. 7.5).

■ *Extrapolated to the clinical setting, these findings suggest that a 30% reduction of subendo-cardial blood flow may not cause detectable alterations in left ventricular contractile function, even when assessed from the extent and peak velocity of systolic regional wall thickening. This small reduction of subendocardial perfusion, particularly when accompanied by an increase in subepicar-dial perfusion, may also be undetectable by myocardial scintigraphy.* ■

7.2.3 Effect of a coronary artery stenosis on exercise tolerance in conscious dogs

In dogs with chronically implanted flowmeters and pressure transducers, and with a left cir-cumflex coronary artery stenosis, reduction of mean transmural blood flow during exercise by 29 and 53% was shown to cause, respectively, a mild degree of dysfunction that reduced

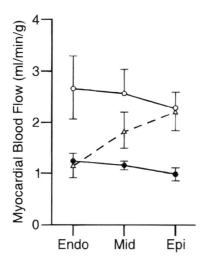

Fig. 7.6 Effect of reduction of coronary blood flow, during exercise, on its transmural distribution. A 30% reduction of total coronary blood flow during exercise lowers flow to resting levels in the subendocardium (Endo), but has no effect on the subepicardium (Epi); the effect is intermediate in the midwall (Mid): ●, at rest; ○, control exercise, △, exercise with coronary stenosis. Systolic thickening is reduced by 29%. (Modified from ref. 11.)

systolic thickening slightly below resting levels (see Fig. 7.6) and a moderate degree of dysfunction that reduced systolic thickening to less than 50% of resting levels (whereas in the normally perfused wall, systolic thickening increased by 20%). Severe regional dysfunction developed during exercise for an 80% reduction of mean flow and a 65% decrease of subepicardial flow compared with the normally perfused wall.[11] Thus, during exercise, left ventricular dysfunction becomes obvious only when subepicardial flow also decreases. This degree of flow reduction can also be easily detected by myocardial scintigraphy. During dipyridamole-induced blood flow "steal," ischemic regional wall motion dysfunction develops in the presence of increased subepicardial blood flow (which is the actual cause of subendocardial blood flow steal and ischemia) (see Ch. 6).

7.3 PRECONDITIONING, STUNNING, AND HIBERNATION

Coronary reperfusion is the prerequisite for the survival of reversibly injured ischemic myocytes, but it may accelerate their death by rapid cell swelling and disruption of the sarcolemma.[2] The response of the myocardium and of the coronary microvessels to less prolonged or severe ischemia varies.

A short episode of myocardial ischemia can reduce the effects of a new episode of ischemia occurring during the subsequent hours; this is termed *"preconditioning."* A prolonged but reversible episode of ischemia can leave a residual impairment of left ventricular function persisting for days; this is known as *"stunning."* In addition, clinical observations have suggested that chronic flow reduction, without detectable metabolic signs of ischemia, can be associated with persistent loss of contractile function, or *"hibernation,"* which is reversed when coronary flow is reestablished following bypass surgery or angioplasty.

7.3.1 Preconditioning

This term was introduced by Reimer et al[13] to define a natural protective mechanism of the heart against ischemia. A reduction of myocardial necrosis was observed in dogs when persistent coronary occlusion followed one or more brief periods of ischemia. The duration of ischemia sufficient to provide preconditioning is shorter than that necessary to produce stunning. Preconditioning can significantly reduce infarct size (or delay cell necrosis) but the duration of the protection provided is short, only 1–2 h.[14,15] The protective role of transient ischemic episodes with regard to the effects of subsequent persistent coronary occlusion was confirmed in other species in isolated hearts,[16–18] as well as in patients during spontaneous episodes of ischemia[19] and angioplasty.[20] Preconditioning also reduces reperfusion arrhythmias.[18] The mechanisms responsible for the myocardial protection provided by preconditioning may be multiple; a reduction of energy consumption similar to that caused by calcium antagonists does not appear to be a sufficient explanation. Increased release of adenosine,[21] and activation of ATP-sensitive potassium channels[22] are not mutually exclusive mechanisms of preconditioning. Increased synthesis of heat shock proteins[23] does not explain the very rapid development of preconditioning within minutes, but could account for protection after some hours, as time is necessary for their synthesis (for details see the review by Lawson and Downey in reference 24).

■ *Although the beneficial effects of preconditioning are very short-lived, the existence of natural mechanisms of myocardial protection from ischemia may open the way to novel therapeutic strategies.*[25,26] ■

7.3.2 Stunning

The term "stunning" was introduced by Braunwald and Kloner[27] to define the persistent postischemic contractile dysfunction of the normally perfused myocardium, originally described in dogs by Heyndrickx et al[28] a few years earlier. Postischemic stunning includes not only systolic but also diastolic[29,30] dysfunction. It can be observed:

a. following sudden coronary occlusion, lasting only 10–15 min or after repeated shorter periods of occlusion
b. after ischemia caused by increased demand in both experimental animals[31] and patients[32,33]
c. at the periphery of infarction, after global flow reduction and after extracorporeal circulation.

The spontaneous recovery of cardiac contractile function may take hours or days, depending on the severity and duration of ischemia,[34] but contraction can be transiently restored by inotropic stimuli such as postextrasystolic potentiation or β-adrenergic drugs.[35] In stunned myocardium the delayed recovery of contractile function is associated with normal, average myocardial perfusion and oxygen consumption, although with considerable regional heterogeneity.[36]

It is not clear to what extent stunning represents a gradual physiologic recovery from the ischemic insult or a consequence of a reperfusion-induced injury, which could delay or reduce the benefits of reperfusion.[37–41] Agents that reduce stunning may either accelerate normal recovery or prevent some unfavorable aspects of reperfusion: the acceleration of normal recovery would be clinically desirable when global residual ventricular contractile function is critically reduced; a reduction of reperfusion-induced injury would be desirable in all cases.

The mechanisms responsible for postischemic mechanical stunning are probably multiple. Besides the immediate damage, ischemic cellular injury modifies genetic programing: for example, in some animal models, following reversible ischemia, changes can be observed in the interstitial collagen matrix and in myosin expression.[42–44] Thus, the delayed recovery following ischemic injury is also the result of a modified gene expression which takes time to revert to the preischemic state. Intracellular calcium overload, altered function of the sarcoplasmic reticulum, decreased sensitivity of the myofilaments to calcium, excitation–contraction uncoupling,[45] and slow resynthesis of the adenosine nucleotide pool have also been proposed, as has microvascular damage with leukocyte activation, which is more prominent when microvascular stunning is severe.[46] The production of free radicals by the myocytes, endothelial cells, and granulocytes may be a common pathway leading to an initial phase of calcium overload in the myocytes. The effects of pharmacologic intervention with calcium antagonists and antioxidants on postischemic mechanical stunning have produced detectable beneficial effects in experimental preparations.[47]

In general, the effects of intervention are most marked in isolated hearts, in which most variables can be controlled. The effects become less evident as experimental conditions become closer to human pathologic conditions. Any benefits will, therefore, be hard to demonstrate in humans, because the biologic response to the ischemic injury is likely to vary in different individuals and to be influenced by the actual cause of ischemia.

■ *Although the consequences of myocardial ischemia may be reduced by preventing specific forms of reperfusion injury, by far the greatest benefit is obtained from reducing the duration or severity of ischemia. Thus, reperfusion and improvement of the supply–demand ratio are still the major therapeutic goals. There would be more scope for therapeutic agents that are capable of reducing the irreversible consequences of ischemia, i.e. cell necrosis and fatal arrhythmias, than for those that accelerate spontaneous improvement of contractile postischemic dysfunction.* ■

7.3.3 Hibernation

This descriptive term was introduced by Rahimtoola[48] to define the recovery of myocardial contraction of kinetic segments of the ventricular wall following successful surgical revascularization. The intuitive interpretation of this observation was teleologic: a reduced contractile activity developed in order to balance ("match") a chronic reduction of oxygen availability. In this way a "smart heart" would prevent a discrepancy between demand and supply, hence avoiding irreversible tissue damage.

This intriguing concept was proved valid by acute animal experiments showing progressive adaptation of regional contractile function to *gradual flow reduction* in conscious dogs[49] as well as in neonatal[50] and adult pig hearts, but only over a period of hours.[51,52] In the pig model, during the period of matched low blood flow and reduced contraction, dobutamine can reestablish near-normal contractile function, but only at the expense of detectable signs of ischemia.[53] In these acute experiments, contraction matching induced by low blood flow appears to be related to a mechanism of contractile dysfunction differing from that observed during ischemia and in reperfused stunned myocardium.[54] Compared with normal myocardium, acutely hibernating myocardium appears to exhibit a marked decrease in cytosolic Ca^{2+} concentration during systole in the presence of normal intracellular pH and inorganic phosphate levels and myofilament sensitivity to Ca^{2+} (see Table 7.1).

The experimental demonstration of acute hibernation does not, in itself, explain the clinical observation of recovery of contractile function following coronary revascularization, which prompted the use of the term "hibernating myocardium," for the following reasons.

First, the concept of hibernation as a matched reduction of contractile function to low blood flow, can be assumed to operate in the clinical setting *only* when it is possible to exclude the presence of either ischemia or stunning, both of which could also be responsible for reversible regional contractile dysfunction of the myocardial wall. Normal blood flow to a segment of the left ventricular wall of normal thickness but with no systolic thickening, is a clear indication of stunning. Reduced blood flow, which is frequently detected in non-contractile myocardial segments,[55] indicates hibernation only when transient, silent ischemia can be excluded. In turn, a chronically reduced blood flow in areas of preserved wall thickness and metabolism could be due to a critical stenosis or to persistent small ves-

Table 7.1 Loss of regional contractile function

	Parameter					
Cause*	Wall thickness	Myocardial blood flow	P_i	pH	Activator Ca^{2+}	Ca^{2+} sensitivity
Ischemia	=	↓↓	↑	↓	↑	↓
Necrosis	=	↓↓	↑	↓↓		
Scar	↓↓	↓↓↓				
Stunning	=	=	=	=	↑	↓
Acute hibernation	=	↓	=	=	↓↓	=

*The causes of loss of regional myocardial contractile function can be multiple. Fibrous scars can be identified because of the marked reduction of diastolic wall thickness. Stunning is associated with normal perfusion. Ischemia and necrosis are characterized by low flow associated with signs of ischemia (low pH and elevated inorganic phosphate [P_i]). A reduced sensitivity to Ca^{2+} is common to ischemia and stunning. A decreased activator Ca^{2+} is characteristic of acute hibernation. There is no information on chronic hibernation

sel dysfunction. A reduction of resting flow requires an approximate 90% reduction in the vessel diameter (a 99% reduction in lumen) (see Fig. 6.2). A stenosis of such severity is unlikely to remain patent for weeks or months and causes a large transstenotic pressure gradient which, over similar periods, should cause sufficient collateral development to maintain adequate resting flow. Thus, this chronic reduction of perfusion is most likely attributable to either chronic inappropriate constriction of prearteriolar vessels or resetting of the metabolic regulation of vasomotor tone in arteriolar vessels.

Second, the matched reduction of flow and contractile function leaves the hibernating myocardium vulnerable to recurrent ischemic episodes whenever adrenergic stimulation reestablishes contraction.[53] It is difficult, therefore, to envisage the possibility that such a precarious equilibrium between low flow and reduced contraction could remain stable over periods of weeks or months.

■ *Hibernating myocardium with hypoperfusion, but with no metabolic signs of ischemia, is unlikely to remain stable and occasional episodes of ischemia, followed by stunning, may be common. Chronic hypoperfusion can be caused by greater than 90% diameter stenosis and extremely poor development of collaterals, by inappropriate constriction of small coronary vessels, or by resetting of the mechanisms that match coronary perfusion to myocardial metabolism at the arteriolar level.* ■

7.4 DEVELOPMENT OF MYOCARDIAL NECROSIS

Following coronary occlusion, ischemic myocytes neither die instantaneously nor all die at the same time: mildly ischemic myocytes may survive indefinitely with biologic and functional adaptations. Experimental coronary artery occlusion in previously normal animal hearts has provided valuable information on the time course of the development and extent of myocardial infarction (MI) and mechanisms of myocardial cell necrosis, on the limitation of infarct size, and on post-MI ventricular remodeling.

7.4.1 Development and extension of infarction

In anesthetized dogs killed at successive time intervals following ligation and reperfusion of a major coronary artery, focal cell necrosis has been shown to begin after about 20 min and to become confluent in subendocardial layers after about 40 min, gradually reaching subepicardial layers with a progressive wave front at about 3 h. By this time necrosis has developed, on average, to about 90% of its full extent, which occurs when ligation is released after 6 h.[56] This wavefront of necrosis is an expression of the transmural gradient of susceptibility to flow reduction in the left ventricular wall. It is determined not only by the transmural gradient of flow that develops when coronary perfusion pressure is critically reduced relative to ventricular systolic pressure, but also by the greater susceptibility of subendocardial regions to ischemia, independent of flow reduction, because of their greater metabolic activity (see Ch. 4).

The extension of the MI depends on the anatomic area at risk, i.e. the area vascularized by the occluded vessel, as well as on collateral blood flow and on the duration of the occlusion; it is also increased by ventricular hypertrophy. In dogs, no MI develops if the anatomic area at risk corresponds to less than 25% of the left ventricular myocardium (see Fig. 7.7). Infarction extends to a much greater fraction of the subendocardial than epicardial layers of the vascular area at risk (see Fig. 7.8).[57]

The development of necrosis is slower in unanesthetized animals, which have lower heart rates and sympathetic tone and, hence, lower myocardial oxygen consumption and a lesser degree of impaired perfusion (see Fig. 7.9).[58]

The precise mechanisms of ischemic cell death are not known, but a series of subcellular and cellular alterations, contributing to and accelerating cell death, have been identified.

In the dog, mild, ultrastructural myocytic changes can be identified after coronary occlusion lasting 15 min, but no striking sudden change marks the transition to irreversible cell death. The earliest signs of irreversible injury are represented by reduction of glycogen granules, disruption of the sarcolemma, swelling of mitochondria with accumulation of amorphous matrix

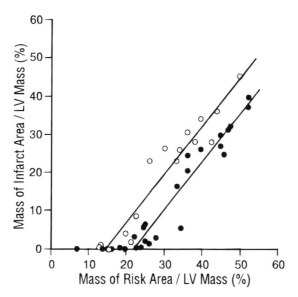

Fig. 7.7 Relation between myocardial mass at risk and infarct size. The infarct size increases linearly with the size of the vascular bed occluded (myocardial mass at risk) and the relation is displaced to the left of normal (●) in the presence of myocardial hypertrophy (○). In dogs, owing to the presence of collaterals, no MI develops when the vascular area at risk involves less than 25% of the ventricular myocardium in the normal heart and 15% in the hypertrophied heart. (Modified from ref. 57.)

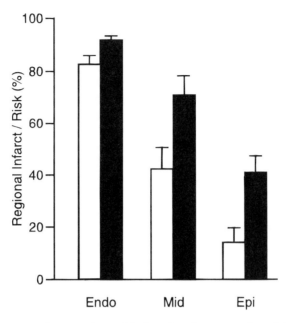

Fig. 7.8 Transmural extension of infarction in normal and hypertrophied hearts. After 3 h occlusion followed by reperfusion in normal hearts (□), over 80% of the area at risk is infarcted in the subendocardium (Endo), but only 10% in the subepicardium (Epi). In hypertrophied hearts (■) receiving the same treatment, the fraction of the area at risk that becomes infarcted is greater also in the subepicardium. (Modified from ref. 57.)

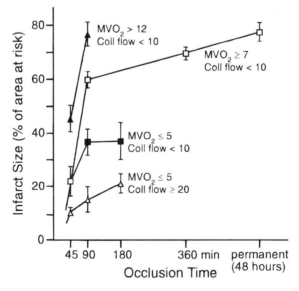

Fig. 7.9 Influence of myocardial demand and collateral flow on the development of myocardial infarction. The infarct involves only a small fraction of the area at risk after 3 h occlusion followed by reperfusion, when myocardial oxygen consumption (MVO_2) is low and collateral (Coll) blood flow high. Infarction involves about 80% of the area at risk after only 90 min occlusion when collateral blood flow is low and MVO_2 high or when the occlusion is permanent. (Modified from ref. 58.)

densities, and aggregation of nuclear chromatin. The ultimate causes of irreversible cell death are the depletion of high-energy phosphates and the accumulation of catabolites (H^+, free radicals, inorganic phosphate, ammonia, fatty acyl derivatives, etc.).

Myocardial necrosis is associated with severe microvascular injury (swelling of the endothelium and plugging by granulocytes). Sudden coronary reopening after 15–30 min occlusion is followed by restoration of flow above preocclusion level, but is followed by markedly reduced flow when it occurs after 60–90 min: this is termed the *no reflow phenomenon*.[59] Capillary compression by swollen myocytes and plugging by white or red cells and fibrin is responsible for the lack of reflow. Activation and injury to the endothelium can be caused by free radicals, cytokines, complement activation, and fibrin-derived peptides. It is unclear whether microvascular injury is merely a secondary phenomenon that accelerates the death of irreversibly injured myocytes, or whether it contributes independently to the extent of myocardial necrosis as part of cytokine- and free radical-induced injury to the microvasculature of nonirreversibly injured myocardium.[60,61]

7.4.2 Limitation of infarct size

The time course of the development of MI following sudden coronary ligation indicates that the most effective means of limiting infarct size is reperfusion of the occluded artery: the shorter the duration of occlusion, the more limited the infarction. Thus, the only long-term means of limiting infarct size is the restoration of CBF. Short-term interventions aimed at limiting infarct size are useful in order to allow more time for the development of collateral blood flow or for the reopening of the obstructed coronary artery. In patients, coronary artery occlusion is very often intermittent in the early hours of MI[62] and the development of adequate collateral blood flow may be rapid in the presence of preexisting interarterial anastomoses. Thus, interventions that delay irreversible cell damage can also be useful in patients when they allow cells to survive until flow is restored either by recanalization of the infarct-related artery or by increased collateral flow.

Considerable debate developed in the 1970s about the existence of an ischemic "border zone" at the periphery of the infarction, which could be saved by invasive intervention. However, the territories of distribution of infarct- and non-infarct-related arteries[63] are so well delineated in most animal species that an appreciable twilight zone of overlapping vascularization cannot be identified. If the extent of necrosis is reduced, this occurs within the vascular territory of distribution of the infarct-related artery, particularly with a lesser progression of the wavefront of necrosis from the subendocardium to the subepicardium.

In the case of *persistent coronary artery occlusion,* limitation of infarct size is based on reduction of the hemodynamic, neural, and biologic mechanisms that either contribute to the worsening of the discrepancy between myocardial oxygen consumption and oxygen supply or accelerate cell necrosis. Experiments in isolated perfused hearts, as well as in anesthetized animals, have shown that cell necrosis may be reduced also in the absence of reperfusion, but in these short-term studies it is not clear whether myocardial necrosis was actually reduced or was simply delayed.

In the case of *early coronary reopening,* infarct size could be further reduced by interventions that limit the possible occurrence of acute reperfusion damage to cells not already irreversibly injured. In isolated hearts, sudden reoxygenation of severely ischemic myocardium causes alterations that are preventable by pharmacologic intervention. Free radical produc-

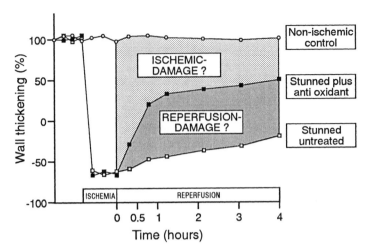

Fig. 7.10 Estimated extent of reperfusion damage. In isolated hearts, treatment with antioxidants reduces the extent of reperfusion damage, estimated from the reduction in wall thickening. The effect of antioxidants is less obvious in intact animals with infarction, possibly because of the buffering effect of blood perfusion. (Modified from ref. 41.)

tion and cytosolic Ca^{2+} overload, resulting from the sudden availability of oxygen and blood flow, could cause extensive additional injury to nonirreversibly damaged myocardium, which can be prevented by antioxidants (see Fig. 7.10)[41] and reduced by Ca^{2+} antagonists administered before reperfusion.[64,65]

■ *Demonstration of the beneficial effects produced by reducing myocardial reperfusion injury in patients has not yet been achieved and will be difficult, first, because the determinants of myocardial response to ischemia are multiple and may differ considerably among patients, and second, because methods for assessment of infarct size that are more precise than those available to assess the effects of thrombolysis, are not available.* ■

7.4.3 Postinfarction ventricular wall repair and remodeling

Necrosis of a segment of the left ventricular wall not only requires post-MI repair, as there is a loss of contractile elements, but also causes profound disruption of the physiologic contraction synergy of the unaffected ventricular wall, which is based on sliding of the three layers of muscle fibers that course at different angles within the wall (see Fig. 2.1). Adaptive changes, with fibrosis of the necrotic area, cause a redistribution of systolic and diastolic tensile stress in adjacent segments of the wall, with consequent hypertrophy of residual myocardial cells, and lead to changes in the shape of the ventricular cavity, with reorganization of the regional sequence of electric activation and of the sequence and magnitude of regional contraction and relaxation. Enlargement of the ventricular cavity increases the tension required by the ventricular wall to develop a given systolic pressure, but the tension is reduced by thickening of the unaffected wall because of hypertrophy (according to the law of Laplace; see Ch. 2). Systolic hypertension is poorly tolerated by enlarged ventricles in the absence of hypertrophy.

Stretching of the necrotic segment can cause expansion of the infarcted segment of the wall. The extent of structural and functional changes in the ventricular wall depends on the size and also on the location of the MI, on regional and global loading conditions in the ventricular wall, and on the biologic response of myocardial tissue.

The postinfarction repair process

Dead cardiac myocytes must be removed, and ultimately replaced by scar tissue. Removal of dead cells depends on lysosomal proteases and lipases released and activated by dead myocytes and, especially, on the influx of inflammatory cells (mainly polymorphonuclear neutrophils and macrophages). The inflammatory reaction that develops in response to ischemia[61] and to the death of myocytes includes intense activation of cytokines, of components of the complementary pathway, of kinins, and of lipooxygenases that can amplify the initial repair reaction and, possibly, cause injury to myocytes and microvessels not irreversibly damaged.

In patients, coagulation necrosis becomes detectable within 6–12 h at the center of non-reperfused infarcts. Contraction bands of necrosis can be detectable as early as 1 h in reperfused infarctions and, sometimes, at the periphery of nonreperfused infarctions also.[66] The influx of neutrophils becomes detectable within 10–20 h and begins to subside within 4–5 days when macrophages become more prominent. After 10 days a peripheral rim of granulation tissue has appeared around the infarct. Necrotic myocardium, including its reticular framework, is removed and replaced by granulation tissue with new capillaries and fibroblasts. Infarct size is the major determinant of the area of scarring, which, when the infarction is small, may be smaller than the volume of necrotic myocardium that it has replaced, owing to shrinkage of the scar tissue. Removal of the necrotic tissue takes from 3 to 6 weeks and the process of infarct repair is completed by 3–6 months, depending on the size of the infarct. The scar tissue, once formed, is resistant to further deformation (see Table 7.2).[67]

Infarct extension[68] is caused by necrosis of adjacent reversibly damaged segments of the wall because ischemia lasts longer, becomes more extensive and severe, or recurs.

Infarct expansion is a gradual, passive process caused by the disruption of myocardial cells and tissue loss within the necrotic zone leading to thinning and stretching of the wall. It is

Table 7.2 Pathologic dating of infarct

Week	Time	Appearance*
1	<5–6 h	Light M: 'wavy fibers' Electron M: mitochondrial swelling
	>5–6 h	Gross: Normal macroscopic appearance Light M: Coagulative necrosis (hyaline change, striations, eosinophils)
	1–4 days	Gross: pale myocardium Light M: neutrophil infiltrate
	>5 days	Light M: invasion of capillaries, fibroblasts, macrophages and myocytolysis
2		Gross: reddish-purple in peripheral areas of infarct Light M: muscle fiber removal and invasion of granulation tissue
3		Light M: by start of week 3 no neutrophils remaining, few eosinophils, but many pigmented macrophages and plasma cells
4–12		Gross: pale gray → gray-white Light M: gradual ↑ connective tissue → vascularity → scar

Modified from ref. 67

* "Gross" refers to gross macroscopic appearance; "Light M" refers to light microscopic appearance; "Electron M" refers to electron microscopic appearance

most common at the apex and develops during the first few weeks after the acute episode, but may progress over the following 2–3 months until the fibrous scar becomes compact. It is exacerbated by increased myocardial work load, which increases stretching of the weakened necrotic segment; it is reduced by preservation of subepicardial layers of myocardium and may be opposed by organization of mural endocardial thrombus. When necrosis involves a large segment of the ventricular wall, including subepicardial layers, a sustained increase in afterload and treatment with steroid anti-inflammatory drugs during the early weeks of infarction may favor infarct expansion, particularly in the elderly. Conversely, when the extension of necrosis is small, no expansion develops, and, ultimately, shrinkage of the fibrous scar may even reduce the segment length of the infarcted wall.

Post-MI ventricular remodeling

The global process of remodeling includes infarct expansion and lengthening of the noninfarcted segments caused by increased end-systolic and end-diastolic volume. Disruption of the normal pattern of regional development of tensile stress, and contraction and relaxation of the myocardial fiber bundles in the different transmural layers of the ventricular wall, together with the development of myocardial hypertrophy, produce a gradual restructuring of the ventricular wall and cavity. Post-MI ventricular remodeling is influenced by infarct site and size, by infarct healing, and by ventricular wall stress. In rats, the size of the infarct is a major determinant of the increase in left ventricular volume at 4 months (see Fig. 7.11).[69]

Enlargement of the left ventricle, with remodeling of the cavity, can be minimized by interventions that reduce infarct size, that either maintain subepicardial perfusion or reduce ventricular afterload and preload, and that have favorable consequences on the healing process and formation of scar tissue. The repair process of myocardial necrosis, and subsequent remodeling, involves elongation, sliding, and hypertrophy of surviving myocytes, which increase in volume by about 30% in rats (see Fig. 7.12).[70] It also involves profound changes in the interstitium and microvasculature, but the intercapillary distance increases in hypertrophied myocardium. Postnecrotic repair is impaired by anti-inflammatory agents,

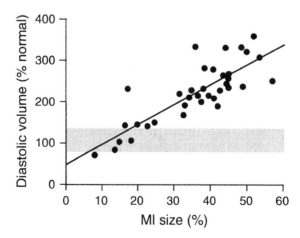

Fig. 7.11 Effect of infarct size on ventricular dilation. In rats 4 months after infarction the diastolic ventricular volume is increased linearly with the percentage of the total myocardium involved by the infarction (MI). Shaded area represents normal ventricular volume. (Modified from ref. 69.)

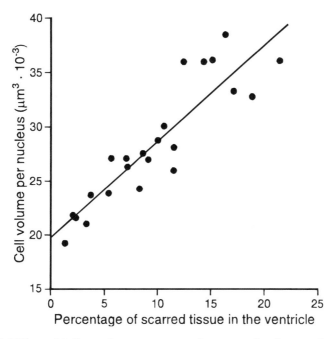

Fig. 7.12 Effect of infarct size on myocyte hypertrophy. In rats, the volume of
myocytes increases in proportion to the size of the postinfarction scar as a result of
compensatory hypertrophy. (Modified from ref. 70.)

which cause a greater degree of expansion of the infarcted area. Administration of nitrates
and of angiotensin-converting enzyme (ACE) inhibitors can attenuate infarct expansion and
reduce left ventricular enlargement (see Fig. 7.13).[69] Besides reducing afterload, long-term
ACE inhibition may also have direct beneficial effects on both the remodeling process and
the coronary vasculature, possibly by reducing local tissue production of angiotensin II and
other growth factors.

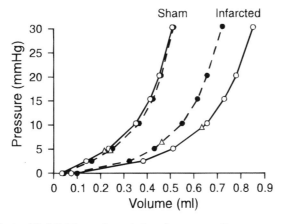

**Fig. 7.13 Effect of inhibition of angiotensin-converting enzyme on ventricu-
lar pressure/volume curves in infarcted rats.** Compared with untreated rats (○),
the curve is displaced to the left and the operating end-diastolic pressure (△) is much
lower in captopril-treated animals (●). No effect is seen in controls (Sham).
(Modified from ref. 69.)

■ *Reduction of ventricular volume by the remodeling process contributes to the improvement of prognosis because ventricular enlargement has unfavorable effects on wall tension, particularly when afterload is high or when it increases acutely (see Ch. 2).* ■

7.5 DEVELOPMENT OF FATAL ARRHYTHMIAS

Myocardial ischemia causes electrophysiologic changes favoring the development of arrhythmias that can be fatal in some cases. Fatal arrhythmias are exceptional during mild transient ischemic episodes, but can develop after the onset, or soon after the termination, of some episodes of transmural ischemia, and occur more frequently in acute MI. Myocardial scarring can also predispose to reentry circuits and ventricular fibrillation (VF). Arrhythmias occurring during acute ischemia and MI are mostly represented by VF and, less often, by A–V block and asystole. In anesthetized experimental animals, and also in isolated perfused hearts, arrhythmias are particularly common immediately after sudden reperfusion, but in patients reperfusion arrhythmias are rare (see Ch. 10).

7.5.1 Electrophysiologic changes caused by ischemia

Ischemia causes a diminution of resting membrane potential, which is responsible for a depression of the T–Q segment on the surface ECG leads. It is followed, within seconds, by diminution of action potential, which is responsible for the elevation of the ST segment, the rate of upstroke, and the duration of the action potential, which may be recognizable also on precordial ECG leads (see Fig. 7.14). The refractory period of ischemic cells is initially shortened, but after a few minutes of ischemia it becomes longer than in adjacent nonischemic cells. Conduction of the electric impulse also increases initially, but decreases after a few minutes until it becomes blocked or fractionated.

The electrophysiologic changes that develop during ischemia are caused by a combination of events: these are the lowering of tissue PO_2, the increase of PCO_2, and the increase

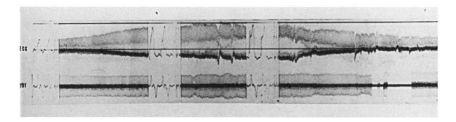

Fig. 7.14 Changes of TQ baseline and ST-segment during episodes of ischemia caused by occlusive spasm. Slow playback of the precordial ECG lead V_4 and of left ventricular dP/dt recorded in the coronary care unit during a spontaneous episode of myocardial ischemia caused by coronary artery spasm in a patient with variant angina. The lack of reduction of dP/dT was most likely caused by the simultaneous increase in systolic blood pressure. The slow speed allows detection of the progressive drop of the TQ baseline and subsequent elevation of the ST-segment. This was a very consistent pattern in most patients, which therefore, although recorded with a standard DC electrode, suggests that progressive diastolic depolarization, followed by reduction of the action potential, are the first consequences of ischemia. In the bottom tracing, as usual the changes in dP/dt precede the ECG changes. (See also epicardial ECG in Figure 6.10.)

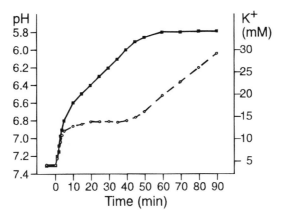

Fig. 7.15 Rate of change of interstitial myocardial pH and K⁺ concentration following sudden coronary occlusion. Within 5 min the pH (■) drops to about 6.8 and K⁺ (○) concentration increases about threefold. Thus, membrane potential and cellular electrolyte exchange are greatly disrupted very soon after the interruption of blood flow. (Modified from ref. 71.)

of phosphate, adenosine, free fatty acids, free fatty acid esters, phospholipids, and, in particular, of K⁺ and H⁺ (see Fig. 7.15).[71]

Arrhythmias may develop because of increased automaticity due to triggered activity precipitated by early or delayed depolarization, and because of reentry circuits, which are favored by the development of conduction delay, fractionation, undirectional block, and regional variability in the duration of the refractory period, and which can be caused by acute ischemia or by chronic alterations.

7.5.2 Ischemia-related arrhythmias in animal models

The development of ischemia-related tachyarrhythmias varies in different animal models of ischemia. VF is much less common, following coronary occlusion, in unanesthetized dogs resting quietly than in anesthetized dogs, and it occurs most frequently in pigs. The incidence of VF is increased by sympathetic stimulation and decreased by vagal stimulation.[72] The onset and mechanisms of arrhythmias vary according to the time that elapses from the onset of myocardial ischemia.

In the early phase after the onset of ischemia (3–30 min in anesthetized dogs), VF occurs frequently if the area of ischemia is sufficiently large.[73] After this initial period, ventricular ectopics are common but VF is rare.

In a late phase (after 72 h), spontaneous arrhythmias occur less frequently, but VF can occur in response to premature ventricular stimulation, indicating the persistence of reentry circuits, which, when activated by an appropriately timed extra stimulus, can cause VF.[74] Late arrhythmias originate from either the periphery of the infarcted area or the postinfarction scar, where asynchronous fragmented conduction predisposes to reentry circuits.[75,76] The onset of arrhythmias may also be favored by interruption, and subsequent regeneration, of nerve fibers by myocardial necrosis.[77]

Reperfusion arrhythmias occur within a few seconds of reperfusion in isolated perfused rabbit hearts[78] and VF is most frequent within 15 min after coronary reperfusion in anesthetized dogs.[79] Free radicals are suspected of favoring the development of reperfusion arrhythmias in isolated perfused hearts.[41]

The reasons for the consistent development of reperfusion arrhythmias in isolated hearts, in anesthetized animals (compared with their rarity in quiet, resting unanesthetized dogs, and following the resolution of spasm or during thrombolysis in man) are not clear.

■ *As the incidence, and probably the mechanisms, of arrhythmias vary considerably according to the animal model used, application of the findings to patients should be cautious. Furthermore, the drugs that are effective in preventing ischemia-induced arrhythmias in animal models, may not necessarily be effective in preventing fatal arrhythmias in patients. The ideal drug should interrupt potential reentry circuits, at the same time preventing ectopic triggering stimuli and reducing the rate of ventricular tachycardia and its degeneration into fibrillation.* ■

7.6 ADRENERGIC MECHANISMS IN MYOCARDIAL ISCHEMIA

Myocardial ischemia can induce important alterations in sympathetic neurotransmission, as well as changes in adrenoreceptor density and postreceptor signal transduction. Activation of both myocardial β-adrenoreceptors and coronary α-adrenoreceptors can contribute to exacerbation of myocardial ischemia and to malignant tachyarrhythmias. Infarction can cause interruption of sympathetic and vagal-mediated afferent responses in noninfarcted myocardium.[77]

7.6.1 Sympathetic and adrenergic activation during myocardial ischemia

Myocardial ischemia excites sensory endings of both the vagal (inhibitory) and the sympathetic (excitatory) sensory fibers that innervate the heart.[80] During short episodes of ischemia lasting less than 10 min, the increase in the myocardial concentration of norepinephrine is moderated by both adenosine release, which inhibits release of exocytotic norepinephrine, and reuptake. However, after ischemia lasting 20 min, concentrations of extracellular myocardial norepinephrine may reach levels 1000 times higher than plasma concentrations.[81] Intense stimulation of β-adrenoreceptors can cause not only transmural blood flow "steal" and exacerbate subendocardial ischemia, but also direct myocite injury (see 6.3).[82] Reflex cardio/cardiac reflex causing α_1 and α_2-adrenergic receptor-mediated coronary constriction may exacerbate ischemia,[83,84] but this effect is controversial,[85] possibly reflecting the different levels of basal constriction of subepicardial and subendocardial vessels in the experimental models used.

7.6.2 Adrenergic mechanisms triggering ischemia-related arrhythmias

The most convincing experimental evidence for a major role of sympathetic nerves in the genesis of VF is provided by the failure of dogs with chronically established cardiac denervation to develop VF during acute MI.[86] Conversely, in dogs, VF is not prevented by acute denervation. The different responses of chronic and acute denervated animals may be due to their myocardial catecholamine content, which is very markedly reduced in the former and minimally reduced in the latter (see Fig. 7.16). The deleterious effect of sympathetic hyperactivity, and the protective effect of vagal activation, on the onset of VF, has been documented in several experimental conditions. In particular, dogs with old MI and a high vagal tone are less susceptible to VF during exercise and acute ischemia than are animals with low vagal tone.[92] In dogs with acute coronary occlusion, the fibrillation threshold was also reduced by the β_1-adrenergic blocker, metoprolol, and by the α_1 adrenoceptor blocker, prazosin.[94]

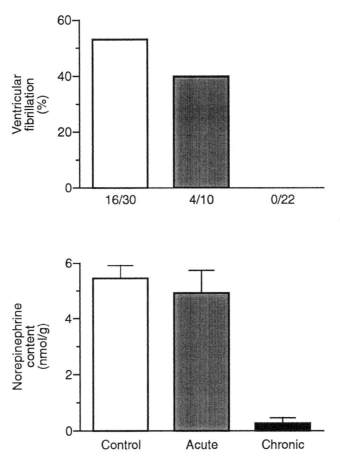

Fig. 7.16 Effect of acute and chronic denervation on the incidence of ventricular fibrillation during acute coronary occlusion. In dogs, ventricular fibrillation during acute coronary occlusion (□) is totally prevented by chronic cardiac denervation (0/22, ■), which is associated with a massive decrease of myocardial norepinephrine content. It is not decreased significantly by acute denervation (4/10, ■), which fails to reduce myocardial norepinephrine content compared with controls (16/30). (Modified from ref. 86.)

■ *The demonstration that, in some models, blockade of adrenergic mechanisms can reduce the incidence of fatal arrhythmias in acute ischemia and MI, is convincing. What remain to be established are reliable ways of identifying the patients in whom this adverse response to myocardial ischemia has an important role.* ■

REFERENCES

1. Jennings RB, Reimer KA, Hill ML, Mayer SE. Total ischemia in dog hearts in vitro. I. Comparison of high energy phosphate production, utilization and depletion, and of adenine nucleotide catabolism in total ischemia in vitro vs. severe ischemia in vivo. Circ Res 1981;*49*:892.

2. Reimer KA, Jennings RB, Hill ML. Total ischemia in dog hearts, in vitro. II. High energy phosphate depletion and associated defects in energy metabolism, cell volume regulation and sarcolemmal integrity. Circ Res 1981;*49:*901.

3. Bolli R. Oxygen-derived free radicals and postischemic myocardial dysfunction ("stunned myocardium"). J Am Coll Cardiol 1988;*12:*239.

4. Krause SM, Jacobus WE, Becker LC. Alterations in cardiac sarcoplasmic reticulum calcium transport in the post-ischemic "stunned" myocardium. Circ Res 1989;*65:*526.

5. Bolli R, Triana FJ, Jeroudi MO. Prolonged impairment of coronary vasodilation after reversible ischemia. Circ Res 1990;*67:*332.

6. Kim YD, Fomsgaard JS, Heim KF et al. Brief ischemia–reperfusion induces stunning of endothelium in canine coronary artery. Circulation 1992;*85:*1473.

7. Bishop VS, Kaspar RL, Barnes GE et al. Left ventricular function during acute regional myocardial ischemia in the conscious dog. J Appl Physiol 1974;*37:*785.

8. Serruys PW, Wijns W, van den Brand M et al. Left ventricular performance, regional blood flow, wall motion and lactate metabolism during transluminal angioplasty. Circulation 1984;*70:*24.

9. Maseri A, Mimmo R, Chierchia S, Marchesi C, Pesola A, L'Abbate A. Coronary artery spasm as a cause of acute myocardial ischemia in man. Chest 1975;*68:*625.

10. Gregg De, Bedynek JL Jr. Compensatory changes in the heart during progressive coronary artery stenosis. In: Maseri A, Lesch M, Klassen GA (eds) Primary and Secondary Angina Pectoris. Grune and Stratton, New York, 1978, p. 3.

11. Gallagher KP, Matsuzaki M, Osakada G, Kemper WS, Ross J Jr. Effect of exercise on the relationship between myocardial blood flow and systolic wall thickening in dogs with acute coronary stenosis. Circ Res 1983;*52:*716.

12. Vatner SF. Correlation between acute reductions in myocardial blood flow and function in conscious dogs. Circ Res 1980;*47:*201.

13. Reimer KA, Murry CE, Yamasawa I, Hill ML, Jennings RB. Four brief periods of ischemia cause no cumulative ATP loss or necrosis. Am J Physiol 1986;*251* (Heart Circ Physiol 20):306.

14. Murry CE, Jennings RB, Reimer KA. Preconditioning with ischemia: a delay of lethal cell injury in ischemic myocardium. Circulation 1986;*74:*1124.

15. Murry CE, Richard VJ, Jennings RB, Reimer KA. Myocardium protection is lost before contractile function recovers from ischemic preconditioning. Am J Physiol 1991;*260* (Heart Circ Physiol 29):H796.

16. Li GC, Vasquez BS, Gallagher KP, Lucchesi BR. Myocardial protection with preconditioning. Circulation 1990;*82:*609.

17. Conen MV, Liu GS, Downey JM. Preconditioning causes improved wall motion as well as smaller infarcts after transient coronary occlusion in rabbits. Circulation 1991;*84:*341.

18. Hagar JM, Hale SL, Kloner RA. Effect of preconditioning ischemia on reperfusion arrhythmias after coronary artery occlusion and reperfusion in the rat. Circ Res 1991;*68:*61.

19. Ovize M, Kloner RA, Hale SL, Przyklenk K. Coronary cyclic flow variations "precondition" ischemic myocardium. Circulation 1992;*85:*779.

20. Deutch E, Berger M, Kussmaul WG, Hirshfeld JW Jr, Herrmann HC, Laskey WK. Adaptation to ischemia during percutaneous transluminal coronary angioplasty: clinical, hemodynamic, and metabolic features. Circulation 1990;*82:*2044.

21. Liu GS, Thornton J, Winkle DM, Stanley AWH, Olsson RA, Downey JM. Protection against infarction afforded by preconditioning is mediated by A1 adenosine receptors in rabbit heart. Circulation 1991;*84:*350.

22. Gross GJ, Auchampach JA. Blockade of ATP-sensitive potassium channels prevents myocardial preconditioning in dogs. Circ Res 1992;*70:*223.

23. Yellon DM, Latchman DS. Stress proteins and myocardial protection. J Mol Cell Cardiol 1992;*24:*113.

24. Lawson CS, Downey JM. Preconditioning: state of the art myocardial protection. Cardiovasc Res 1993;*27:*542.

25. Walker DM, Yellon DM. Ischemic preconditioning: from mechanism to exploitation. Cardiovasc Res 1992;*26:*734.

26. Mullane K. Myocardial preconditioning. Part of the adenosine revival. Circulation 1992;*85:*845.
27. Braunwald E, Kloner RA. The stunned myocardium: prolonged, postischemic ventricular dysfunction. Circulation 1982;*66:*1146.
28. Heyndrickx GR, Millard RW, McRitchie RJ et al. Regional myocardial function and electrophysiological alterations after brief coronary occlusion in conscious dogs. J Clin Invest 1975;*56:*978.
29. Przyklenk K, Patel B, Kloner RA. Diastolic abnormalities of postischemic "stunned" myocardium. Am J Cardiol 1987;*60:*1211.
30. Charlat ML, O'Neill PG, Hartley CJ et al. Prolonged abnormalities of left ventricular diastolic wall thinning in the "stunned" myocardium in conscious dogs: time course and relation to systolic function. J Am Coll Cardiol 1989;*13:*185.
31. Homans DC, Laxson DD, Sublett E, Lindstrom P, Bache RJ. Cumulative deterioration of myocardial function after repeated episodes of exercise-induced ischemia. Am J Physiol 1989;*256:*H1462.
32. Kloner RA, Alloen J, Cox TA, Zheng Y, Ruiz CE. Stunned left ventricular myocardium after exercise treadmill testing in coronary artery disease. Am J Cardiol 1991;*68:*329.
33. Mathias P, Kent NZ, Blevins RD, Cascase P, Rubinfire M. Coronary vasospasm as a cause of stunned myocardium. Am Heart J 1987;*113:*383.
34. Patel B, Kloner RA, Przyklenk K, Braunwald E. Postischemic myocardial "stunning": a clinically relevant phenomenon. Ann Intern Med 1988;*108:*626.
35. Becker LC, Levine JH, DiPaula AF et al. Reversal of dysfunction in postischemic stunned myocardium by epinephrine and postextrasystolic potentiation. J Am Coll Cardiol 1986;*7:*580.
36. Stahl LD, Weiss HR, Becker LC. Myocardial oxygen consumption, oxygen supply/demand heterogeneity, and microvascular patency in regionally stunned myocardium. Circulation 1988;*77:*865.
37. Braunwald E, Kloner RA. Myocardial reperfusion: a double-edged sword? J Clin Invest 1985;*76:*1713.
38. Becker LC, Ambrosio G. Myocardial consequences of reperfusion. Prog Cardiovasc Dis 1987;*30:*23.
39. Bolli R. Mechanisms of myocardial "stunning". Circulation 1990;*82:*723.
40. Opie LH. Reperfusion injury and its pharmacologic modication. Circulation 1989;*80:*1049.
41. Hearse DJ. Stunning: a radical re-view. Cardiovasc Drugs Ther 1991;*5:*853.
42. Zhao M, Ahang H, Robinson TF et al. Profound structural alterations of the extracellular collagen matrix in postischemic ("stunned") but viable myocardium. J Am Coll Cardiol 1987;*10:*1322.
43. Charney RH, Takahashi S, Zhao M, Sonnenblick EH, Eng C. Collagen loss in the stunned myocardium. Circulation 1992;*85:*1483.
44. Schaper W. Molecular mechanisms in "stunned" myocardium. Cardiovasc Drugs Ther 1991;*5:*925.
45. Laster SB, Becker LC, Ambrosio G, Jacobus WE. Reduced aerobic metabolic efficiency in globally "stunned" myocardium. J Mol Cell Cardiol 1989;*21:*419.
46. Mullane K, Engler R. Proclivity of activated neutrophils to cause post-ischemic cardiac dysfunction: participation in stunning? Cardiovasc Drugs Ther 1991;*5:*915.
47. Opie LH. Postischemic stunning: the case for calcium as the ultimate culprit. Cardiovasc Drugs Ther 1991;*5:*895.
48. Rahimtoola SH. The hibernating myocardium. Am Heart J 1989;*117:*211.
49. Ross J Jr. Myocardial perfusion–contraction matching. Implications for coronary heart disease and hibernation. Circulation 1991;*83:*1076.
50. Downing SE, Chen V. Myocardial hibernation in the ischemic neonatal heart. Circ Res 1990;*66:*763.
51. Fedele FA, Gerwitz H, Capone RJ et al. Metabolic response to prolonged reduction of myocardial blood flow distal to a severe coronary artery stenosis. Circulation 1988;*78:*729.
52. Pantely GA, Malone SA, Rhen WS et al. Regeneration of myocardial phosphocreatine in pigs despite continued moderate ischemia. Circ Res 1990;*67:*1481.
53. Schulz R, Guth BD, Pieper K, Martin C, Heusch G. Recruitment of an inotropic reserve in mod-

erately ischemic myocardium at the expense of metabolic recovery. A model of short-term hibernation. Circ Res 1992;*70:*1282.

54. Marban E. Myocardial stunning and hibernation. The physiology behind the colloquialisms. Circulation 1991;*83:*681.

55. Uren NG, Camici PG. Hibernation and myocardial ischemia: clinical detection by positron emission tomography. Cardiovasc Drugs Ther 1992;*6:*273.

56. Reimer KA, Jennings RB. The "wavefront phenomenon" of myocardial ischemic cell death. II. Transmural progression of necrosis within the framework of ischemic bed size (myocardium at risk) and collateral flow. Lab Invest 1979;*40:*633.

57. Dellsperger KC, Marcus ML. Effects of left ventricular hypertrophy on the coronary circulation. Am J Cardiol 1990;*65:*1504.

58. Schaper W. Residual perfusion of acutely ischemic heart muscle. In: Schaper W (ed) The Pathophysiology of Myocardial Perfusion. Elsevier, Amsterdam, 1979.

59. Kloner RA, Ganote CE, Jennings RB. The "no-reflow" phenomenon after temporary coronary occlusion in the dog. J Clin Invest 1974;*54:*1496.

60. Rowland FN, Donovan MJ, Picciano PT, Wilner GD, Kreutzer DL. Fibrin-mediated vascular injury. Identification of fibrin peptides that mediate endothelial cell retraction. Am J Pathol 1984;*117:*418.

61. Crawford MH, Grover FL, Kolb WP et al. Complement and neutrophil activation in the pathogenesis of ischemic myocardial injury. Circulation 1988;*78:*1449.

62. Hackett D, Davies G, Chierchia S, Maseri A. Intermittent coronary occlusion in acute myocardial infarction. Value of combined thrombolytic and vasodilator therapy. N Engl J Med 1987;*317:*1055.

63. Factor SM, Okun EM, Kirk ES. The histological lateral border of acute canine myocardial infarction. Circ Res 1981;*48:*640.

64. Ferrari R, Visioli O. Protective effects of calcium antagonists against ischaemia and reperfusion damage. Drugs 1991;*42:*14.

65. Nayler W. The molecular basis for the use of calcium antagonists in ischaemic heart disease. Drugs 1992;*43:*21.

66. Baroldi G. Different types of myocardial necrosis in coronary heart disease: a pathophysiologic review of their functional significance. Am Heart J 1975;*89:*742.

67. Robbins S, Angell M. Myocardial infarction. In: Robbins S, Angell M (eds) Basic Pathology, 2nd Edition. WB Saunders, Philadelphia. 1976, p. 296.

68. Hutchins GM, Bulkley BH. Infarct expansion versus extension: two different complications of acute myocardial infarction. Am J Cardiol 1978;*41:*1127.

69. Pfeffer JM, Pfeffer MA, Braunwald E. Influence of chronic captopril therapy on the infarcted left ventricle of the rat. Circ Res 1985;*57:*84.

70. Anversa P, Beghi C, Kikkawa Y, Olivetti G. Myocardial infarction in rats: infarct size, myocyte hypertrophy, and capillary growth. Circ Res 1986;*58:*26.

71. Gettes LS. Effect of ischemia on cardiac electrophysiology. In: Fozzard HA, Haber E, Jennings RB, Katz AM, Morgan HE (eds) The Heart and Cardiovascular System. Raven Press, New York 1986;*2:*1317.

72. Malliani A, Schwartz PJ, Zanchetti A. Neural mechanisms in life-threatening arrhythmias. Am Heart J 1980;*100:*705.

73. Schwartz PJ, Billman GE, Stone HL. Autonomic mechanisms in ventricular fibrillation induced by myocardial ischemia during exercise in dogs with healed myocardial infarction. Circulation 1984;*69:*790.

74. Mehra R, Zeiler RH, Gough WB, El-Sherif N. Reentrant ventricular arrhythmias in the late myocardial infarction period. 9. Electrophysiologic–anatomic correlation of reentrant circuits. Circulation 1983;*67:*11.

75. Kimura S, Basset AL, Kohya T et al. Automaticity, triggered activity, and responses to adrenergic stimulation in cat subendocardial Purkinje fibers after healing of myocardial infarction. Circulation 1987;*75:*651.

76. Vracko R, Thorning D, Frederickson RG. Fate of nerve fibers in necrotic, healing, and healed rat myocardium. Lab Invest 1990;*63:*490.

77. Zipes DP. Influence of myocardial ischemia and infarction on autonomic innervation of heart. Circulation 1990;*82:*1095.

78. Tanaka K, Hearse DJ. Reperfusion-induced arrhythmias in the isolated rabbit heart: characterization of the influence of the duration of regional ischemia and the extracellular potassium concentration. J Mol Cell Cardiol 1988;*20:*201.

79. Reimer KA, Jennings RB. Effects of reperfusion on infarct size: experimental studies. Eur Heart J 1985;*6 (Suppl E):*97.

80. Malliani A. Cardiocardiac excitatory reflexes during myocardial ischemia. In: Heusch G, Ross J Jr (eds) Adrenergic mechanisms in myocardial ischemia. Steinkopff Verlag, Darmstadt, 1990.

81. Schömig A, Richardt G. Cardiac sympathetic activity in myocardial ischemia: release and effects of noradrenaline. In: Heusch G, Ross J Jr (eds) Adrenergic mechanisms in myocardial ischemia. Steinkopff Verlag, Darmstadt, 1990.

82. Gallagher KP. Transmural steal with isoproterenol and exercise in poststenotic myocardium. In: Heusch G, Ross J Jr (eds) Adrenergic mechanisms in myocardial ischemia. Steinkopff Verlag, Darmstadt, 1990.

83. Jones CE, Gwirtz PA. α_1-Adrenergic coronary constriction during exercise and ischemia. In: Heusch G, Ross J Jr (eds) Adrenergic mechanisms in myocardial ischemia. Steinkopff Verlag, Darmstadt, 1990.

84. Seitelberger R, Guth BD, Heusch G, Ross J Jr. α_2-Adrenergic coronary constriction in ischemic myocardium during exercise. In: Heusch G, Ross J Jr (eds) Adrenergic mechanisms in myocardial ischemia. Steinkopff Verlag, Darmstadt, 1990.

85. Feigl EO. The paradox of adrenergic coronary vasoconstriction. Circulation 1987;*76:*737.

86. Ebert PA, Vanderbeek RB, Allgood RJ, Sabiston Jr DC. Effect of chronic cardiac denervation on arrhythmias after coronary artery ligation. Cardiovasc Res 1970;*4:*141.

87. Janse MJ, Schwartz PJ, Wilms-Schopman F, Peters JG, Durrer D. Effects of unilateral stellate ganglion stimulation and ablation on electrophysiologic changes induced by acute myocardial ischemia in dogs. Circulation 1985;*72:*585.

88. Schwartz PJ, Stone HL, Brown Am. Effects of unilateral stellate ganglion blockade on the arrhythmias associated with coronary occlusion. Am Heart J 1976;*92:*589.

89. Schwartz PJ, Vanoli E. Cardiac arrhythmias elicited by interaction between acute myocardial ischemia and sympathetic hyperactivity: a new experimental model for the study of antiarrhythmic drugs. J Cardiovasc Pharmacol 1981;*3:*1251.

90. Schwartz PJ, Billman GE, Stone HL. Autonomic mechanism in ventricular fibrillation induced by myocardial ischemia during exercise in dogs with a healed myocardial infarction. An experimental preparation for sudden cardiac death. Circulation 1984;*69:*780.

91. Lombardi F, Verrier RL, Lown B. Relationship between sympathetic neural activity, coronary dynamics, and vulnerability to ventricular fibrillation during myocardial ischemia and reperfusion. Am Heart J 1983;*105:*958.

92. Schwartz PJ, Vanoli E, Stramba-Badiale M, De Ferrari GM, Billman GE, Foreman RD. Autonomic mechanisms and sudden death. New insight from the analysis of baroreceptor reflexes in conscious dogs with and without a myocardial infarction. Circulation 1988;*78:*969.

93. Haverkamp W, Gülker H, Hindricks G, Breithardt G. Effects of β-blockade on the incidence of ventricular tachyarrhythmias during acute myocardial ischemia: experimental findings and clinical implications. Basic Res Cardiol 1990;*85 (Suppl I):*293.

94. Willber DJ, Lynch JJ, Montgomery DG, Lucchesi BR. Alpha-adrenergic influences in canine ischemic sudden death: effects of alpha-1 adrenoceptor blockade with prazosin. J Cardiovasc Pharmacol 1987;*10:*96.

Major pathogenetic components and time course of ischemic heart disease

CHAPTER 8

The variable chronic atherosclerotic background

INTRODUCTION

The term "atherosclerosis" is commonly used to describe almost any raised lesion involving the intimal layer of the wall of epicardial coronary arteries, regardless of its nature or pathogenetic and etiologic mechanisms. However, "fatty streaks" involving the intima, Monckeberg's sclerosis characterized by medial calcification, and arteriolosclerosis characterized by either intimal fibromuscular proliferative thickening or medial hyperplasia, are usually considered separately. Atherosclerotic lesions can be induced by a variety of stimuli, ranging from a lipid diet in normal animals to immunologic reactions taking place in the transplanted hearts of children. The general term of "atherosclerosis" is justified by the frequent association of atherosclerotic lesions of roughly similar morphology with the development of ischemic syndromes, but it prevents the search for the specific role of individual atherogenic stimuli and the variable response of the arterial wall in the development of the lesions and of their thrombotic or vasoconstrictor potential.

In patients with ischemic heart disease (IHD) the intimal involvement is focal rather than uniformly diffuse, producing individual lesions known as "plaques." The term "atheroma" is derived from the Greek "athera" (gruel) and was originally applied to plaques with a central core of yellow fluid. However, over 95% of smaller plaques in human coronary arteries are composed only of ground substance and fibrous tissue in variable proportions and show no "atheroma" (see below). Although the lesions broadly described as atherosclerotic have variable histologic features and varied origins, they are generally classified into only two types—fibrous or complicated plaques.

Fibrous plaques are typically characterized by a fibrous cap covering a raised lesion composed of fibrous tissue of variable density, with or without a deep core of extracellular lipids and cellular debris. They have four histologic features that occur in variable proportions:

1. Intimal proliferation of smooth muscle cells (SMCs) with occasional and variable accumulation of macrophages.
2. Accumulation of large amounts of collagen and ground substance.
3. Variable accumulation of extracellular and intracellular lipids (usually only in larger lesions).
4. Possible formation of cellular debris and calcium deposits, smooth muscle atro-

phy, intimal and adventitial perineural inflammatory cell infiltrates, and neovascularization, all of which are present only in larger lesions.

Any one of these four features may predominate in different individuals and also in different lesions in the same individual, producing a whole spectrum of lesions with different characteristics, and, possibly, with very different origins and clinical consequences.
Complicated plaques probably originate from some types of fibrous plaques. They are characterized by one or more of the following features:

a. a broken cap
b. an intraplaque hemorrhage, and/or
c. a superimposed mural thrombus in various stages of organization.

The variable features and evolution of plaques, first, depend on the nature of the noxious stimuli that initiate the lesion (chemical, physical, or inflammatory); second, reflect the local response of the coronary arterial wall to such noxious stimuli and to the repair process; and third, are affected by the interaction of the individual lesion with blood constituents, which strongly influence the lesion's progression and outcome.

Only stenosing plaques persistently limit coronary flow, but nonflow-limiting atherosclerotic lesions may also occasionally and unpredictably interfere with coronary blood flow (CBF) if they have vasomotor or thrombotic potential.

The lipid theory, most popular in the United States, proposes that atherosclerotic plaques originate from fatty streaks and are caused by excessive deposits of cholesterol. Although this is most likely the case in young individuals with familial hypercholesterolemia, there is no conclusive evidence that this applies to all or most plaques in most individuals.

This chapter summarizes the information obtained from postmortem and angiographic studies and examines the vasomotor and thrombotic ischemic potential of coronary atherosclerotic lesions and the mechanisms of atherogenesis.

8.1 POSTMORTEM AND ANGIOGRAPHIC FINDINGS

The relationship between coronary atherosclerosis and ischemic manifestations should be evaluated, first, by comparing the severity of atherosclerotic involvement in the coronary arteries of individuals with no history of IHD who died of noncardiac causes with that of patients who died of IHD; second, by assessing the severity of coronary atherosclerosis in the various ischemic syndromes, and third, by correlating the evolution of ischemic manifestations with that of coronary atherosclerotic lesions.

Angiographic and postmortem data are somewhat complementary. Angiographic data, examined by the patient's physician, can easily be correlated not only with the ischemic manifestations but also with their evolution and may provide information on vasomotor abnormalities; they cannot, however, provide accurate information on the extent of coronary atherosclerosis or data on histologic alterations. Postmortem data provide a precise account of the anatomic and histologic lesions at the time of death, but usually cannot be accurately correlated with antemortem symptoms and signs of ischemia and their evolution in time, nor can they provide information on abnormalities of coronary thrombotic tendency and vasomotion during life. Intracoronary echocardiography, a technique now in a rapid phase of development, may provide an invasive research tool for mapping in vivo the coronary lumina of major coronary branches and the involvement by atherosclerotic plaques relative to the internal elastic lamina, and for assessing the local vasomotor potential. Endarterectomy specimens can provide valuable local histologic information.

8.1.1 Assessment of stenosis severity and wall remodeling

The extent of the involvement of the coronary intimal surface by raised fibrous plaque can be assessed either *post mortem,* by examining arteries that are cut open either longitudinally or in cross-sections at regular distances (usually 5 mm) apart, or at *angiography,* by estimating for each coronary segment the fraction of the luminal profile that exhibits stenoses or wall irregularities. There are traditional differences in the way that stenosis severity is expressed at autopsy and angiography: at autopsy, stenoses are expressed as the percentage reduction in the luminal area caused by subintimal plaque; at angiography, they are expressed as percentage reduction in diameter in relation to an adjacent "normal" reference segment. Both methods have inherent limitations, as discussed below, but even when they are both correct, 50, 70 and 90% diameter stenoses would correspond respectively to 75, 91 and 99% luminal area stenoses, simply because of the quadratic relationship between diameter (2r) and area (πr^2) of a circle (see Table 8.1). In addition to these purely geometric differences, there are other sources of error in the estimate of stenosis severity with both techniques, and a major difference related to wall and lumen remodeling at the site of plaques (see below).

Postmortem measurements

With this technique, the severity of the stenosis may be overestimated when the coronary arteries are not fixed at "physiologic" distending pressure or when remodeling with compensatory dilation of the atherosclerotic vessel wall at the site of the plaque is significant (see below). Comparisons between arteriography in vivo and autopsy findings consistently underestimate the severity of the stenosis in vivo,[1] largely owing to compensatory remodeling of the lumen.

Table 8.1 Geometric relation between diameter and area of a stenotic vessel (expressed as a percentage)*

Flow-limiting	Percentage Reduction Caused by Stenosis	
	In diameter	In area
No	10	19
	20	36
	30	51
	40	64
	50	75
Yes	60	84
	70	91
	80	96
	90	99

*The percentage of a stenosis is usually expressed as a percentage reduction of diameter in angiographic studies and of area in postmortem studies. The percentage reduction is greater for area than for diameter because of the quadratic relation between diameter and area of a circle

Angiographic measurements

With this technique, the severity of the stenosis may be underestimated when the reference diameter is also stenosed, when the X-ray beam is not perpendicular to the longitudinal axis of the vessel, or when the maximal narrowing is superimposed on other branches.

Conversely, the severity of organic stenoses may be overestimated when peristenotic vasomotor tone is increased and when stenoses are very severe or occur in small vessels. The overestimation of severe stenoses derives from the limited resolution of radiographic techniques, which prevents the visualization of stenotic segments below 0.3 mm in diameter, even under optimal geometric conditions: thus, a 90% stenosis of a 3 mm diameter vessel will appear in the image as an interruption of the vessel, even under ideal filming conditions.

Remodeling of the vessel wall at the site of plaques

Recent quantitative morphometric studies indicate that the development of atherosclerotic subintimal plaque is associated with remodeling and compensatory dilation of the arterial wall (see Fig. 8.1). Thus, until the plaque occupies about 40% of the internal elastic laminal area, appreciable reduction of the lumen is prevented by expansion of the atherosclerotic segment towards the outside of the wall.[2] A 90% area stenosis calculated morphometrically from the ratio of the residual lumen to the area included within the internal elastic lamina may, therefore, correspond to a 60% area stenosis (less than 40% diameter reduction) relative to the normal lumen calculated from angiography (see Fig. 8.2). The relationship between the morphologic features of plaques and their ischemic potential is discussed in section 8.2.

■ *These observations indicate that, on the one hand, angiographically normal segments may have sizeable subintimal plaques and, on the other, that even severe stenoses seen postmortem may not be flow limiting. The prevalence, mechanisms and significance of remodeling have so far received scant attention.* ■

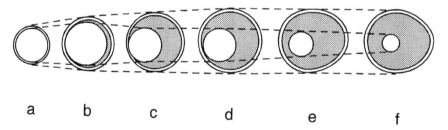

a   b   c   d   e   f

Fig. 8.1 Remodeling of the lumen associated with growth of atherosclerotic plaques. The area encircled by the internal elastic lamina increases progressively at the site of a plaque compared with that of proximal normal segments. Thus, initially, the lumen at the site of the plaque actually increases above normal, and becomes reduced compared with the proximal normal segment only when the plaque occupies a very considerable fraction of the area encircled by the internal elastic lamina. In sections b and c, the lumen is dilated compared with that in section a. In section f, although the reduction in area of the internal elastica lamina looks impressive, the diameter of the original lumen (a) is reduced by only 48%. The reasons for the early remodeling with dilation of the lumen are not known: they may be very prevalent in some patients and in some segments of artery to give rise to local arterial ectasia. (Modified from ref. 2.)

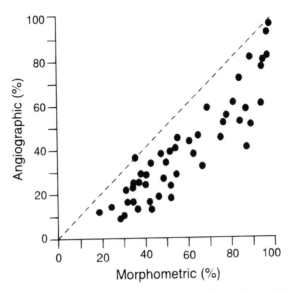

Fig. 8.2 Relation between morphometric and angiographic postmortem measurements of area of stenosis. Morphometric measurements overestimate to a variable degree the actual reduction of the lumen because of the remodeling process described in Fig. 8.1. A 90% area stenosis measured at postmortem examination may correspond to a 75% or less luminal area stenosis (i.e. to a 50% or less diameter stenosis). (Modified from ref. 1.)

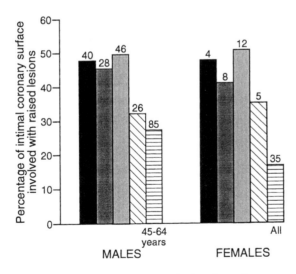

Fig. 8.3 Percentage of coronary artery intimal surface covered by raised fibrous plaque in fatal ischemic syndromes and in controls. About 50% of the intimal surface area is covered by raised lesions in individuals with old (▨), or recent (▨), or recent and old (■) MI. Only about 30% of the intima is covered by plaque in sudden coronary deaths which occur as the very first manifestation of IHD (◩). This percentage is similar to that found in individuals who died violently (▤). The differences between men and women are not significant. Numbers above columns are numbers of individuals. (Modified from ref. 4.)

8.1.2 Coronary atherosclerosis in "control" subjects dying of noncardiac causes

As stated in the introductory chapter, individuals who died of noncardiac causes have, on average, less extensive and less severe coronary atherosclerosis than patients who died of IHD. However, in most industrialized countries the vast majority of individuals over the age of 50 who died accidentally, without symptoms or signs of IHD, exhibit extensive coronary artery raised fibrous plaques, as well as flow-limiting stenoses.

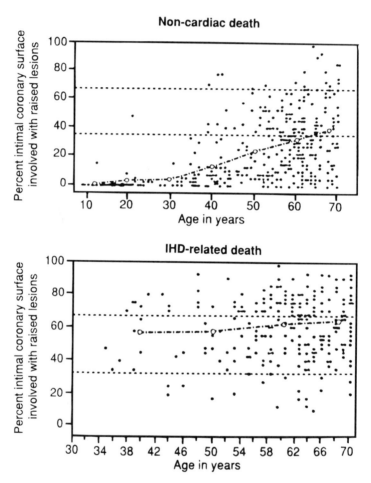

Fig. 8.4 **Percentage of the intimal surface of the major coronary arteries covered by raised fibrous plaque in patients dying of IHD and in controls.** Data from the Oslo study, one of the centers involved in the International Atherosclerosis Project; the results from the other centers were similar. The percentage of the intimal surface of the coronary arteries covered by raised fibrous plaques in patients dying of IHD **(A)** was, on average, higher than that found in individuals dying of noncardiac causes **(B),** but there is considerable overlap between the two groups (Mean values are indicated by open circles connected by dashed lines.) Many patients in the IHD group had less than one-third of the intimal surface of the coronary artery covered by plaque; conversely, many individuals in the control group had more than two-thirds of the intimal surface covered by plaque. Some individuals have no plaques, even in old age, indicating that the process is not an inevitable consequence of aging. (Modified from ref 5.)

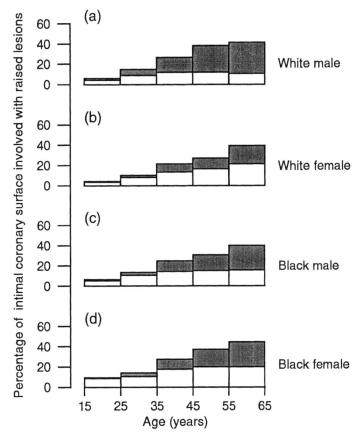

Fig. 8.5 Relation between raised fibrous plaques and fatty streaks in (a) white males, (b) white females, (c) black males, and (d) black females. The average percentage of the coronary intima covered by raised fibrous plaques (■) and by fatty streaks (□) varies considerably with age, gender, and race. The reasons for this variability are not known. On average, only 60% of the intima is macroscopically normal but a large dispersion of individual values about the mean is to be expected on the basis of the data presented in Fig. 8.4. (Modified from ref. 6.)

8.1.2.1 *Extent of raised fibrous plaque*

In the Pooling Project,[3] coordinated, prospective postmortem studies from different countries consistently demonstrated that in major epicardial coronary artery branches the percentage of the intimal surface covered by raised fibrous plaque, first, increases progressively with age up to the sixth decade of life, second, is, on average, higher in populations with a greater incidence of IHD, and third, can be relatively low in some individuals who died of IHD and, conversely, can be very high in others who died of noncardiac causes.

Average percentage values of intima covered by raised fibrous plaque are higher in patients with recent or old infarctions than in those in whom sudden death was the first manifestation of IHD, in which the average values were similar to those in individuals who died violently (see Fig. 8.3).[4]

Although the percentage of the intimal surface covered by plaque was found, on average, to be lower in controls than in patients with IHD in all age-groups, the overlap was quite large: many patients who died of IHD had less than one-third of the intimal surface of major epicardial coronary arteries covered with plaque, whereas many "controls" had more than

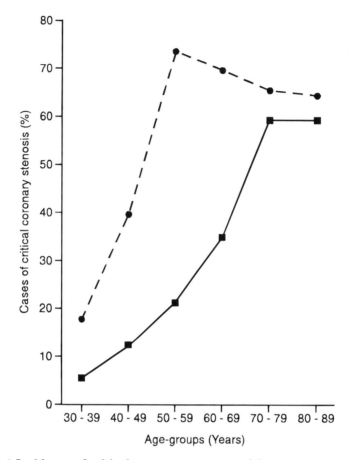

Fig. 8.6 Incidence of critical coronary stenoses with age at autopsy. In 1200 cases of in-hospital mortality (600 men (dashed line) and 600 women (continuous line) subdivided into six groups of 100 unselected cases per decade for both men and women, the percentage of cases with at least one critical coronary stenosis increases with age but then plateaus. About 60% of men had at least one critical coronary stenosis by the sixth decade; the same percentage is reached only in the seventh decade in women. (Modified from refs. 9 and 10.)

two-thirds covered with plaque (see Fig. 8.4). Extensive raised fibrous plaque is less common in nonindustrialized countries with a low incidence of IHD.[5]

In patients with IHD and in control subjects, in addition to raised fibrous plaque, another 10–20% of the intima was found to be covered by "fatty streaks," with considerable variability associated with age, gender, and race (see Fig. 8.5).[6]

Flow-limiting stenoses

The presence of flow-limiting stenoses in individuals who died of noncardiac causes is documented in a large series of studies.[3,4,7,8] Stenoses were shown to increase with age up to the sixth decade of life, with a trend similar to that of raised plaque covering the coronary intima, and to occur earlier in men than in women (see Fig. 8.6).[9,10] The lack of increase in the extent of coronary atherosclerosis after the age of 65 is consistent with the fact that the incidence of angina pectoris in the general population plateaus at the age of 60, but is in sharp contrast with the exponential increase in mortality from myocardial infarction (MI) after this age (see Ch. 11). Compared with individuals who died of noncardiac causes or violently, the number of coronary stenoses greater than 50% in diameter was found to be similar,[4] or only slightly higher,[8] in individuals in whom sudden ischemic cardiac death (SICD) was the first manifestation of IHD, or in those with their first MI (see Fig. 8.7A,B). It is possible that some individuals with extensive coronary fibrous plaque and/or flow-limiting

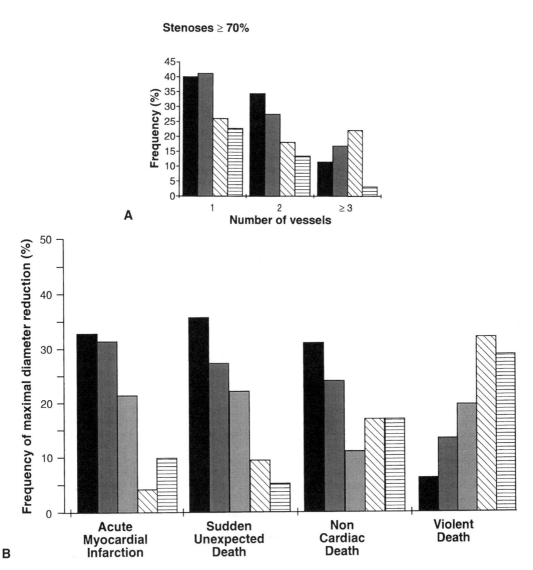

Fig. 8.7 Number and severity of coronary stenoses in acute IHD death and in controls. (A) The number of cases with more than 70% diameter stenoses in one, two, or three vessels is similar in acute MI (■), unexpected SICD (■) (witnessed within 15 min of the onset of symptoms) and in noncardiac death (◳), but is lower in violent death (▤) (occurring, in general, in younger individuals). **(B)** The maximal diameter reduction (■, ≥90%; ■, 80–89%; ■, 70–79%; ◳, 50–69%; ▤, <50%) found in any of the major coronary arteries was also on average similar in acute MI, SICD and noncardiac death, but was significantly lower in violent death. (Modified from ref. 8.)

stenoses who died of noncardiac causes might have experienced episodes of silent or unrecognized myocardial ischemia during life: they were, nevertheless, asymptomatic and did not die of IHD.

For obvious reasons, coronary arteriography during life cannot be performed in "control" subjects, but coronary stenoses are found much less frequently in patients with valvular heart disease than in those with clinical manifestations of IHD. However, in the Coronary Artery Surgery Study (CASS) about 20% of 20 000 patients with angina severe enough to justify angiography[11] were found to have no flow-limiting stenoses, or even had angiographically normal coronary arteries; although a number of these patients may have had extracardiac causes for their symptoms, at least some could have had myocardial ischemia.

■ *Thus, in most individuals above the age of 50 with no signs of IHD, only a fraction of the coronary artery intimal surface is macroscopically normal. A sharp contrast exists between the exponential increase in IHD mortality and the lack of increase of coronary atherosclerosis after the age of 65.* ■

8.1.3 Severity of coronary atherosclerosis in the various ischemic syndromes

In general, postmortem and angiographic studies that specifically consider the features of coronary atherosclerosis in a selected ischemic syndrome—such as MI, angina pectoris, or SICD—also include patients with histories of other ischemic syndromes. Studies of SICD usually include a mixture of patients who previously had displayed chronic stable or unstable angina and/or infarction; patients with MI include patients with a history of chronic stable or unstable angina, and studies of chronic stable angina include patients with a history of MI. It is not surprising, therefore, that the conclusions of the vast majority of postmortem and angiographic studies that followed such broad inclusion criteria, are that the severity of coronary atherosclerosis and the number of major coronary artery branches with flow-limiting stenoses are similar in patients with chronic stable angina, unstable angina, MI, and SICD.

Histological sections of the main coronary artery branches, 5 mm in length, obtained from unselected patients with each of the syndromes mentioned above, usually exhibit very extensive coronary lesions.[12] However, the extent of the involvement may vary from multivessel coronary stenoses (more common in older patients with a long history of IHD) to a few flow-limiting stenoses (more frequently found in patients below the age of 40 with very recent onset of IHD). In general, autopsy material is likely to include patients who were more vulnerable to ischemic insults, i.e. those with extensive left ventricular damage and the most extensive coronary artery disease, and hence with a long, composite history of IHD.

In order to establish a more precise correlation between the features of the coronary atherosclerotic background and the specific ischemic syndromes recognized clinically, it is essential to consider "pure" subsets of patients, i.e. those who can be studied at the time of their very first presentation of IHD.

Chronic stable angina

Angiographic studies in a selected group of patients with a history of uncomplicated chronic stable angina of 2–15 years' duration and no signs of infarction showed that the number of stenoses and total occlusions, as well as the extent of detectable atherosclerosis in the main coronary arterial segment, were nearly twice those found in patients with their

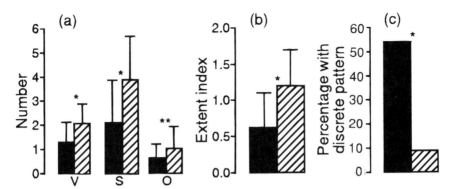

Fig. 8.8 Angiographic assessment of coronary atherosclerosis in patients with unheralded MI as the very first manifestation of IHD and in those with uncomplicated chronic stable angina of about 5 years' duration. The (a) severity (number of vessels with critical stenosis [V], number of stenoses [S], and occlusions [O]), (b) extent (average score of each coronary segment in terms of the length involved by atheroma), and (c) pattern (diffuse versus discrete segmental coronary atherosclerotic involvement) were significantly greater in uncomplicated angina (◪) than in MI (■). (Modified from ref. 13.)

first unheralded MI (see Fig. 8.8).[13] These data are consistent with postmortem findings in patients with chronic stable angina with no signs of old MI, which confirm that total coronary occlusion is quite common in the absence of distal myocardial scars, and show that many vessels exhibit multichanneled stenoses resulting from recanalized thrombi.[14] Some thrombotic occlusions, recanalized by newly formed channels, appear to have occurred at the site of only mild stenoses without causing MI (see Fig. 8.9). Thus, in patients with stable angina, severe coronary stenoses can be present for years and total thrombotic occlusion may develop with no evidence of MI, and later be gradually recanalized by newly formed channels.

De novo unstable angina

In unselected patients with unstable angina, postmortem and angiographic studies show that the severity of stenoses is comparable to that found in patients with chronic stable angina, but the frequency of irregular stenoses, compatible with plaque rupture and thrombosis, is much higher. (A review of the subject by Fuster is contained in reference 15.) Patients in whom unstable angina was the very first manifestation of IHD can only be studied angiographically because, if they die, they become cases of either acute MI or SICD, which may occur soon after the onset of acute coronary occlusion. Angiography in such patients shows that the coronary atherosclerotic background is characterized much more frequently by a single-vessel flow-limiting stenosis, largely resulting from an organized local thrombus, than by severe multivessel coronary disease, as is the case in complicated chronic stable angina or in patients with a long composite history of IHD.[16]

Acute MI as the first manifestation of IHD

The study of such patients allows the extent of the atherosclerotic background that predisposes to the development of acute coronary occlusion to be assessed, without the confounding effects of lesions that could previously have been responsible for either chronic stable angina or other infarctions.

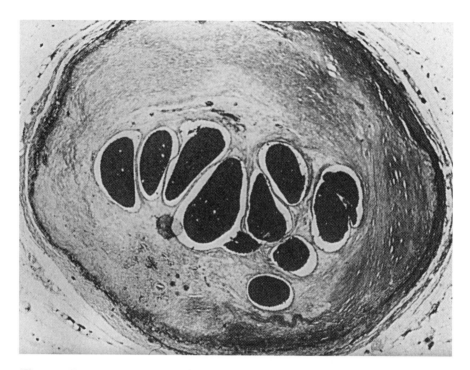

Fig. 8.9 Recanalized thrombus in a histologic section of a coronary artery from a patient with chronic stable angina. A very large section of the lumen is replaced by multiple channels resulting from the recanalization of a massive thrombus that formed at the site of a mild stenosis. (Modified from ref. 14.)

In patients younger than 60 years of age, angiographic studies show that a strong prevalence of single-vessel disease[13] and mild residual coronary stenosis after thrombolysis is fairly common, not only in patients with their first MI (see Fig. 8.10),[17] but also in other groups of unselected patients. Thus, in acute MI occurring as the very first manifestation of IHD, as in de novo unstable angina, severe coronary stenoses or extensive angiographically detectable nonstenosing coronary atherosclerosis (which usually characterizes chronic stable angina) do not appear to be necessary prerequisites for the development of the first sudden acute coronary occlusion.

The angiographic observation that MI can be unrelated to flow-limiting stenoses is in keeping with postmortem studies, such as the Pooling Project,[3] and others.[4,7,8,18] Even angiographically normal coronary arteries are found in about 5–10% of cases and this percentage increases to 25% in individuals younger than 35 years of age.[19–21] This previously puzzling finding can now be explained by the angiographic demonstration that arteries found to be occluded soon after the onset of symptoms of acute MI, undergo very early spontaneous recanalization in 40–50% of cases (see Ch. 9).

Sudden ischemic cardiac death

Sudden death may occur at variable stages in the course of the clinical manifestations of IHD; it is the very first presentation of IHD in about 15% of individuals and is the last event in about 50% of patients with established IHD, independent of their degree of functional

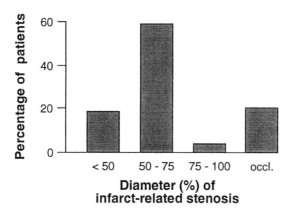

Fig. 8.10 Severity of residual stenosis at the very end of intracoronary thrombolysis in patients with their first MI. The residual stenosis is less than 50% in diameter in about 20% of cases and less than 75% in about 60% of cases; occl., occluded. This may represent an overestimate of the preexisting stenosis if not all the thrombus was lysed. (Modified from ref. 17.)

cardiac impairment (i.e. NYHA Classification Classes I–IV) (see Ch. 24). The most common postmortem anatomical substratum in the total number of SICD patients with known IHD is, therefore, heavily biased in favor of the severe extensive coronary disease typical of patients in NYHA Classes III or IV, who have by far the highest total mortality rate and who represent the largest fraction of the total. However, at postmortem examination in previously healthy individuals in whom SICD was the very first manifestation of IHD, and which was preceded within not more than 1 h by the onset of ischemic cardiac pain, the severity of coronary atherosclerosis is similar to that found in controls dying of noncardiac causes or presenting with infarction out of the blue, and overlaps, to some extent, with the findings in individuals dying from noncardiac causes or accidentally (see Figs 8.3 and 8.7).

■ *Thus, SICD, which represents the most dramatic cardiac response to acute myocardial ischemia, usually develops in individuals with a relatively mild coronary atherosclerotic background when it is the very first manifestation of IHD, and in patients with severe left ventricular dysfunction and a severe atherosclerotic background when it is the last event of a composite history of IHD.* ■

8.1.4 Discrepancies between initial severity or progression of coronary stenoses and ischemic manifestations

Repeated angiographic studies in patients with established IHD, who either exhibited worsening of symptoms and the development of new infarctions or remained quite stable, show a marked discrepancy between initial severity or progression of angiographically demonstrated coronary artery stenoses and ischemic manifestations. The isolated development of new severe lesions and the obvious rapid progression of some mild or moderate stenoses, even to occlusion, with no changes occurring in the majority of other severe flow-limiting stenoses, were recognized in very early repeated angiographic studies,[22–24] and suggested a nonlinear progression of coronary atherosclerosis, with a dominant role of very localized alterations. In patients who underwent coronary arteriography three times,[25] progression of residual lesions was found to be a highly unpredictable process (see Fig. 8.11), not related

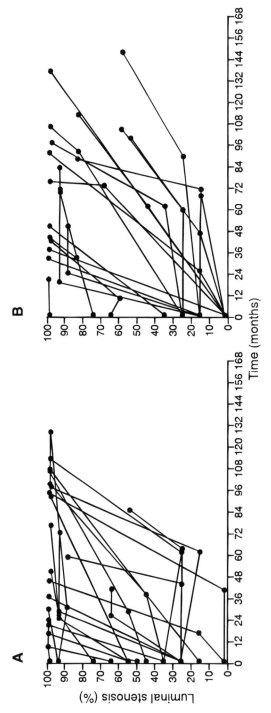

Fig. 8.11 Progression of luminal stenoses (%) in patients undergoing coronary arteriography on three occasions. The progression of stenoses in the right (**A**) and circumflex (**B**) coronary arteries was quite variable and not necessarily time dependent. Some severe stenoses remained unchanged over several years; other, minimal, stenoses became occluded in about 1 year. Stenosis progression was often, but not necessarily, associated with the development of MI. (Modified from ref. 25.)

significantly to known risk factors and often, but not necessarily always, associated with the development of MI and, hence, probably with an acute coronary thrombosis.

In patients who presented with unstable angina, repeated angiography showed progression of stenoses in 76% of cases, but progression was also observed in 31% of patients who remained stable; conversely, no detectable progression was seen in about one-quarter of unstable cases.[26] In addition, the analysis of angiograms performed before MI demonstrated that it was impossible to predict from the severity of coronary stenoses which artery would be the culprit, as most often it had only a minimal or mild stenosis, whereas more severe stenoses were present in other arteries (see Fig. 8.12A).[27,28] Moreover, following MI, progression of culprit coronary stenoses occurs only in some cases and not necessarily the most severe (see Fig. 8.12B). Progression of stenoses observed after either the onset of instability or MI is most likely related to incomplete lysis of recently formed thrombi. Thus, progression of the stenosis of the culprit vessel is often part of the process associated with the development of instability or infarction, rather than being its cause.

Retrospective analysis of angiograms performed at variable time intervals before the development of MI does not identify the future infarct-related artery, as infarction develops more often distal to minor plaques than distal to flow-limiting stenoses.

Ambrose et al[29] found that the median stenosis of the infarct-related artery was 48%. On average, it was 34% in those who developed a Q-wave MI and 80% in those who developed a nonQ-wave MI. Little et al[27] found that in 66% of patients the artery that subsequently occluded had a less than 50% stenosis on the postinfarct angiogram. They also observed that in only 34% of patients did the infarction occur due to occlusion of the artery that had previously contained the most severe stenosis. Giroud et al[30] found that 52% of the coronary artery segments responsible for a future MI were stenosed less than 20%, and 26% were stenosed between 21 and 50%. In only 23% of patients was MI related to the most severe stenosis.

At the other extreme, repeated angiographic examination shows that significant progression of coronary artery obstructions and total occlusion may develop with no evidence of myocardial ischemia and with no clinically detectable deterioration of symptoms and signs of ischemia or MI. Although irregular complex lesions are more likely to progress and be associated with the development of infarction than are smooth lesions,[31] they may remain stable for years or may progress without detectable ischemic manifestations (whereas, as discussed above, unstable angina or infarction may develop in the absence of gradual stenosis progression).

Stenoses may not necessarily progress, even when they are the site of reported occlusive spasm in patients with variant angina.[32]

In 103 stenoses measured by computerized angiography, Kaski et al[33] found that over an average interval of 15 months, progression was of similar proportions whether the initial presentation was acute MI, unstable angina, or chronic stable angina; 60% of complicated stenoses remained unchanged; 40% of patients who became unstable showed no stenosis progression, and 19% of patients who remained stable developed coronary occlusion at the site of a preexisting stenosis with no evidence of MI.

Crake et al[34] found that, in patients with chronic effort-related angina who remained stable and exhibited no changes in effort tolerance, obvious exacerbation of lesions and development of total occlusion may be common. In a study of 27 patients who underwent repeated angiography after intervals of 27 ± 1.3 months, according to various research protocols, 11 had obvious progression of coronary stenoses (eight to total occlusion or subocclusion) and, in five others, stenoses progressed in the absence of any clinical signs of instability. The development

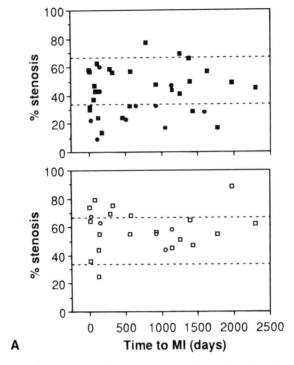

Fig. 8.12 The infarct-related artery cannot be identified from a coronary angiogram performed before the MI. (A) No relation can be seen between the severity of coronary stenoses in the infarct-related artery (indicated by closed symbols in the top panel), and the time interval between the angiogram and the MI. The MI often did not develop in the territory of the artery with the most severe stenoses (which are indicated in the lower panel by open symbols. (Data in squares from ref. 27 and in circles from ref. 28.) **(B)** The changes in stenosis severity after MI compared with the angiogram taken before the infarction. The variable progression of the stenosis is most likely related to a variable degree of incorporation of thrombus into the plaque, but in some cases no stenosis progression was detectable. Mean values are indicated by a dash. (Modified from ref. 28.) *(Figure continues.)*

of occlusion was not correlated with the initial severity of the lesion. Six new lesions developed in patients who exhibited progression but none developed in those who did not (see Fig. 8.13A,B).

A very gradual progression to occlusion with a parallel development of collaterals could explain the absence of unstable phases and of worsening of effort tolerance. However, as reported in 8.1.3, histologic studies in patients with pure forms of chronic stable angina[14] often show vessels where a thrombosis has been recanalized by multiple channels at the site of mild stenoses. Occlusion, therefore, may also have been thrombotic and failed to cause infarction because of the presence of preexisting collaterals.

8.1.5 Conclusions

In general, even the most careful postmortem examination confined to the epicardial coronary arteries cannot produce conclusive evidence as to whether or not the patient had chronic IHD.

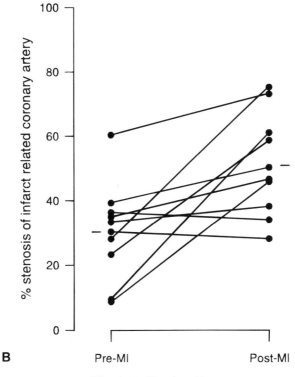

B Pre-MI Post-MI

Fig. 8.12 *(Continued.)*

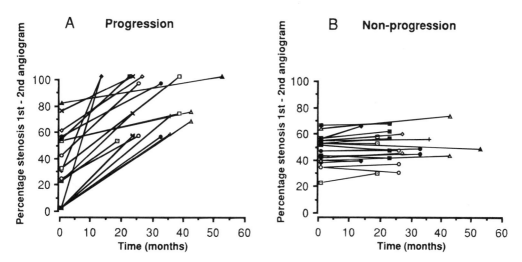

Fig. 8.13 Dissociation between stenosis progression and ischemic manifesta-tions in patients with chronic stable angina. In a group of patients with chronic stable angina who remained stable and in whom no changes in either exercise toler-ance or ventricular function were observed, stenosis progression up to occlusion was found in some lesions **(A)** but not in others **(B)** at the time of repeated angiography. The progression of stenoses and the development of new lesions was related neither to their initial severity nor to the time interval between the two angiograms (the sec-ond of which was performed purely for research purposes). In another group of patients included in the same study, no stenosis progression and no new lesions were observed, but neither patients with progression nor those without could be identified on the basis of known risk factors. (Modified from ref. 34.)

Postmortem studies cannot tell when and why the plaque originated; or, had the patient not died, which plaque would have grown; or if, when, and how it would have caused myocardial ischemia. At the time of the very first presentation of IHD there is a fairly weak correlation between the severity of coronary atherosclerosis and that of ischemic manifestations. The first reason for this is the broad overlap in the extent of coronary atherosclerosis observed in patients who died of IHD and in controls. The second factor is the mild degree of coronary stenosis frequently observed in patients who died from acute MI or SICD, when these events were the very first manifestations of IHD. This contrasts sharply with the extent and severity of coronary atherosclerosis observed in patients who present with uncomplicated chronic effort-related angina of many years' duration. The third reason is the lack of progression of coronary atherosclerosis observed in some patients with IHD who develop unstable angina and/or infarction, and conversely the obvious progression observed in others with chronic effort-related angina who remain stable. Finally, there is an obvious discrepancy between the exponential increase in the rate of mortality from IHD and the lack of progression of coronary atherosclerosis after the age of 65.

These conclusions are not new and are in line with those reached by Mitchell and Schwartz in 1963[7] and by Baroldi in 1978[8] in their postmortem studies.

"The factor that marks out these patients, (those with acute MI), therefore, is not the severity of coronary stenosis alone but the presence of coronary thrombosis. It is often suggested that wall disease must be present for a thrombus to form, but the main evidence for this concept is the rarity with which thrombosis occurs in a normal vessel. However, if one postulates that stenosis and thrombosis are not related, but are both age-dependent phenomena, thrombosis would thus be rare in normal arteries, for patients at risk from thrombosis would be unlikely to have normal arteries."[7]

■ *Although, in general, ischemic stimuli are more likely to occur in individuals with extensive, rather than limited coronary atherosclerosis, the lack of a close correlation between coronary atherosclerosis and ischemic manifestations points to a major role of occasional ischemic stimuli that cause the acute manifestations of IHD.* ■

8.2 ISCHEMIC POTENTIAL OF ATHEROSCLEROTIC PLAQUES

Each plaque may grow at a very variable rate to form a flow-limiting coronary stenosis that chronically limits the possible increase of flow and is only partly compensated for by the development of a collateral circulation. However, the ischemic potential of plaques depends not only on the severity of the reduction of the coronary lumen that they cause, but also on their propensity to become the site of local vasoconstriction and thrombosis. This propensity may be related to the origin and composition of a particular plaque, or to a predisposition to the localization of occasional inflammatory triggers of instability (toxic, immunologic, viral) (see Ch. 9).

The chronic limitation of flow is a *constant, stable* alteration and, therefore, it causes a predictable limitation of flow, modulated only by the behavior of distal and collateral vessels. The dynamic tendency to develop coronary constriction and thrombosis is *occasional* and hence causes an unpredictable impairment of flow. Both flow-limiting and minimally obstructive plaques may undergo vasoconstriction and/or thrombosis as a result of dynamic alterations to the endothelial lining and/or to the other layers of the wall.

Plaques exhibiting a dynamic modulation of the residual lumen by changes of peristenotic vasomotor tone may:

a. remain stable over a period of months and years, as is typically the case of some patients with chronic mixed stable angina

b. become associated with thrombosis or occlusive spasm over periods of days or weeks in some patients with unstable or variant angina, or

c. develop sudden persistent occlusion, typically in patients with acute MI.

Plaques exhibiting dynamic stenosis are not necessarily associated with a tendency to evolve towards persistent coronary occlusion. The morphology and composition of plaques may provide some clues to their flow-limiting potential, as well as to their possible acute thrombotic or vasomotor potential.

■ *In patients with and without flow-limiting stenoses and with either chronic stable or unstable angina, residual coronary flow reserve can be modulated, not only by changes in the stenotic lumen, but also by abnormal constriction of distal small coronary vessels (see Ch. 9).* ■

8.2.1 Morphology and composition of plaques

Not only the extent of lumen reduction, but also the morphology and composition of plaques, may contribute to their ischemic potential. Angiographically, a clinically useful classification of coronary stenoses, with a general histologic counterpart, is based on their morphology and has been described by Ambrose et al.[35] *Concentric stenoses* are usually fibrotic but can also be lipid rich and, when severe, are associated with considerable medial smooth muscle atrophy. *Eccentric stenoses with smooth borders* often have a disease-free wall arc length with preserved smooth muscle;[36] thus, the size of their residual lumen can be dynamically modulated by vasomotor stimuli. *Eccentric stenoses with irregular borders* correspond to complex lesions resulting from plaque fissures and/or fresh or organized mural thrombi. *Irregular plaques* are more susceptible to thrombosis at an early stage of their formation but may also remain stable for months and years.[33] The correspondence between angiographic and histopathologic aspects is not absolute: the sensitivity and specificity of angiography postmortem in detecting complicated plaques on the basis of irregular borders or intraluminal lucencies was found to be 88 and 79%, respectively;[37] obviously angiography in vivo is likely to have a lower sensitivity and specificity. In addition, occlusive thrombi recanalized by multiple channels, that cannot be detected by angiography, are found relatively often, even in the absence of signs of infarction.[14,38]

As a baseline to a better understanding of their ischemic potential, stenosing plaques can be classified into four types:

a. fixed flow-limiting stenoses (mostly concentric and severe)

b. stable plaques with vasomotor potential (mostly mild and eccentric with or without irregular borders)

c. unstable plaques with high thrombotic potential (mostly irregular)

d. potentially unstable plaques (often causing only mild stenoses).

The presence of detectable calcium deposits at the site of a plaque neither implies a flow-limiting stenosis nor excludes the possibility of local vasomotion. Thrombosis may form at the site of all plaques but only types b, c, and d above can undergo local vasoconstriction. The composition of plaques is discussed in 8.3.1.

8.2.2 Vasomotor potential of plaques: fixed and dynamic stenoses

The local vasomotor potential of plaques varies considerably. At one extreme, irregular stenoses, recently formed from the organization of a mural thrombus, in a previously near-normal vessel, are the most likely to retain a preserved arc of intact media and, therefore,

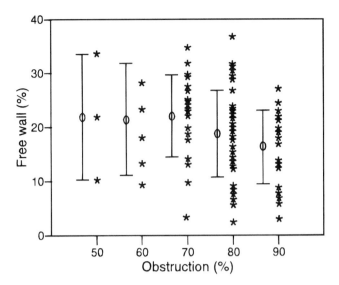

Fig. 8.14 Relation between the disease-free arc and severity of coronary stenosis. For area stenoses greater than 50% the percentage of the arc with preserved structure is, on average, about 20% but with considerable individual variations. Area stenoses less than 50% have a greater vasomotor potential. (Modified from ref. 36.)

have considerable vasomotor potential. At the other extreme, multichanneled recanalized thrombi are unlikely to have any vasomotor potential because the newly formed channels are surrounded by dense fibrous tissue. In between these two extremes are chronic smooth eccentric and concentric stenoses.

Studies carried out postmortem suggest that, on average, the potential for dynamic vasomotor changes is greatest in chronic mild eccentric stenoses and least in flow-limiting stenoses, particularly when they are concentric. This is confirmed by angiographic studies (see Ch. 9).

The percentage of concentric and eccentric stenoses at postmortem examination varies in different studies because the proportion of eccentric plaques becomes lower with increasing stenosis severity. Up to 70% of stenoses were found to be eccentric in one histologic study of 200 coronary artery segments.[39] Conversely, in another study, only 30% of 2121 stenoses were found to be eccentric (40% of stenoses with less than 70% diameter reduction and 13% with more than 70% diameter reduction).[40] In a study of patients with chronic stable angina, stenoses with an arc of normal vessel wall occupying more than 16% of the circumference were found in 15% of 448 lesions with stenoses more than 75% in diameter and in 44% of 693 plaques causing a 30–50% diameter stenosis.[14] In the same study, 20% of patients had no eccentric plaques, while in 7% all plaques were eccentric. In general, as the segment of free wall arc decreases with the severity of the stenosis, medial atrophy increases, but the relation between severity of stenosis and the arc free of disease is extremely variable (see Fig. 8.14).

Fixed flow-limiting stenoses

As discussed in Chapter 6, only plaques that reduce the lumen by about 70% of its original diameter limit flow by causing a critical transstenotic pressure gradient, which lowers the driving pressure at the origin of arterioles. Further reductions of the residual diameter beyond about 70%, caused by plaque growth or intraluminal thrombosis, increase the transstenotic pressure gradient exponentially. The length of the stenosis and the presence of multiple stenoses in series have lesser effects on the amount of flow limitation.

Stable plaques resulting in a critical, but *fixed*, limitation of coronary flow cause myocardial ischemia with a stable predictable pattern; ischemia develops only when (and every time that) myocardial oxygen consumption exceeds the residual flow reserve and the compensatory capacity of collaterals. A fixed limitation of coronary flow may be caused by chronic total occlusions, or by concentric or eccentric, regular or irregular rigid plaques that have no vasomotor potential because of peristenotic smooth muscle atrophy and/or plaque rigidity. They are associated with a very stable and predictable onset of angina and signs of ischemia.

Stable plaques with vasomotor potential

Such plaques (both flow-limiting and nonflow-limiting) may cause ischemia with a chronic but less predictable pattern, because the residual lumen can be modulated by the vasomotor tone of the surrounding smooth muscle. Plaques with vasomotor potential are usually eccentric, smooth, or irregular, with compliant segments of wall and preserved muscular media. In patients with such plaques, the increase in myocardial oxygen consumption that is tolerated without the development of ischemia is maximal, and may even be totally normal when coronary vasomotor tone is minimal; however, it decreases in proportion to the degree of lumen reduction caused by constrictor stimuli.

When the plaque occupies a large fraction of the lumen, when the constrictor stimuli are intense, and when the compliance of the stenotic segment is well preserved, ischemic episodes can occur even at rest; however, in these extreme cases, the lumen reduction should be at least 90%. In patients with chronic stable IHD, the vasomotor potential of stenoses, assessed angiographically from both the maximal coronary dilation obtained after administration of nitrates, and the maximal constriction obtained after administration of ergonovine, is quite variable. It is greatest in eccentric stenoses with regular or irregular borders, but can be detected even in some concentric stenoses (see Ch. 9). Plaques with vasomotor potential may remain stable for years.

Unstable plaques with vasomotor potential

In unstable plaques with vasomotor potential, intense local smooth muscle constriction may result from disruption or local activation of the endothelium and from mural thrombi. Mural thrombi in nonrigid coronary segments with preserved media can amplify geometrically the constrictor effect of increased vasomotor tone (see Ch. 9).

8.2.3 Unstable plaques with thrombotic potential

Mural thrombosis, sometimes stratified with layers of different ages, is the most commonly recognized feature of unstable active plaques. Thrombi are often, (but not necessarily always) found over fissures, ulcerations, or plaque hemorrhage; however, some plaque fissures are not associated with mural thrombi, and, conversely, some mural thrombi are not associated with any plaque fissure. At angiography the residual lumen often presents grossly irregular contours, and may undergo dynamic changes as luminal thrombus is deposited and either lyses or fragments, embolizing downstream branches, or contributes to rapid plaque growth by becoming organized. Before mural thrombi are covered by endothelial cells, they may represent a site of further thrombosis. Alterations in unstable plaques do not appear limited to the luminal surface, but extend to the adventitia where perineural infiltrates of inflammatory cells are often observed. Although irregularity of the stenosis, thrombosis, plaque fissure, inflammatory cellular infiltrates, and peristenotic smooth muscle contraction bands are all most commonly present in unstable plaques, they may also be found in patients with chronic IHD and, occasionally, even in controls, and are not detectable in all cases of unstable angina (see Ch. 9).

■ *Thus, irregular stenoses detectable angiographically may be markers of the instability, but are not necessarily its cause. They result from thrombosis or an ulcerated plaque, but at angiography cannot be dated and, hence, may also represent just the longstanding consequence of a previously unstable lesion which healed and remained stable for years. It is likely that other elusive pathogenetic factors, as yet unidentified, play a major part in initiating plaque instability.* ■

Potentially unstable plaques

During stable phases of IHD, the existence of a specific type of plaque with the propensity to become unstable is speculative. The rupture of a highly thrombogenic plaque may be sufficient, in itself, to precipitate sudden occlusive thrombosis, but it does not explain fully the frequent stuttering evolution of unstable angina (see Ch. 9). Some plaques with a very thin fragile fibrous cap covering a large pool of extracellular lipids are thought to represent potentially unstable plaques because they are more likely to fissure.[41] In such plaques, fissure occurs at the border of the plaque cap, where macrophage-derived foam cells appear to be concentrated; enzymatic degradation by monocytes or other inflammatory cells has been proposed as one of the possible causes of plaque fissure, because collagen and glycosaminoglycan concentrations are reduced in ruptured plaques.[42]

A careful analysis of published results indicates not only that coronary plaque fissure can be found in 10–25% of controls who died of noncardiac causes (and hence it must be a relatively frequent event in individuals with severe coronary atherosclerosis), but also that more than one fissured plaque can often be found in different coronary branches of unstable patients. The frequent observation of multiple plaque fissures in patients who died as a result of acute ischemic syndromes suggests the possible presence of specific precipitating factors of plaque fissure. The segments of plaques which have the thinnest fibrous caps and are exposed to the highest tensile stress are obviously those most likely to fissure when, for example, inflammatory stimuli cause enzymatic digestion of intracellular matrix and collagen (see Ch. 9). Activation of the endothelium caused by inflammatory cytokines, can cause local thrombosis and vasoconstriction also without plaque fissure.

■ *The development of either instability or infarction is an occasional rare event, even in patients with the most severe coronary atherosclerosis. Such occurrences cannot be fully explained by any of the morphologic features identified so far, because such features are not detectable in all unstable patients, and are also observed occasionally in patients with chronic IHD and, more rarely, even in controls.* ■

8.3 PATHOGENESIS OF THE ATHEROSCLEROTIC BACKGROUND

The pathogenesis of atherosclerotic lesions has long been debated. In 1844, von Rokitansky[43] was impressed by the observation of mural thrombi and suggested that atherosclerotic obstructions were composed of organized thrombi. In 1856, Virchow,[44] observing lipid deposits, proposed the "infiltration" theory. He dismissed von Rokitansky's "encrustation" hypothesis because the localized intimal thickenings were subendothelial and "hence could not be derived from surface deposits." Nearly a century later, Duguid[45] succeeded in reviving

interest in the possible role of thrombosis in plaque formation, by showing a gradual evolution from masses that are clearly surface deposits to those covered by endothelium, and a gradual subsequent organization of fibrin-stained bands with infiltration by SMCs and lipids. Although Duguid's findings were extensively confirmed (for reviews of the topic see references 15 and 46), the lipid deposition hypothesis became more widely accepted as a result of:
a.   the alterations found in patients with familial hypercholesterolemia
b.   the positive correlation between cholesterol levels and IHD mortality
c.   the development of animal models of hypercholesterolemia.
   Since then, the emphasis on the pathogenesis of "atherosclerosis as an overgrowth of and degenerative change in the intima of arteries" has remained and is not surprising, as Duguid stated that "this view is so firmly established that we have come to regard it as a ruling principle."[45]

A review of available data indicates that both Virchow and von Rokitansky were correct in their observations, but mistaken in their postulation of a single mechanism for all lesions in all patients.

Any theory on atherogenesis should account for the following:

a.   the most prevalent histologic features of human atherosclerotic plaques
b.   the relationship between plaque localization and blood rheology
c.   the very first human lesions and the pattern of their progression
d.   the available information on the arterial wall response to potentially atherogenic stimuli
e.   the variety of potential atherogenic stimuli.

8.3.1 Histologic features

Raised fibrous plaques are subintimal, i.e. inside the internal elastic lamina; they often protrude only slightly into the lumen because of the remodeling of the wall, and are associated with alterations in the media and adventitia. In humans, over 95% of small plaques are composed of fibrous tissue.

The major component of plaques appears to be a combination of dense acellular and cellular fibrous tissue, with much smaller portions being composed of pultaceous debris, calcium, foam cells with and without inflammatory infiltrates, and inflammatory infiltrates without foam cells. Plaque composition varies as a function of the degree of luminal narrowing. In the study from the Pathology Institute of the National Heart, Lung, and Blood Institute of Bethesda, Maryland, USA, linear increases were observed in the mean percentage of dense fibrous tissue (from 5 to 50%), calcific deposits (from 1 to 10%), pultaceous debris (from 0 to 10%), and inflammatory infiltrates without significant numbers of foam cells (from 0 to 5%), and a linear decrease was observed in the mean percentage of cellular fibrous tissue (from 94 to 22%) in sections narrowed from 25% to more than 95% in cross-sectional area. Small plaques composed predominantly of cellular fibrous tissue had no foam cells (see Fig. 8.15).[47]
   A study by Baroldi et al[40] on 2121 coronary artery stenotic sections gave similar results. It showed that, when their internal thickness measured more than 300 μm and less than 600 μm, the plaque was fibrous without foam cells in 96 and 50%, respectively. On average, the frequency of lipid deposits and atheroma increased progressively with increasing lumen stenosis. Ground substance (mainly proteoglycans), collagen, atheroma, neovascularization, and intimal and/or adventitial inflammatory cell infiltrates were all found to be present in only the most severe stenoses. Increased intimal thickness was usually associated with decreased

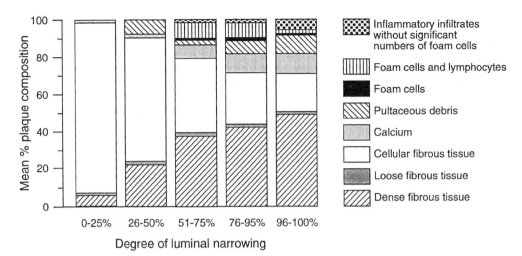

Fig. 8.15 Composition of atherosclerotic plaques as a function of the area stenoses they produce. The smallest plaques are composed of cellular fibrous tissue, with a small proportion of loose and dense fibrous tissue. Pultaceous debris and calcium are present in stenoses greater than 25%, but foam cells, lymphocytes, and inflammatory cell infiltrates are present only in plaques reducing the lumen by more than 50%. The composition of human atherosclerotic plaques found in this study is similar to that found in a previous study,[40] but differs markedly from the composition of atherosclerotic plaques in cholesterol-fed animals, in which foam cells are very prevalent in smaller lesions. (Modified from ref. 47.)

medial thickness, indicative of smooth muscle atrophy. No foam cells were noted in lesions less than 300 μm in thickness. Calcification, even when severe, was frequently associated with only mild stenoses. Inflammatory cell infiltrates were found more frequently in stenoses occupying more than 50% of the luminal area and were less common in fibrous plaques. In smaller plaques, inflammatory infiltrates were found in the adventitia surrounding the nervous structures related to the plaque.

The features of coronary atherosclerotic plaques described in the above studies are similar to those of femoral artery plaques as studied by Ross et al,[48] for which "A general and prominent feature of most of the lesions . . . . . was the fibrous nature of the plaque and the relative absence of lipid-filled atheromatous centers."

Immunohistochemical features

In humans, a high proportion of small, fibrous, and also fibrolipid plaques present histologic features indicative of the presence of thrombus buried below the endothelium. Histologically identifiable layers of fibrin separated by layers of fibrous tissue can be found in a large proportion of fibrous and fibrolipid plaques, even when they are barely visible to the naked eye.[46] Their thrombotic nature is confirmed by staining in discrete bands using antifibrin and antiplatelet antibodies. In one study, immunohistochemical evidence of incorporated thrombus was found in 71% of coronary plaques in patients with coronary occlusions and in 28% of patients without total occlusions. Such mural thrombi and microthrombi become covered with the endothelium and are eventually replaced by collagen, SMCs, ground substance, and lipids, in variable combinations, so that after about 6 months the thrombotic origin of these plaques is no longer recognizable, even by immunohistochemical techniques, because the antigens have been gradually degraded. The very frequent presence of fibrinogen, fibrin, and their degradation products in atherosclerotic plaques has been confirmed using monoclonal antibodies.[49]

Variability in plaque composition in the same patient

In a study of patients with chronic stable angina,[14] about 60% of plaques causing stenosis greater than 75% of the luminal area were found to be fibrous. The percentage was even higher in less severe stenoses; lipid plaques represented a tiny minority of those causing a mild stenosis and about 40% of those causing a greater than 75% cross-sectional area stenosis. In about 15% of patients all plaques were fibrous; another 15% had only lipid plaques. In 33% of patients, no plaques with large pools of lipids were found. Between these extremes, individual patients were found to have variable proportions of both fibrous and lipid plaques, suggesting differences in the local response to the atherogenic stimuli, or in the type of stimuli.

At present, unfortunately, no information is available about the relationship between the composition of plaques and antemortem serum cholesterol levels, lipid profiles, and other risk factors in individual patients.

Neovascularity of plaques

The normal human intima is avascular and becomes vascularized only when its thickness increases critically because of the atherosclerotic process.[50] Deep intimal vessels derive from vasa vasorum;[51] more superficial vessels may derive from ingrowth of capillaries from overlying organized mural thrombus.[52] Vessel rupture within a plaque was proposed as a cause of coronary artery thrombosis over 50 years ago,[53] and separated from plaque fissure 30 years ago by Constantinides,[54] but the frequency with which plaque fissure and intraplaque hemorrhage are found below the thrombi is still debated among pathologists (see Ch. 9).

■ *Thus, in humans, the vast majority of raised fibrous plaques are composed of fibrous tissue, in which detectable residues of buried thrombi or diffuse fibrin are common, and a variable, usually small, component of extracellular lipid. Foam cells and a deep central pool of lipids, absent in all small plaques, are present only in some of the largest plaques, most of which show significant neovascularization. The presence of calcium deposits is not indicative of flow-limiting stenoses. That different types of plaque are frequently found in the same individual suggests:*

a.   *an important role of different local stimuli*
b.   *major differences in the local response or*
c.   *that the same stimulus may have occurred at different times under different circumstances.* ■

8.3.2 Blood rheology and localization of plaques

Atherosclerotic plaques form only on the arterial side of the circulation in large elastic or muscular arteries and saphenous vein aortocoronary bypass grafts, and are found in the pulmonary circulation only in the presence of chronic pulmonary hypertension. In the arterial system, sites of initial plaque formations are represented by areas of low wall/blood shear stress.[55,56] The increased tendency of plaques to form at sites of high blood pressure, but of low rather than high wall/blood shear stress, suggests that the deposition of bloodborne substances and particles, with an increased residence time, has a more important role than merely mechanical damage to the vessel wall in sites of high shear stress with secondary local platelet adhesion and activation.

Furthermore, intimal thickening and the putative precursors of atherosclerotic plaques (i.e. fatty streaks and gelatinous lesions) (see 8.3.3) are more prevalent in areas of low shear stress. Substances accumulating in the arterial wall at the sites of low shear stress include not only low-density lipoprotein (LDL)-cholesterol and fibrinogen, but also immune complexes, toxins, and viruses. The fate of the deposits and their rate of removal depend on adequate local drainage in the lymphatic system and vasa vasorum, among other factors.

■ *Thus, deposition of physiologic or pathologic substances and particles carried by blood, and inadequate adventitial clearance, both contribute to the local accumulation of potentially atherogenic stimuli at sites of low shear stress.* ■

8.3.3 Initial intimal lesions in humans

In humans, an individual atherosclerotic lesion can be viewed by the histopathologist at only one point in its natural history. The events leading up to that point and those that may follow it can thus only be the result of an imaginative reconstruction. For example, the intimal thickening and fatty streaks observed in the first and second decades of life and seen at the site of fibrous plaques in the third and fourth decades, cannot be taken as definite proof that the latter derive from the former, as is currently proposed.[57] In addition, the extent to which findings in hypercholesterolemic animals can be extrapolated to humans is limited, as they represent the response of a previously healthy animal exposed to sustained, extremely high levels of a single, potentially atherogenic, stimulus. Experimental lipid-induced atherosclerosis is not considered, by some investigators, to be an adequate model of human disease.[58,59]

Within these constraints, two types of lesions are considered as possible candidates for the origin of raised fibrous plaques in humans: these are *fatty streaks* and *gelatinous lesions*.

Fatty streaks are yellow, poorly demarcated and only slightly raised. This morphologic, merely descriptive, lesion represents a very heterogeneous entity.[60,61] Some fatty streaks are composed of SMCs and macrophage-derived foam cells; others contain mostly extracellular lipid and are found in about 40% of infants, and also in populations that tend not to develop atherosclerosis.

Most fatty streaks are composed of extracellular lipids and of foam cells containing mostly cholesterol oleate; the latter is practically absent in extracellular and plasma lipids and also in lipid plaques, where cholesterol is predominantly esterified with linoleate.[61,62] These foam cells must, therefore, result from intracellular esterification of cholesterol with oleate, a process that probably differs from that involved in plaque formation. However, it is possible that, in some individuals with cholesterol levels similar to those found in experimental animal models, the composition and evolution of fatty streaks could also be similar.

Thus, although the macroscopic appearance of fatty streaks is the same in animals and humans, their composition in humans usually differs from that found in hypercholesterolemic animals, in which fatty streaks composed of macrophage-derived foam cells appear to be the most common lesions, are caused exclusively by extremely high blood concentrations of cholesterol, and evolve gradually into fibromuscular plaques (see below).

Gelatinous lesions are translucent elevations[60,61] (already described by Virchow) composed of extracellular matrix with widely spaced collagen bundles and SMCs, with large quantities of fibrinogen (three- or fourfold greater than that found in the normal intima), and sometimes with perifibrous lipid in variable but small quantities (mostly in the form of LDL).[62]

In normal intima, concentrations of fibrin and fibrinogen are very low; in early gelatinous lesions, levels of fibrinogen clearly exceed those of fibrin. However, the apparently normal intima of a hypertensive hypercholesterolemic individual may contain twice as much LDL as that found in gelatinous lesions in individuals with low serum cholesterol levels. In lipid-rich gelatinous regions, fibrin becomes a major plaque component and is associated with increased concentrations of LDL, which appear to be bound at the collagen–fibrin interface. Fibrin deposits, recognized by antifibrin antibodies in the large majority of very early lesions, present either a uniform diffuse pattern, suggestive of a transformation within the wall of fibrinogen diffused from the blood, or well-defined strands, suggestive of organized mural microthrombi, as confirmed by the associated presence of platelet antigens. Defective platelet adhesion, as in von Willebrand's disease, is associated with resistance to the atherosclerotic process.[63] A recent review emphasizes the frequent occurrence of microthrombi in otherwise normal segments of coronary arteries.[64]

■ *There appears to be no sound scientific basis, therefore, for the dispute over whether the initial lesion of human atherosclerosis is represented only by fatty streaks or only by gelatinous lesions. Both may result in raised fibrous plaques and have a variable prevalence in different individuals and in different lesions.* ■

Progression of initial lesions

In humans, the most common evolution of initial lesions, whatever they may be, is obviously towards intercellular matrix production, leading to fibrous or fibromuscular plaques, which are the most common (over 95%) among small plaques. In contrast to what is observed in experimental hypercholesterolemic animals,[65,66] in the very large majority of individuals only a tiny minority of smaller plaques have foam cells. Only some of the larger plaques develop a deep central atheromatous core. Furthermore, foam cells in a subendothelial location appear to be very rare in human raised fibrous plaques and are found only at the borders of the atheromatous core and at the edges of some large plaques that reduce the lumen by more than 50%. The situation is likely to be different in patients with marked elevation of serum cholesterol levels (i.e. in the range observed in hypercholesterolemic animal models). Inflammatory infiltrates also appear only in larger plaques (see 8.2.1).

Extraluminal expansion of the plaque

Planimetry of the area defined by the internal elastic lamina indicates an expansion of the wall towards the outside as the intimal thickness increases with maintenance of a normal-size lumen (see Figs 8.1 and 8.2). In some cases, angiography shows a marked ectasia of the lumen (see Fig. 8.16), suggesting that weakening of the structure of the coronary wall may be an important, yet variable, component of the atherosclerotic process in humans. This pathogenetic component, which implies digestion and remodeling of the supporting structure of the wall, has so far, received little attention. In some patients this ectasia can be reminiscent of the alterations that are characteristic of Kawasaki disease, for which viral, inflammatory, autoimmune, or toxic origins are postulated.[67,68]

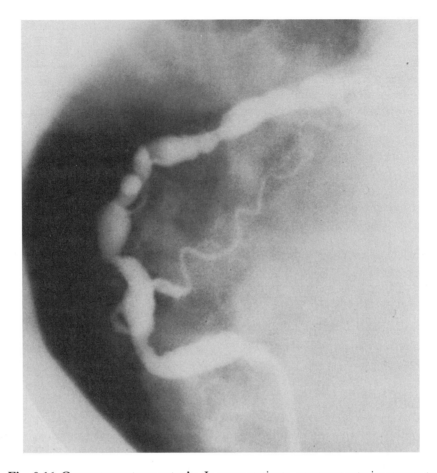

Fig. 8.16 Coronary artery ectasia. In some patients, coronary arteries appear to be diffusely or segmentally ectatic. This obvious alteration in a 56-year-old patient with chronic angina and no known risk factors may be one extreme of the remodeling process that is described in Fig. 8.1, alternatively, in some cases, coronary ectasia is reminiscent of the pattern of coronary dilation observed in Kawasaki disease in children.

Rapid versus gradual reduction of the coronary lumen

The progression of stenoses can be assessed only by repeated coronary angiography. As discussed in 8.1.4, a comparison of repeated angiographic studies has shown that the reduction is typically focal and occurs irrespective of the severity of the initial lumen reduction; it can be obvious at the site of one or two plaques and totally undetectable at all other sites. Newly formed, isolated plaques also become detectable at one or two sites, often with no detectable (even minimal) new wall irregularities in the other coronary segments.[69] The development and progression of the lumen reduction caused by plaques (and observed in only some plaques and not in others with similar—or even greater—initial stenosis) are only weakly correlated with the time interval between successive angiographic studies, suggesting that the progression proceeded in sporadic steps, rather than as a continuous and gradual process.

Postmortem studies have shown that a sudden growth of plaques occurs because of incorporation into the intima of large mural thrombi, intraintimal thrombosis or hemorrhage (see Fig. 8.17).[70]

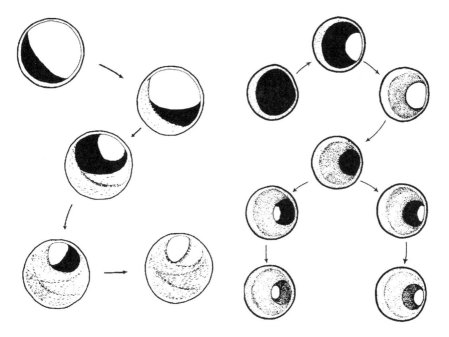

Fig. 8.17 Schematic diagram illustrating rapid plaque growth from the organization of thrombi. Mural thrombi can become organized and form successive crescents on the plaque. Occlusive thrombi can partially recanalize. (Modified from ref. 70.)

■ *In patients with known IHD, the development and progression of coronary stenoses thus seem to occur more often as occasional, local, thrombosis-related processes than as a diffuse, gradual, time-dependent process.* ■

8.3.5 The arterial wall response to noxious stimuli

In recent years, cellular and molecular biological techniques have provided insight into the mechanisms involved in cell-to-cell interaction (between endothelial cells, monocytes, platelets, and SMCs), as well as those involved in chemotaxis, cell proliferation, and matrix production in response to a wide variety of noxious stimuli in the arterial wall (see review by Ross in reference 71). Although the process begins as a physiologic repair of the insult, it subsequently evolves toward a pathologic alteration because of the severity of the insult and its persistence or recurrence.

The initial response of the arterial wall is essentially similar for a wide variety of noxious stimuli.[72,73] These can be:

a. mechanical, such as balloon denudation of the endothelium, air drying, or other injuries
b. chemical, such as exposure to oxidized LDL, fibrin, and homocysteine
c. immunologic
d. toxic or viral.

The response is also similar when the endothelium is intact, but blood and lymphatic exchanges at the adventitial side are prevented by local banding with either a plastic cuff or a cellophane film.[73]

In all cases, the response of the local arterial wall is proliferative, characterized by:

a. migration of SMCs from the media into the intima
b. rapid proliferation of SMCs within the intima
c. massive production of collagen and extracellular matrix, predominantly gly-cosaminoglycans
d. accumulation of lipid when blood cholesterol levels are elevated.

The proliferative response is triggered by a variety of growth factors and vasoconstrictors, which have variable time courses from days to weeks,[74] opposed by heparin, heparan sulfate, and vasodilators such as endothelial-derived relaxing factors (EDRFs), and modulated by various cytokines.[71]

Migration of SMCs

Migration of SMCs from the media into the intima can be observed during growth and as a response to hypertension and to intimal injury. A variable number of SMCs are present in the intima of adults but are absent in childhood and experimental animals. Several chemotactic factors that stimulate migration of SMCs and macrophages have been identified, among them oxidized LDL, fibrin and leukotriene B$_4$. In order for SMCs to migrate, they must digest the intercellular matrix.[75]

Proliferation of SMCs

Growth factors stimulate proliferation of only those SMCs that are in a "synthetic" state, but not of those that are in a contractile phenotypic state. In humans, the SMC phenotype in the "synthetic" state is found not only in the intima but also sparsely within the media.

Growth factors, such as platelet-derived growth factor (PDGF) and epidermal growth factor, are released by activated platelets and are also produced by fibroblasts (fibroblast-derived growth factor), endothelium and SMCs. SMC proliferation is inhibited by heparin-like mole-cules and by EDRF produced by the endothelium.

Matrix production

In the synthetic state, SMCs produce types I and II collagen, glycosaminoglycans, and other components of the intercellular space.

Limited replicative life-span

Based on the demonstration in vitro that the number of passage generations of cultured cells is inversely related to the age of the donor, SMCs cultured from human plaques appear to behave like senescent cells, as they soon lose their capacity to multiply.[48] Death of SMCs can initiate the formation of the central necrotic core of plaques.

Regardless of the initial noxious stimulus, cholesterol may accumulate in a plaque as a result of multiple processes when its blood level is elevated. These processes include:

a. direct deposition of extracellular lipids from LDL
b. intracellular lipid accumulation in SMCs and macrophages, both of which may even-tually transform into foam cells filled with cholesterol (which is the most prevalent, early alteration in hypercholesterolemic animal models and possibly, in patients with familial hypercholesterolemia)
c. accumulation in extracellular pools, typically observed at the base of some of the larger plaques and derived from extracellular lipids, cell debris and dead foam cells.

In general, in human atherosclerotic plaques, the proliferative response with matrix production predominates in small lesions. Foam cells with degenerative and inflammatory components become evident only in larger plaques.

■ *The much greater prevalence of foam cell accumulation and degenerative and inflammatory processes in larger, rather than smaller, lesions suggests that these components are more important in the late, rather than in the early, stages of plaque formation.* ■

8.3.6 Atherogenic stimuli

Although the explosion of cellular and molecular biology is providing very fine details about the growth factors, cytokines and vasoregulatory molecules that participate in the cascade of events that follows injury to the arterial wall, much less information is available on the actual nature and prevalence of the various atherogenic stimuli in humans. Yet this information is at least as important as that on the derangement of the local vessel wall repair mechanisms in response to atherogenic stimuli.

Animal studies show that in the initial phases of the wall response, very high levels of LDL-cholesterol cause a considerable accumulation of foam cells, whereas, in the absence of hypercholesterolemia, nonlipid noxious stimuli predominantly cause SMC proliferation and matrix formation without foam cells. Nonlipid atherogenic stimuli include:

a. mechanical injury, caused by arterial blood pressure and flow
b. fibrin deposition, by insudation into the wall of fibrinogen or by microthrombi formation
c. chemical stimuli, such as those caused by tobacco smoking or homocysteine
d. immunologic stimuli
e. viral stimuli.

In the later phases of plaque development, vicious cycles can develop during which some initially fibrous plaques are infiltrated by lipids when their blood levels are elevated; conversely, intense SMC proliferation may develop in some, initially predominantly lipid, plaques.

Regardless of the initial stimulus, mutagens may cause monoclonal SMC proliferation. According to studies by Benditt and Benditt,[76] many foci of SMCs in plaques are monoclonal in response to a variety of stimuli. Hence, these cells could originate from a local somatic mutation, although a local "natural selection" mechanism of a single original SMC cannot be excluded. The finding of a transforming gene in human atherosclerotic plaques would be consistent with the possibility of monoclonal proliferation. Furthermore, impairment of tissue exchange at the adventitial side may enhance SMC migration into the intima, local proliferation, and matrix production in the absence of hypercholesterolemia and of any damage to the intima.[73]

Lipid noxious stimuli

The prevailing emphasis on lipid atherogenic stimuli is related to the very convincing evidence that elevated blood levels of cholesterol are associated with increased mortality from IHD, and to the production of atherosclerotic lesions in experimental animals with induced or spontaneous hypercholesterolemia.

In animals with chronic hyperlipidemia, cholesterol deposition and oxidation of LDL results in toxic injury to the endothelium, altering its permeability and causing adhesion of monocytes and T lymphocytes. Monocytes entering the subendothelial space become macrophages, take up oxidized LDL (eventually becoming foam cells), and release a variety of cell growth regulators.[71] LDL accumulation is reduced by high-density lipoprotein and increased by lipoprotein(a) (Lp(a)) and is also influenced by the local rates of drainage via adventitial lymphatics and blood vessels.

In vitro, oxidized LDL is a chemotactic stimulus for SMCs and macrophages (not yet proven in man); it also is mitogenic for SMCs, activates macrophages and stimulates antibody formation.[77] Ultimately, at the site where cholesterol-laden macrophages emerge from the intima, platelet adhesion and activation cause release of PDGF, which further stimulates SMC proliferation. The factors that control LDL accumulation within the intima and subsequent oxidization are incompletely known, but antioxidants such as vitamins C and E have a protective effect against LDL oxidation.

In humans, however, postmortem studies show that the extent of coronary atherosclerosis is only weakly correlated to elevated levels of cholesterol during life (see Ch. 12) and that the majority of initial plaques have no foam cells.

■ *Thus, the demonstrated causal role of elevated cholesterol levels in IHD may not necessarily be related only to their atherogenic effects.* ■

Mechanical injury caused by arterial blood pressure and flow

The importance of mechanical injury related to arterial blood pressure and flow can be assessed by considering:

a. the results of experimental mechanical vascular injury
b. the preferential location of initial lesions in arterial branches
c. the correlation between arterial blood pressure levels and extension of coronary atherosclerosis in postmortem studies.

Experimental, mechanical vascular injury. Fuster et al[15] distinguished three types of severity of vascular injury:

a. type I, functional alterations to the endothelial cells without substantial morphologic changes
b. type II, endothelial denudation and intimal damage with intact elastic lamina
c. type III, damage extending to the media.

The analysis below suggests that mechanical injury caused by arterial blood pressure and flow is not likely, per se, to be an important determinant of the extent of atherosclerosis in humans, but mural thrombi related to types II and III injury or to strong local thrombogenic stimuli can be major determinants of rapid plaque formation and growth.

As quiescent endothelium represents an anatomic and functional barrier, its removal could represent an atherogenic stimulus. In animals, however, areas of the endothelium gently denuded without deep intimal injury are rapidly covered by a monolayer of adhering, but not aggregating, platelets not associated with SMC migration and proliferation. SMC migration and proliferation occur only when regenerated endothelium is removed a second time and is followed by the formation of fibrin–platelet thrombus, or when the injury to the intima is so severe that the internal elastica lamina is disrupted. In both cases, the resulting mural platelet thrombus is covered rapidly with endothelial cells and invaded by proliferating SMCs.[64] In rabbits, severe thrombocytopenia and antiplatelet serum reduce SMC proliferation following intimal injury.[78,79] The importance of adhesion of platelets to strands of von Willebrand factor is suggested by resistance to the development of atherosclerotic-like lesions in pigs with von Willebrand's disease in the homozygous state.[62] Platelet deficiency may not be relevant when the atherogenic stimuli are not associated with endothelial damage.

Thrombus formation associated with deep intimal or subintimal damage can cause atherosclerotic plaques that later become indistinguishable from those caused initially by lipid accumulation. In experimental arterial thrombi, new vascular channels develop within days of injury, connecting the deeper layers of the thrombus with the main arterial lumen. Large numbers of both SMCs and monocytes can be seen in mural thrombi within about 3 weeks of their formation. SMCs may also derive from intimal mesenchymal cells rather than from SMCs that have migrated into the thrombus from the media. After 2 months, a central core of atheroma with foam cells can be detected in some plaques. Platelet-rich pulmonary artery emboli in cholesterol-fed rabbits, but not in those on a normal diet, became complex fibrolipid lesions with fibrous caps overlying basal lipid-rich pools. The SMCs within organized thrombi were also found to acquire cell populations with monoclonal characteristics. Thus, experimentally induced mural thrombi can gradually develop all the features of atherosclerotic plaques, but endothelial denudation is insufficient per se to initiate the process of plaque formation, unless it is associated with the formation of a mural thrombus.

Preferential location of initial atherosclerotic lesions. The preferential location of plaques at sites of low, rather than high, shear stress indicates that deposition of LDL, immune complexes, fibrinogen, viruses, and toxic bloodborne potentially atherogenic stimuli at these sites seems to be a common prerequisite for the initial formation of plaques. The subsequent fate of initial lesions depends on local clearance, on the local tissue response, and on blood–endothelial interaction.

Relation of hypertension to the extent of coronary atherosclerosis. The extent of coronary atherosclerosis assessed at postmortem examination does not appear to correlate with the levels of arterial blood pressure during life, suggesting that other atherogenic stimuli predominate over the mechanical stimuli caused by elevated arterial blood pressure (see Ch. 12).

■ *The close positive correlation between IHD mortality and blood pressure levels is thus not mediated by a greater extent of coronary atherosclerosis.* ■

Injury caused by chemical stimuli

Chemical stimuli include, for example, products derived from tobacco smoking and homocysteine,[80] which can initiate fibrin deposition and intimal arterial wall lesions. Blood levels of homocysteine were found to be elevated in about 30% of adults with coronary peripheral or cerebral vascular diseases in relation to genetic causes[81] and environmental causes such as folic acid or vitamin B_{12} deficiency.[82] Although endothelial damage was observed on electron-microscopic examination of the umbilical cord arteries of infants whose mothers smoked during pregnancy,[83] postmortem studies failed to show a relationship between tobacco smoking and extent of coronary atherosclerosis (see Ch. 12), suggesting that other atherogenic stimuli are more important than smoking.

■ *Thus, the positive correlation between smoking and IHD mortality is also not mediated by a greater extent of coronary atherosclerosis.* ■

Injury caused by fibrin and fibrinogen degradation products

Fibrin causes SMC migration and proliferation and binds thrombin, which is itself a major growth factor; fibrin degradation products generated by plasmin stimulate synthesis of DNA and collagen and are chemotactic.[84,85] Thrombin and fibrin degradation products are chemotactic for macrophages.[86] The lipoprotein Lp(a), which is structurally related to plasminogen,[87] may be sequestered in the arterial wall by binding to fibrin and, in turn, may block plasminogen binding and clearance of fibrin. Fibrin present in gelatinous lesions can derive from microthrombi or from transformation in situ of fibrinogen accumulated in the wall.

1. Fibrinogen deposition depends on its rate of filtration from the blood through the endothelial barrier at sites of low shear stress; its subsequent fate depends on its rate of removal through the adventitia and on its transformation to fibrin within the wall.
2. Fibrin deposition over morphologically normal endothelial cells can derive from local activation of the endothelium by toxic immunologic and viral stimuli, causing local expression of tissue factor and thrombin formation.

Immunologic stimuli

The role of immunologic stimuli in atherogenesis[88,89] has been confirmed in patients. Evidence of an in situ immune-mediated hypersensitivity reaction was found in cellular infiltrates in different types of atherosclerotic lesion.[90] This line of research is now beginning to receive appropriate attention.[91]

In transplanted hearts, the distribution of atherosclerotic lesions—uniformly diffuse around the lumen and along its length, rather than in discrete plaques—suggests a uniform distribution of the target antigen. In the other common forms of atherosclerosis, the localization of T lymphocytes in distinct lesions (i.e. the plaques) suggests that the target antigens are confined to some components of the plaque. The much greater frequency with which inflammatory cell infiltrates are found in large, rather than in small, plaques suggests that they have a complicating, rather than a primary, pathogenetic role. Complement activation[92] and T lymphocytes[93] have been detected in human atherosclerotic plaques. An immunologic component of atherosclerosis may be related to LDL oxidation, as immunoglobulin-bound lipoprotein levels were found to be elevated in the circulating blood of patients with familial and non-familial hypercholesterolemia, but it may also have a primary role.[94-96]

Immune complex deposition, which is likely to occur throughout life at sites of either low shear stress or turbulence created by stenoses, could contribute to the development of atherosclerotic lesions by producing local inflammatory and procoagulant changes.[97,98] Circulating immune complexes specific to *Chlamydia pneumoniae* were detected in 41% of patients with chronic IHD and in 15% of controls.[99] In patients with atherosclerotic peripheral vascular disease, a high degree of prevalence of cytotoxic autoantibodies against monocytes and endothelial cells has also been reported.[100]

■ *The significance of the immunologic component in coronary atherosclerotic plaques is still unclear, but it deserves attention because signs of inflammation are a characteristic feature of plaques, particularly in unstable angina (see Ch. 9).* ■

Infectious agents

The possibility that a viral or bacterial infection may initiate and contribute to the progression of atherosclerosis has received much less attention than other, more widely recognized, risk factors. Yet viral infection was shown to cause atherosclerosis in animals and several studies have demonstrated the presence of viral DNA and *Chlamydia pneumoniae* in a high percentage of human atherosclerotic plaques, giving a prevalence of these putative risk factors comparable to that of known proven risk factors (see Ch. 12).

Herpesvirus was shown to cause atherosclerosis in animals[101,102] and to have proinflammatory and procoagulant effects on human endothelium.[103] The presence of cytomegalovirus antigen and nucleic acids has been demonstrated in a high percentage of human atherosclerotic plaques.[104–107] The plaque localization of the virus could be part of a widespread presence of histologically occult cytomegalovirus occurring via endothelial cell infection.[107]

Chlamydia pneumoniae infection was also shown to be associated with the development of MI and coronary atherosclerosis.[108] This organism is classified as a bacterium, but it grows only intracellularly and is a common cause of mild respiratory infections (see Ch. 9). Following the demonstration of a serologic association of *C. pneumoniae* infection with acute MI and chronic IHD in both retrospective and prospective studies, the organism was recently demonstrated in a high proportion of coronary plaques at postmortem and in those removed by arterectomy. *C. pneumoniae* was not described until the early 1980s, and as Spodick suggested in an editorial review,[109] a wide variety of infectious agents could be candidates for a pathogenetic component in IHD.

■ *The high degree of frequency with which evidence of cytomegalovirus and* Chlamydia *infection can be obtained in patients with coronary atherosclerosis, is not yet proof of their pathogenetic roles in atherogenesis. They are not found in all patients and are found also in unaffected controls in the same way as causal risk factors for IHD. Coronary localization or reactivation of dormant infectious agents could trigger local coronary inflammatory reactions with the sudden growth of an atherosclerotic plaque, as well as with an acute phase of instability.* ■

Development of vicious circles

Whatever the initial stimulus, vicious circles can develop that enhance the rate of plaque growth. First, lipids tend to accumulate in some of the initially fibrous or fibromuscular plaques (irrespective of the original cause of SMC proliferation) to a greater extent when their blood levels are elevated, and oxidized LDL stimulates smooth muscle proliferation and matrix production and causes migration of monocytes and T lymphocytes into the subendothelial space. Second, micro- and macrothrombi can form over fibrous and fibrolipid plaques (in response to platelet aggregation or mechanical, chemical, autoimmune or viral activation of the endothelium), become incorporated into the plaque and cause further SMC proliferation. Third, mechanical or inflammatory injury can cause plaque fissure and intraplaque or mural thrombosis resulting in rapid plaque growth and, possibly, in unstable phases of IHD. Finally, the variable rate of wall remodeling determines the extent to which plaques cause flow-limiting stenoses.

The local response to injury may be modulated by the hemostatic system (for example, von Willebrand factor), the fibrinolytic system (for example, tissue-plasminogen activator [t-PA] and plasminogen activator inhibitor-1 [PAI-1] balance), by antioxidants (for example, vitamins A and E) as well as by the central nervous system (as suggested by some experimental studies).[110]

■ *All these different stimuli, acting continuously or in bouts over the years, can do so in various combinations and temporal sequences with variable rates of local vascular and systemic response and repair. This lifelong protracted and extremely variable alternation and sequence of different atherogenic stimuli, together with local response and repair, causes atherosclerotic lesions with different ischemic potential and cannot be reproduced adequately by introducing a single atherogenic stimulus in animal models.* ■

8.3.7 Theories of atherogenesis

There is now general agreement that the development of human atherosclerotic plaques is the result of a local response of the arterial wall to noxious stimuli that initiate SMC proliferation and, at some stage in some lesions, also initiate a large deposition of lipids. However, there are still two major theories in contention regarding the nature of the noxious stimuli responsible for this process. One theory, based on epidemiologic observations and findings in lipid-fed experimental animals, postulates that the primary cause of human atherosclerosis is deposition of lipid in the vessel wall and that the initial lesion is represented by fatty streaks. The other theory maintains that the disease is essentially a response of the vessel wall to a variety of injuries and that the deposition of lipid, when present, may be a secondary phenomenon. There is an increasing tendency to merge these two views, so that they remain in contention only for those who believe that in order for one theory to be correct the other must be incorrect.[72]

Evolution of hypotheses

As available information has been examined more critically, the hypotheses that have been proposed in order to explain atherogenesis have become more complex, but, at the same time, more comprehensive.

In 1976, on the basis of their studies in hypercholesterolemic animals, Ross and Glomset[65] proposed that injury to the endothelium was the initiating event in atherogenesis. Ten years later, Ross[66] updated this hypothesis because of the accumulation of information regarding the possible interaction between endothelial cells, macrophages, and SMCs. This modified "response-to-injury" hypothesis of atherogenesis suggests that SMC proliferation can result from at least two causes:

a.   interaction of SMCs with monocytes and platelets
b.   direct stimulation of SMCs by growth factors released by endothelial cells and autogenous growth factors released by SMCs themselves.

In 1992, based on their studies of experimental vascular injury, Fuster and colleagues proposed a broader theory,[15] taking into account the micro- and macrothrombotic aspects, which are much more prevalent in human disease than in hypercholesterolemic animal models. As reported in 8.3.6, they proposed that the local response, the extent of platelet deposition and the size of the thrombus are proportional to the severity of the vessel wall injury defined as types I, II and III injury.

Both Ross and Fuster broadly accept the proposition that the initial lesion from which plaques develop is represented by fatty streaks. This theory was developed in detail by Stary[57] on the basis of analogies of the sites at which fatty streaks are found in infants, children, and adolescents with those at which fibrous plaques are found in adults, and it "became widely accepted in the scientific community, particularly in the United States, because it fitted well epidemiologic data."[111] There is no *direct* evidence in humans for this hypothesis which does not take into account the varied composition of this macroscopically descriptive entity, the possible origin of plaques from gelatinous lesions and the fibrous composition, without foam cells, of at least 95% of small plaques in humans.

A general theory of atherogenesis must take due account of the following facts:

1. Atherogenesis is not inevitably related to aging, as the coronary arteries in some individuals belonging to different communities with both high and low prevalence of IHD remain practically free from raised fibrous plaque until old age (see Fig. 8.4).
2. Over 95% of plaques occupying less than 25% of the lumen are composed of fibrous tissue and have no foam cells (see Fig. 8.15).
3. Remodeling of the arterial wall at the site of plaques, in general prevents reduction of the lumen until the plaque occupies about 40% of the space limited by the internal elastic lamina (an apparent 40% lumen reduction).
4. Development and progression of angiographically detectable stenoses occurs rapidly and unpredictably, often as a consequence of a local proliferative response or of acute ischemic stimuli leading to thrombus formation.

The variable origin and evolution of the atherosclerotic background

It seems rather simplistic to attribute the wide variety of atherosclerotic lesions found in the majority of adults to any single initial lesion or pathogenetic mechanism. At any given point in time the amount of atherosclerosis present in any individual reflects the overall balance between the varied noxious stimuli (listed in 8.3.6) that acted until that time and the local wall physiologic repair processes and their pathologic derangement.

Throughout life, the arterial wall is submitted to a process of wear and tear caused not only by the continuous pulsatile changes in blood pressure and flow and continuous inflow of macromolecules from the bloodstream, but also by occasional chemical, viral, and immunologic insults. Physiologic wear and tear and occasional wall damage caused by any kind of noxious stimuli *are continuously repaired* but, in general, the efficiency of the repair reponse decreases progressively with age. Stimuli that are noxious to the coronary arteries are, therefore, more likely to be better tolerated in younger individuals with nearly intact arterial walls than in middle-aged individuals with previously healed lesions and a reduced ability to repair. When the damage exceeds the local repairability and is associated with abnormal blood composition or abnormal handling of macromolecules by the wall, initial lesions and raised fibrous plaques develop and progress at very variable speeds, depending also on the local endothelial interaction with blood components. After their development, some initial lesions and, perhaps, even some initial raised fibrous plaques, may heal or remain stable; others may progress at variable rates towards the formation of major plaques and complex lesions.

A composite theory of atherogenesis

Atherosclerosis should be considered as a multifactorial pathologic process that is related to the waxing and waning over the years of a variety of atherogenic stimuli acting on the "physiologic" wear-and-tear and repair processes of the arterial wall.

Some stimuli (such as elevated levels of serum cholesterol or homocysteine) may act very gradually over long periods; others (such as viral infections or immune complex deposition) may act occasionally over short periods. Atherogenic stimuli may be combined and their local effects may be influenced by antioxidants (such as vitamins C and A), by the thrombotic–fibrinolytic balance and by the efficiency of the repair process in all the wall components, (including the media and adventitia), which, in turn, determine the local remodeling of the coronary artery lumen.

The localization and growth of a plaque is influenced by the following:

a.   the local accumulation in the vessel wall of material carried by the blood
b.   its local drainage from the vessel wall
c.   the balance of growth factors and their inhibitors that have the physiologic task of optimizing the repair response
d.   the extent of its derangement.

Healed lesions may represent sites of predilection for plaque formation in response to new atherogenic stimuli.

Raised fibrous plaques may derive either from gelatinous lesions or from some types of fatty streaks, but this sequence of progression is not necessarily the only one and it is impossible to establish precisely the time of origin, the course of progression, and the type of initial lesion from which they originated. Statistically, vasoconstriction and thrombosis are more likely to develop in the presence of a strong atherosclerotic background, but the development of lesions with ischemic vasomotor and thrombotic potential may not be a random process.

Complex lesions are likely to be derived from some raised fibrous plaques, but it is not known whether this is a random event or whether it is related to the specific pathogenetic mechanisms of some plaques that are not present in others.

Rapid plaque growth due to thrombosis may be the result of acute ischemic stimuli caused by local chemical, immunologic or viral insults producing local inflammation, activation of the endothelium and, possibly, favoring the fissure of plaques.

■ *Thus, the atherosclerotic background is not only a predisposing factor for acute ischemic stimuli, but is also a possible consequence of acute ischemic stimuli leading to thrombosis or to a rapid proliferative response, and is hence a marker of a susceptibility to ischemic stimuli.* ■

The elucidation of the potential atherogenic role of endothelial cells, monocytes, T lymphocytes, mast cells, and SMCs, and of the various factors stimulating or inhibiting cell interaction and multiplication, may represent a promising approach to the treatment and prevention of atherogenesis.[71] However, the primary physiologic functions of these cells and cell regulators are to protect the vascular wall from noxious stimuli and to repair the damage caused by such stimuli. As in the case of fever, which is a beneficial general reaction that enhances defense mechanisms, the intended protective mechanism may itself become a disease entity when the noxious stimuli are either too strong or too prolonged, or when the response becomes abnormal.

As the atherogenic stimuli and the derangements in the local wall repair response that cause atherosclerotic plaques are multiple, their prognostic implications can be varied. The etiological factors of atherosclerosis must also be multiple and composite, with causative and protective genetic mechanisms interacting with causative and protective environmental factors (see Ch. 12).

■ *The control and prevention of atherosclerosis requires not only a clear understanding of the derangement of the protective mechanisms, but also the precise identification of prevailing atherogenic stimuli and of their prevalence in different groups of individuals.* ■

REFERENCES

1. Stiel GM, Stiel LSG, Schofer J, Donath K, Mathey DG. Impact of compensatory enlargement of atherosclerotic coronary arteries on angiographic assessment of coronary artery disease. Circulation 1989;*80:*1603.
2. Glagov S, Weisenberg E, Karins CK, Stankunavicius R, Kolettis GJ. Compensatory enlargement of human atherosclerotic coronary arteries. N Engl J Med 1987;*316:*1371.
3. McGill HC, Arias-Stella J, Carbonell LM et al. General findings of the international atherosclerosis project. Lab Invest 1968;*18:*38.
4. Rissanen V. Coronary atherosclerosis in cases of coronary death as compared with that occurring in the population. Ann Clin Res 1975;*7:*412.
5. Solberg LA, Strong JP. Risk factors and atherosclerotic lesions. Arteriosclerosis 1983;*3:*187.
6. Strong JP, Restrepo C, Guzm n. Coronary and aortic atherosclerosis in New Orleans. Lab Invest 1978;*39:*364.
7. Mitchell JRA, Schwartz CJ. The relation between myocardial lesions and coronary artery disease. Br Heart J 1963;*25:*1.
8. Baroldi G. Coronary stenosis: ischemic or non-ischemic factor? Am Heart J 1978;*96:*139.
9. White NK, Edwards JE, Dry TJ. The relationship of the degree of coronary atherosclerosis with age in man. Circulation 1950;*1:*645.
10. Ackermann RF, Dry TJ, Edwards JE. Relationship of various factors to the degree of coronary atherosclerosis in women. Circulation 1950;*1:*1345.
11. Kemp HG, Kronmal RA, Vliestra RE, Frye RL. Seven year survival of patients with normal or near normal coronary arteriograms: a CASS registry study. J Am Coll Cardiol 1986;*7:*479.
12. Roberts WC. Qualitative and quantitative comparison of amounts of narrowing by atherosclerotic plaques in the major epicardial coronary arteries at necropsy in sudden coronary death, transmural acute myocardial infarction, transmural healed myocardial infarction and unstable angina pectoris. Am J Cardiol 1989;*64:*324.
13. Bogaty P, Brecker SJ, White SE et al. Comparison of coronary angiographic findings in acute and chronic first presentation of ischemic heart disease. Circulation 1993;*87:*1938.
14. Hangartner JRW, Charleston AJ, Davies MJ, Thomas AC. Morphological characteristics of clinically significant coronary artery stenosis in stable angina. Br Heart J 1986;*56:*501.
15. Fuster V, Badimon L, Badimon JJ, Chesebro JH. The pathogenesis of coronary artery disease and the acute coronary syndromes. N Engl J Med 1992;*326:*242.
16. Cianflone D, Ciccirillo F, Buffon A et al. Comparison of coronary angiographic findings in patients with stable angina, unstable angina or acute myocardial infarction as the initial presentation of ischemic heart disease: pathogenetic implications. Am J Cardiol 1995 (in press).
17. Hackett D, Davies G, Maseri A. Pre-existing coronary stenoses in patients with first myocardial infarction are not necessarily severe. Eur Heart J 1988;*9:*1317.
18. Crawford T, Crawford MD. Prevalence and pathological changes of ischaemic heart-disease in a hard-water and in a soft-water area. Lancet 1967;*1:*229.
19. Betriu A, Castaner A, Sanz GA et al. Angiographic finding 1 month after myocardial infarction: a prospective study of 259 survivors. Circulation 1982;*65:*1099.
20. DeWood MA, Notske RN, Simpson CS et al. Prevalence and significance of spontaneous thrombolysis in transmural myocardial infarction. Eur Heart J 1985;*6:*33.
21. Eliot RS, Baroldi G, Leone A. Necropsy studies in myocardial infarction with minimal or no coronary luminal reduction due to atherosclerosis. Circulation 1974;*49:*1127.
22. Rafflenbeul W, Smith LR, Rogers WJ, Mantle JA, Rackley CE, Russell RO. Quantitative coronary arteriography. Coronary anatomy of patients with unstable angina pectoris reexamined 1 year after optimal medical therapy. Am J Cardiol 1979;*43:*699.
23. Singh RN. Progression of coronary atherosclerosis. Br Heart J 1984;*52:*451.
24. Rafflenbeul W, Nellessen U, Galvao P, Kreft M, Peters S, Lichtlen P. Progression and regression of coronary artery disease as assessed with sequential coronary angiography. Z Kardiol 1984;*73:*33.
25. Bruschke A, Kramer J, Bal E, Haque I, Detranto R, Goormastic M. The dynamics of progres-

sion of coronary atherosclerosis studied in 168 medically treated patients who underwent coronary arteriography three times. Am Heart J 1989;*117*:296.

26. Moise A, Th roux P, Tapymans Y et al. Unstable angina and progression of coronary atherosclerosis. N Engl J Med 1983;*309*:685.

27. Little WC, Constantinescu M, Applegate RJ et al. Can coronary angiography predict the site of a subsequent myocardial infarction in patients with mild-to-moderate coronary artery disease? Circulation 1988;*78*:1157.

28. Hackett D, Verwilghen J, Davies G, Maseri A. Coronary stenoses before and after acute myocardial infarction. Am J Cardiol 1989;*63*:1517.

29. Ambrose JA, Tannenbaum MA, Alexopoulos D et al. Angiographic progression of coronary artery disease and the development of myocardial infarction. J Am Coll Cardiol 1988;*12*:56.

30. Giroud D, Li JM, Urban P, Meier B, Rutishauser W. Relation of the site of acute myocardial infarction to the most severe coronary arterial stenosis at prior angiography. Am J Cardiol 1992;*69*:729.

31. Ellis S, Alderman EL, Cain K, Wright A, Bourassa M, Fisher L. Morphology of left anterior descending coronary territory lesions as a predictor of anterior myocardial infarction: A CASS registry study. J Am Coll Cardiol 1989;*13*:1481.

32. Kaski JC, Tousoulis D, McFadden E, Crea F, Pereira WI, Maseri A. Variant angina pectoris: the role of coronary spasm in the development of fixed coronary obstructions. Circulation 1992;*85*:619.

33. Kaski JC, Tousoulis D, Pereira WI, Crea F, Maseri A. Progression of complex coronary artery stenosis in patients with angina pectoris: its relation to clinical events. Coronary Artery Disease 1992;*3*:305.

34. Crake T, Tousoulis D, Kaski JC, Maseri A. Stability of symptoms in chronic angina pectoris in spite of severe coronary stenosis progression. Submitted for publication.

35. Ambrose J, Winters S, Arora R. Angiographic evolution of coronary artery morphology in unstable angina. J Am Coll Cardiol 1986;*7*:472.

36. Saner HE, Gobel FL, Salomonowitz E, Erlien DA, Edwards JE. The disease-free wall in coronary atherosclerosis: its relation to degree of obstruction. J Am Coll Cardiol 1985;*6*:1096.

37. Levin DC, Fallon JT. Significance of the angiographic morphology of localized coronary stenosis: histopathologic correlations. Circulation 1982;*66*:316.

38. Kragel AH, Gertz SD, Roberts WC. Morphologic comparison of frequency and types of acute lesions in the major coronary epicardial arteries in unstable angina pectoris, sudden coronary death and acute myocardial infarction. J Am Coll Cardiol 1991;*18*:801.

39. Vlodaver Z, Edwards JE. Pathology of coronary atherosclerosis. Prog Cardiovasc Dis 1971;*14*:256.

40. Baroldi G, Mariani F, Silver MD, Giuliano G. Correlation of morphological variables in the coronary atherosclerotic plaque with clinical patterns of ischemic heart disease. Am J Cardiovasc Path 1988;*2*:159.

41. Richardson P, Davies M, Born G. Influence of plaque configuration and stress distribution on fissuring of coronary atherosclerotic plaques. Lancet 1989;*2*:941.

42. Tracy R, Devaney K, Kissling G. Characteristics of the plaque under a coronary thrombus. Virchows Arch [A] 1985;*405*:411.

43. von Rokitansky K. In: Handbuch der Pathologischen Anatomie, 2. Braunm ller and Seidel, Vienna, 1844.

44. Virchow R. Gesammelte Abhandlungen zur wissenchtlichen Medicin. Meidinger, Frankfurt, 1856, p.496.

45. Duguid JB. Thrombosis as a factor in the pathogenesis of coronary atherosclerosis. J Path Bact 1946;*58*:207.

46. Woolf N. Thrombosis and atherosclerosis. In: Bloom AL, Thomas DP (eds) Thrombosis and Haemostasis. Churchill Livingstone, Edinburgh, 1981, p.527.

47. Kragel AH, Reddy SG, Wittes JT, Roberts WC. Morphometric analysis of the composition of coronary arterial plaques in isolated unstable angina pectoris with pain at rest. Am J Cardiol 1990;*66*:562.

48. Ross R, Wight TN, Strandness E, Thiele B. Human atherosclerosis. I. Cell constitution and characteristics of advanced lesions of the superficial femoral artery. Am J Pathol 1984;*114:*79.
49. Bini A, Fenoglio JJ Jr, Mesa-tejada R, Kudryk B, Kaplan KL. Identification and distribution of fibrinogen, fibrin, and fibrin(ogen) degradation products in atherosclerosis: use of monoclonal antibodies. Arteriosclerosis 1989;*9:*109.
50. Geiringer E. Intimal vascularisation and atherosclerosis. J Pathol Bacteriol 1951;*63:*201.
51. Barger AC, Beeuwkes R, Lainey LL, Silverman KJ. Hypothesis: vasa vasorum and neovascularisation of human coronary arteries: a possible role in the pathology of atherosclerosis. N Engl J Med 1983;*310:*175.
52. Crawford T, Levene C. The incorporation of fibrin in the aortic intima. J Pathol Bacteriol 1952;*64:*523.
53. Paterson JC. Vascularisation and haemorrhage of the intima of arteriosclerotic coronary arteries. Arch Path 1936;*22:*313.
54. Constantinides P. Plaque fissures in human coronary thrombosis. J Atherosclerol Res 1966;*61:*1.
55. Sabbah HN, Khaja F, Hawkins ET et al. Relation of atherosclerosis to arterial wall shear stress in the left anterior descending coronary artery of man. Am Heart J 1986;*112:*453.
56. Glagov S. Zarins C, Giddens DP, Ku ND. Hemodynamics and atherosclerosis. Arch Pathol Lab Med 1988;*112:*1018.
57. Stary H. Evolution and progression of atherosclerotic lesions in coronary arteries of children and young adults. Arteriosclerosis 1989;*9:*1.
58. Stehbens WE. An appraisal of cholesterol feeding in experimental atherogenesis. Prog Cardiovasc Dis 1986;*29:*107.
59. Stehbens WE. Vascular complications in experimental atherosclerosis. Prog Cardiovasc Dis 1986;*29:*221.
60. Haust MD. The morphogenesis and fate of potential and early atherosclerotic lesions in man. Human Pathol 1971;*2:*1.
61. Smith EB. The pathogenesis of atherosclerosis. In: Julian DG, Cann AJ, Fox KM, Hall RJC, Poole-Wilson PA (eds). Diseases of the Heart. Baillière Tindall, London, 1989, p.1067.
62. Smith EB. Molecular interactions in human atherosclerotic plaques. Am J Pathol 1977;*86:*665.
63. Fuster V, Bowie E, Lewis J, Fass DN, Owen C Jr, Brown A. Resistance to arteriosclerosis in pigs with von Willenbrand's disease: spontaneous and high-cholesterol diet-induced arteriosclerosis. J Clin Invest 1978;*61:*722.
64. Woolf N, Davies M. Interrelationship between atherosclerosis and thrombosis. In: Fuster V, Verstraete M (eds). Thrombosis in Cardiovascular Disorders. WB Saunders, Philadelphia, 1992, p.41.
65. Ross R, Glomset JA. The pathogenesis of atherosclerosis. N Engl J Med 1976;*295:*369.
66. Ross R. The pathogenesis of atherosclerosis—An update. N Engl J Med 1986;*314:*488.
67. Burns JC, Huang AS, Newburger JW et al. Characterization of the polymerase activity associated with cultured peripheral blood mononuclear cells from patients with Kawasaki disease. Pediatr Res 1990;*27:*109.
68. Abe Y, Nakano S, Nakahara T et al. Detection of serum antibody by the antimitogen assay against streptococcal erythrogenic toxins. Age distribution in children and the relation to Kawasaki disease. Pediatr Res 1990;*27:*11.
69. Haft J, Haik B, Goldstein J, Brodyn N. Development of significant coronary artery lesions in areas of minimal disease. A common mechanism for coronary disease progression. Chest 1988;*94:*731.
70. Fulton WFM. Coronary thrombotic occlusion in myocardial infarction and thrombus in the pathogenesis of atherosclerosis. In: Carlson LA et al (eds) International Conference on Atherosclerosis. Raven Press, New York, 1978, p.75.
71. Ross R. The pathogenesis of atherosclerosis: a perspective for the 1990s. Nature 1993;*362:*801.
72. Campbell GR, Chamley-Campbell JH. Invited review: the cellular pathobiology of atherosclerosis. Pathology 1981;*13:*423.
73. Booth RFG, Martin JF, Honey AC, Hassall DG, Beesley JE, Moncada S. Rapid development of atherosclerotic lesions in the rabbit carotid artery induced by perivascular manipulation. Atherosclerosis 1989;*76:*257.

74. Fagin JA, Forrester JS. Growth factors, cytokines and vascular injury. Trends Cardiovasc Med 1992;*2:*90.
75. Sperti G, van Leeuwen RTJ, Quax PHA, Maseri A, Kluft C. Cultured rat aortic vascular smooth muscle cells digest naturally produced extracellular matrix. Involvement of plasminogen-dependent and plasminogen-independent pathways. Circ Res 1992;*71:*385.
76. Benditt EP, Benditt JM. Evidence for a monoclonal origin of human atherosclerotic plaques. Proc Nat Acad Sci USA 1973;*70:*1753.
77. Steinberg D, Parthasarathy S, Carew TE, Khoo JC, Witztum JL. Modifications of low-density lipoprotein that increase its atherogenicity. New Engl J Med 1989;*320:*915.
78. Friedman RJ, Stemerman MB, Wenz B et al. The effect of thrombocytopenia on experimental arteriosclerotic lesion formation in rabbits. J Clin Invest 1977;*60:*1191.
79. Moore S, Friedman RJ, Singal DP et al. Inhibition of injury induced thromboatherosclerotic lesions by anti-platelet serum in rabbits. Thromb Haemost 1976;*35:*70.
80. Harker LA, Ross R, Slichter SJ et al. Homocystine-induced arteriosclerosis: The role of endothelial cell injury and platelet response in its genesis. J Clin Invest 1976;*58:*731.
81. Boers GHJ, Smal AGH, Trijbels FJM et al. Heterozygosity for homocysteinuria in premature peripheral and cerebral occlusive arterial disease. New Engl J Med 1985;*313:*725.
82. Clarke R, Daly L, Robinson K et al. Hyperhomocysteinemia: An independent risk factor for vascular disease. N Engl J Med 1991;*324:*1149.
83. Asmussen I. Ultrastructure of human umbilical arteries from newborn children of smoking and non-smoking mothers. Acta Path Microbiol Immunol Scand. Sect A 1982;*90:*375.
84. Smith EB. Fibrinogen, fibrin and fibrin degradation products in relation to atherosclerosis. Clin Haematol 1986;*15:*355.
85. Smith EB, Alexander KM, Massie IB. Insoluble "fibrin" in human aortic intima. Quantitative studies on the relationship between insoluble "fibrin", soluble fibrinogen and LD-lipoprotein. Atherosclerosis 1976;*23:*19.
86. Bar-Shavit R, Wilner GD. Mediation of cellular events by thrombin. Int Rev Exp Pathol 1986;*29:*213.
87. Brown MS, Goldstein JL. Plasma lipoproteins: teaching old dogmas new tricks. Nature 1987;*330:*113.
88. Minick CR, Alonso DR, Rankin L. Role of immunologic arterial injury in atherogenesis. Thromb & Haemos 1978;*39:*304.
89. Lopes-Virella MF, Virella G. Immunological and microbiological factors in the pathogenesis of atherosclerosis. Clin Immunol Immunopathol 1985;*37:*377.
90. Van der Wal AC, Das PK, Bentz Van de Berg D, Van der Loos CM, Becker AE. Atherosclerotic lesions in humans. In situ immunophenotypic analysis suggesting an immune mediated response. Lab Invest 1989;*61:*166.
91. Libby P, Hansson GK. Biology of Disease. Involvement of the immune system in human atherogenesis: current knowledge and unanswered questions. Lab Invest 1991;*64:*5.
92. Seifert PS, Messner M, Roth I, Bhakdi S. Analysis of complement C3 activation products in human atherosclerotic lesions. Atherosclerosis 1991;*91:*155.
93. Emeson EE, Robertson AL Jr. T-Lymphocytes in aortic and coronary intimas. Their potential role in atherogenesis. Am J Pathol 1988;*130:*369.
94. Beaumont JL, Doucet F, Vivier P, Antonucci M. Immunoglobulin-bound lipoproteins (Ig-Lp) as markers of familial hypercholesterolemia, xanthomatosis and atherosclerosis. Atherosclerosis 1988;*74:*191.
95. Criqui MH, Lee ER, Hamburger RN, Klauber MR, Coughlin SS. IgE and Cardiovascular Disease. Results from a population-based study. Am J Med 1987;*82:*964.
96. Korkmaz ME, Oto A, Saraçlar Y et al. Levels of IgE in the serum of patients with coronary arterial disease. Int J Cardiol 1991;*31:*199.
97. Høiby N, Döring G, Schiøtz PO. Antibody and immune complexes induce tissue factor production by human endothelial cells. J Immunol 1986;*40:*29.
98. Tannenbaum SH, Finko R, Cines DB. Antibody and immune complexes induce tissue factor production by human endothelial cells. J Immunol 1986;*137:*1532.

99. Linnanmäki E, Leinonen M, Mattila K, Nieminen MS, Valtonen V, Saikku P. Chlamydia pneumoniae-specific circulating immune complexes in patients with chronic coronary heart disease. Circulation 1993;*87:*1130.
100. D'Anastasio C, Impallomeni M, McPherson GA et al. Antibodies against monocytes and endothelial cells in the sera of patients with atherosclerotic peripheral arterial disease. Atherosclerosis 1988;*74:*99.
101. Petrie BL, Adam E, Melnick JL. Association of herpesvirus/cytomegalovirus infections with human atherosclerosis. Prog med Virol 1988;*35:*21.
102. Hajjar DP, Fabricant CG, Minick CR, Fabricant J. Virus-induced atherosclerosis. Herpesvirus infection alters aortic cholesterol metabolism and accumulation. Am J Pathol 1986;*122:*62.
103. Vercellotti GM. Proinflammatory and procoagulant effects of herpes simplex infection on human endothelium. Blood Cells 1990;*16:*209.
104. Melnick JL, Petrie BL, Dreesman GR, Burek J, McCollum CH, DeBakey ME. Cytomegalovirus antigen within human arterial smooth muscle cells. Lancet 1983;*2:*644.
105. Myerson D, Hackman RC, Nelson JA, Ward DC, McDougall JK. Widespread presence of histologically occult cytomegalovirus. Hum Pathol 1984;*15:*430.
106. Hendrix MG, Dormans PH, Kitslaar P, Bosman F, Bruggeman CA. The presence of cytomegalovirus nucleic acids in arterial walls of atherosclerotic and nonatherosclerotic patients. Am J Pathol 1989;*134:*1151.
107. Hendrix MGR, Salimans MM, van Boven CP, Bruggeman CA. High prevalence of latently present cytomegalovirus in arterial walls of patients suffering from grade III atherosclerosis. Am J Pathol 1990;*136:*23.
108. Grayston JT. Chlamydia in atherosclerosis. Circulation 1993;*87:*1408.
109. Spodick DH. Inflammation and the onset of myocardial infarction. Ann Intern Med 1985;*102:*699.
110. Kahn JP, Perumal AS, Gully RJ, Smith TM, Cooper TB, Klein DF. Correlation of type A behaviour with adrenergic receptor density: implications for coronary artery pathogenesis. Lancet 1987;*2:*937.
111. Wissler RW. Principles of the pathogenesis of atherosclerosis. In: Braunwald E (ed). Heart Disease. 2nd Edition. Philadelphia, W B Saunders, 1984.
112. Fulton WFM. The Coronary Arteries. Springfield, Illinois, Charles C Thomas, 1965.

The multiple ischemic stimuli

INTRODUCTION

Ischemic stimuli are the fundamental components of ischemic heart disease (IHD) because without them there would be no ischemic disease. They include all acute *coronary* and *extra-coronary* organic and functional changes that cause, or contribute to cause, a sudden imbalance between myocardial oxygen requirements and coronary blood supply, and hence myocardial ischemia (see Table 9.1).

Coronary ischemic stimuli that suddenly reduce myocardial blood supply include epicardial coronary artery occlusive spasm, dynamic modulation of pliable stenoses, small coronary vessel constriction, and mural or occlusive thrombosis. They can cause a variable degree of impairment of myocardial perfusion and carry an extremely variable prognosis: they can be mild and cause a subliminal reduction of coronary flow reserve that results in ischemia only in the presence of a coincidental increase of myocardial oxygen demand, or they can be so intense as to reduce resting coronary blood flow (CBF) and cause transient or persistent subendocardial or transmural myocardial ischemia. Both mild and intense ischemic stimuli can reflect either chronic stable coronary alterations with no intrinsic evolutive tendency, as in *chronic stable angina,* or coronary lesions that can evolve in the short term towards persistent coronary artery occlusion and infarction, as in *unstable angina.* Any intense coronary ischemic stimulus, when persisting for longer than 30 min, can cause *acute myocardial infarction* (MI); such persistent stimuli, resulting in infarction (whatever their initiating mechanisms), are usually associated with coronary thrombosis.

Extracoronary ischemic stimuli include all changes in cardiac function that increase myocardial oxygen requirements beyond maximal residual coronary flow reserve (which is typically limited by chronic obstructions in epicardial coronary arteries). When ischemia is caused by such stimuli, although the coronary circulation has a reduced flow reserve it does not have an *active acute* role in the development of myocardial ischemia, or at least not initially. Typically, extracoronary stimuli occur in patients with at least one critical coronary artery stenosis. When such stimuli are the only cause of ischemia, patients develop ischemic episodes *only when,* and *each time that,* myocardial oxygen demand exceeds coronary flow reserve (fixed threshold, stable exertional angina). Extracoronary stimuli can cause life-threatening myocardial ischemia only when the ischemia is severe, extensive, and prolonged,

Table 9.1 Causes of Myocardial Ischemia*

Ischemic stimuli	Mechanisms
1. Extracoronary: cause ischemia only when myocardial demand exceeds maximal residual coronary flow reserve	Increased myocardial demand beyond the possibility of coronary blood supply, limited by chronic atherosclerotic stenoses, by fresh thrombi, or by inadequate dilatory response of prearterioles or arterioles
2. Coronary (stable or unstable): cause ischemia also in the absence of increased myocardial demand	Sudden impairment of CBF by occlusive epicardial coronary artery spasm, dynamic stenosis, platelet aggregation, and thrombosis, and by small coronary vessel constriction (prearteriolar or arteriolar)
3. Combination of extracoronary and coronary: cause ischemia during subliminal increases of myocardial demand because of a coincidental transient subliminal reduction of coronary flow reserve by any of the mechanisms listed under (2) above	An occasional combination of a transient, subliminal increase of myocardial demand and a transient subliminal coronary ischemic stimulus, each in itself insufficient to cause myocardial ischemia

* Myocardial ischemia, painful or painless, can be caused by extracoronary stimuli in the presence of flow-limiting stenoses, by stable or unstable coronary stimuli that suddenly reduce coronary blood flow, or by a variable combination of the two

i.e. in patients with proximal coronary artery stenoses not compensated for by collaterals, when the increase in myocardial oxygen consumption far exceeds the possible increase in CBF.

When a large fraction of left ventricular wall becomes ischemic and fails to contract, acute left ventricular failure and fatal arrhythmias may occur, particularly in the presence of previous infarction and/or scar tissue. In general, in the absence of scarring, when the ischemic area is small and the discrepancy between demand and supply is also small, extracoronary ischemic stimuli carry a good prognosis, at least in the short term, because they have no intrinsic evolutive tendency toward sudden persistent coronary occlusion.

This chapter reviews the mechanisms of ischemia caused by extracoronary stimuli and presents the available information on the mechanisms of epicardial coronary artery constriction and spasm, small coronary vessel constriction, and mural and occlusive thrombosis. It discusses the association of ischemic stimuli causing acute MI and, finally, indicates rational therapeutic principles.

9.1 ISCHEMIA CAUSED BY EXTRACORONARY ISCHEMIC STIMULI

Extracoronary stimuli generally cause only subendocardial myocardial ischemia, usually characterized by ST-segment depression on the ECG, because coronary flow reserve distal to flow-limiting stenoses is much lower in subendocardial than in subepicardial layers. The development of ischemia produces a vicious hemodynamic cycle which, unless interrupted, progressively exacerbates the condition.

Distal to flow-limiting stenoses, myocardial ischemia can develop as a consequence of:

a. increased myocardial metabolic demand
b. subepicardial arteriolar vasodilation caused by drugs
c. severe arterial hypotension.

The effect of ischemic stimuli is enhanced by tachycardia and increased diastolic ventricular pressure (see Chs 4 and 6).

Increased cardiac contractile activity causes metabolically mediated arteriolar dilation and increased blood flow. In the absence of flow-limiting stenoses, perfusion pressure at the origin of arteriolar vessels is normally maintained within an optimal range by flow-mediated vasodilation of prearteriolar vessels. In contrast, flow-limiting stenoses cause a transstenotic pressure gradient that increases exponentially with flow (see 6.1.1). Doubling of flow across a stenosis, therefore, requires more than doubling of the transstenotic pressure gradient, i.e. it requires the reduction of poststenotic coronary pressure by more than one-half.

When metabolic demand increases, flow distal to flow-limiting stenoses can increase more in subepicardial layers, where there is a larger coronary flow reserve, than in subendocardial layers; however, oxygen consumption is greater in subendocardial than in subepicardial layers. During progressive increase of myocardial metabolic demand, poststenotic pressure may become insufficient to perfuse subendocardial layers, and subendocardial flow decreases progressively as subepicardial flow increases above basal (see Fig. 6.4).

Selective vasoconstriction of subepicardial vessels (prearterioles and/or arterioles) would result in both a lesser increase of transstenotic flow and a lesser drop in poststenotic pressure. Conversely, excessive subepicardial vessel dilation would cause a larger decrease in poststenotic perfusion pressure and more severe subendocardial ischemia. Thus, luxury perfusion of subepicardial layers can contribute to myocardial ischemia in subendocardial layers by transmural blood flow "steal" (see 6.1.2).

Pharmacologically induced coronary arteriolar vasodilation can cause, or help to cause, subendocardial ischemia by the hemodynamic mechanisms outlined above. Dipyridamole is the classic vasodilator stimulant which, when given acutely in sufficient doses, can cause subendocardial ischemia distal to flow-limiting stenoses, predominantly by increasing subepicardial blood flow (transmural blood flow steal) (see Chs 6 and 10). Its proischemic effects are potentiated by stimuli that simultaneously increase cardiac contractile activity and heart rate. Other vasodilator drugs may also cause luxury perfusion of subepicardial layers—directly, by increasing subepicardial perfusion, or indirectly, by opposing subepicardial vasoconstrictor mechanisms (see Ch. 6).

Acute arterial hypotension can cause subendocardial ischemia distal to flow-limiting stenoses when the poststenotic pressure that is required to maintain flow becomes too low to perfuse the subendocardial layers. The deleterious effects of acute arterial hypotension are potentiated by increased cardiac contractile activity, by tachycardia, and by drugs that cause dilation or prevent constriction of subepicardial vessels, thus resulting in transmural blood flow steal.

Paradoxical proischemic effects of nifedipine and, less frequently, nitrates have been very occasionally reported in association with a fall in arterial blood pressure in patients with severe effort-related angina. These hypotension-related ischemic effects may be potentiated by transmural myocardial blood flow steal.

9.1.1 General concepts of residual coronary flow reserve

As discussed in Chapter 6, a 75% diameter stenosis allows CBF to increase about threefold above resting values (when resting flow is not elevated). This increased flow should allow the heart rate/blood pressure product to increase at least twofold during exercise without causing ischemia (see Ch. 4).

As discussed in Chapters 4 and 6, for a given coronary stenosis, resting poststenotic pressure depends on:

a. resting CBF across the stenosis
b. collateral blood flow
c. systemic blood pressure.

Transstenotic flow depends on myocardial blood flow per gram of tissue and on the total amount of tissue perfused. The conditions that increase resting myocardial oxygen consumption or reduce the oxygen content of arterial blood (anemia or hypoxia), therefore, increase resting CBF and hence reduce resting coronary poststenotic pressure and residual coronary flow reserve. (In the presence of a 50% reduction of hemoglobin concentration, resting blood flow approximately doubles.) In addition, doubling of myocardial mass by hypertrophy causes doubling of resting transstenotic flow. In a patient with severe hypertrophy and severe anemia, resting coronary flow through a stenosis can be increased fourfold and doubling of resting myocardial oxygen consumption would require an eightfold increase in transstenotic flow, and a greater than eightfold decrease in poststenotic coronary pressure.

Adequate *collateral blood flow* is compatible with a normal effort test, even in the presence of a total proximal occlusion of the left anterior descending or right coronary arteries.

A decrease in *systemic blood pressure* can decrease coronary flow reserve because of the consequent reduction of coronary poststenotic pressure. Conversely, an increase in systemic

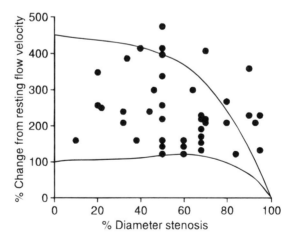

Fig. 9.1 Lack of relationship between stenosis severity and coronary flow reserve in patients. No relationship exists between the severity of coronary stenoses and peak hyperemic response following transient coronary occlusion at the time of bypass surgery. The continuous lines indicate the relationship between resting flow and flow reserve observed in dogs (see Ch. 6). Some vessels with moderate stenoses have a very reduced coronary flow response, which may be due to distal vessel dysfunction. (Modified from ref. 1.)

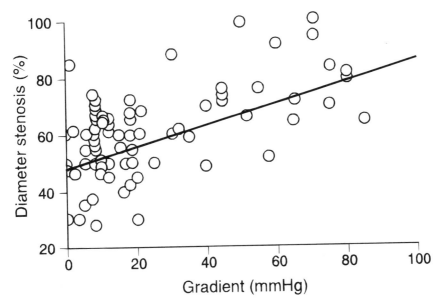

Fig. 9.2 Variable relation between coronary stenosis and transstenotic pressure gradient. Measurements obtained during coronary arteriography indicate, for example, that the same pressure gradient of 20 mmHg can be found in stenoses ranging from 30 to 70% diameter reduction. Large gradients across mild stenoses may be caused either by very high basal flow or by dynamic stenoses; small gradients across severe stenoses may be caused either by low transstenotic flow or by high collateral flow (which increases poststenotic pressure). (Modified from ref. 2.)

blood pressure should increase residual coronary flow reserve according to the findings obtained in experimental animals; however, this effect is not easily detectable in patients and has not been studied in depth.

In patients with multiple stenoses, the stenosis that determines the level of the residual coronary flow reserve is that with the lowest poststenotic pressure, independent of the size of the distal myocardial territory. When ischemia develops distal to one stenosis, the subsequent positive feedback mechanism described below may impair perfusion distal to other subcritical stenoses and cause an extension of ischemia.

As indicated in Chapter 6, in experimental animals acute reduction of the coronary diameter by about 90% (a 99% lumen stenosis) is required to reduce basal resting flow, and in chronic conditions such a severe stenosis is usually compensated for by the development of collaterals that prevent ischemia from occurring in resting conditions. For the same levels of resting flow and aortic pressure, the residual coronary flow reserve can be dynamically reduced by transient constriction or thrombosis at the level of a stenosis, by reduction of collateral flow, or by inappropriate constriction of distal vessels.

In sharp contrast to the results of animal studies, measuring coronary flow reserve in patients at the time of bypass surgery reveals the lack of any correlation between the severity of coronary stenoses and coronary flow reserve (see Fig. 9.1).[1] This large variability is unlikely to be due to measurement errors and probably results from the variable compensation provided by collateral blood flow and from small coronary vessel dysfunction (see 9.3.2). These pioneering findings were confirmed subsequently during cardiac catheteriza-

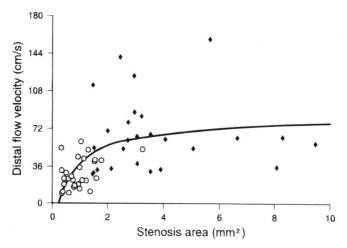

Fig. 9.3 Wide variation in the relation between coronary stenosis severity and distal flow velocity during vasodilation. The flow response during a vasodilator stimulus is very weakly correlated to the stenotic area. A low flow response may be due to either the severity of the stenosis or an inadequate dilator stimulus of resistive vessels. When the limitation of flow is caused by the severity of the stenosis, the transstenotic pressure gradient should be very large. (Modified from ref. 3.)

tion: the transstenotic pressure gradient was very weakly correlated not only with the diameter of stenosis (see Fig. 9.2)[2] but also with the distal hyperemic flow velocity (see Fig. 9.3).[3]

9.1.2 Positive and negative feedback mechanisms created by ischemia

The absence of contractile function in an ischemic region causes an impairment of global ventricular contractile function, with dyskinetic asynchronous contraction, increased diastolic pressure, and increased ventricular volume. The elevated diastolic pressure increases tissue pressure and hence diastolic extracoronary resistance in the inner ventricular wall, which may reduce flow in areas where perfusion pressure is low and subendocardial coronary flow reserve is critically reduced. Increased ventricular volume attributable to incomplete systolic emptying contributes to the increase of both extravascular resistance and oxygen consumption. Myocardial oxygen consumption can also be increased by the elevation of arterial pressure and of heart rate that accompany anginal pain. When ischemia is prolonged it may also impair endothelial function and, hence, the endothelial control of CBF in the ischemic vascular bed. Thus, once initiated, myocardial ischemia (also when caused by extracoronary stimuli), tends to be exacerbated by multiple elements in a vicious cycle. Conversely, transient ischemic episodes may provide protection against subsequent persistent ischemia by preconditioning of the myocardium (see Ch. 7).

9.2 OCCLUSIVE SPASM AND DYNAMIC STENOSIS OF EPICARDIAL CORONARY ARTERIES

It is now generally accepted that an episodic increase of vasomotor tone in a segment of an epicardial coronary artery is not only the cause of variant angina but may also represent a pathogenetic component in other, more common, anginal syndromes.[4-6] Occlusive spasm, as typically observed in variant angina, is fairly rare compared with nonocclusive dynamic stenosis and should, therefore, be considered separately. Occlusive epicardial coronary artery spasm causes transmural ischemia and ST-segment elevation when it reduces flow by at least 50%. An acute reduction of the coronary diameter by about 90% is required in order to cause subendocardial ischemia and ST-segment depression at rest. Lesser degrees of lumen reduction can cause ischemia when resting flow per gram of myocardium is greatly elevated by anemia or hypoxia, or when the myocardial mass is greatly increased by hypertrophy. Thus, the degree of constriction necessary to precipitate ischemia at the site of a 70% diameter stenosis is considerably less than that at the site of a 50% diameter stenosis. The degree of lumen reduction required to cause ischemia is greater in the presence of collaterals, and no detectable ischemia may develop even during occlusive spasm if the collaterals are well developed and function normally (see Ch. 10).

Changing concepts

As reported in a recent review,[7] the concept of coronary artery spasm, proposed by Osler to explain the apparently spontaneous occurrence of some episodes of angina, gradually lost favor after the dogmatic statement by Keefer and Resnik, that the coronary arteries in patients with angina were so severely fibrosed and calcified that it was not possible for them to go into spasm, and also after the classic studies of Blumgart and coworkers. The pendulum swung to an extreme when Pickering stated that spasm was "a resort of the diagnostically destitute." It began to swing in the opposite direction with the clinical reasoning of Prinzmetal et al, who proposed that "increased tonus at the site of an atherosclerotic plaque" was the probable cause of a "variant" form of spontaneous angina characterized by ST-segment elevation; however, at that time they did not dare use the term "spasm"! An occasional angiographic record of spasm was reported by Gensini et al in 1962, but it was not until the early 1970s that the hypothesis of spasm was resurrected by MacAlpin et al to explain the preserved exercise tolerance of patients with Prinzmetal's angina. A "variant of the variant" was then described in some patients with this syndrome, who had no detectable atherosclerotic epicardial coronary artery stenoses. Objective demonstration of spasm in variant angina was first provided in isolated case reports and subsequently by systematic studies; thus, it became a "proved hypothesis."

Consequences of the revival of coronary artery spasm

The proof that angina could be caused by a transient reduction of coronary flow, as well as by an excessive increase of myocardial demand (traditionally the only accepted cause), broke a conceptual barrier. In 1976, we presented our experience and proposed that many other non-variant cases of angina at rest were caused by a transient impairment of coronary blood supply, rather than by an increased demand. At the time, we proposed the term "primary" angina, rather than "vasospastic" angina, to emphasize not just coronary artery spasm as one of the possible causes but the more general concept of a transient impairment of coronary flow.[8] At the time, however, angina not caused by increased myocardial demand was still thought to be so unbelievably rare that it was labeled "Pisa" angina by several leading international cardiologists, and spasm was thought to be "a totally Italian syndrome,"[9] as McGregor recently recalled.[10]

Nowadays, the term "coronary spasm" is often used to indicate any form of coronary vasoconstriction. This generalization may find some justification in the common clinical indication for coronary vasodilator therapy that nonspecifically reduces smooth muscle tone, but it is confusing when trying to identify the actual causes of abnormal vasoconstriction and develop specific forms of preventive treatment. Three facts are now clear.

1. The degree of epicardial coronary artery constriction can vary. At one extreme is the mild, physiologic response to common constrictor stimuli commonly observed in experimental animals; at the other is the severe, segmental constriction leading to total occlusion of a major coronary artery, typically observed in patients with variant angina.

2. The effects of constrictor stimuli depend on their intensity and on the reactivity of the smooth muscle (see Ch. 5), as well as on the severity and anatomic features of stenoses and basal tone. The rigidity and smooth muscle atrophy of athero-

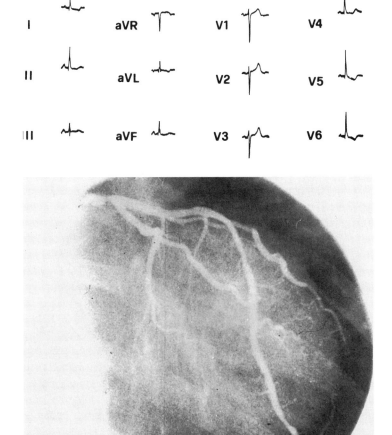

A

Fig. 9.4 Diffuse rather than focal coronary constriction in a patient with variant angina. Compared with basal (**A**), ergonovine (**B**) caused diffuse constriction with typical angina and ST-segment depression. A diffuse constrictor response is fairly rare in Caucasian patients, but is observed more frequently in Japanese patients. This patient had spontaneous angina with ST-segment elevation and a negative exercise test. (Modified from ref. 11.) *(Figure continues.)*

sclerotic plaques considerably limit the constrictor response of chronic coronary stenoses. Endothelial function has a profound influence on coronary tone (see Chs 1 and 5).

3. The mechanisms responsible for the occlusive spasm that typically recurs in patients with variant angina over weeks or months without causing infarction, may differ from those that occur very occasionally and cause acute MI, and certainly differ from those of stable dynamic but nonocclusive stenoses that recur over months or years in patients with chronic stable angina.

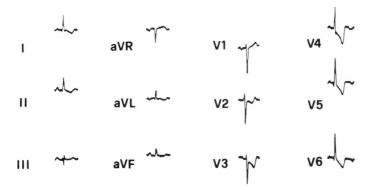

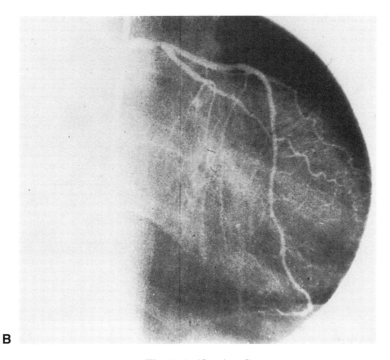

Fig. 9.4 *(Continued)*.

9.2.1 Different degrees and patterns of coronary vasoconstriction

In response to vasoconstrictor stimuli, epicardial coronary arteries can undergo uniform mild diffuse constriction, occlusive segmental spasm, and also intermediate degrees of constriction at the site of organic stenoses.

"Physiologic" coronary constriction

As discussed in Chapter 6, epicardial coronary arteries in animals respond to a variety of common constrictor stimuli with a uniform reduction in diameter not exceeding 20–30%, which fails to cause a pressure gradient. The constrictor response depends on basal tone, as vessels that are maximally dilated in the basal state can constrict more in response to constrictor stimuli: in patients who do not have variant angina, the reduction in epicardial coronary artery diameter in response to the administration of ergonovine is usually diffuse and quite mild, not exceeding 30%. As this fairly uniform, mild to moderate degree of constriction is usually observed in both animal and human coronary arteries, it can be considered within the "physiologic" range. However, the identification of an abnormal constrictor response may not be straightforward because, for example, some patients with variant angina exhibit intense (greater than 30% reduction in diameter) diffuse constriction of all coronary artery branches rather than segmental occlusive spasm, during spontaneous or induced ischemic episodes[11,12] (see Fig. 9.4). Yet similar diffuse constriction may also be observed occasionally in response to ergonovine, in the absence of both angina and ischemic ECG changes, in patients with no clinical features of variant angina (see Fig. 9.5).[13] Abnormal diffuse coronary vasomotion is rare, at least among Caucasians, as it was observed in only 40 of 2758 patients after the ergometrine test.[12]

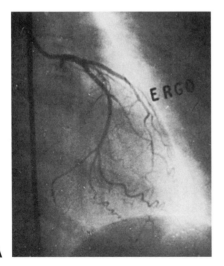 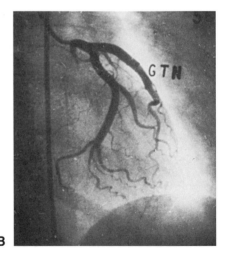

A   B

Fig. 9.5 Diffuse coronary vasoconstriction in a patient with atypical chest pain. Ergonovine caused diffuse coronary constriction (**A**) compared with the angiogram taken after administration of nitrates, in the absence of pain and ECG changes (**B**). This rather extreme case indicates the difficulty of defining normal and abnormal coronary vasomotion. (Modified from ref. 13.)

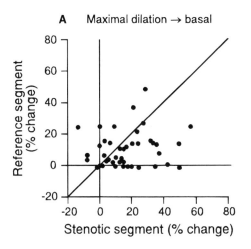

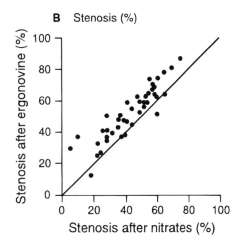

Fig. 9.6 Variability of basal vasomotor tone in moderate coronary stenoses compared with reference segments. **(A)** In stenotic segments with a basal diameter reduction of 20–70%, the dilation observed following administration of nitrates is proportional to that observed in the angiographically normal adjacent reference segment in only a minority of cases; some stenoses dilated much more than reference segments, probably because their basal vasomotor tone was greater; others dilated much less, possibly because they were already dilated in the basal state or had a reduced vasomotor potential. **(B)** The percentage stenosis calculated as the ratio of stenosed to reference segments is, on average, greater during a constrictor stimulus than during maximal dilation, indicating that the vasomotor response to constrictor stimuli is, on average, greater in stenotic than in reference segments. (Modified from ref. 14.)

Dynamic coronary stenoses

Between the physiologic degree of constriction observed in normal coronary arteries in response to common constrictor stimuli, and occlusive segmental spasm in patients with variant angina, intermediate degrees of coronary constriction can be observed at the site of organic coronary stenoses in patients with chronic stable angina and in those with unstable angina. In patients with chronic stable angina, stenotic and atherosclerotic coronary segments can develop constriction (but without causing vessel closure) in response to stimuli that normally cause vasodilation (see Ch. 5 and 9.2.5). This abnormal response to vasoactive stimuli does not have the same cause or the same clinical significance as occlusive spasm (see below). In addition, the vasomotor response of coronary stenoses depends on their basal tone, which may not necessarily be related to that of the adjacent angiographically normal segment (see Fig. 9.6A,B). The basal tone can only be assessed by comparing an angiogram taken in basal conditions with one taken after maximal coronary dilation. In patients who do not have variant angina, when a vasoconstrictor stimulus such as ergonovine or ergometrine is given, the stenoses that constrict the most are often those that dilate the least when intracoronary nitrates are administered, and vice versa (see Fig. 9.7).[14] In general, distal and eccentric stenoses have a greater potential for vasomotor reactivity than proximal and concentric stenoses[15–17] (see Fig. 9.8).

Unfortunately, the dynamic vasomotor potential of very tight stenoses, which would have the most dramatic hemodynamic effects, cannot be measured as accurately as that of mild

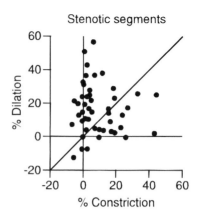

Fig. 9.7 Constrictor and dilator response of stenoses from basal state. Compared with basal, the percentage constriction of stenoses following the administration of ergonovine is, on average, greater in those stenoses that dilate less following nitrates and smallest in those that dilate more, as observed in normal coronary segments (see Ch. 5). Stenoses that are more constricted in the basal state have a greater potential to dilate than to constrict further. (Modified from ref. 14.)

or moderate stenoses because of the limited resolution of the radiographic images. For example, small changes in diameter of a 75% stenosis of a 2 mm artery cannot be measured even by automatic computerized analysis because its basal diameter (0.5 mm) is close to the limits of the geometric resolution of radiographic equipment, even under favorable imaging conditions.

Occlusive epicardial coronary artery spasm

The degree of constriction that characterizes occlusive spasm, as typically observed in the rare syndrome of variant angina, can easily be distinguished angiographically from lesser forms of epicardial coronary constriction.[7] Occlusive segmental spasm should be considered as a separate entity because it is usually localized, and because only when increased vasomotor tone causes occlusion of the vessel, with interruption of blood flow, does the ST segment become elevated; blood stasis predisposes to the development or extension of coronary thrombosis, to potentially fatal arrhythmias, and, when persistent, to myocardial

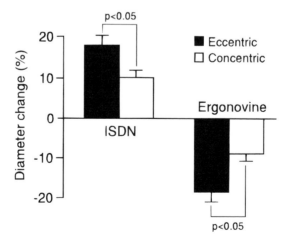

Fig. 9.8 Vasomotor response of concentric and eccentric stenoses. In patients with chronic stable angina, eccentric stenoses (■) exhibit, on average, significantly larger constrictor and dilator responses ($P < 0.05$) than concentric stenoses (□). ISDN, isosorbide dinitrate. (Modified from ref. 15.)

necrosis. These complications are not inevitable consequences of occlusive coronary artery spasm, as they are fairly rare in patients with variant angina even when they have frequent episodes of transmural ischemia (see Ch. 19).

9.2.2 Limited geometric amplification of constriction in chronic stenoses

Theoretically, even a mild constriction of an epicardial coronary artery could cause a critical reduction of the lumen, or total occlusion at the site of an intimal plaque that occupies a significant fraction of the lumen. This concept, originally proposed by MacAlpin,[18] can be grasped intuitively by considering that a vessel in which the lumen is uniformly reduced by 50% by a constrictor stimulus could become occluded at the site where a plaque occupies 50% of the lumen. However, the geometric magnification of the reduction of the lumen produced in normal segments by vasoconstriction can take place only if the plaque does not increase the rigidity of the wall and does not cause smooth muscle atrophy. The rigidity and smooth muscle atrophy of atherosclerotic coronary segments increases with the severity of the stenosis (see Ch. 8). Angiographic studies in patients with chronic stable angina indicate also that mild and moderate stenoses constrict to a much lesser extent than predicted by the geometric amplification theory from the constriction observed in the adjacent reference segment (see Fig. 9.9A,B), whereas in patients with variant angina they constrict more than predicted (see Fig. 9.10). The theory of geometric amplification may apply when the lumen is occupied by a fresh thrombus in a previously normal vessel without impairing its wall compliance, but this hypothesis lacks confirmation.

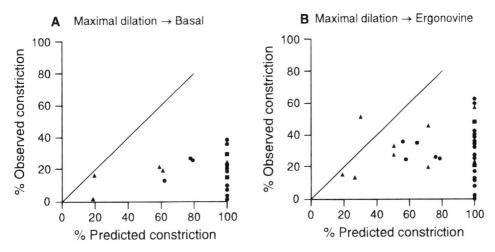

Fig. 9.9 Limited geometric amplification of constriction in chronic stenoses. The degree of constriction at the site of stenosis (■, severe; ●, moderate; ▲, mild) is consistently smaller than predicted from the degree of constriction observed in the adjacent reference segment on the basis of the geometric theory. **(A)** Compared with the maximal dilation following administration of nitrates, many stenotic segments should become occluded in the basal state if the same amount of constriction observed in reference segments was amplified geometrically by the subintimal plaque at the site of the stenosis. **(B)** Following ergonovine administration, all but one stenosis constricted less than predicted from the constriction observed in reference segments. Thus, in chronic stenoses, the predicted geometric amplification of constriction by subintimal plaques is limited by smooth muscle atrophy and wall rigidity. (Modified from ref. 14.)

■ *At the site of chronic plaques, therefore, segmental occlusive spasm of an epicardial coronary artery can develop either in response to very efficacious abnormal constrictor stimuli or, in the presence of local hyperreactivity, to constrictor stimuli. Vasoconstriction within a "physiologic" range could cause total occlusion only at the site of a normal or near-normal segment of the wall in which a considerable fraction of the lumen is occupied by fresh or recently organized thrombus.* ■

9.2.3 Mechanisms of occlusive segmental spasm in variant angina

A distinctive clinical feature of variant angina is the frequent recurrence of occlusive epicardial coronary artery spasm for weeks or months, even several times a day. It is this recurrence that allows the mechanisms of spasm to be studied in this syndrome. As discussed in a recent review,[7] spasm in variant angina cannot be attributed to either a dysfunction of the parasympathetic or α-adrenergic sympathetic autonomic nervous systems or an imbalance between local production of prostacyclin and thromboxane A_2, as initially suggested by some investigators. Furthermore, geometric magnification of a degree of constriction within the "physiologic" range does not explain the segmental vessel occlusion that occurs in variant angina, because spastic segments often constrict more than predicted by the geometric theory (see Fig. 9.10).[19] A local coronary artery hyperreactivity to a wide variety of normal constrictor stimuli has been shown to be the fundamental alteration underlying occlusive spasm. The causes of segmental coronary hyperreactivity responsible for occlusive coronary artery spasm in patients with variant angina are not clear.

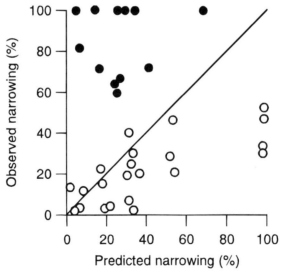

Fig. 9.10 Enhanced constrictor response of spastic segments in variant angina. Following administration of ergonovine, the constrictor response of spastic segments is much greater than that predicted by the geometric theory in patients with variant angina (●), in contrast to patients who do not have variant angina (○). Thus, in variant angina, the constrictor response of spastic segments is markedly enhanced. (Modified from ref. 19.)

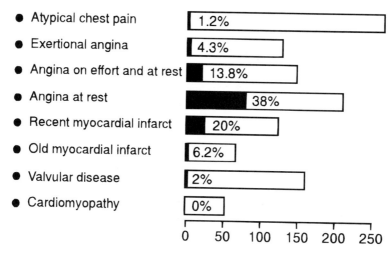

- Atypical chest pain — 1.2%
- Exertional angina — 4.3%
- Angina on effort and at rest — 13.8%
- Angina at rest — 38%
- Recent myocardial infarct — 20%
- Old myocardial infarct — 6.2%
- Valvular disease — 2%
- Cardiomyopathy — 0%

0   50   100   150   200   250

Fig. 9.11 Frequency of provoked coronary arterial spasm in 1089 patients undergoing coronary arteriography. The frequency of ergometrine-induced spasm is greatest in patients with angina at rest and recent MI, and is very low in patients with atypical chest pain, exertional angina, old MI, valvular disease, and cardiomyopathy. Thus, a localized coronary artery hyperreactivity to ergometrine, similar to that observed in patients with variant angina, is common only in acute ischemic syndromes. (Modified from ref. 20.)

A review of available data indicates that the cause of the local hyperreactivity cannot be attributed merely to any of the following:

1. *Atherosclerotic plaques or cholesterol deposits;* these are extremely common, whereas the syndrome of variant angina is very rare.
2. *Critical coronary stenoses;* these are also fairly common. Ergonovine induces ischemia in only a very few patients with chronic stable exertional angina, i.e. those with severe stenoses and positive exercise tests at very low work loads, but never with ST-segment elevation. After administration of ergonovine, occlusive spasm has been detected in a minority of patients with chronic effort angina or old MI and flow-limiting coronary stenoses[20] (see Fig. 9.11).
3. *Endothelial dysfunction;* this cannot be the only cause, first, because endothelial denudation and massive platelet deposition in previously normal arteries cause only a 30% diameter reduction (see Ch. 6); second, because total occlusion has never been reported in endothelial denuded coronary arteries; and third, because atheroma and fatty streaks are fairly common in epicardial coronary arteries and spasm is *very* rare. Finally, spasm in some patients may occur occasionally over periods of weeks or months; in others it may occur persistently for years without changes occurring in the severity of the underlying stenosis.
4. *The type of lesions responsible for segmental coronary hyperreactivity in the miniature swine model;* in this model, spasm can be predictably elicited by histamine or serotonin (5-HT), but not by ergonovine.

In patients with variant angina, the cause of the local coronary hyperreactivity should be compatible with the following observations:

1. In some patients the exaggerated local response can either persist practically unchanged for months or years, or it can wane within weeks or months.
2. In some patients, coronary artery spasm can be induced by handgrip (with a delay of about 30 s) and the cold pressor test (with a delay of about 1 min), suggesting that it may respond to a neural trigger, but an exclusive neural origin can be excluded because spasm has also been observed in transplanted human hearts.
3. In the same patient, spasm can be caused by a variety of drugs (such as ergonovine, histamine, dopamine, acetylcholine, and 5-HT) acting on different receptors.
4. Spasm can also be caused by increasing the arterial blood pH to 7.65–7.70.
5. The histologic finding of fibromuscular hyperplasia at the site of coronary artery spasm, reported in some cases, could be a possible anatomic substratum for recurrent segmental spasm, but other patients have typical atherosclerotic plaques, and still others no detectable atherosclerosis (for review see references 7 and 13).

■ *The multiplicity of possible triggers and the possible persistence of local hyperreactivity for months or years in some patients, without macroscopic growth of the plaque lesion, would seem more compatible with a postreceptor alteration of signal transduction in local smooth muscle cells (SMCs) than with an alteration of the local endothelial lining.* ■

9.2.4 Coronary occlusive spasm in other acute ischemic syndromes

Occlusive coronary artery spasm may also be demonstrated in some patients who do not have the clinical syndrome of variant angina, but who present with unheralded acute MI or who suffer sudden ischemic cardiac death (SICD).[21,22] The largest systematic study in patients with IHD was performed by Bertrand et al[20] in 1089 patients, in whom the ergometrine test was performed during coronary arteriography.

This study showed that ergometrine (a substance very similar to ergonovine and used more widely in France) induced occlusive spasm in only 1% of patients with "atypical chest pain," in 4% of those with chronic stable exertional angina, and in 6% of those with old MI, but in as many as 38% of patients with rest angina and in 20% of those with recent MI (see Fig. 9.11). In *some* of the patients with recent MI the spasm occurred in a nonculprit artery. Although the pathophysiologic implications of a positive ergometrine test are not clear, the results of this study indicate that a local coronary hyperreactivity to ergometrine, similar to that encountered in variant angina, seems to be fairly rare in patients with stable angina, old infarction, and atypical chest pain, but may occur more frequently in patients with the acute coronary syndromes of infarction and angina at rest. Persistent, intense smooth muscle constriction would be consistent with the postmortem report of contraction bands found in the smooth muscle surrounding plaques in patients with unstable angina,[23] and with reports of spasm persisting post mortem.[24,25] Occlusive epicardial coronary artery spasm (which is often quite resistant to dilator drugs) was also reported in the immediate period after bypass surgery, and occlusive spasm was also detected in aortocoronary bypass grafts. The differences in clinical presentation suggest that the nature of the local coronary alteration responsible for the occasional spasm observed in some acute coronary syndromes may not be exactly the same as that responsible for the more chronic course typically observed in patients with variant angina.

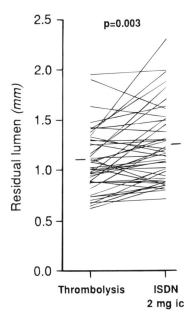

Fig. 9.12 Vasodilator response of infarct-related stenoses at the very end of intracoronary thrombolysis. Following intracoronary injection of isosorbide dinitrate (ISDN; 2 mg), most residual stenoses dilated ($P = 0.003$), some very considerably. This response occurred in spite of the very large doses of sublingual, intravenous, and intracoronary nitrates that all patients received during the last hour. Thus, constriction at the site of the infarct-related stenosis may be reduced only by very high doses of locally administered dilators because of the intensity of either the constrictor stimuli or the constrictor response. (Modified from ref. 26.)

The possible existence of localized coronary smooth muscle hyperreactivity in acute coronary syndromes, whatever its cause, is intriguing and appears to be worth exploring. Some recently recanalized infarct-related stenoses show the potential to dilate (often to a considerable extent) after administration of intracoronary nitrates (see Fig. 9.12),[26] and hence also to constrict. In such cases, the degree of constriction produced by thromboxane A_2, 5-HT, and thrombin would be greatly amplified geometrically at the site of fresh mural thrombi. The presence of local coronary hyperreactivity may be one of the coincidental crucial factors in the transition from a nonocclusive platelet–fibrin mural thrombus to an occlusive red thrombus.

9.2.5 Mechanisms of dynamic coronary stenosis in chronic stable angina

The mechanisms of dynamic modulation of coronary stenoses in patients with chronic stable angina obviously differ from those responsible for spasm in patients with variant angina, as the former:

a. have predominantly diurnal rather than nocturnal or early morning distribution of ischemic attacks
b. may have a positive cold pressor test but usually have a negative hyperventilation test (they do not develop ST-segment elevation), which is in contrast to patients with variant angina
c. have a positive ergonovine test only rarely (in the presence of severe reduction of effort tolerance) and never with ST-segment elevation.[7,13]

Thus, the reactivity of smooth muscle at the site of stenoses is not enhanced by the same mechanisms that operate in variant angina. Constriction may be caused by an abnormal response to the physiologic stimuli that cause vasodilation in the presence of normal endothelial function, or by pathologic neural or humoral constrictor stimuli.

As discussed in Chapters 1 and 6, endothelial dysfunction can abolish the dilator effect of vasoactive stimuli, leaving their direct constrictor effect unopposed. Several studies have shown that, in patients with angiographically detectable atherosclerosis, and even in older individuals or in those with risk factors for IHD, intracoronary infusion of acetylcholine causes coronary constriction rather than dilation. A similar response was also reported during exercise stress testing, during handgrip and cold pressor tests, and following intracoronary infusion of 5-HT: conversely, a normal dilator response was observed during intracoronary infusion of substance P and calcitonin gene-related peptide. (A review of the subject is contained in reference 27.)

Defective flow-mediated dilation can explain ischemic episodes caused by increased myocardial oxygen demand, but episodes of coronary constriction occurring at rest or during minimal efforts that are usually well tolerated, and the paradoxical constriction that occurs during handgrip and cold pressor tests, cannot be explained simply by defective flow-mediated vasodilation, as there is no increase in flow. Thus, they must be caused by abnormal vasoconstrictor humoral or neural mechanisms,[28] by vasoconstrictor substances released by resident cells in the arterial wall,[29] or by an enhanced smooth muscle constrictor response. The possibility that the dynamic impairment of CBF may not be related to endothelial dysfunction alone is suggested, first, by the high prevalence of both raised fibrous plaques and fatty streaks in normal individuals, which indicates that chronic endothelial dysfunction may often be attenuated by compensatory mechanisms, and, second, by the frequent waning of ischemic symptoms and signs in patients with chronic stable angina and angiographically detectable coronary atherosclerosis.

9.3 SMALL CORONARY VESSEL CONSTRICTION

The possibility that, in patients with IHD, impairment of CBF could also occur at the level of distal rather than proximal coronary vessels received little consideration until recently.[30] This is not surprising, as epicardial coronary artery stenoses, spasm, and dynamic modulation of stenoses by vasomotor tone or by intravascular plugging provide such readily available and plausible mechanisms for the development of ischemia.

That ischemia can be caused by constriction of small coronary vessels was demonstrated not only by pharmacologic studies in animals (see Ch. 6) and patients, but also by other clinical studies. The clinical importance of distal coronary vasomotion is suggested by studies in the following:

a. in selected patients with chronic stable angina, in whom the development of myocardial ischemia could not be attributed to epicardial coronary artery stenoses, thrombosis, or spasm
b. in patients after successful coronary angioplasty
c. in nonstenotic arteries of patients with IHD and coronary stenoses in other coronary arteries
d. in patients with syndrome X.

It is not yet known precisely where the abnormal constriction of small vessels takes place, nor what mechanisms are involved. Small vessel constriction typically causes predominantly subendocardial ischemia with ST-segment depression.

9.3.1 Pharmacologic studies in humans

Intracoronary infusion, not only of neuropeptide Y (NPY) and of large doses of acetylcholine in patients with angiographically normal coronary arteries, but also of 5-HT in patients with coronary stenoses and chronic stable angina, indicates that myocardial ischemia can be caused by constriction of small coronary vessels at both angiographically visible and invisible sites.

Studies in patients with angiographically normal coronary arteries showed that the intracoronary infusion of NPY can cause massive ischemia, with extremely slow dye progression, but without detectable epicardial coronary artery constriction.[31] Distal, rather than proximal, constriction of arterial coronary vessels is consistent with animal studies that show that NPY causes constriction only of vessels less than 0.5 mm in diameter. Large doses of acetylcholine caused ischemia with diffuse constriction of secondary and tertiary branches, but with minimal proximal epicardial coronary artery constriction (see Fig. 9.13A–D).[32]

Studies in patients with coronary stenoses showed that the intracoronary infusion of 5-HT caused myocardial ischemia, with only small reductions in the caliber of stenotic segments, but with diffuse constriction of secondary and tertiary branches, and with reduced filling of collateral vessels (see Fig. 9.14A–C).[33] The dose of 5-HT that caused ischemia is within the range that can be produced in coronary vessels by intracoronary platelet activation. The constriction of distal vessels is not blocked by ketanserin (a $5-HT_2$-receptor blocker),[34] suggesting that distal vessel constriction may be mediated by other types of 5-HT receptors (this is also the case in epicardial coronary artery spasm, which cannot be blocked by ketanserin; see Ch. 20).

9.3.2 Clinical studies in patients with chronic stable angina

In patients with coronary artery stenoses, the demonstration of the modulation of residual coronary flow reserve by distal coronary vasoconstriction is difficult, as the change in the caliber of stenoses represents a readily available scapegoat for any dynamic impairment of blood flow. However, the possible role of small coronary vessels can be evaluated in special clinical models of IHD in which the interference of dynamic epicardial coronary stenoses can be excluded.

Patients with a single coronary occlusion, no other stenoses and no evidence of old infarction can present very wide variations in the ischemic threshold during both ambulatory Holter monitoring and standardized exercise stress testing following administration of nitrates and ergonovine (see also Ch. 10).[35] Coronary angiography following ergonovine has shown an obvious reduction in collateral filling of the occluded vessel in the absence of any evidence of epicardial coronary artery spasm. In this clinical model of chronic stable angina, therefore, the large degree of variability in ischemic threshold (which is comparable to that observed in unselected groups of patients with chronic stable angina) cannot be attributed to dynamic modulation of the residual lumen at the site of critical stenoses and must be caused by constriction of distal coronary vessels. The angiographic data do not provide any indication of the site of impairment of flow, which could be before the origin of collaterals, in the collaterals themselves, or in the vessels fed by the collaterals.

Patients with single vessel disease and persistent ischemia following successful coronary angioplasty represent another clinical model of IHD, in which the role of distal coronary vessel constriction can be assessed without the confounding element of a stenosis (which has been dilated). The evidence for a persistent reduction of the dilator response of resistive vessels, and for residual myocardial ischemia following successful coronary angioplasty, is provided by exercise stress testing and by studies performed using intracoronary Doppler flow measurements and positron emission tomography (PET) following administration of different pharmacological dilator stimuli. Signs of myocardial ischemia were demonstrated by regional defects of thallium uptake during stress myocardial scintigraphy[36,37] and also by the appearance of ischemic ST-segment changes, which cannot be attributed to spasm at the site of the dilated segment because the ergonovine test was found to be consistently negative.[38]

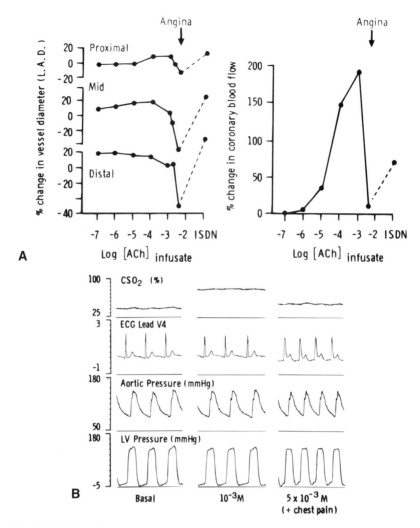

Fig. 9.13 Ischemic response to high doses of acetylcholine in patients with atypical chest pain and angiographically normal coronary arteries. As the concentration of acetylcholine in the infusate was increased, the arterial segments that initially dilated began to constrict, but flow continued to increase (calculated from the coronary sinus A–V difference using the indirect Fick principle) up to 10^{-3} M (**A**). At 5.10^{-3} M, signs of ischemia appeared with elevation of both the ST segment and end-diastolic ventricular pressure (**B**), but coronary sinus oxygen saturation remained above basal, which is indicative of inhomogenous, luxury perfusion in some segments of myocardium. *(Figure continues.)*

The reduced vasodilator response of resistive vessels was attributed to a vascular adaptation to decreased poststenotic pressure.[39]

A markedly reduced coronary flow response to administration of intracoronary papaverine and to systemic administration of dipyridamole was demonstrated by intracoronary Doppler flow velocity measurements[40–43] and by PET flow measurements.[44,45] In the majority of patients, the vasodilator response returned gradually towards normal over a period of 3 months (see

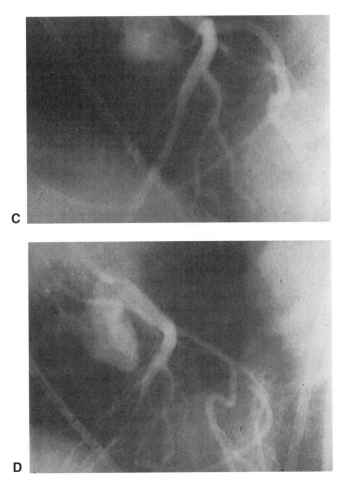

Fig. 9.13 *(Continued)* Compared with control (**C**), the ischemic changes were associated with diffuse constriction of secondary and tertiary branches (**D**). (From data presented in ref. 32.)

Fig. 9.15).[44] As the reduced vasodilator response to dipyridamole could not be improved by high doses of intracoronary nitroprusside,[45] it does not appear to be caused simply by the deficient production of endothelial nitric oxide by prearteriolar vessels (in which case nitrates would have an enhanced dilator effect) (see Ch. 5).

The observations that a reduced dilator response is not detectable in all patients immediately after angioplasty (see Fig. 9.16), may regress or persist, and may be present in adjacent, nonstenosed arteries (see next section), suggest that it may be due not only to a remodeling of distal vessels related to the presence of the stenosis, or to the acute effects of angioplasty, but could also be part of an independent dysfunction of resistive coronary vessels, which may be exacerbated by the presence of the stenosis.

Patients with single vessel disease and reduced vasodilator response in nonstenosed coronary arteries represent another example of small coronary vessel dysfunction. Recent studies by PET and by Doppler flow measurements demonstrate a reduced dilator response to dipyridamole in the vascular territory perfused by angiographically normal arteries, in

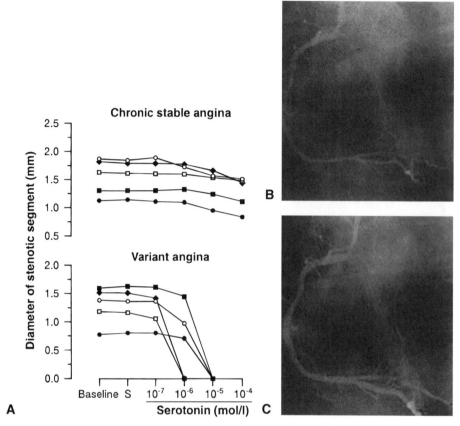

Fig. 9.14 Constriction of distal vessels and ischemia caused by 5-HT.
Intracoronary infusion of 5-HT caused occlusive spasm at 10^{-6} M or 10^{-5} M in patients with variant angina, but it caused only very mild constriction of stenotic segments at 10^{-4} M in patients with chronic stable angina and stenoses of comparable severity (**A**). However, ischemia also developed in stable patients because of small vessel constriction, which was indicated by diffuse constriction of secondary and tertiary branches and reduced filling of collaterals (**B**) compared with basal (**C**). (From data presented in ref. 33.)

patients with single vessel disease and chronic stable angina (performed by different groups using different methods: PET and ^{15}O-labeled water by Uren et al;[46] PET and NH_4 by Sambuceti et al[47]), and also in patients with recent MI and single-vessel disease (see Fig. 9.17).[48]

Patients with syndrome X comprise a spectrum of patients presenting with angina pectoris that is sufficiently typical and severe to justify coronary angiography—which shows a normal coronary arteriogram. These patients form a heterogeneous group, with no clinical features of variant angina and no demonstration of epicardial coronary artery spasm (see Ch. 16 and 18). The presence of transient "ischemic" ECG changes during anginal attacks indicates that the pain has a cardiac, although not necessarily ischemic, origin. Some of these patients do, however, have myocardial ischemia, because they have positive results on myocardial scintigraphy and either reduction of oxygen saturation or lactate production in the coronary sinus during angina induced by exercise or pacing (see Fig. 18.2).[49] Many of

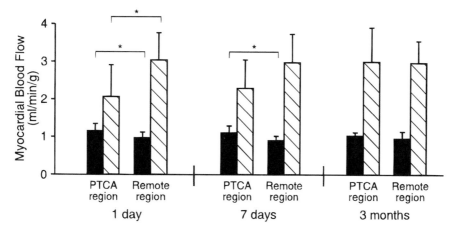

Fig. 9.15 Gradual improvement of coronary flow response after successful percutaneous transluminal coronary angioplasty (PTCA). The coronary vasodilator response to dipyridamole assessed by positron emission tomography and ^{15}O-labeled water improved gradually during the first week after successful percutaneous transluminal coronary angioplasty (PTCA) and became similar to that in the control region at 6 months: ■, basal state; ◳, flow at peak dipyridamole effect. Asterisks indicate significant differences (* $P < 0.01$). (Modified from ref. 44.)

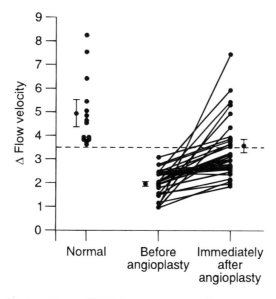

Fig. 9.16 Variable effect of PTCA on coronary flow response. Following successful PTCA, the flow response to intracoronary papaverine increased markedly in some patients, but remained below the normal range in the majority: Δ = change from basal. The immediate normalization of the flow response in some patients indicates that the reduced response observed in the majority is not attributable solely to the effects of the chronic reduction of poststenotic pressure. (Modified from ref. 40.)

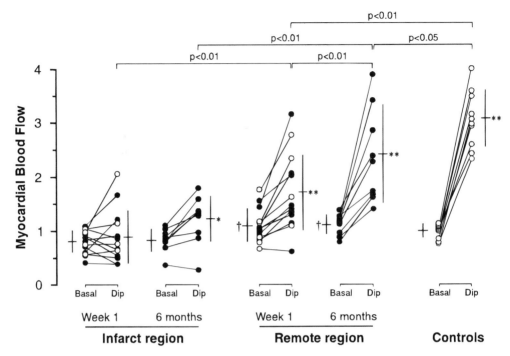

Fig. 9.17 Reduced coronary flow response of nonstenosed, noninfarct-related arteries. Regional myocardial blood flow (in ml/min/g) at peak dipyridamole effect (Dip) in the infarcted and remote regions in study patients at 1 week was much lower than in the control group; the difference was less at 6 months. Patients who underwent study at 1 week only are shown with open circles. Thus, the myocardium perfused by nonstenosed arteries also has a very reduced vasodilator response in the early postacute phase. (Modified from ref. 48.)

them also have a reduced vasodilator response to pacing, particularly after ergonovine, and to dipyridamole. A reduced vasodilator response detected by the coronary sinus thermodilution technique is consistent with an increased myocardial oxygen extraction (see Fig. 9.18).[50] As these alterations cannot be attributed to dynamic stenoses of epicardial coronary arteries, a dysfunction of resistive vessels must be postulated (see Ch. 18).

■ *Thus, constriction of distal coronary vessels may be a frequent component of the impairment of coronary flow reserve in patients with IHD, independent of atherosclerotic coronary stenoses, and could be one of the explanations for the variable relationship between the severity of coronary stenoses, the impairment of coronary flow reserve, and anginal symptoms.* ■

9.3.3 Site and mechanisms of abnormal constriction of small coronary vessels

Myocardial ischemia caused by distal vessel constriction can result from dysfunction of either prearteriolar or arteriolar vessels. Ischemia occurring during increased myocardial activity can be explained by either inadequate flow-mediated coronary dilation or active constriction; ischemia occurring at rest and during either emotion or very light physical activity that is usually well tolerated (i.e. in the absence of increased myocardial oxygen consumption) can be caused only by active constriction of prearteriolar or arteriolar vessels.

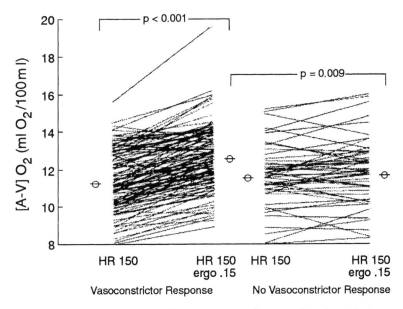

Fig. 9.18 Reduced coronary flow response is associated with increased myocardial oxygen extraction in patients with microvascular angina. In patients who, following administration of ergonovine (ergo .15), exhibited a smaller flow increase (vasoconstrictor response) during pacing at a heart rate of 150 (HR 150), myocardial oxygen extraction increased, compared with those who exhibited no vasoconstrictor response. As expected from the argument presented in Chapter 4, the demonstration of an increased oxygen extraction associated with a reduced flow response strengthens the argument that a microvascular dysfunction is a cause of angina in at least some of these patients. (Modified from ref. 50.)

The sites and mechanisms of small coronary vessel dysfunction are difficult to investigate, not only because the only way to assess coronary resistive vessels in humans is by measuring flow, which provides information only on total coronary resistance, but also because the alterations responsible for ischemia caused by small vessel constriction are unlikely to be present or reproducible in experimental animals.

The causes of small coronary vessel dysfunction are commonly attributed to atherosclerosis,[51] but they may also be due to neurohumoral alterations or to vascular remodeling associated with systemic diseases such as hypertension or vasculitis.

Prearteriolar constriction or inadequate dilation could cause a critical reduction in pressure at the origin of arterioles, which cannot be compensated for by maximal arteriolar dilation; thus, ischemia ensues, most frequently occurring in the subendocardial layers where flow is more critically dependent on perfusion pressure and where oxygen consumption is higher (see Ch. 4). When the degree of prearteriolar constriction is not uniform, myocardial ischemia could be patchily distributed and may not be sufficient to cause detectable abnormalities of regional contractile function. The patchy distribution of ischemia due to coronary microvascular dysfunction may be an exaggeration of the physiologic spatial and temporal heterogeneity of myocardial perfusion (see Ch. 4). An increased release of adenosine distal to constricted arterioles may cause pain even in the absence of ischemia. Thus, pain may occur in the presence of increased flow through adjacent arterioles (distal to nonconstricted prearterioles), as a result of adenosine overflow from adjacent areas distal to constricted arterioles (see also Ch. 18).[52]

Dysfunction of prearteriolar vessels can be due to the following:

a.   inadequate flow-mediated vasodilation, related to endothelial dysfunction (which would explain ischemic episodes occurring when myocardial metabolic activity and, hence, flow demand, increase)
b.   abnormal neurogenic vasoconstriction, abnormal constrictor stimuli derived from cells in the vessel wall or carried by the blood, or hyperreactivity of the smooth muscle
c.   organic alterations such as perivascular fibrosis or medial hypertrophy.

■ *When constrictor mechanisms act at the level of prearteriolar vessels, they cannot be directly opposed locally by ischemic metabolites, in the same way as constriction occurring in large epicardial arteries cannot be opposed by ischemic metabolites.* ■

Arteriolar constriction or inadequate dilation could cause ischemia when the adequate matching of flow to myocardial metabolism is prevented either by dysfunction of the physiologic mechanisms that match blood supply to myocardial metabolic needs or by active local constriction that prevents these mechanisms from operating normally.

When operating in arteriolar vessels, the possible constrictor mechanisms (listed above for prearteriolar vessels), need to be strong enough to overcome locally the dilator effects of ischemic metabolites; also, arteriolar dysfunction can be patchily distributed.

9.4 CORONARY ARTERY THROMBOSIS

Coronary artery thrombosis is the acute alteration most commonly detected in patients with unstable angina, acute MI or SICD. In each of these syndromes, thrombosis may be associated with other ischemic stimuli, such as increased myocardial demand, coronary artery spasm, dynamic coronary stenoses, and distal coronary vasoconstriction. Neither the causes of thrombosis nor the mechanisms that cause thrombi to grow and produce acute MI are precisely known. In order to analyse the local coronary alterations that may trigger the initial thrombotic process and favor the development of large mural thrombi and their progression to acute coronary occlusion, it would be useful to review the mechanisms of thrombosis as a repair process, the features of coronary thrombi, and the histologic features of plaques at the site of thrombi in acute ischemic syndromes. Usually, recurrent transient ischemic episodes in unstable patients are characterized by ST-segment depression and only occasionally by its elevation (which is the common alteration in the early phases of infarction and in variant angina).

9.4.1 Thrombosis as a repair process

As discussed in Chapter 6, in animal models occlusive thrombosis does not develop in response to a mechanical injury to a normal vessel, and only in the presence of an acutely induced flow-limiting stenosis can platelet adhesion and aggregation cause occlusion. In the absence of a critical stenosis only very intense thrombogenic stimuli, such as a copper coil, or very persistent stimuli, such as a continuous electric current, can cause vessel occlusion within minutes or within 1 h respectively.

Thus, only at the site of a severe stenosis can local vessel wall damage cause rapid occlusive thrombosis as part of the physiologic reparative response.

Lesser thrombogenic stimuli may occur in coronary arteries without causing symptoms or signs of myocardial ischemia. According to the observations of Rokitansky and Duguid, such stimuli are dealt with by a process of physiologic repair which tends to restore the continuity of the vessel wall with the minimum necessary selective activation of the hemostatic systems in situ, contributing to rapid progression of atherosclerotic plaques without necessarily causing ischemia (see Ch. 8). The repair process to minor wall injuries or thrombogenic stimuli may become "nonphysiologic" and lead to total vessel occlusion in the presence of a prothrombotic state or an enhanced local coronary vasoconstrictor response.

In patients with unstable angina, local thrombosis associated with coronary vasoconstriction develops intermittently as an occlusive or subocclusive process that may cause repeated transient episodes of impairment of blood flow occurring over periods of days or weeks, and may ultimately either cause acute MI or heal. This "stuttering" evolution of coronary thrombosis is more suggestive of recurrent thrombogenic stimuli (like the intermittent application of an electric current in the dog model) than of a process of physiologic repair of a single initial injury. This possibility is supported by the composition of thrombi and by some features of the plaques found beneath the thrombi.

9.4.2 Frequency and features of coronary thrombi in acute ischemic syndromes and pathogenetic implications

Angiographic and angioscopic studies in unstable patients showed evidence of thrombosis in a higher proportion of those who had suffered a recent ischemic episode than in those who had had no episodes of ischemia in the preceding days (for review see reference 53). Thus, the discrepancies found in different autopsy reports may be due not only to the accuracy with which thrombi are researched, but also to their variable growth and lysis, which differ according to the inclusion criteria of the material studied.

Patients who die of IHD are classified as having had unstable angina, acute MI or SICD, according to descriptive criteria. Most patients in the SICD or unstable angina groups died of arrhythmias occurring during or at the end of an episode of severe, potentially reversible, myocardial ischemia, or during the first hours of infarction, when histologic evidence of myocardial necrosis was not yet available; however, others with old infarction may have died during arrhythmias not associated with ischemic episodes.[54] Patients with acute MI may also have died of cardiac rupture, pump failure, or reperfusion arrhythmias. The pathogenetic components that caused the fatal episode in these varied conditions are not necessarily the same, and it will be impossible to draw precise conclusions about the frequency of thrombosis unless the patients studied are classified according to the features and time course of symptoms before death, rather than according to purely descriptive terms.

The frequency with which coronary thrombi occur both in patients dying from acute IHD and in those dying from noncardiac causes, as well as their composition, have important pathogenetic implications.

Frequency of coronary thrombi in acute IHD deaths

At autopsy, the finding of coronary thrombi in unstable angina, SICD and acute MI is high, but variable in different reports. Thrombi are invariably present and occlusive in patients dying of pump failure after the onset of infarction, and are often mural and nonocclusive in patients who died suddenly, within 1h of the onset of symptoms. In a classic review,[55] Chandler discusses the variable relationship of thrombi with plaque hemorrhage and fissure, the frequently observed multilayered appearance of thrombi, and the frequent report of multiple thrombi in different coronary arteries.

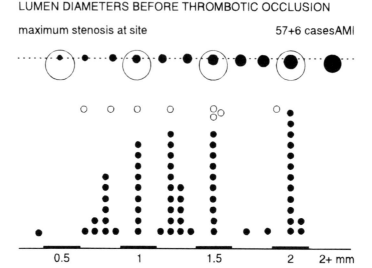

LUMEN DIAMETERS BEFORE THROMBOTIC OCCLUSION

maximum stenosis at site   57+6 casesAMI

0.5   1   1.5   2   2+ mm

Fig. 9.19 Frequency of acute thrombosis in noninfarct-related arteries. The lumen diameters before thrombotic occlusion at the site of maximum stenosis in 63 cases of acute MI (AMI) are represented schematically by the black dots within the open circles: in 22% of cases the lumen was 2 mm, reducing the diameter by about 50%. The open circles indicate thrombosis found in noninfarct-related branches at the site of stenoses, the size of which is indicated on the abscissa: 13% of patients had two acute thrombi in two different arterial branches, indicating the presence of multiple thrombogenic sites. (Modified from ref. 60.)

The distinction between occlusive and nonocclusive thrombi may sometimes be difficult to make and thus they are also defined as "major" and "minor." In a mixed series of 100 individuals, some with and some without previously known IHD, who died within 6 h of the onset of symptoms and who thus were defined as cases of "sudden death," Davies and Thomas[56] found major thrombi in 37% of patients and minor thrombi in 47%. In a controlled series, Baroldi et al[57] found occlusive and nonocclusive thrombi in 55 and 24%, respectively, of 100 acute MI patients, in 30 and 14% of 50 patients with chronic IHD, in 8.8 and 13.7% of 102 previously healthy individuals who died suddenly in the presence of witnesses within 15 min of the onset of chest pain, and in 25.4 and 14.1% of 106 previously healthy individuals who died suddenly without prodromal symptoms of chest pain. Kragel et al[58] found a similar frequency of intraluminal thrombus (29%) in unstable angina and SICD (within 3 h of the onset of symptoms), but a significantly higher frequency (69%) in acute transmural MI at least 6 h from the onset of symptoms. They found that the thrombus was composed almost entirely of platelets and was nonocclusive in the patients with unstable angina and SICD, and that it was composed entirely of fibrin and was occlusive in the patients with infarction.

In patients who died during a period of unstable angina, 81% of coronary thrombi were found to have a multilayered appearance, being composed of thrombotic material of different ages, which is indicative of successive, discrete episodes of mural thrombosis occurring over periods of days or weeks.[59] Another intriguing observation that has failed to receive appropriate attention is the finding of multiple fresh thrombi in separate coronary branches in up to 10% of cases of acute MI or SICD (see Fig. 9.19).[55,56,60-62]

Frequency of coronary thrombi in noncardiac deaths

Thrombi are very occasionally found in individuals dying accidentally outside hospital, but are not exceptional in noncardiac deaths occurring in hospital, being found in nine of 132 hearts of patients who died in hospital from noncardiac causes with no ischemic manifesttion; of these, one heart had two thrombi in different coronary arteries.[63]

Pathogenetic implications of the composition of thrombi

As discussed in Chapter 8, coronary thrombi are frequently, but not exclusively, found at the site of plaque fissure or hemorrhage.

The composition of thrombi found post mortem in the coronary arteries that were specifically examined in the study by Davies[64] provides clues to the mechanisms of their formation:

1. Thrombi inside fissured plaques are composed almost exclusively of platelets (this indicates that such thrombi cannot be postmortem artefacts as platelets can accumulate only in flowing blood).
2. Mural thrombi extending from the fissure to the lumen are composed of platelets and fibrin.
3. Occlusive thrombi at the site of noncritical stenoses and distal to very severe stenoses are composed of fibrin and red cells with few platelets, as are thrombi that form in veins. Conversely, occlusive thrombi at the site of very critical stenoses are composed of platelets and fibrin.

This information suggests that intraplaque thrombi form gradually in flowing blood, with an initial selective deposition of platelets within the discontinuity of the wall, followed by a much more obvious activation of the hemostatic system, with deposition of large amounts of fibrin together with platelets as the thrombus begins to occupy the lumen of the vessel. The initial phase of mural thrombosis involving the formation of fibrin in a "white mural thrombus" must occur fairly gradually, as it accumulates many more platelets than red cells. As in the animal model of coronary thrombosis induced by electric wire, continuing accumulation of platelets is likely to require a persistent thrombogenic stimulus much weaker than that provided by a copper coil. Under such a weak stimulus the thrombus may stop growing, and may not become occlusive if the stimulus is interrupted or if platelet activation is inhibited or reduced (see Ch. 6).

As platelet emboli are found in small vessels distal to mural thrombi, fairly tenuous platelet adhesion and aggregation must occur episodically in both intrafissure and mural thrombi in response to episodic thrombotic stimuli. The growth of white mural thrombi must be largely self-limiting, although they represent a very thrombogenic surface, because nonocclusive thrombi are frequently found at the postmortem examination of patients who died from unstable angina and those who suffered sudden death within 1 h of the onset of symptoms, as well as on angiography. However, as some white mural thrombi are composed of layers of different ages, their growth must recur in phases separated by days or even weeks, most likely as a result of recurrent weak thrombogenic stimuli (similar to the electric wire model in the dog).

Occlusive thrombi at the site of flow-limiting stenoses may be platelet rich, like those produced in the dog model developed by Folts et al (see Ch. 6) as a result of acute local

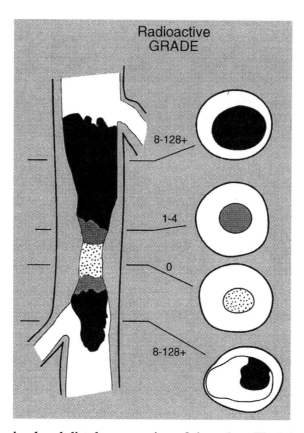

Fig. 9.20 Proximal and distal propagation of thrombus. The injection of [121]I-labeled fibrinogen at the time of hospital admission for acute MI allowed the detection of a thrombus that had formed subsequent to the time of injection, by its radioactivity. In a series of 38 cases in which death occurred after the administration of the radioactive fibrinogen, thrombus extension was found in 23 cases on either side of the central cold occlusion indicated by the stippled area (which, therefore, was formed before the injection, as in this figure); in seven cases the whole thrombus was radioactive, indicating formation after the injection, and in another seven the thrombus was not totally occlusive. (Modified from ref. 66.)

endothelial injury and of shear stress-induced platelet aggregation. Conversely, occlusive thrombi at the site of a noncritical stenosis, when containing red cells and platelets in approximately the same proportion as those found in a clot or in flowing blood, must form either very rapidly as a result of very intense local thrombogenic stimuli (as in the animal model of copper coil-induced coronary thrombosis—see Ch. 6) or in stagnant blood.

The greater frequency of occlusive thrombi being found in patients with transmural MI may not necessarily be related only to a larger fissure or to plaque hemorrhage (see 9.4.3), but also to blood stasis and enhanced local thrombotic tendency. Elegant studies using ^{125}I-labeled fibrinogen[65,66] have shown that extension and, possibly, even formation of the occlusive thrombus, occurs after hospital admission for acute MI (see Fig. 9.20). In patients with acute MI or unstable angina, occlusive thrombi are most common at the site of stenoses of more than 95% area (estimated from the area limited by the internal elastic lamina).

The presence of multiple thrombi in different coronary arteries suggests the simultaneous presence of multiple sites of vascular injury, which are unlikely to be merely the result of purely mechanical causes occurring by chance at the same time.

9.4.3 Features of plaques at the site of thrombi

A specific therapeutic and preventive approach to coronary thrombosis requires the identification of the causes not only of the strong thrombogenic stimuli that are associated with the sudden development of occlusive thrombi, but also of the weak waxing and waning thrombogenic stimuli responsible for mural platelet thrombi and their frequently multilayered appearance. Unfortunately, the nature of the coronary lesions at the site of coronary thrombi in fatal acute IHD has received specific attention only in recent years and no absolute distinctive features of stenosis severity, plaque fissure, or histologic composition have emerged so far. All the features considered so far as putative causes or at least markers of instability, although much more prevalent in unstable patients, are not present in all cases and can be found sometimes also in stable patients and even in controls, suggesting that they do not represent either an essential or a sufficient component of the instability.

Stenosis severity

The severity of the stenosis has received considerable attention as a cause of coronary thrombosis because occlusive thrombi are most often found at the site of histologically defined severe stenoses, which does not necessarily imply that they are flow limiting (see Figs 8.1 and 8.2). On the one hand, animal models indicate that endothelial disruption can cause occlusive platelet thrombi at the site of an acute flow-limiting stenosis; on the other, irregular stenoses are found in about 70% of unstable patients, but many severe stenoses, even those with irregular borders, may remain stable for years and, conversely, the infarct-related artery often has no flow-limiting or irregular stenosis (see Ch. 8).

Plaque fissure

The dramatic picture of a ruptured plaque, with intrafissure thrombus protruding to occlude the coronary lumen, can provide readily available evidence that rupture of a thrombogenic plaque may in itself be a possible cause of occlusive thrombosis. However, an isolated plaque fissure occurring at random as a result of abnormal local mechanical stress is unlikely to be a sufficient cause of prolonged phases of unstable angina, for the following reasons:

a. fissures or plaque hemorrhage were not identified beneath coronary thrombi in 25–53% of patients with cardiac ischemic death
b. fissures were also found in 10–17% of individuals dying from noncardiac causes
c. the simple fissure of a plaque does not explain easily the common waxing and waning of ischemic manifestations over days or weeks in unstable patients
d. multiple plaque fissures are quite common in patients who died from acute cardiac ischemic syndromes, which makes the possibility of a purely random mechanical rupture rather unlikely (see also below).

Percentage of plaque fissure found at the site of coronary thrombosis. No plaque fissures or intraplaque hemorrhages were found under coronary mural thrombi in 25% of cases by Davies,[64] and in 53% by Kragel et al,[58] who reported plaque hemorrhage with no evidence of fissure in 26% of thrombi (more frequently in cases of infarction than in cases of unstable angina or SICD).

The distinction between intraplaque hemorrhage and plaque fissure with thrombosis may not be easy but it reflects different pathogenetic mechanisms. Intraplaque hemorrhage derives from rupture of neoformed vessels within the plaque: it can, therefore, contain only red cells and platelets in the same proportion as that in circulating blood. It is unlikely that it can directly cause further encroachment of the lumen by enlargement of the plaque, as pressure is higher within the vessel than in the neoformed intraplaque vessels. However, intraplaque hemorrhage could stimulate local vasoconstriction and thrombosis. Conversely, plaque fissure, by allowing free communication of flowing blood with the intraplaque surface, allows the deposition of platelets, white cells, fibrin, and, when large, also of red cells (in which case it may be confused with a hemorrhage when neither the platelet thrombus nor the wall discontinuity are identified).

Fissured atherosclerotic plaques in non-cardiac deaths. Plaque fissures were found in 9% of unselected controls[56] and in 17% of individuals with coronary risk factors, who died from noncardiac causes.[64] Discrepancies between thrombosis and plaque fissure were also observed in hospital noncardiac deaths.[63]

Waxing and waning of ischemic episodes. This is so typical of unstable angina that a period of 1–2 months from the onset or sudden worsening of symptoms is an accepted definition. The simple fissure of a plaque, with its weak thrombogenic stimulus causing a platelet thrombus, cannot be considered in itself a plausible explanation for this long-lasting instability.

Simultaneous fissure of multiple plaques in unstable patients. The finding of more than one fissured plaque in the same patient is common in cases of fatal acute coronary syndromes. A total of 103 fissured plaques was found by Falk in 47 patients[67] and a total of 111 was found by Davies and Thomas in 76 patients.[56] The simultaneous presence of multiple fissured plaques in some patients with fatal acute IHD indicates that fissuring is unlikely to be merely a random event caused by mechanical stress or occlusive spasm or by plaque hemorrhage due to rupture of neoformed vessels.[68] It suggests, rather, that multiple fissures may be caused by a diffuse process such as an inflammatory response due to immune, infectious, or toxic stimuli. Digestion of the matrix by proteolytic enzymes released by inflammatory cells is more likely to weaken critically those segments of the plaque that have thin, as opposed to thick, fibrous caps.[69] The presence of a gene for stromelysin was demonstrated in plaques by in situ hybridization and its activation could contribute to disruption of the plaque capsule.[70]

Histologic features of unstable plaques

In the same way that the severity, morphology, and even the fissuring of plaques are not entirely distinctive features of unstable plaques, histologic findings are also not entirely specific features of instability. Coronary atherosclerotic plaques in patients with coronary thrombi are characterized by the presence of foam cells, macrophages, mast cells,[71] and inflammatory cells.[72–74] Inflammatory cells, including B and T lymphocytes,[75] were found in both the intima[76] and the surrounding adventitial nerves in patients with unstable angina.[77,78]

These inflammatory features also are not exclusive to patients with acute ischemic syndromes as they can be found (although in lower proportions) in unselected patients and even in individuals who died of noncardiac causes.[63] As discussed in Chapter 8, the presence of inflammatory cell infiltrates appears to be related to the size of the plaque (i.e. only to those plaques greater than 300 μm in thickness[79] or occupying more than 50% of the area encircled by the internal elastica).[80] Not even the study of growth factors, oncogene products, and proliferative cell markers seems capable of providing a clear separation between stable and unstable plaques and stable and unstable patients.[81] Contraction bands in the SMCs surrounding coronary plaques, suggestive of intense vasoconstriction, have also been described in patients with unstable angina[23] but are also not entirely specific to unstable patients. SMC proliferation has been proposed as a possible mechanism of instability.[82] However, it can not, by itself, be a cause of instability, since SMC proliferation is also present in patients with restenosis after percutaneous transluminal coronary angioplasty, who exhibit no signs of instability. Moreover, SMC proliferation does not explain the typical waxing and waning of symptoms in unstable angina.

The relation between thrombosis, plaque fissure and histologic features was examined specifically in 20 patients who had died of acute MI. A deep intimal rupture extending into the lipid core was encountered in 12 plaques, whereas eight had superficial erosions only, of which three showed fibrocellular lesions without clear lipid cores. In each instance macrophages and, to a lesser extent, T lymphocytes were the dominant cells at the immediate site of either rupture or superficial erosion: these sites, moreover, were characterized by abundant expression of HLA-DR antigens on both inflammatory cells and adjacent SMCs, suggesting an active inflammatory reaction.[83] These alterations do not, however, appear to be specific to plaques underlying fresh thrombi, as the same group of investigators demonstrated, by in situ immunophenotypic analysis, an immune-mediated hypersensitive reaction (in association with the development of atherosclerosis) in segments of aortic and coronary specimens in unselected patients, with lesions of variable severity—from fatty streaks, to diffuse intimal thickening, to raised fibrous plaques.[84]

In addition, endoarterectomy specimens obtained from patients with unstable angina or with non-Q-wave MI were found to have significantly larger macrophage-rich areas than those obtained from patients with chronic stable angina, but clusters of macrophages were also found in specimens obtained from stable patients.[84a]

The incomplete specificity for acute ischemic syndromes of stenosis severity, plaque fissure, histologic features of plaques, and cellular alterations examined so far, suggests that the development of the instability and the progression towards infarction may require the simultaneous presence of multiple pathogenetic components, one of which is represented by an inflammatory reaction.

9.4.4 Activation of the endothelium in the absence of plaque fissures

In the absence of plaque fissures, the coronary endothelium can be injured and/or activated by a variety of noxious stimuli that may be mechanical, anoxic, chemical, immunologic, or infectious.[85,86] As discussed in Chapter 1, activated endothelium produces powerful vasoconstrictor substances, exposes adhesive receptors for leukocytes, and becomes thrombogenic. Diffuse endothelial injury and activation may involve more than one coronary artery segment but be more intense or have greater effects in areas of turbulent flow, such as stenoses, where mural thrombosis and vasoconstriction may develop preferentially.

Mechanical injury caused by high shear stress was considered sufficient to dislodge the endothelium at the site of very severe stenoses.[87] This hypothesis is compatible with the acute experimental model of Folts (see Ch. 6), but contrasts with the fact that many critical flow-limiting stenoses remain stable for years in patients with chronic effort-related angina. However, shear stress-induced endothelial damage may become a localizing and intensifying factor of diffuse endothelial activation attributable to other noxious stimuli.

Ischemia and anoxia due to interruption of blood flow can cause gaps between adjacent endothelial cells where platelets become deposited.[88] Thus ischemia may amplify endothelial injuries caused by other noxious stimuli (see 7.1.1).

Chemical stimuli such as oxidized low-density lipoprotein, homocysteine, and endotoxin can produce endothelial activation and injury, but should act acutely, rather than chronically, in order to account for the acute activation of the endothelium.

Immunologic injury can be caused either by specific antibodies directed against cell surface antigens or by sensitized lymphocytes. In addition, circulating immune complexes may cause injury, particularly where there is disturbed blood flow (i.e. caused by stenoses): an immunoglobulin E-mediated response to an allergen in cigarette smoke has been proposed as a cause of endothelial injury in hypersensitive smokers;[89] *Chlamydia pneumoniae*-specific circulating immune complexes have been detected in patients with IHD;[90] antibodies and immune complexes have been shown to induce tissue factor production in endothelial cells.[91,92] Immunologic stimuli acting acutely may cause endothelial leukocyte adhesion[93] and initiate thrombosis.

Infectious injury may be mediated by viruses such as cytomegalovirus and herpesvirus, or by bacteria such as *Chlamydia pneumoniae,* which may be responsible for the formation of atheroma (see Ch. 8 and 9.5.3). The sudden reactivation of a dormant infectious agent in the coronary arteries, caused by toxic, infectious, physical, or psychological stimuli, could be a powerful stimulus for endothelial activation.

No information is yet available on the actual role and incidence of these various potential noxious stimuli, but they are not mutually exclusive and can potentiate each other.

Although the specific stimuli responsible for activating the coronary endothelium are still unknown, a growing body of evidence indicates that inflammation may be an important component of unstable angina by favoring plaque fissure and by becoming a localizing factor for thrombosis and vasoconstriction.

9.4.5 Evidence of inflammation in unstable angina

The possible role of inflammatory components, suggested by the histologic demonstration of intraplaque and perivascular inflammatory cell infiltrates in unstable coronary plaques, is consistent with observations reported at the time of cardiac surgery and is supported by several studies that provide evidence of systemic markers of inflammation.

Signs of perivascular inflammation at the time of bypass surgery

An intriguing observation that was made at the time of bypass surgery has received insufficient attention—the report of red streaks with perivascular inflammatory infiltrates along one or more coronary artery branches in 21 of 200 patients with unstable angina.[78] Patients with the red streaks were indistinguishable clinically from those without. In some patients, the involvement of long segments of coronary artery and of multiple coronary arteries, including those that were angiographically normal, indicates a diffuse process, not localized to the site of a single coronary plaque. The finding of multivessel involvement by red streaks could explain the puzzling observation of signs of myocardial ischemia (detected by

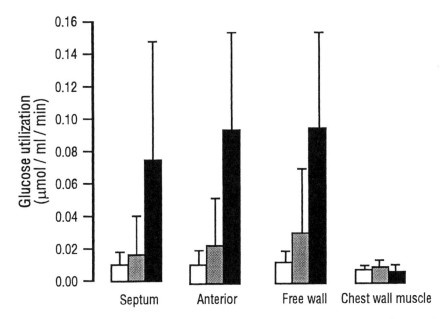

Fig. 9.21 Diffuse increase of myocardial uptake of fluorodeoxyglucose in patients with unstable angina. Compared with controls (□) and with patients with chronic stable angina (▨), in patients with unstable angina and single-vessel disease (■), the myocardial metabolic rate for glucose was increased not only in the myocardium perfused by the culprit vessel but also in regions perfused by angiographically normal vessels. Glucose utilization by the chest wall muscles was similar in patients and in controls. The increased myocardial glucose uptake may be caused by previous episodes of ischemia or by other abnormalities not limited to the territory perfused by the culprit vessels. (Modified from ref. 94.)

increased ^{18}F-labeled deoxyglucose uptake on PET scanning), distal not only to culprit stenoses, but also to angiographically normal arteries in unstable patients with single-vessel disease (see Fig. 9.21).[94]

Systemic markers of inflammation

An inflammatory component in unstable angina is provided by four independent lines of evidence.

First, in patients with unstable angina in whom platelet production of thromboxane A_2 was blocked by low-dose aspirin, Vejar et al[95] found that urinary excretion of the thromboxane A_2 metabolite, 11-dehydro-thromboxane B_2, was often much higher than that found during coronary angioplasty in stable patients, who were on a similar dose of aspirin[96] (see Fig. 9.22). This observation suggests the possible origin of this metabolite from inflammatory cells, in which thromboxane A_2 production by the inducible cyclooxygenase 2 was only partially and transiently inhibited by the low-dose aspirin (which was sufficient instead to block platelet cyclooxygenase and platelet thromboxane production irreversibly). In addition, in unstable patients, high urinary excretion levels of this metabolite (with and without aspirin treatment) were often not associated with the occurrence of painful or painless ischemic episodes. Conversely, no increase in urinary thromboxane metabolites was observed during some painful or painless ischemic episodes (see Fig. 9.23). The finding of a dissociation

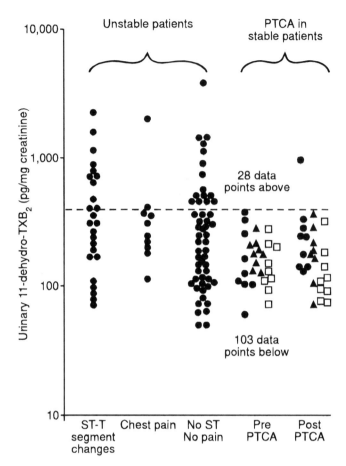

Fig. 9.22 Evidence of extraplatelet production of thromboxane A$_2$ in unstable angina. Following blockade of platelet thromboxane A$_2$ synthesis by aspirin, excretion of one of its metabolites (11-dehydro-TXB$_2$) was elevated in many urine samples from patients with unstable angina but, except in one case, not in stable patients following PTCA (dashed line = 2SD above mean for individuals on aspirin). In unstable patients, urinary excretion was not correlated with the occurrence of ischemic episodes. (Doses of aspirin; ●, 75 mg/day; ▲, 300 mg/day; ■, 300 mg/day plus 1000 mg i.v.) Extraplatelet synthesis of thromboxane A$_2$ may be common in unstable angina, possibly because of activation of inducible cyclooxygenase-2 in inflammatory cells, and is not necessarily associated with ischemic episodes. (Modified from refs. 95 and 96.)

between urinary excretion of thromboxane A$_2$ metabolites and anginal episodes in unstable angina was also reported by Fitzgerald et al,[97] who attributed the discrepancy to silent ischemia, but this interpretation was not supported by continuous ECG recording.[95] In addition, the elevated urinary excretion of leukotrienes D$_4$ and E$_4$ in patients with unstable angina[98] is consistent with the existence of a systemically detectable inflammatory component in this syndrome, which may not be only a consequence of ischemia and reperfusion injury.

Second, a significant neutrophil activation was inferred by Mehta et al[99] and by Dinerman et al,[100] in patients with unstable angina, from the 15-fold higher values of a neutrophil elastase-derived fibrinopeptide compared with those in controls and stable patients. The authors

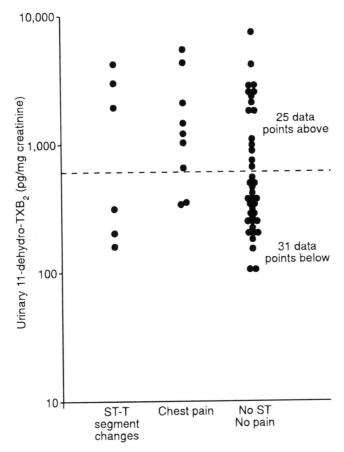

Fig. 9.23 Dissociation of urinary excretion of thromboxane metabolites from ischemic episodes in unstable angina. In patients with unstable angina not treated with aspirin, urinary excretion of a thromboxane A_2 metabolite was elevated considerably, but no relation was observed with the occurrence of painful or painless ischemic episodes during the urine collection periods. Dashed line = 2 SD above mean for individuals not on aspirin. (Modified from ref. 95.)

attributed the elastase release by granulocytes to their activation during reflow into the ischemic myocardium, but granulocyte interaction with activated endothelium, independent of ischemia, could be an alternative explanation. Increased expression of neutrophil and monocyte adhesion molecules was observed by Mazzone et al during the passage of these cells through the coronary circulation (see Fig. 9.24A,B),[101] owing to endothelial activation either secondary to ischemic injury or primary.

Third, activation of monocytes by lymphocytes in unstable (but not in stable) patients, and limited to the acute phase of the instability, was reported by Neri Serneri et al (see Fig. 9.25),[102] who proposed that unstable angina is associated with an acute transient bout of inflammation, with lymphocyte activation triggered by unknown factors. These findings are supported by an increased procoagulant activity in circulating monocytes[103] and by the elevation of circulating monocytes–macrophages with expressed T_3 DR major histocompatibility complex class II antigen.[104] They are also compatible with the abundant expression of HLA-DR antigens on both inflammatory cells and adjacent smooth muscle cells in plaques beneath thrombi.[83]

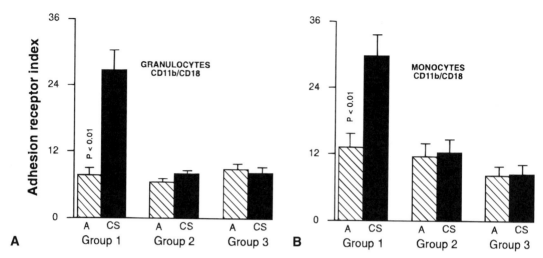

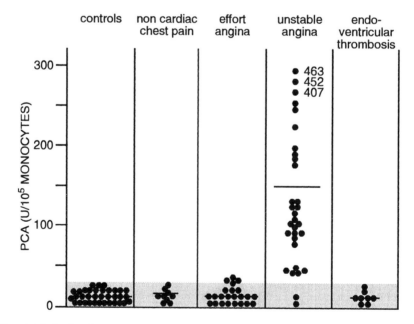

Fig. 9.24 Expression of adhesion receptors in granulocytes and monocytes during their passage through the coronary circulation in unstable angina. CD11/CD18 adhesion receptor expression is higher in granulocytes (**A**) and monocytes (**B**) sampled from the coronary sinus (CS) than in those sampled from the aorta (A) in unstable patients (group 1), but not in stable patients (group 2) or controls (group 3). Thus, in unstable patients, leukocyte activation occurs during their passage through the coronary circulation. The activation can be secondary to ischemic injury or primary. (Modified from ref. 101.)

Fig. 9.25 Activation of monocytes by lymphocytes in unstable patients. During the active phase of the disease, lymphocytes sampled in peripheral blood can activate monocytes to increase their procoagulant activity (PCA). No activation is induced by lymphocytes in other conditions or during remissions. The cause of lymphocyte activation is unknown. (Modified from ref. 102.)

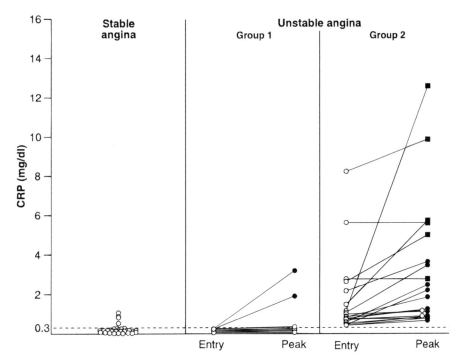

Fig. 9.26 Systemic inflammation in unstable angina indicated by elevation of acute-phase proteins and its relationship to short-term prognosis. Individual concentrations of C-reactive protein (CRP) in patients with either stable (left) or unstable angina (entry and peak) separated according to CRP at entry less than 0.3 mg/dl (middle) and more than 0.3 mg/dl (right). The broken line represents the upper limit in 90% of normal subjects. Symbols indicate patients' outcome: ●, urgent coronary revascularization, PTCA or coronary artery bypass graft (CABG), ■, acute MI or death. Prognosis was significantly worse in patients with CRP values more than 0.3 mg/dl at entry, and most severe in those with values more than 1.0 mg/dl at entry. (Modified from ref. 106.)

Finally, increased blood levels of an acute-phase protein (C-reactive protein, CRP) were reported by Berk et al in patients with unstable angina, but no evidence was provided that the elevation was not secondary to myocardial necrosis.[105] This latter possibility was excluded by Liuzzo et al,[106] who observed that not only CRP but also serum amyloid A protein (SAA) were elevated on admission in all unstable patients who had complicated courses, in the absence of any detectable evidence of myocardial necrosis. This study also showed that all patients with acute MI who had a history of unstable angina were found to have elevated values of acute-phase proteins on admission, in the absence of elevation of serum markers of myocardial necrosis (see Figs 9.26–9.28). In contrast, many patients presenting with unheralded infarction had normal blood levels of CRP and SAA, suggesting that the precipitating causes of unheralded infarction may differ from those responsible for the progression to infarction from unstable angina. The absence of an associated elevation of troponin-T, which is a very sensitive index of myocardial cell necrosis,[107] should rule out the possibility that the acute-phase response is caused by myocardial necrosis. Thus, the elevation of acute-phase proteins is likely to originate from some toxic, immunologic, or inflammatory stimulus causing coronary endothelial and inflammatory cell activation (see 9.5.3).

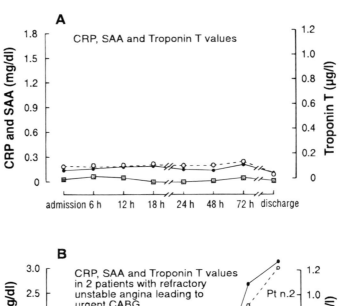

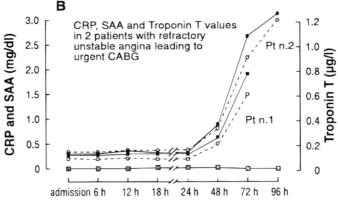

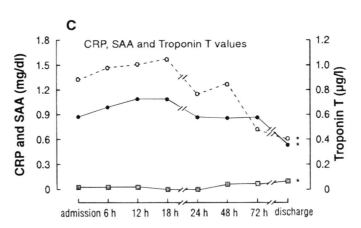

Fig. 9.27 Time course of acute-phase proteins in unstable angina in relation to prognosis. C-reactive protein (CRP) (●), serum amyloid A (SAA) protein (○) and troponin T (▦) after admission to the CCU in uncomplicated patients (**A**) and in two patients in whom CRP and SAA protein increased together with worsening symptoms (**B**). The values remained elevated in patients with a complicated course (**C**). Group data are expressed as median (CRP and SAA) and mean (troponin T). Data at discharge do not include patients with MI, those who underwent emergency CABG, or those who died. (Modified from ref. 106.)

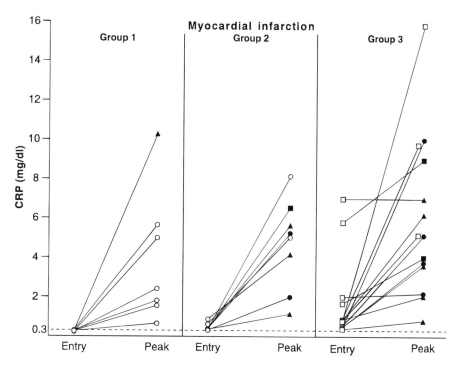

Fig. 9.28 Values of C-reactive protein in patients with acute MI (entry and peak). All patients had normal values of collective phosphokinase and troponin T on admission. They were separated into three groups according to the value of C-reactive protein (CRP) on entry and to a history of unstable angina prior to the onset of acute MI. Patients in groups 1 and 2 had no previous history of unstable angina; group 1 had normal values of CRP at entry and group 2 had elevated values. Group 3 patients had previous histories of unstable angina. Symbols indicate patients' outcome: ▲, recurrence of angina; ●, urgent coronary revascularization, PTCA or CABG; ■, reinfarction. All patients with a history of unstable angina (□) had CRP values more than 0.3 mg/dl at entry. The peak values observed in patients with infarction are similar to those observed in some patients with unstable angina who had evidence of necrosis. These findings confirm the observation that elevated levels of CRP or SAA in unstable angina can be predictive of acute MI, but indicate also that in a minority of patients the development of MI may occur independent of elevated levels of acute-phase proteins, suggesting the existence of different pathogenetic mechanisms. (Modified from ref. 106.)

Elevated levels of CRP and SAA imply an increased hepatic synthesis of these proteins, stimulated by interleukin-1 (IL-1) and interleukin-6 (IL-6). The precise origin of IL-1 and IL-6 is still unknown, but endotoxin and tumor necrosis factor, for example, can induce IL-1 gene expression in adult vascular endothelial cells.[108]

A persistent inflammatory state involving the endothelium could also be responsible for the persistent activation of blood coagulation indicated by the persistently high blood levels of fibrinopeptide A,[109,110] which, as this has a half-life of only about 5 min, implies a continuous generation of thrombin.

■ *Although the inflammatory stimuli are still unknown, these multiple, independent lines of evidence converge to demonstrate the presence of a systemically detectable inflammatory state in unstable patients,[111,112] which may not be a direct consequence of myocardial ischemia as it is not detectable in patients with variant angina and frequent ischemic episodes.[113]* ■

9.4.6 Conclusions

Coronary thrombosis is undoubtedly the most obvious common denominator in unstable angina, MI, and fatal IHD, but the occasional finding of coronary thrombi in noncardiac deaths, and of rapid angiographic progression of stenoses in patients with no evidence of instability, indicates that, under certain circumstances, coronary thrombosis may develop with no detectable ischemic manifestations.

Plaque fissure and rupture are common but not a necessary or sufficient substrate for triggering unstable angina. Some ruptured plaques may be highly thrombogenic and cause rapid thrombotic occlusion (like the copper coil dog model of coronary thrombosis), but most fissured plaques are not highly thrombogenic if they allow the formation of intrafissure and mural platelet thrombi (like the electric wire dog model of coronary thrombosis). Indeed, plaque fissuring must be a fairly common event in patients with extensive coronary atherosclerosis if it can be found so frequently in unselected cases of individuals with mild atherosclerosis dying from noncardiac causes. How frequently multiple fissures occur in patients with unstable angina and whether they are larger in patients with infarction remains to be established.

The not uncommon dissociation between plaque fissure and mural and occlusive thrombosis, and the frequent finding of superimposed layers of thrombi of different ages and of recurring ischemic episodes in unstable angina, suggest the presence of recurring, weak thrombogenic stimuli, most often (but not necessarily) associated with fissured plaques.

The frequent presence of multiple plaque fissures and the absence of detectable fissures under some thrombi suggest that a diffuse activation of coronary endothelium or of the whole arterial wall may be a common feature of instability and of acute MI (see Fig. 9.17). Accumulating evidence converges to suggest that inflammation may cause local endothelial activation and, possibly, plaque fissure, leading to episodic thrombogenic and vasoconstrictor stimuli that are important components of the onset, waxing, and waning of unstable angina and of its evolution towards infarction. Fissures could represent a consequence of the inflammatory process and determine its most obvious coronary localization (just as bacterial endocarditis is usually localized only on one valve). Nevertheless, inflammation, too, does not appear to be an entirely specific feature of unstable plaques.

■ *No information is yet available on the causes of inflammation, on its systemic or coronary localization, or on the additional elusive components that, in association with inflammation, contribute to cause the instability, but these novel lines of research may open the way to new types of therapeutic and preventive strategies.* ■

9.5 ACUTE ISCHEMIC STIMULI RESPONSIBLE FOR MYOCARDIAL INFARCTION

Myocardial infarction is the major cause of irreversible cardiac damage and of ischemia-related fatal arrhythmias. Only some patients with unstable angina develop MI and in many cases MI is not preceded by a phase of unstable angina. The ischemic stimuli that cause infarction deserve, therefore, to be analysed separately because their precise understanding is the major challenge for research in the treatment and prevention of IHD.

Research into the pathogenetic mechanisms of infarction is difficult because it is a very rare event, even in patients with very diffuse or with very severe angiographically detectable coronary atherosclerotic lesions, and because it usually develops as the very first manifestation of IHD in apparently healthy individuals. Identification of the pathogenetic mechanisms of infarction is also difficult for two reasons: first, because they are multiple, as an infarction develops as a result of a massive, persistent reduction of myocardial blood flow through a major coronary artery, caused by thrombus, spasm, embolus, distal vessel constriction, or any combination of these factors; second, because the causes of a single mechanism of persistent interruption of CBF, such as coronary thrombosis or occlusive spasm, can be multiple.

In humans, infarction can be transmural (usually associated with the development of Q waves on the ECG), or nontransmural (usually not associated with the development of Q waves). Based on animal studies, the transmural or nontransmural distribution of myocardial necrosis depends on the duration of the occlusion, on the level of myocardial oxygen consumption and on the presence and function of collaterals (discussed in Ch. 10). In patients, therefore, the general pathogenetic mechanisms initiating transmural and nontransmural MI are often likely to be the same, the different outcomes being related to the modulatory factors defined above.

When infarction occurs suddenly and unheralded, its causes can be studied only after its symptoms have brought the patient to medical attention. Unstable angina is a clinically recognizable precursor of infarction, but an unstable phase cannot be identified in about 70% of cases of infarction (see Ch. 11). Some patients may have a mild, unrecognized or totally silent unstable ischemic phase, but the onset of infarction seems to be totally abrupt in a substantial number of patients. The causes of infarction with abrupt onset and of that preceded by unstable angina are not necessarily the same.

The very infrequent occurrence of MI, even in patients with the most severe and extensive coronary atherosclerosis, can be explained only by either a single cause, which has an extremely low probability of occurring, or, (more likely) by the simultaneous coincidental occurrence of rather rare unfavorable pathologic events, which concur to cause a sudden persistent coronary artery occlusion. The following analysis serves as a basis for identifying future lines of research into the pathogenetic mechanisms of acute coronary occlusion (see Fig. 9.29) and into their etiologic components.

The simultaneous occurrence of a variable combination of several pathogenetic mechanisms that contribute to cause a sudden persistent coronary artery occlusion is fairly unlikely and can explain the rarity of the event. In statistical terms, the probability of developing a sudden coronary occlusion (P) can be defined as the probability of the simultaneous occurrence of the following:

a. a thrombogenic stimulus, T (P_T)
b. a vasoconstrictor stimulus, V (P_V)
c. an enhanced thrombotic response, ET (P_{ET})
d. an enhanced vasoconstrictor response, EV (P_{EV})

(where P_T, P_V, P_{ET} and P_{EV} are much smaller than 1 and may vary considerably in different individuals). Assuming the independence of these different pathogenetic mechanisms, $P = P_T \cdot P_V \cdot P_{ET} \cdot P_{EV}$.

Not only may the individual roles of these pathogenetic mechanisms (T, V, ET and EV), and the probability of their occurrence at the same time, vary considerably among different individuals, but their etiologies may also vary. A thrombogenic stimulus, T, may be caused by a mechanical rupture of a plaque or by endothelial activation due to an inflammatory response (the stimuli causing an inflammatory response can also be multiple). A vasoconstrictor stimu-

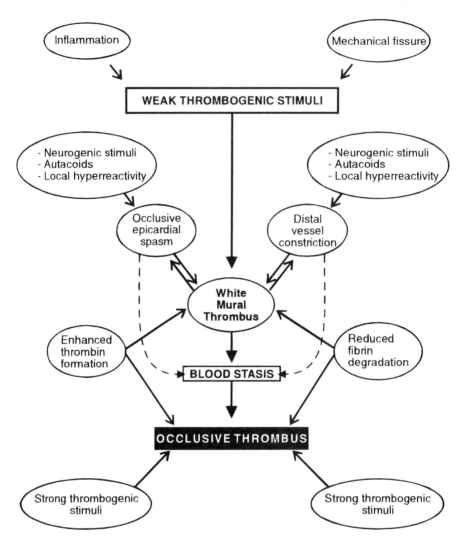

Fig. 9.29 Vicious circles leading to the formation of a thrombus at the site of coronary occlusion. An occlusive red thrombus can form rapidly within minutes at the site of a highly thrombogenic injury (as in the copper coil dog model). An occlusive white thrombus can form only very gradually at the site of a weak, persisting thrombogenic stimulus (as in the electric wire dog model). In the presence of a mural thrombus, occlusive thrombosis may be the result of vicious circles, in which proximal or distal coronary constriction creates blood stasis, with consequent formation of an occlusive red thrombus. The triggers of the vicious circle and the "gain" of its components can have a variable importance and prevalence in different groups of patients. For example, an enhanced thrombotic tendency can be caused, on the one hand, by all the alterations that lead to an enhanced thrombin formation and, on the other, by all the alterations that reduce fibrinolysis.

lus, V, may be represented by epicardial coronary artery spasm or by intense small vessel constriction (the causes of spasm and small vessel constriction may also be multiple). An
enhanced thrombotic response, ET, may be caused by increased activation of thrombosis or
by a reduced activation of fibrinolysis (the causes of which can also be multiple). An enhanced
vasoconstrictor response, EV, may be represented by smooth muscle hyperreactivity or by an
endothelial dysfunction in epicardial coronary arteries or in small coronary vessels (which can
have multiple causes).

Finally, the size of the infarction caused by the sudden interruption of coronary blood
flow is determined not only by the location, intermittence, and duration of the interrupted
flow, but also by the extent of interarterial anastomoses and of collateral vessel development
and function.

■ *Thus, not only can the roles of the various pathogenetic components involved in the vicious circle leading to sudden persistent coronary occlusion and their etiologies be multiple, but also the compensatory role of collaterals can vary. The causes of infarction may have different prevalences
according to age, gender, race, and geographic area, as well as to clinical presentation.* ■

9.5.1 Angiographic findings in the initial phases of infarction

Angiographic studies in the early hours of infarction have provided six fundamental observations that apply to those patients who are most commonly studied soon after hospitalization.

First, total or subtotal occlusion of the infarct-related artery is the rule in the first few
hours after the onset of symptoms.[114] Within 2–4 h after the onset of symptoms, complete
occlusion of a major epicardial coronary artery branch is found in about 90% of patients
and subtotal occlusion in the remaining 10%. Thrombus is frequently detected at the time
of emergency bypass surgery[114] and on angioscopy (being more frequently white in unstable angina and red in acute MI).[115] After MI the acute occlusion recanalizes spontaneously
within 24 h in 35% of patients[114] and within 2–3 weeks in about 50% of patients.[116]

■ *The paradox of patent infarct-related coronary arteries that has puzzled pathologists[117] for
decades is explained, therefore, by the spontaneous recanalization of the occluded vessel.* ■

Second, both the rate and the extent of spontaneous recanalization are markedly
increased by thrombolytic therapy. Following thrombolysis, recanalization occurs within 90
min in about 75% of patients. In the recanalized arteries, the infarct-related stenosis often
presents with irregular contours, which is compatible with an incompletely lysed thrombus
and/or with a ruptured atherosclerotic plaque. The residual stenosis at the very end of
thrombolysis may dilate markedly in response to high doses of intracoronary nitrates in a
substantial percentage of cases (see Fig. 9.12)[26] and gradually remodels over days or weeks.
Some of the remaining 25% of arteries that fail to recanalize following thrombolytic therapy are found to have done so 24 h later.

■ *The large increase in the speed and percentage of recanalization of the culprit artery following
thrombolysis, in sharp contrast to the limited and slow rate of spontaneous recanalization, proves
beyond any doubt the very prevalent role of thrombosis as a cause of persistent epicardial coronary
occlusion. Recanalization may fail to occur because of the characteristics of the thrombus, because of
the intensity or persistence of the thrombogenic stimulus, or because of the local coronary vasoconstrictor component.* ■

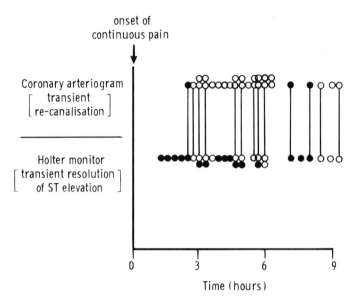

Fig. 9.30 Coronary occlusion is often intermittent in acute MI even during intracoronary infusion of streptokinase. Electrocardiographic evidence (i.e. return of ST-segment elevation to baseline) (●) and angiographic demonstration (○) of patency observed during Holter monitoring in patients enrolled in a study of the efficacy of intracoronary streptokinase. The abscissa shows the time from the onset of symptoms. Coronary angiography performed during the time that the ST segment was returning to baseline consistently showed patency of the infarct-related stenosis. Intermittent reopening of the occluded vessel can be observed at variable intervals from the onset of symptoms. (Modified from ref. 26.)

The third fundamental point is that coronary occlusion is a very dynamic process and may be intermittent, even when the pain is apparently continuous. During the first 5–6 h after the onset of symptoms, the infarct-related coronary artery may exhibit occasional spontaneous transient recanalization in over 60% of cases and may reocclude in spite of intracoronary infusion of streptokinase and nitrates (see Fig. 9.30).[26,118] This observation is consistent with the frequent history of intermittent chest pain and with the occasional transient return to baseline of the elevated ST segment during continuous ECG monitoring,[119] even in cases where the pain was reported as continuous[118] (see Figs. 9.31 and 9.32). In some cases, irreversible reocclusion occurs during intracoronary infusion of streptokinase in spite of high doses of intracoronary nitrates.[26,118]

■ *Initially, therefore, the occlusion that eventually leads to infarction often develops dynamically: when it is preceded by a phase of unstable angina, the culprit coronary artery is predominantly open, but it may occlude from time to time over periods of days or weeks; subsequently, during the initial hours of the infarction, it is predominantly occluded, but may open occasionally. In some cases, however, the thrombogenic and vasoconstrictor stimuli may be so strong that they cannot be opposed by the intracoronary infusion of thrombolytic and dilator agents.* ■

Fourth, only some of the patients with unstable angina and angiographically demonstrable thrombus develop infarction, and they do so after very variable time intervals.

■ *Although most patients with unstable angina have mural thrombi, only a minority develop infarction. Whether the different outcome is related to the intensity of the thrombogenic stimuli, to the response of the hemostatic system, or to the coronary vasomotor response is not known.* ■

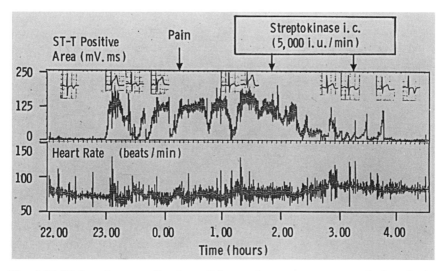

Fig. 9.31 Delayed onset of pain and intermittent coronary occlusion during the very early phases of infarction. In a patient in whom infarction developed during Holter monitoring, the onset of pain followed the onset of ST-segment elevation, and continued when the ST segment returned intermittently to baseline. The time course of intermittent reocclusions during streptokinase infusion, with gradual elevation of the ST segment and an abrupt decline, are the mirror image of the cyclic flow oscillations observed in Folts' animal model (see Ch. 6), suggesting gradual platelet plugging and fragmentation. (Modified from ref. 118.)

Fifth, as discussed in Chapter 8, an occlusion often develops at the site of a nonflow-limiting preexisting stenosis, which may also have smooth rather than irregular borders, and can even occur in angiographically normal arteries. The residual coronary artery stenosis in the infarct-related artery is not necessarily severe or irregular and the culprit stenosis cannot be predicted from analysis of preinfarction angiograms.

■ *Neither the severity of the stenoses nor the presence of irregular borders per se, therefore, represent sufficient or necessary prerequisites for the development of infarction.* ■

Finally, in the very early phases of infarction, immediate dilation of the artery by angioplasty may not be associated with restoration of flow: the contrast medium exhibits a slow runoff or total stagnation, as if flow were blocked distal to the stenosis. Occasionally, the contrast in the distal vessel may have a mottled appearance, which is suggestive of very diffuse intravascular clotting, possibly caused by diffuse endothelial activation; such a finding has been reported formally.[120]

■ *Distal vessel constriction and diffuse endothelial activation may therefore be two of the components that contribute to the development of infarction.* ■

9.5.2 Multiple pathogenetic mechanisms of sudden persistent interruption of coronary blood flow

The conclusions of the previous section, that dynamic thrombosis develops in acute MI in arteries with both severe and mild stenoses, indicate the need for analysis of the pathogenetic components of the vicious cycle outlined in Figure 9.29 in relation to the severity of flow-limiting coronary stenoses. Analysis of the possible mechanisms of sudden persistent

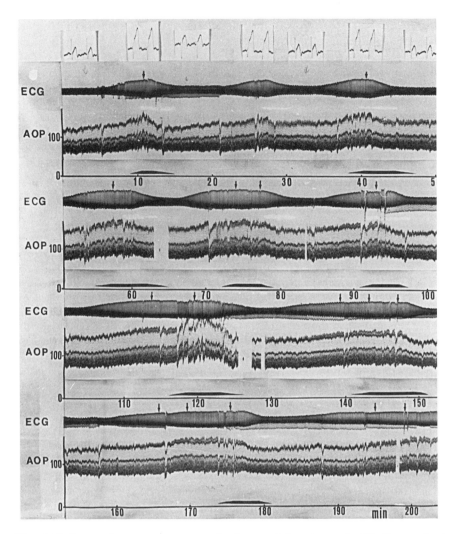

Fig. 9.32 Intermittent coronary occlusion evolving towards MI. In a patient with variant angina, a small anteroseptal MI developed during ECG and aortic pressure (AOP) monitoring in CCU. The ischemic episodes gradually became more prolonged, with a progressively delayed onset of pain, until the final irreversible episode which was not associated with pain. Arrows indicate nitroglycerin administration: the onset and duration of pain are indicated at the bottom of the tracing. The recurrent transient ischemic episodes that preceded the final irreversible episode were characterized, not only by a gradual increase, but also by a gradual decrease of the ST segment, suggesting a mechanism of occlusion differing from that observed in the case described in Figure 9.31. (Modified from ref. 119.)

occlusion in angiographically normal vessels at one extreme, and at the site of severe flow-limiting stenoses at the other, should help define also the variable mixture of these two extreme mechanisms involved in the occlusion of vessels with nonflow-limiting and of moderately flow-limiting stenoses. For each of these prevailing mechanisms, the etiologic components can be multiple.

Infarction distal to very severe stenoses

Lesser thrombogenic stimuli are sufficient to cause thrombotic occlusion at the site of severe flow-limiting stenoses, according to both the animal model described by Folts and to the frequent lack of plaque fissures under thrombi at the site of severe stenoses. In dogs, endothelial damage or activation at the site of very severe stenoses, together with high shear stress, can produce occlusive platelet plugs without enhanced thrombotic tendency; such occlusion may be prevented by inhibiting platelet function.

In patients, the same mechanisms may operate, but they appear to occur very seldom as patients with very critical stenoses can remain stable for years. As most chronic severe stenoses have lost their vasomotor potential, a local vasoconstrictor component is unlikely (see 8.2). In addition, when occlusion develops at the site of a severe chronic preexisting stenosis, collateral blood flow should be sufficient to provide protection, at least from transmural MI, unless the collateral vessels were insufficiently developed or were constricted, or unless diffuse small vessel constriction occurs. The observed higher frequency of preexisting, severe flow-limiting stenoses in patients with non-Q-wave infarction than in those without, is consistent with this hypothesis;[121] however, occasional development of a transmural MI in the presence of a very severe preexisting stenosis remains puzzling and must be due to inadequate collateral development or function. This is in sharp contrast to the postmortem observation of old thrombi, recanalized by multiple channels, at the site of mild or moderate stenoses without signs of infarction in some patients with chronic stable angina (see Fig. 8.9). In such cases, collaterals must have been present in spite of the fact that the stenoses were not critical and must have been functional.

■ *Thus, the development of infarction at the site of severe preexisting chronic coronary stenoses does not require intense local thrombogenic stimuli or an enhanced thrombotic response, and occlusion can be caused by a platelet thrombus. It is unlikely to have a local spastic component, but requires a reduced development or function of collaterals or intense distal vessel constriction.* ■

Infarction distal to angiographically normal arteries

Acute persistent coronary occlusion in coronary arteries without preexisting detectable flow-limiting stenosis may result from the following:

1. It may be caused by a highly thrombogenic local stimulus, such as a large fissure of a small but highly thrombogenic plaque, or a strong local inflammatory response to toxic, immunologic, or infective stimuli, even in the absence of any abnormality of either the hemostatic system or the coronary vasoconstrictor response (this case would be similar to that of a normal dog in which a copper coil or an electric wire is inserted in a normal coronary artery).
2. It may result from lesser coronary thrombogenic stimuli occurring simultaneously with a marked displacement of the hemostatic equilibrium towards thrombosis (a prothrombotic state).
3. It may be attributable to occlusive epicardial coronary artery spasm or intense distal coronary vessel constriction causing prolonged blood flow stasis.

Local thrombogenic stimuli. There is no conclusive evidence that, in humans, the extent of thrombosis depends on the severity of the mechanical injury to the vessel wall, as observed in previously normal vessels in animals. A major component of the local thrombus growth is therefore likely to be related to the local thrombogenicity, rather than the extent of the vessel wall injury. A very intense, local thrombogenic stimulus (similar to the copper coil in the dog model) would be indicated by a totally red fibrin thrombus, but not by just the proximal or distal extension of an originally occlusive platelet thrombus (see Fig. 9.20). A weak persistent thrombogenic stimulus (similar to the electric wire model in the dog) would be suggested by a white thrombus, and its layered appearance would suggest an intermittent stimulus.

The possible role of "prothrombotic" states. The displacement of the thrombotic/thrombolytic equilibrium towards thrombosis may modulate the speed and growth of mural thrombi and transform the local coronary repair process of mild thrombogenic stimuli into an occlusive thrombosis. Increased thrombotic activity or decreased fibrinolytic activity could occur only days or hours before the development of coronary artery thrombosis in response to inflammatory or neural systemic stimuli: for example, platelet activation can be caused by emotional stress.[122] A detectable prothrombotic state in patients with acute MI or unstable angina may also be a consequence of the ischemic stimuli. There is some evidence that a prothrombotic state may be present months or years before the development of acute coronary events, but it is not clear whether this prothrombotic state has a causal role or is just a marker of other pathogenetic components of IHD (see Ch. 12). Platelet antiaggregants, heparin, and vitamin K inhibitors reduce the thrombotic risk not only by correcting prothrombotic states but also by reducing the normal hemostatic repair response to the local coronary injury and thrombogenic stimuli; hence, they reduce the gain of one of the feedback mechanisms of acute persistent coronary occlusion.

Coronary constriction and blood flow stasis as a component of thrombus growth. The development of CBF stasis in the presence of even a minimal intraplaque or mural thrombus would represent a very powerful combination of stimuli for thrombus growth and for the development of an occlusive red thrombus. In patients with variant angina, occlusive epicardial coronary artery spasm does not usually cause coronary thrombosis because it can recur several times a day for weeks, with recurrent episodes of ST-segment elevation lasting even 10–15 min. Although activation of thrombin formation during transient occlusive coronary artery spasm has been reported,[123,124] the rarity of infarction in patients with variant angina and frequent transient ischemic episodes indicates the need for unusually persistent constrictor stimuli,[125,126] or for additional pathogenetic components of persistent, rather than transient, interruption of CBF, such as the formation of small mural thromboses.[119] At the site of mural thrombi the generation of thrombin and the release of 5-HT and thromboxane A_2 by platelets stimulates local and distal coronary vasoconstriction, particularly when the endothelium is activated, for example, by inflammatory cytokines or anoxia. Persistent occlusive spasm at the site of mural thrombosis can result from a local enhanced vasoconstrictor response, such as that demonstrable in variant angina,[7] but CBF can also be interrupted by intense constriction of hyperreactive small vessels distal to a mural thrombus, such as an exaggerated response to 5-HT and to other vasoconstrictor substances.

Blood stagnation in the presence of a mural thrombus prevents the continuous dilution and removal of the activators of thrombin and the continuous supply of inhibitors of thrombin and of fibrinolytic components, and anoxia causes endothelial activation; thus, an occlusive thrombus may develop. When the vasoconstrictor stimuli are exhausted and the vascular smooth muscle relaxes, flow may not be restored if a red thrombus occludes the lumen. Strong constrictor stimuli or enhanced constrictor response were shown to result in severe epicardial coronary constriction persisting postmortem.[24,25]

In most patients with infarction and angiographically normal coronary arteries, no predisposing factors can be found; such patients often have a history of cigarette smoking and, in women, also the use of oral contraceptives, but rarely do they have histories of hyperlipidemia, diabetes or hypertension. In a few patients, abnormalities of the coagulation or fibrinolytic systems, predisposing to thrombosis, have been identified but the causes of the localization of thrombosis in the coronary artery are totally unknown. Munitions workers, following withdrawal of exposure to nitroglycerin,[127] develop angina and infarction due to coronary artery spasm, but the precise causes of the persistent, rather than reversible, coronary spastic occlusion observed in most individuals exposed to the same stimulus, are not known. Cocaine abuse may also cause acute MI, possibly through coronary artery vasoconstriction.[128] The sudden occlusion of a normal coronary artery may cause only a small MI in those patients with well-developed interarterial anastomoses (see Ch. 10).

■ *The occurrence of infarction in patients without angiographically detectable coronary artery stenoses must be caused by very strong local thrombogenic or constrictor stimuli or by their combination with enhanced thrombotic tendency and/or enhanced coronary vasoconstrictor response. These same types of mechanisms could have a lower threshold for precipitating infarction in the presence of coronary stenoses. Both the etiologic components of the vicious circle that leads to persistent coronary occlusion and the "gain" of its components may vary in different groups of patients.* ■

9.5.3 Predisposing and precipitating events

When MI is caused simply by the fissure of a highly thrombogenic plaque occurring at random, it could be facilitated by sudden bursts of raised arterial blood pressure during intense effort or emotion, but only a very few patients report acute events immediately preceding the onset of symptoms. When infarction is not simply the result of such a randomly occurring purely mechanical plaque fissure, it may be preceded by predisposing factors, as suggested by reports of intense acute or chronic psychological distress, unusual fatigue, vital exhaustion or of influenza-like symptoms that led to the patient consulting a doctor during the preceding weeks for noncardiac symptoms. Analysis of the events that preceded infarction and of the circumstances during which symptoms began could provide clues useful for the reconstruction of prevailing pathogenetic components in selected groups. This reconstruction is made difficult by the subjective nature of symptoms, by their prevalence among individuals who do not develop infarction, and by the likelihood that the triggers of infarction may vary according to age, gender, ethnic group, and geographic location.

So far, the search for predisposing and precipitating factors has usually included, indiscriminately, male and female patients of any age, race and geographic location.

Circumstances in which symptoms appear

In about 50% of cases the attack begins at rest without any detectable immediate precipitating cause; in about 10% of cases, infarction occurs during sleep. In 35% of cases the onset of symptoms occurs during ordinary daily activities; only in 5% of cases is it preceded by strenuous exercise. The occurrence of MI during heavy physical exertion is virtually confined to those patients who do not exercise regularly.[129] In some cases, infarction develops during general surgery. Infarction has also been reported soon after strokes and transient ischemic attacks. Very occasionally, infarction occurs during extremely intense systemic and hemodynamic stimulation, such as serum sickness, allergic reactions, wasp stings, pulmonary embolism, hypoglycemia, and thoracic trauma. It may also occur following cocaine abuse and administration of ergot derivatives in young individuals without risk factors or coronary atherosclerosis. The mechanisms by which some unusual precipitating events cause infarction in some individuals but not in others, even in the absence of a detectable atherosclerotic background, are not clear; however, the very fact that they can do so suggests that much less intense stimuli of a similar type could be sufficient in the presence of severe coronary athero-sclerosis.

Psychological distress

Frequent clinical observations suggest that infarction, particularly among young individuals, develops during a particularly stressful period of life with which they are unable to cope.[130–136] The limited sensitivity of psychological distress as a marker of risk depends on the difficulty in quantifying it (as the intensity of distress is also influenced by personality type and level of social support) and on the prevalence of other predisposing and precipitating factors, in different communities, social groups, and age-groups. The limited specificity depends on the simultaneous coincidental presence of other predisposing and precipitating factors that are required to cause infarction.

Subclinical infections

Several reports suggest the possibility that MI occurs more frequently during bacterial or viral epidemics.[137–142] The evidence for such an association is particularly difficult to collect in cases of subclinical infections or of acute reactivation of dormant herpesvirus, *Chlamydia pneumoniae* or cytomegalovirus (see Ch. 8), unless objective diagnostic markers can be identified and appropriately controlled studies performed. A prospective controlled study failed to find evidence for Coxsackie B virus infections in acute MI,[143] but the variable incidence of positive findings and their specificity depends on the prevalence of the infectious agent considered in the groups studied. A variety of infectious agents[140] may predispose to infarction, but this predisposition may occur only in some individuals, under some circumstances, in some geographic regions.

Vital exhaustion

A fairly common but nonspecific complaint is that of unusual fatigue (vital exhaustion) in the weeks preceding the infarct.[144] This complaint may be related to psychological distress and depression or to subclinical infection. These two conditions may be related, as psychological stress reduces immunologic defenses.[145]

Elevation of acute-phase proteins

The recent observation of elevated blood levels of CRP and SAA in unstable angina with a complicated course, and in cases of infarction preceded by a history of unstable angina,[106] is an objective marker of an inflammatory response that could be due to toxic, immunologic, or infectious stimuli responsible for activation of the coronary vascular endothelium and of inflammatory cells. Endothelial activation causes a local vasoconstrictor and thrombotic tendency with expression of adhesive molecules, which leads to activation of monocytes and granulocytes. Activated granulocytes and monocytes release cytokines responsible for hepatic synthesis of acute-phase proteins.[146,147] Interleukin-1 can also be produced in response to stress,[148,149] together with nerve growth factor.[150]

The common absence of elevated levels of CRP and SAA in patients with infarction not preceded by unstable angina is suggestive of possible differences in the triggering stimuli of these two forms of presentation. The relation between these markers of inflammation, subclinical viral infections, and vital exhaustion is still unknown.

Circadian distribution of infarction

When expressed per hour, the onset of symptoms is more frequent during the morning (from 06.00 to 1200 h) than during the other hours of the day,[151,152] but obviously most infarctions occur during the remaining 18 h (see Fig. 9.33A,B). Thus, the factors responsible for the slight-

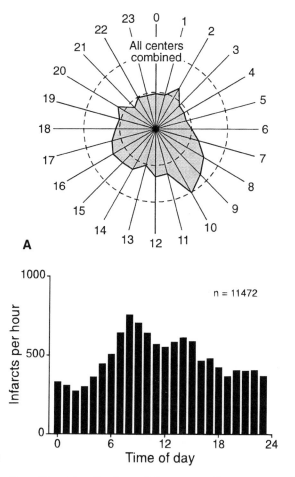

A

B

Fig. 9.33 Circadian distribution of the onset of symptoms of MI. An increase in the morning incidence of the onset of symptoms was observed in both the World Health Organization multicenter study (**A**) (modified from ref. 151), and in the GISSI-2 study (**B**) (modified from ref. 152). The European findings are similar to those obtained in the USA and reported in ref. 153. Although the development of MI is more common in the morning hours, the majority of cases occur during the remaining 24 h.

ly higher frequency of infarction during the morning hours have only a modulatory role. They can be related to a wide variety of physiologic parameters with a circadian variability, with peaks or troughs coinciding with the morning hours. Not only adrenergic tone, procoagulant activity, and coronary vasomotor tone,[153] but also fibrinolytic activity (see Fig. 9.34)[154] and a variety of humoral and metabolic parameters have a similar circadian distribution.[155] The observed associations are, therefore, either not necessarily causal or not necessarily the only causes of the morning excess of infarctions.

Psychological distress, unusual fatigue, influenza-like symptoms, vital exhaustion, heavy physical exertion, and elevated levels of acute-phase proteins may be associated with alterations that influence coronary vasomotion and hemostatic and immunologic reactivity, pre-

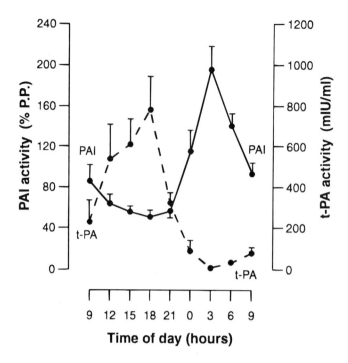

Fig. 9.34 Circadian distribution of fibrinolytic components. The circadian distribution of tissue-type plasminogen activator (t-PA) and plasminogen activator inhibitor (PAI) activity in plasma indicates a reduced fibrinolytic potential in the morning hours, which is another of the many modulatory factors that, together with platelet aggregability and adrenergic tone, may favor the morning excess of infarction (% P.P., percentage of pooled plasma). (Modified from ref. 154.)

disposing to coronary endothelial activation and plaque fissure and enhancing the thrombotic and vasoconstrictor response.

■ *The lack of specificity of the predisposing factors investigated so far reflects the need for the coincidental presence of multiple, unfavorable conditions that contribute to the precipitation of MI only when they occur simultaneously. The lack of sensitivity of predisposing factors indicates that these are not the same in all patients. As the etiologic components that may initiate the pathogenetic mechanisms of the vicious circle described in Figure 9.29 and the factors that may influence the "gain" of the pathogenetic mechanisms are multiple, it is necessary to try to define their prevalence in homogeneous groups of patients.* ■

9.5.4 Conclusions

The observation of a frequently lesser extent of atherosclerosis in patients presenting with infarction as the first manifestation of IHD than in those presenting with chronic stable angina suggests that infarction may not be a random event occurring when atherosclerosis has reached a critical threshold. The beneficial effects of thrombolytic therapy, aspirin, and heparin clearly demonstrate the very prevalent role of thrombosis among the causes of infarction, but a number of questions still remain.

The failure of prompt restoration of blood flow with any intravenous thrombolytic therapy in at least 20% of cases (even when thrombolytic therapy is given early and directly into the culprit coronary artery) may be due either to the intensity of the thrombogenic stimulus or to the features of the hemostatic or vasomotor response.

The observation of platelet fibrin mural, rather than of occlusive, thrombi in many patients dying suddenly in the first few hours after the onset of symptoms, indicates a rather weak local thrombogenic stimulus and leaves unsolved the question of the precise mechanisms of the sudden interruption of CBF.

For patients who present with unstable angina and an intermittent clinical evolution towards persisting coronary occlusion of the coronary artery lesions (over a period that may range from hours to several weeks), it seems reasonable to postulate the waxing and waning of either weak thrombogenic stimuli or intense vasoconstriction in epicardial arteries or in distal vessels. The nature of the coronary lesions responsible for such fluctuations is unknown and unlikely to be related primarily, or solely, to a fissured plaque. In such patients, evidence for the possible role of local inflammatory stimuli is fairly strong, but the causes of the inflammatory process may be multiple and are not precisely known. The lower prevalence of increased values of acute-phase proteins in patients with unheralded MI, compared with those in whom infarction was preceded by unstable angina, suggests a possible difference in the precipitating events in these two subgroups.

The frequent reports of severe fatigue and vital exhaustion suggest that they could be markers of subclinical infections or of toxic or immune alterations (that may be responsible for the occurrence of coronary inflammation and activation of the endothelium, with consequent thrombogenic and vasoconstrictor stimuli, as well as the occurrence of a pro-thrombotic state). The profound distress resulting from the inability to cope with stressful situations could also influence, either chronically or acutely, both the nervous and immune responses and hence could trigger or potentiate coronary vasoconstrictor and thrombogenic stimuli. The relationship of vital exhaustion to psychological distress, infections, and blood levels of acute-phase proteins should be explored specifically. As similar complaints are common in other organic diseases, the mechanisms of their association with the coronary circulation (as the target organ) should be investigated. The prevalence of psychological distress, vital exhaustion, and subclinical infections as predisposing factors of infarction may vary according to age, gender, and cultural and ethnic grouping, as well as to the mode of presentation of the infarction.

■ *As stated repeatedly, acute MI is an extremely rare event in the life of a patient with even the most severe coronary atherosclerosis and it occurs most commonly in individuals with no previous history of IHD. Very rare events can be precipitated only by very rare single causes or by multiple, independent, unfavorable events that must coincide in order to initiate and potentiate the components of the vicious circle illustrated in Figure 9.29. The etiologic component and "gain" of the various pathogenetic mechanisms may vary in different subgroups of patients.* ■

9.6 RATIONAL THERAPEUTIC PRINCIPLES

Ischemic stimuli can be multiple in the same syndrome and in different syndromes of IHD and can develop unpredictably in variable succession during the life of any individual patient. For this reason, generalized forms of treatment and prevention that are valid for the multiple stimuli capable of causing myocardial ischemia do not exist. The only currently available, broadly applicable, but nonspecific preventive approach is the control of known risk factors (see Chs. 12 and 13). Specific therapeutic and preventive strategies to prevent ischemic episodes call for both the identification of the prevailing types of ischemic stimuli that require treatment in a particular subgroup of patients, and a precise knowledge of their causes.

Extracoronary stimuli are the most extensively studied and, for these, specific forms of treatment are available. Vasoconstrictor and thrombotic stimuli are less clearly understood and, therefore, their therapeutic and preventive strategies are less specifically targeted.

9.6.1 Extracoronary stimuli

In the presence of a limited coronary flow reserve caused by atherosclerotic plaques, the most radical treatment is the removal of the stenosis by appropriate revascularization procedures. Other possibilities are as follows:

a. improvement of residual coronary flow reserve by reducing basal myocardial oxygen demand (i.e. by correcting hypertension, hyperkinetic circulatory states, hyperthyroidism, fever, tachyarrhythmias) or by improving basal oxygen supply (i.e. by correcting anemia and hypoxia)
b. limitation of physical effort
c. use of drugs that allow the heart to work more economically (i.e. to perform its pump function using less oxygen with lower heart rate, end-diastolic volume, systolic pressure, and velocity of contraction)
d. a novel, complementary pharmacologic approach could be the use of drugs that limit luxury perfusion of subepicardial layers in order to maintain higher levels of poststenotic pressure and hence improve subendocardial perfusion.

9.6.2 Coronary vasoconstriction

The only therapy currently available for the treatment and prevention of coronary vasoconstrictor stimuli, whatever their cause, is based on the use of vasodilators, of which nitrates and calcium antagonists are the most widely used. Their beneficial clinical effects are well established but present inherent limitations.

First, vasodilators affect only one of the complex mechanisms that control vasomotor tone (see Ch. 5). The mechanism that is disrupted and impairs blood flow may vary in different vascular beds and in different segments of the same vascular bed (large arteries, prearterioles, arterioles, veins). Interorgan and within-organ segmental differences in vasomotor control may be enhanced in disease states and are more obvious in some individuals than in others, as shown by the development of hypotension or headache in response to nitrates or dihydropyridines in some individuals but not in others. The doses that are required to prevent or relieve abnormal segmental coronary vasoconstriction may, therefore, vary considerably with both the intensity of the stimulus and the constrictor response. In addition, doses of drugs that are usually sufficient to produce systemic and coronary dilation may be insufficient to prevent constriction or to cause relaxation of the involved segment when either the local constrictor stimuli are intense or when the constrictor response is greatly enhanced. This is the case with epicardial coronary artery spasm, refractory to large doses of vasodilators, reported after coronary bypass surgery or the administration of ergonovine, and also in some patients with variant angina (see Ch. 20).

Second, as the control mechanisms of coronary vasomotor tone in conductive coronary arteries and prearteriolar and arteriolar vessels differ markedly, the causes of epicardial coronary artery spasm, dynamic coronary stenosis, and distal coronary vessel constriction are also likely to differ. It should not be surprising, therefore, that the chronic administration of nitrates and calcium antagonists causes an 80% reduction in the number of attacks in variant angina, but a less than 50% reduction in those occurring in chronic stable angina, and has no convincing effect on those occurring in syndrome X (see Chs. 17, 18, and 20).

Finally, in order to prevent occasional episodes of segmental coronary constriction, vasodilators persistently reduce the vasomotor tone of the whole body and, thus, could induce a reflex increase of tone in the coronary vascular bed.

■ *It is essential, therefore, to reach a better understanding of the varied mechanisms of abnormal coronary constriction, in order to develop therapeutic agents capable of preventing them by counteracting the specific local alteration. Adequate prevention of inappropriate coronary vasoconstriction would allow patients with coronary stenoses to use the maximum residual coronary flow reserve available and, hence, to experience only a fixed-threshold effort-induced angina. It would cure totally those patients in whom vasoconstriction is the only cause of angina.* ■

9.6.3 Prevention of coronary thrombosis

The prevention of coronary thrombi that cause or contribute to unstable angina, acute MI, and the sudden progression of coronary artery stenoses should be based, not only on the prevention of local thrombogenic stimuli, but also on the limitation of thrombus growth beyond the requirements of its physiologic repair function.

At present, the prevention and treatment of coronary thrombosis is based on the use of antithrombotic and fibrinolytic drugs, because local coronary thrombogenic stimuli are very poorly understood. The incidence of thrombosis secondary to the fissure of an atherosclerotic plaque can be reduced only by preventing plaque fissure or plaque formation. The incidence of thrombosis not secondary to a plaque fissure can be reduced only by first identifying the local stimuli that cause the endothelial denudation or activation responsible for thrombosis; the search for such inflammatory or toxic stimuli has, so far, received little attention.

The prevention of "excessive" thrombus growth can be achieved by correcting chronic or acute prothrombotic states (when present), by reducing the normal thrombotic activity or by enhancing the normal fibrinolytic activity. Administration of aspirin, heparin, and other drugs that reduce blood levels of vitamin K-dependent components of the hemostatic system has been found to reduce markedly the incidence of infarction in different circumstances. Administration of various types of thrombolytic drugs to patients with acute MI has been found to reduce mortality and infarct size substantially. These studies have proved convincingly, not only that reduction of the hemostatic response can prevent and limit infarction, but also that in acute MI, when a fresh occlusive thrombus is present, enhancement of fibrinolytic activity can reestablish flow and reduce myocardial ischemia and necrosis. Although antithrombotic and fibrinolytic therapy is successful, it has certain drawbacks that are outlined below.

First, in order to prevent or limit thrombus growth that may occur occasionally and unpredictably in a segment of a coronary artery, long-term antithrombotic therapy reduces the hemostatic efficiency in the whole vascular bed. The greater its efficacy in preventing and limiting coronary thrombosis, the greater the inhibition of hemostasis and the greater the risk of bleeding at other sites in the body where thrombosis may occur merely as a physiologic repair process. However, in a substantial number of cases, treatment with aspirin, heparin, antivitamin K drugs, and their combinations is not sufficient to prevent infarction, possibly because of the intensity of the local thrombogenic stimuli, and/or the contributory role of coronary vasoconstriction. With the antithrombotic regimens used so far, which have confirmed partial but significant beneficial effects, the benefits outweigh the risks of bleeding in most circumstances, but this may not be the case with more aggressive approaches.

Second, in order to favor the lysis of thrombi that interrupt or contribute to the interruption of flow through a major coronary artery and that cause persistent myocardial ischemia, thrombolytic drugs are used in acute MI that also increase the lysis of other thrombi that may provide physiologic hemostatic plugs. Nevertheless, in 20% of cases, and irrespective of the thrombolytic agent used, coronary recanalization is not achieved promptly, even when the drug is injected directly into the culprit artery soon after the onset of symptoms, and, in 50% or more of cases, full patency (TIMI Grade 3) is not achieved at 90 min.[156] The failure to achieve prompt recanalization may be due to the characteristics of the local thrombogenic stimuli, to the composition of the thrombi, or to the prevalence of local coronary vasoconstrictor components. Despite these drawbacks, the benefits of fibrinolytic therapy in acute MI, like the preventive effects of antithrombotic therapy, largely outweigh the risks of bleeding.

Finally, newer approaches, such as the blockade of platelet adhesive receptors, the inhibition of thrombin by antithrombins, and the use of more selective thrombolytic agents, could be advantageous if they were found to be more efficacious and to carry a lower risk of bleeding. Drugs aimed at preventing coronary thrombosis may have different effects on thrombi developing at the site of severe flow-limiting stenoses than on those developing in noncritically stenosed segments. Thrombi that occlude severe flow-limiting stenoses are predominantly composed of platelets and thus are prevented more efficiently by antiplatelet drugs than by heparin (at least in animal models). Thrombi occurring in nonstenosed arteries are composed mainly of fibrin and are thus more efficiently prevented by antithrombin than by antiplatelet drugs.

■ *More rational, specifically targeted preventive approaches should come from a better understanding of the nature and prevalence of the triggers that initiate and potentiate the components of the vicious circle that lead to thrombosis, to interruption of CBF and to acute MI.* ■

REFERENCES

1. White CW, Wright CB, Doty DB et al. Does visual interpretation of the coronary arteriogram predict the physiologic importance of a coronary stenosis? New Engl J Med 1984;*310:*819.
2. Kern MJ, Donohue TJ, Aguirre FV et al. Assessment of angiographically intermediate coronary artery stenosis using the Doppler Flowire. Am J Cardiol 1993;*71:*26D.
3. Serruys PW, Di Mario C, Meneveau N et al. Intracoronary pressure and flow velocity with sensor-tip guidewires: a new methodologic approach for assessment of coronary hemodynamics before and after coronary interventions. Am J Cardiol 1993;*71:*41D.
4. Epstein SE, Talbot TL. Dynamic coronary tone in precipitation, exacerbation and relief of angina pectoris. Am J Cardiol 1981;*48:*797.
5. Brown BG. Coronary vasospasm: observations linking the clinical spectrum of ischemic heart disease to the dynamic pathology of coronary atherosclerosis. Arch Intern Med 1981;*141:*716.
6. Willerson JT, Hillis LD, Winniford M, Buja M. Speculation regarding mechanisms responsible for acute ischemic heart disease syndromes. J Am Coll Cardiol 1986;*8:*245.
7. Maseri A, Davies G, Hackett D, Kaski JC. Coronary artery spasm and coronary vasoconstriction: the case for a distinction. Circulation 1990;*81:*1983.
8. Maseri A. Preface. In: Maseri A, Klassen G, Lesch M (eds) Primary and Secondary Angina Pectoris. New York, Grune and Stratton, 1978, p. xiii.
9. Round Table Discussion. Perspectives and guidelines in the investigation and treatment of

patients with angina pectoris. In: Maseri A, Klassen G, Lesch M (eds) Primary and Secondary Angina Pectoris. New York, Grune and Stratton, 1978, p. 439 & 443.

10. McGregor M. Mechanisms of transient myocardial ischemia. Can J Cardiol 1986;*1*:53A.

11. Maseri A, L'Abbate A, Pesola A et al. Coronary vasospasm in angina pectoris. Lancet 1977;*1*:713.

12. Lablanche JM, Deturck R, Fourrier JL, Gommeaux A, Bertrand ME. Abnormal diffuse coronary vasomotion. Eur Heart J 1989;*10*:111.

13. Maseri A. Role of coronary artery spasm in symptomatic and silent myocardial ischemia. J Am Coll Cardiol 1987;*9*:249.

14. El-Tamimi H, Maseri A, Bertrand M. Study of the vasomotor response of human stable coronary artery stenoses. 1995. Submitted for publication.

15. Kaski JC, Tousoulis D, Haider AW, Gavrielides S, Crea F, Maseri A. Reactivity of eccentric and concentric coronary stenoses in patients with chronic stable angina. J Am Coll Cardiol 1991;*17*:627.

16. Tousoulis D, Kaski JC, Bogaty P et al. Reactivity of proximal and distal angiographically normal and stenotic coronary segments in chronic stable angina pectoris. Am J Cardiol 1991;*67*:1195.

17. Kaski JC, Tousoulis D, Gavrielides S et al. Comparison of epicardial coronary artery tone and reactivity in Prinzmetal's variant angina and chronic stable angina pectoris. J Am Coll Cardiol 1991;*17*:1058.

18. MacAlpin RN. Contribution of dynamic vascular wall thickening to luminal narrowing during coronary arterial constriction. Circulation 1980;*61*:296.

19. Freedman B, Richmond DR, Kelly DT. Pathophysiology of coronary artery spasm. Circulation 1982;*66*:705.

20. Bertrand ME, La Blanche JM, Tilmant PY et al. Frequency of provoked coronary arterial spasm in 1089 consecutive patients undergoing coronary arteriography. Circulation 1982;*65*:1299.

21. Dalen JE, Ockene IS, Alpert JS. Coronary spasm, coronary thrombosis and myocardial infarction: a hypothesis concerning the pathophysiology of acute myocardial infarction. Am Heart J 1982;*104*:1119.

22. Myerburg RJ, Kessler K, Mallon SM et al. Life-threatening ventricular arrhythmias in patients with silent myocardial ischemia due to coronary artery spasm. New Engl J Med 1992;*326*:1451.

23. Factor SM, Cho S. Smooth muscle contraction bands in the media of coronary arteries: a postmortem marker of antemortem coronary spasm? J Am Coll Cardiol 1985;*6*:1329.

24. El-Maraghi NRH, Sealey BJ. Recurrent myocardial infarction in a young man due to coronary arterial spasm demonstrated at autopsy. Circulation 1980;*61*:199.

25. Roberts WC, Curry RC, Isner JM et al. Sudden death in Prinzmetal's angina with coronary spasm documented by angiography. Am J Cardiol 1982;*50*:203.

26. Hackett D, Davies G, Chierchia S, Maseri A. Intermittent coronary occlusion in acute myocardial infarction: value of combined thrombolytic and vasodilator therapy. N Engl J Med 1987;*317*:1055.

27. Maseri A, Crea F. Segmental control of vascular tone in the coronary circulation and pathophysiology of ischemic heart disease. J Appl Cardiovasc Biol 1991;*2*:163.

28. Berkenboom G, Abramowicz M, Vandermoten P, Degre SG. Role of alpha-adrenergic coronary tone in exercise-induced angina pectoris. Am J Cardiol 1986;*57*:195.

29. Kalsner S, Richards R. Coronary arteries of cardiac patients are hyperreactive and contain stores of amines: a mechanism for coronary spasm. Science 1984;*223*:1435.

30. Maseri A. Coronary vasoconstriction: visible and invisible. New Engl J Med 1991;*325*:1579.

31. Clarke JG, Davies GJ, Kerwin R et al. Coronary artery infusion of neuropeptide Y in patients with angina pectoris. Lancet 1977;*1*:1057.

32. Newman CM, Maseri A, Hackett DR, El-Tamimi HM, Davies GJ. Response of angiographically normal and atherosclerotic left anterior descending coronary arteries to acetylcholine. Am J Cardiol 1990;*66*:1070.

33. McFadden EP, Clarke JG, Davies GJ, Haider AW, Kaski JC, Maseri A. Effect of intracoronary serotonin on coronary vessels in patients with stable and variant angina. New Engl J Med 1991;*324*:648.

34. McFadden EP, Bauters C, Lablanche JM et al. Effect of ketanserin on proximal and distal coronary constrictor responses to intracoronary infusion of serotonin in patients with stable angina, patients with variant angina and control patients. Circulation 1992;*86:*187.

35. Pupita G, Maseri A, Kaski JC et al. Myocardial ischemia caused by distal coronary constriction in stable angina pectoris. New Engl J Med 1990;*323:*514.

36. Powelson SW. Discordance of coronary angiography and 201-thallium tomography early after transluminal coronary angioplasty. J Nuc Med 27 1986;*6:*900.

37. Manyari DE, Knudtson M, Kloiber R, Roth D. Sequential thallium-201 myocardial perfusion studies after successful coronary angioplasty: delayed resolution of exercise-induced scintigraphic abnormalities. Circulation 1988;*77:*86.

38. El-Tamimi H, Davies GJ, Crea F, Sritara P, Hackett D, Maseri A. Inappropriate constriction of small coronary vessels as a possible cause of a positive exercise test soon after successful coronary angioplasty. Circulation 1991;*84:*2307.

39. Fishell TA, Bausback KN, McDonald TV. Evidence for altered epicardial coronary artery autoregulation as a cause of distal coronary vasoconstriction after successful percutaneous transluminal coronary angioplasty. J Clin Invest 1990;*86:*575.

40. Wilson RF, Johnson MR, Marcus ML et al. The effect of coronary angioplasty on coronary flow reserve. Circulation 1988;*77:*873.

41. Kern MJ, De Ligonul U, Vandormael M et al. Impaired coronary vasodilator reserve in the immediate postcoronary angioplasty period: analysis of coronary artery flow velocity indexes and regional cardiac venous efflux. J Am Coll Cardiol 1989;*13:*860.

42. Zijlstra F, den Boer A, Reiber JH, van Es GA, Lubsen J, Serruys PW. Assessment of immediate and long-term functional results of percutaneous transluminal coronary angioplasty. Circulation 1988;*78:*15.

43. Segal J, Kern MJ, Scott NA et al. Alterations of phasic coronary artery flow velocity in humans during percutaneous coronary angioplasty. J Am Coll Cardiol 1992;*20:*276.

44. Uren NG, Crake T, Lefroy DC, de Silva R, Davies GJ, Maseri A. Delayed recovery of coronary resistive vessel function after coronary angioplasty. J Am Coll Cardiol 1993;*21:*612.

45. Uren NG, Crake T, Lefroy DC, Davies GJ, Maseri A. Altered resistive vessel function after coronary angioplasty is not due to reduced production of nitric oxide. 1995. Submitted for publication.

46. Uren NG, Marraccini P, Gistri R, de Silva R, Camici PG. Altered coronary vasodilator reserve and metabolism in myocardium subtended by normal arteries in patients with coronary artery disease. J Am Coll Cardiol 1993;*22:*650.

47. Sambuceti G, Parodi O, Marcassa C et al. Alteration in regulation of myocardial blood flow in one-vessel coronary artery disease determined by positron emission tomography. Am J Cardiol 1993;*72:*538.

48. Uren NG, Crake T, Lefroy DC, de Silva R, Davies GJ, Maseri A. Reduced coronary vasodilator response in infarcted and normal myocardium after myocardial infarction. New Engl J Med 1994;*331:*222.

49. Crake T, Canepa-Anson R, Shapiro LM, Poole-Wilson PA. Continuous recording of coronary sinus oxygen saturation during atrial pacing in patients with coronary artery disease and with syndrome X. Br Heart J 1988;*89:*31.

50. Cannon RO III. Microvascular angina. Cardiovascular investigations regarding pathophysiology and management. Med Clinics of N America 1991;*75:*1097.

51. Zeiher AM, Drexler H, Wollschläger, Just H. Modulation of coronary vasomotor tone in humans. Circulation 1991;*83:*391.

52. Maseri A, Crea F, Kaski JC, Crake T. Mechanisms of angina pectoris in Syndrome X. J Am Coll Cardiol 1991;*17:*499.

53. Fuster V, Badimon L, Badimon JJ, Chesebro JH. The pathogenesis of coronary artery disease and the acute coronary syndromes. New Engl J Med 1992;*326:*310.

54. Davies MJ, Bland JM, Hangartner JRW, Angelini A, Thomas AC. Factors influencing the presence or absence of acute coronary artery thrombi in sudden ischaemic death. Eur Heart J 1989;*10:*203.

55. Chandler AB. Mechanisms and frequency of thrombosis in the coronary circulation. Thrombosis Res 1974;*4*:3.

56. Davies MJ, Thomas A. Thrombosis and acute coronary lesions in sudden cardiac ischemic death. New Engl J Med 1984;*310*:1137.

57. Baroldi G, Falzi G, Mariani F. Sudden coronary death: a postmortem study in 208 selected cases compared to 97 "control" subjects. Am Heart J 1979;*98*:20.

58. Kragel AH, Gertz SD, Roberts WC. Morphologic comparison of frequency and types of acute lesions in the major coronary epicardial arteries in unstable angina pectoris, sudden coronary death and acute myocardial infarction. J Am Coll Cardiol 1991;*18*:801.

59. Falk E. Unstable angina with fatal outcome: dynamic coronary thrombosis leading to infarction and/or sudden death. Circulation 1985;*71*:699.

60. Fulton WFM. The morphology of coronary thrombotic occlusions relevant to thrombolytic intervention. In Kaltenbach M et al (eds). Transluminal coronary angioplasty and intracoronary thrombolysis. Springer-Verlag, Berlin, 1982, p. 244.

61. Qiao JH, Fishbein MC. The severity of coronary atherosclerosis at sites of plaque rupture with occlusive thrombosis. J Am Coll Cardiol 1991;*17*:1138.

62. Arbustini E, Grasso M, Diegoli M et al. Coronary atherosclerotic plaques with and without thrombus in ischemic heart syndromes: a morphologic immunohistochemical and biochemical study. Am J Cardiol 1991;*68*:36B

63. Arbustini E, Grasso M, Diegoli M et al. Coronary thrombosis in non-cardiac death. Cor Art Dis 1993;*4*:751.

64. Davies MJ. Macroscopic or microscopic view of coronary thrombi. Circulation 1990;*82*:1138.

65. Erhardt L, Unge G, Bowman G. Formation of coronary arterial thrombi in relation to onset of necrosis in acute myocardial infarction in man. Am Heart J 1976;*91*:592.

66. Fulton W. Coronary thrombosis in myocardial infarction. In: Hjalmarson Å, Wilhelmsen L (eds) Acute and long-term medical management of myocardial ischaemia. Proceedings of a conference held in Copenhagen, Denmark, September 8–9, 1977, arranged by Medical Department I, Sahlgrenska University Hospital, Göteborg, Sweden, in collaboration with AB Haessle, Mölndal.

67. Falk E. Plaque rupture with severe pre-existing stenosis precipitating coronary thrombosis. Characteristics of coronary atherosclerotic plaques underlying fatal occlusive thrombi. Br Heart J 1983;*50*:127.

68. Barger AC, Beeuwkes R, Lainey LL, Silverman KJ. Hypothesis: vasa vasorum and neovascularisation of human coronary arteries: a possible role in the pathology of atherosclerosis. New Engl J Med 1983;*310*:175.

69. Richardson P, Davies M, Born G. Influence of plaque configuration and stress distribution in fissuring of coronary atherosclerotic plaques. Lancet 1989;*2*:941.

70. Henney AM, Wakeley PR, Davies MJ et al. Localization of stromelysin gene expression in atherosclerotic plaques by in situ hybridization. Proc Natl Acad Sci USA 1991;*88*:8154.

71. Promerance A. Peri-arterial mast cells in coronary atheroma and thrombosis. J Path Bact 1958;*76*:55.

72. Schwartz CJ, Mitchell JRA. Cellular infiltration of the human arterial adventitia associated with atheromatous plaque. Circulation 1962;*26*:73.

73. Gown AM, Tsukada T, Ross R. Human atherosclerosis. Immuno-histochemical analysis of cellular composition of human atherosclerotic lesions. Am J Pathol 1986;*125*:191.

74. Manion WC. Inflammations of the arterial wall and vasovasorum: their role in the pathogenesis of atherosclerosis and arterial occlusion. In: James TN, Keys JW (eds) Myocardial Infarction. Little, Brown, Boston, 1963, p.255.

75. Hansson GK, Holm J, Jonasson L. Detection of activated T lymphocytes in the human atherosclerotic plaque. Am J Pathol 1989;*135*:169.

76. Sato T. Increased subendothelial infiltration of the coronary arteries with monocytes/macrophages in patients with unstable angina. Atherosclerosis 1987;*68*:191.

77. Kochi K, Takebayashi S, Hikori T, Nobuyoshi M. Significance of adventitial inflammation of the coronary artery in patients with unstable angina: results at autopsy. Circulation 1985;*71*:709.

78. Wallash E, Weinstein GS, Franzone A, Clavel A, Rossi PA, Kreps E. Inflammation of the coronary arteries in patients with unstable angina. Texas Heart Institute J 1986;*16:*105.

79. Baroldi G, Silver MD, Mariani F, Giuliano G. Correlation of morphological variable in the coronary atherosclerotic plaque with clinical patterns of ischemic heart disease. Am J Cardiovasc Path 1988;*2:*159.

80. Kragel AH, Reddy SG, Wittes JT, Roberts WC. Morphometric analysis of the composition of coronary arterial plaques in isolated unstable angina pectoris with pain at rest. Am J Cardiol 1990;*66:*562.

81. Arbustini E, Grasso M, Diegoli M, Concardi M, Porcu E, Specchia G. Expression of growth factors and oncogene products in human normal and atherosclerotic coronary arteries with and without thrombosis. Pathol Res Pract 1993;*189:*637.

82. Flugelman MY, Virmani R, Correa R et al. Smooth muscle cell abundance and fibroblast growth factors in coronary lesions of patients with nonfatal unstable angina. A clue to the mechanism of transformation from the stable to the unstable clinical state. Circulation 1993;*88:*2493.

83. van der Wal AC, Becker AE, van der Loos CM, Das PK. Site of intimal rupture or erosion of thrombosed coronary atherosclerotic plaques is characterized by an inflammatory process irrespective of the dominant plaque morphology. Circulation 1994;*89:*36.

84. van der Wal AC, Das PK, van de Berg DB, van der Loos CM, Becker AE. Atherosclerotic lesions in humans—*in situ* Immunophenotypic analysis suggesting an immune mediated response. Lab Invest 1989;*61:*166

84a. Moreno PR, Falk E, Palacios IF, Newell JB, Fuster V, Fallon JT. Macrophage infiltration in acute coronary syndromes. Implications for plaque rupture. Circulation 1994;*90:*775.

85. Majno G, Joris I. Endothelium 1977: A review. Adv Exp Med Biol 1978;*104:*169.

86. Harker LA, Schwartz SM, Ross R. Endothelium and arteriosclerosis. Clin Haematol 1981;*10:*283.

87. Mustard JF, Packham MA, Kinlough-Rathbone RL. Mechanisms in thrombosis. In: Bloom AL, Thomas DP (eds.) Haemostasis and Thrombosis. Churchill Livingstone, New York, 1981, p.503.

88. Bhawan J, Joris I, De Girolami V et al. Effect of occlusion on large vessels: I. A study of the rat carotid artery. Am J Pathol 1977;*88:*355.

89. Becker CG, Levi R, Zavecz JH. Induction of IgE antibodies to antigen isolated from tobacco leaves and from cigarette smoke condensate. Am J Pathol 1979;*96:*249.

90. Linnanmäki E, Leinonen M, Mattila K, Nieminen MS, Valtonen V, Saikku P. Chlamydia pneumoniae-specific circulating immune complexes in patients with chronic coronary heart disease. Circulation 1993;*87:*1130.

91. Höiby N, Döring G, Schiötz PO. The role of immune complexes in the pathogenesis of bacterial infections. Annu Rev Microbiol 1986;*40:*29.

92. Tannenbaum SH, Finko R, Cines DB. Antibody and immune complexes induce tissue factor production by human endothelial cells. J Immunol 1986;*137:*1532.

93. Patarroyo M, Makgoba MW. Leucocyte adhesion to cells in immune and inflammatory responses. Lancet 1989;*2:*1139.

94. Araujo LI, Camici P, Spinks TJ, Jones T, Maseri A. Abnormalities in myocardial metabolism in patients with unstable angina as assessed by positron emission tomography. Cardiovasc Drugs Ther 1988;*2:*41.

95. Vejar M, Fragasso G, Hackett D et al. Dissociation of platelet activation and spontaneous myocardial ischemia in unstable angina. Thromb Haemost 1990;*63:*163.

96. Ciabattoni G, Ujang S, Sritara P et al. Aspirin, but not heparin, suppresses the transient increase in thromboxane biosynthesis associated with cardiac catheterisation or coronary angioplasty. J Am Coll Cardiol 1993;*21:*1377.

97. Fitzgerald DJ, Roy L, Catella F, FitzGerald GA. Platelet activation in unstable coronary disease. N Engl J Med 1986;*315:*983.

98. Carry M, Korley V, Willerson JT, Weigelt L, Ford-Hutchinson AW, Tagari P. Increased urinary leukotriene excretion in patients with cardiac ischemia: in vivo evidence for 5-lipoxygenase activation. Circulation 1992;*85:*230.

99. Mehta J, Dinerman J, Mehta P et al. Neutrophil function in ischemic heart disease. Circulation 1989;79:549.

100. Dinerman JL, Mehta JL, Saldeen TGP et al. Increased neutrophil elastase release in unstable angina pectoris and acute myocardial infarction. J Am Coll Cardiol 1990;15:1559.

101. Mazzone A, De Servi S, Ricevuti G et al. Increased expression of neutrophil and monocyte adhesion molecules in unstable coronary artery disease. Circulation 1993;88:358.

102. Neri Serneri GG, Abbate R, Gori AM et al. Transient intermittent lymphocyte activation is responsible for the instability of angina. Circulation 1992;86:790.

103. Jude B, Agraou B, McFadden EP et al. Evidence for time-dependent activation of monocytes in the systemic circulation in unstable angina but not in acute myocardial infarction or in stable angina. Circulation 1994;90:1662.

104. Rab ST, Alexander RW, Ansari AA. Evidence for activated circulating macrophage/monocytes in unstable angina. (Abst) J Am Coll Cardiol 1990;15:168A.

105. Berk BC, Weintraub WS, Alexander RW. Elevation of C-reactive protein in active coronary disease. Am J Cardiol 1990;65:168.

106. Liuzzo G, Biasucci LM, Gallimore JR et al. The prognostic value of C-reactive protein and serum amyloid A protein in severe unstable angina. New Engl J Med 1994;331:417.

107. Hamm CW, Ravkilde J, Gerhardt W et al. The prognostic value of serum troponin T in unstable angina. N Engl J Med 1992;327:146.

108. Libby P, Ordovas JM, Aauger KR, Robbins AH, Birinyi KK, Dinarello CA. Endotoxin and tumor necrosis factor induced interleukin-1 gene expression in adult human vascular endothelial cells. Am J Pathol 1986;124:179.

109. Neri Serneri GG, Gensini GF, Carnovali M et al. Association between time of increased fibrinopeptide A levels in plasma and episodes of spontaneous angina: a controlled prospective study. Am Heart J 1987;113:672.

110. Kruskal JB, Commerford PJ, Franks JJ, Kirsch RE. Fibrin and fibrinogen-related antigens in patients with stable and unstable coronary artery disease. N Engl J Med 1987;317:1361.

111. Entman ML, Ballantyne CM. Inflammation in acute coronary syndromes. Circulation 1993;88:801.

112. Buia LM, Willerson JT. Role of inflammation in coronary plaque disruption. Circulation 1994;89:503.

113. Liuzzo G, Biasucci L, Rebuzzi AG et al. C-reactive protein is increased in unstable angina but not in active variant angina: is inflammation in acute coronary syndromes related to ischemia? (Abst.) Circulation 1994;90:I-664.

114. DeWood M, Spores J, Notske R et al. Prevalence of total coronary occlusion during the early hours of transmural myocardial infarction. New Engl J Med 1980;303:897.

115. Mizuno K, Satomura K, Miyamoto A et al. Angioscopic evaluation of coronary-artery thrombi in acute coronary syndromes. New Engl J Med 1992;327:206.

116. Bertrand M, Lefebvre J, Laisne C, Rousseau M, Carre A, Lekieffre J. Coronary arteriography in acute transmural myocardial infarction. Am Heart J 1979;97:61.

117. Roberts WC, Buja OM. The frequency and significance of coronary arterial thrombi and other observations in fatal acute myocardial infarction. Am J Med 1972;52:425.

118. Davies G, Chierchia S, Maseri A. Prevention of myocardial infarction by very early treatment with intracoronary streptokinase. Some clinical observations. New Engl J Med 1984;311:1488.

119. Maseri A, L'Abbate A, Baroldi G et al. Coronary vasospasm as a possible cause of myocardial infarction. A conclusion derived from the study of "preinfarction" angina. New Engl J Med 1978;299:1271.

120. Wilson RF, Lesser JR, Laxon DD, White CW. Intense microvascular constriction after angioplasty of acute thrombotic coronary arterial lesion. Lancet 1989;1:807.

121. Ambrose JA, Tannenbaum MA, Alexopoulos D et al. Angiographic progression of coronary artery disease and the development of myocardial infarction. J Am Coll Cardiol 1988;12:56.

122. Grignani G, Soffiantino G, Zucchella M et al. Platelet activation by emotional stress in patients with coronary artery disease. Circulation 1991;83 (Suppl. II):128.

123. Oshima S, Ogawa H, Yasue H, Okumura K, Matsuyama K, Miyagi H. Increased plasma fibrinopeptide A levels during attacks induced by hyperventilation in patients with coronary vasospastic angina. J Am Coll Cardiol 1989;*14:*150.

124. Irie T, Imaizumi T, Matuguchi T et al. Increased fibrinopeptide A during anginal attacks in patients with variant angina. J Am Coll Cardiol 1989;*14:*589.

125. Buxton AE, Goldberg S, Hirshfeld JW et al. Refractory ergonovine induced coronary vasospasm: importance of intracoronary nitroglycerin. Am J Cardiol 1980;*46:*329.

126. Buxton AE, Goldberg S, Harken A et al. Coronary artery spasm immediately after myocardial revascularization: recognition and management. New Engl J Med 1981;*304:*1249.

127. Lange R, Reid M, Tzesch D et al. Non atheromatous ischemic heart disease following withdrawal from chronic industrial nitroglycerin exposure. Circulation 1972;*46:*666.

128. Lange RA, Cigarroa RG, Yancy CW et al. Cocaine-induced coronary artery vasoconstriction. N Engl J Med 1989;*321:*1557.

129. Curfman GD. Is exercise beneficial—or hazardous—to your heart? N Engl J Med 1994;*329:*1730.

130. Jenkins CD. Recent evidence supporting psychologic and social risk factors for coronary disease. N Engl J Med 1976;*294:*987 and 1033.

131. Haynes SC, Feinleib M, Kannel WB. The relationship of psychosocial factors to coronary heart disease in the Framingham study: eight-year incidence of coronary heart disease. Am J Epidemiol 1980;*111:*37.

132. Carney RM, Rich MW, Freedland KE et al. Major depressive disorder predicts cardiac events in patients with coronary heart disease. Psychosom Med 1988;*50:*627.

133. Dembrosky TM, MacDougall JM, Costa PT Jr, Grandits GA. Components of hostility as predictors of sudden death and myocardial infarction in the Multiple Risk Factor Intervention Trial. Psychosom Med 1989;*51:*514.

134. Rahe RH, Arajärvi H, Arajärvi S, Punsar S, Karvonen MJ. Recent life changes and coronary heart disease in East versus West Finland. J Psychosom Res 1976;*20:*431.

135. Appels A. Mental precursors of myocardial infarction. Br J Psychiat 1990;*156:*465.

136. Byrne DG, Whyte HM. Life events and myocardial infarction revisited: the role of measures of individual impact. Psychosom Med 1980;*42:*1.

137. Bainton D, Jones GR, Hole D. Influenza and ischaemic heart disease—a possible trigger for acute myocardial infarction? Int J Epidemiol 1978;*7:*231.

138. Kron J, Lucas L, Lee TD, McAnulty J. Myocardial infarction following an acute viral illness. Arch Intern Med 1983;*143:*1466.

139. Spodick DH, Flessas AP, Johnson MM. Association of acute respiratory symptoms with the onset of acute myocardial infarction: prospective investigation of 150 consecutive patients and matched control patients. Am J Cardiol 1984;*53:*481.

140. Spodick DH. Inflammation and the onset of myocardial infarction. Editorials. Ann Int Med 1985;*102:*699.

141. Saikku P, Leinonen M, Mattila K et al. Serological evidence of an association of a novel chlamydia, TWAR, with chronic coronary heart disease and acute myocardial infarction. Lancet 1988;*2:*983.

142. Leinonen M, Linnanmäki E, Mattila K, Nieminen MS, Valtonen V, Saikku P. Circulating immune complexes containing chlamydia lipopolysaccharide in acute myocardial infarction. Microb Pathog 1990;*9:*67.

143. Griffiths PD, Hannington G, Booth JC. Coxsackie B virus infections and myocardial infarction. Lancet 1980;*1:*1387.

144. Appels A, Mulder P. Fatigue and heart disease. The association between vital exhaustion and past, present and future coronary heart disease. J Psychosom Res 1989;*33:*727.

145. Kluger MJ. Psychological stress causes development of fever and release of cytokines. In: Genazzani AR, Nappi G, Petraglia F, Martignoni E (eds) Stress and Related Disorders, From Adaptation to Dysfunction. Parthenon Publishing, Carnforth, 1991, p.415.

146. Bornstein DL. Leukocyte pyrogen: a major mediator of the acute phase reaction. Ann NY Acad Sci 1982;*389:*323.

147. Dinarello CA. Interleukin-1. Rev Infect Dis 1984;6:51.
148. Long NC, Otterness I, Kunkel SL, Vander AJ, Kluger MJ. Roles of interleukin-1β and tumour necrosis factor in lipopolysaccharide-fever in rats. Am J Physiol 1990;259:R724.
149. LeMay LG, Vander AJ, Kluger MJ. The effects of psychological stress on plasma interleukin-6 activity in rats. Physiol Behav 1990;47:957.
150. Aloe L, Alleva E, Böhm A, Levi-Montalcini R. Aggressive behavior induces release of nerve growth factor from mouse salivary gland into the bloodstream. Proc Natl Acad Sci USA 1986;83:6184.
151. Myocardial Infarction Community Registers. Results of a WHO International Collaborative Study coordinated by the Regional Office for Europe. Public Health in Europe 5. WHO, Copenhagen, 1979.
152. Ghecchi-Ruscone T, Piccaluga E, Guzzetti S, Contini M, Montano N, Nicolis E on behalf of GISSI-2 Investigators. Morning and Monday: critical periods for the onset of acute myocardial infarction. The GISSI-2 Study experience. Eur Heart J 1994;15:882.
153. Muller JE, Tofler GH, Stone PH. Circadian variation and triggers of onset of acute cardiovascular disease. Circulation 1989;79:733.
154. Andreotti F, Davies GJ, Hackett DR et al. Major circadian fluctuations in fibrinolytic factors and possible relevance to time of onset of myocardial infarction, sudden cardiac death and stroke. Am J Cardiol 1988;62:635.
155. McFadden ER. Circadian rhythms. Am J Med 1988;85 (Suppl IB):2.
156. The GUSTO Angiographic Investigators. The effects of plasminogen activator, streptokinase, or both on coronary-artery patency, ventricular function, and survival after acute myocardial infarction. N Engl J Med 1993;329:1615.

The variable cardiac response to ischemic stimuli

INTRODUCTION

In healthy animals, when a coronary artery is suddenly occluded, the severity of ischemia in the area of the myocardium at risk, the extent of necrosis, and the development of arrhythmias are all influenced, rather predictably, by the level of myocardial oxygen consumption and by the duration of the occlusion. In contrast, in patients who died of acute myocardial infarction (MI), the extent of necrosis in the area at risk can vary from 50 to 90%:[1] even larger differences between area at risk and infarcted area may be observed in those who survived an infarction. Fatal arrhythmias may develop some minutes after the onset of potentially reversible episodes of ischemia or very early after the onset of a small infarction, yet they never develop in many patients with extensive infarction.

The urge to define and treat the average response to coronary obstructions, myocardial ischemia, and acute MI has, so far, limited the amount of interest shown in the variable individual responses to ischemic stimuli and ischemic insults and in the causes of the variability. Yet this variability, rather than occurring at random, may reflect individual differences that may benefit from specific therapeutic and preventive strategies. Two major sources of this variable individual response to ischemic stimuli and insults are presented in this chapter as examples of the magnitude of the problem and of the need for further research: first, the relationship between epicardial coronary artery obstructions, residual coronary flow reserve, and ischemia or infarction may be profoundly influenced by a variable development and function of collateral vessels; second, the myocardial response to a similar ischemic insult can be dramatically influenced by the development of fatal arrhythmias, which may not occur merely randomly, and by the mortality rate from infarction, which varies considerably with gender, and particularly with age, independent of the size of the infarct.

10.1 VARIABLE INDIVIDUAL COLLATERAL RESPONSE TO ISCHEMIC STIMULI

The assessment of the presence of collateral vessels in man is based on postmortem and angiographic studies, neither of which, unfortunately, can provide any information about the degree of compensation provided during ischemic events, as collateral protection depends on whether such vessels developed before or after infarction, and on their function during ischemia.

The protective role of coronary collaterals has been questioned in the past because they were found more frequently in patients with MI than in those without:[2] the greater frequency of persistent coronary occlusion or the presence of very severe stenoses in patients with infarction who are not receiving thrombolytic therapy, together with the subsequent development of collaterals, are likely explanations of this apparent paradox. A protective role, similar to that clearly demonstrated in experimental animals by gradual coronary occlusion (see Ch. 6), was subsequently shown in patients.[3-7] Sudden occlusion of a mild stenosis, in the absence of collaterals, has been proposed to explain the higher frequency of sudden ischemic cardiac death (SICD) than of acute MI in previously totally asymptomatic patients, compared with those with chronic stable angina.[8] However, the protective effect of collaterals depends not only on their anatomic development, but also on their function as related to changes in coronary vasomotor tone, and, as proposed by some, on coronary blood flow "steal."

10.1.1 Variable collateral blood flow reserve

A marked variability in the number and size of angiographically visible collaterals, for a comparable severity of coronary artery obstruction, is a common clinical observation. At one extreme, in some patients with no signs of MI, complete proximal occlusion of a major branch can be compensated for by angiographically visible collaterals to such an extent that maximal predicted heart rate can be attained during effort testing, with no detectable signs of ischemia.[9] Postmortem studies have shown the frequent presence of coronary occlusion with no signs of infarction.[10,11] Even occlusion of the left main coronary artery may be associated with a well-preserved left ventricular function, when epicardial and septal collateral vessels from a dominant right coronary artery perfuse the territories normally supplied by the left anterior descending (LAD) and circumflex arteries.[12] At post-mortem examination patients who had suffered from chronic stable angina were frequently found to have complete coronary occlusion in the absence of any signs of MI;[13] this was also confirmed by angiographic studies.[14] In such patients, the amount of compensation provided by collaterals supplying the occluded artery branch was obviously sufficient to prevent the development of myocardial necrosis and, as recanalized thrombi can also be found at the site of pre-existing mild stenoses (see Ch. 8), compensatory collateral blood flow must have been adequate to prevent infarction, even in the absence of flow-limiting stenoses (as the process of thrombi recanalization by multiple vessels takes several weeks). At the other extreme, occlusion at the site of a very severe flow-limiting stenosis may cause infarction to develop in some patients, and, in others with chronic stable angina, collateral function does not seem to increase progressively as exercise tolerance can remain low for months, with persistent angina, ischemic ST-segment depression and positive myocardial scintigraphy on mild effort.

As discussed in Chapter 6, differences in the number and size of preexisting interarterial anastomoses would seem to be the most plausible explanation for the variable degree of collateral development observed in cross-species studies. However, in patients, the degree of collateral development in response to the development of coronary stenoses or occlusion has not been studied specifically and the causes of the variable amount of compensation provided by collateral development are still speculative. At the time of writing, no information is available about:

a. the frequency of coronary occlusion with no signs of infarction because of very good collateral compensation
b. the mechanisms responsible for the development of infarction in the presence of preexisting severe flow-limiting stenoses
c. the causes of variable collateral development and compensatory function.

The protective role of collateral vessels has been investigated by coronary angiography in patients with chronic stable, unstable, and variant angina, MI, and during acute coronary artery occlusion in patients undergoing percutaneous transluminal coronary angioplasty (PTCA). However, first, angiography at best can define only those vessels greater than 0.3 mm in diameter and second, collaterals become visible only when a sufficient pressure gradient develops to ensure the flow of contrast dye through them (either chronically, because of fixed critical stenoses, or transiently, because of balloon PTCA[15,16] or epicardial coronary artery spasm).[17] In general, patients with coronary occlusion and a good coronary flow reserve have larger and a greater number of visible collaterals and quicker and more intense collateral filling of the occluded vessel than those with low coronary flow reserve.

In patients with chronic stable angina, single-vessel disease, no previous transmural MI, and normal left ventricular function, collateral filling on average is correlated with both the severity of the coronary stenosis and the duration of angina,[16,18] but the individual variability is quite large.

In patients with variant angina, the presence of collaterals is more frequently associated with ST-segment depression than with ST-segment elevation.[19–21] The possible protective role of collaterals during epicardial coronary artery spasm was demonstrated conclusively following ergonovine-induced coronary artery spasm, by a transient visualization of collateral vessels from nonspastic arteries associated with ST-segment depression.[17] Collaterals can also provide protection from ischemia during subocclusive spasm in the absence of organic stenoses (see Fig. 10.1) These findings indicate that during severe coronary artery spasm, flow may become established through preexisting collateral vessels and may prevent transmural myocardial ischemia.

In patients with MI and coronary artery occlusion, well-developed collaterals are associated with a lower incidence of Q waves on the ECG, with dyskinesia at ventriculography and with a better prognosis. In one study, survival rates after 10 years were 51.5% in patients with good collaterals and 34.5% in those with poorly developed collaterals.[6] Hearts with subendocardial infarction have a greater degree of residual flow in the collateral-dependent area than those with transmural infarcts.[22] Collaterals may provide protection from the formation of left ventricular aneurysm.[23,24] In patients in whom thrombolytic therapy failed to induce reperfusion within 90 min of its administration, the presence of angiographically visible coronary collaterals was associated with significantly smaller infarcts than those in patients without collaterals.[7] Significant improvement in regional and global ventricular function was observed in patients with good collaterals and successful reperfusion.[23–25] In addition, other studies have demonstrated a tendency toward improved left ventricular function in patients with well-developed collaterals and no reperfusion.[26,27] It is likely that collateral blood flow maintains myocardial viability in the infarct-related arterial bed, at least in subepicardial layers, for a prolonged period after an acute MI.

More severe preexisting stenoses (80%) were found in patients who developed non-Q-wave infarctions than in those who developed Q-wave infarctions.[28] This difference could be related

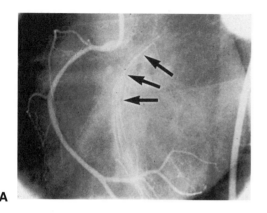
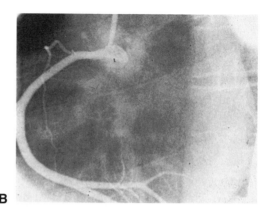

A   B

Fig. 10.1 Appearance of collaterals in the absence of organic stenosis. In a 40-year-old Korean patient with subocclusive spasm of the proximal left anterior descending coronary artery (LAD), injection of dye into the right coronary artery (RC) visualizes the LAD (**A**) in the absence of detectable evidence of ischemia. Collaterals are no longer visible after the proximal LAD spasm was relieved by nitroglycerin (**B**). Thus, in this patient, collaterals were well developed in the absence of organic stenoses; they became functional when a pressure gradient developed between RC and LAD, but were not visualized when it disappeared.

to the presence of preexisting collaterals distal to more severe stenoses, but may also be related to the stronger, possibly more diffuse, thrombogenic stimuli that are required to cause occlusion in the absence of severe stenoses.

In patients undergoing PTCA, coronary artery occlusion by balloon inflation provides a clinical model for the assessment of collateral vessels and their protective role. During balloon inflation, compared with patients without visible collaterals, those with good collaterals show a lesser degree of ECG ST-segment shift, ventricular hypocontractility, reduction in ejection fraction (EF) and less frequent angina.[15,17,29]

In patients, an objective assessment of the degree of compensation provided by collaterals can be provided by the value of intracoronary pressure in the collateralized territory distal to the occlusion, i.e. by the peripheral coronary pressure (PCP). Measurements of PCP obtained by closing the aortocoronary bypass graft after extracorporeal circulation was withdrawn, indicate an average pressure, distal to an acutely occluded mild stenosis, of only 20% of aortic pressure, but of 40 ± 10% of aortic pressure, distal to chronic occlusion. In contrast, PCP was 76 ± 12% of aortic pressure distal to a 70% diameter stenosis and 90 ± 7% distal to a 50% stenosis (see Fig. 10.2).[30] In another study, the protective role of collaterals in chronic coronary artery occlusion (assessed during bypass surgery by measuring PCP in the transiently occluded vein graft) also showed an average value of 40% of aortic pressure, but with a very large scatter from 12 to 80%. In some of these patients (probably those with a high coronary vasomotor tone), collateral blood flow was increased by intra-aortic nitroglycerin when aortic pressure was maintained constant (see Fig. 10.3).[31] These values of postocclusion PCP indicate that the degree of collateral compensation is quite variable, may be influenced by vasomotor changes, and is only partly related to the presence of visible collaterals and to the duration of angina.

■ *The available observations suggest that, when well developed and functional, the collateral circulation can rapidly protect the myocardium at risk of ischemia from the very onset of coronary*

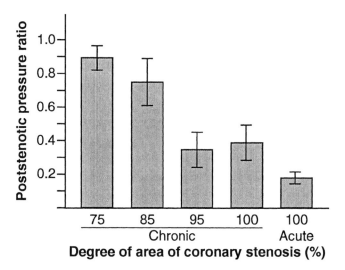

Fig. 10.2 Coronary poststenotic pressure at the time of bypass surgery.
Transient closure of the vein graft allowed the measurement of poststenotic coronary pressure at the end of bypass surgery. Poststenotic pressure distal to area stenoses of 75% (about 50% diameter reduction) was, on average, 90% of aortic pressure, whereas distal to total chronic obstruction, but in the presence of collaterals, it was about 40% of aortic pressure (chronic). Intermediate reduction of aortic pressure was found distal to 85 and 95% area stenoses. When arteries with mild stenoses were occluded transiently (acute) in the absence of visible collaterals, the poststenotic pressure was only 20% of aortic pressure. The difference between pressure distal to a chronic occlusion, as opposed to an acute occlusion, is due to the development of collaterals in the presence of chronic occlusions. Peripheral coronary pressure is a partial index of stenosis severity and of collateral flow compensation as it is influenced markedly by CBF (see Ch. 6). (From data in ref. 30.)

occlusion, but the individual determinants of collateral development and function are still not known. ■

10.1.2 Collateral blood flow "steal"

The phenomenon of subclavian blood flow "steal" from the brain has been deduced from clinical observations. During intense dynamic exercise of the arm, transient deficits in cerebral function were noted in patients with total occlusion of the subclavian artery perfused by collaterals originating from the carotid and vertebral arteries. These deficits were attributed to a critical fall in pressure in the cerebral territory as blood was diverted to the arm.

In analogy to this phenomenon, in the late 1960s Fam and McGregor introduced the concept of collateral blood flow steal for the coronary circulation.[32] They assumed that when arteriolar vessels distal to a critical coronary stenosis were maximally dilated, flow through them was strictly dependent on the perfusion pressure generated by collateral flow. Under these conditions, pharmacologically or metabolically induced coronary dilation could not affect the collateralized vascular bed because it was already maximally dilated, but could cause a decrease in pressure at the origin of collaterals if the upstream resistance in the parent coronary artery was significant.

In patients with coronary occlusion and a good effort tolerance, the arteriolar vessels in the collateralized vascular bed are not maximally dilated at rest and perfusion pressure may not be very low (see Fig. 10.3). Thus, during generalized coronary vasodilation induced by increased myocardial oxygen consumption or by drugs, arteriolar pressure also drops in the collateralized territory. Such a drop in pressure may cause transmural blood flow steal to occur before driving pressure through collaterals is reduced. Blood flow steal from the collateralized territory can, therefore, occur only when collaterals originate distal to a critical coronary artery stenosis and when pressure at their origin decreases during high flow more than pressure at their termination in the collateralized territory. Blood flow steal from collateralized territories can be defined ("lateral steal") in order to separate it from blood flow steal from subepicardial vessels by excessive dilation of subendocardial vessels ("transmural steal").

In a recent study using positron emission tomography (PET), regional myocardial perfusion was measured using ^{15}O-labeled water at rest and during the dipyridamole test, in six patients with single occlusion and angiographically visible collaterals.[33] All patients had a history of chronic stable angina lasting for at least 6 months, none had evidence of previous MI, and all had normal left ventricular function. The exercise stress test was positive in five patients, but in one patient with complete occlusion of a proximal right coronary artery it was negative at maximal predicted heart rate. The dipyridamole test caused myocardial ischemia in all, as evidenced by an increased uptake of ^{18}F-labeled 2-deoxyglucose in the collateralized myocardium immediately after the test. Myocardial ischemia induced by dipyridamole was associated with a smaller increase in average blood flow to the collateralized myocardium than to those

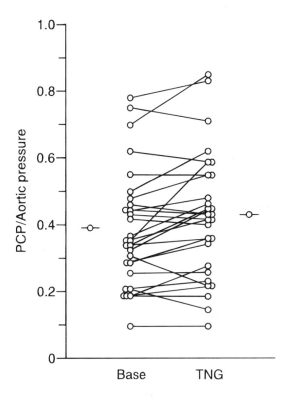

Fig. 10.3 Variability of coronary pressure distal to a total chronic coronary occlusion. In this study the mean peripheral coronary pressure (PCP)/aortic pressure ratio is 40% distal to a total chronic occlusion (similar to that described in Fig. 10.2), but the range varies from 12 to 80% as a result of very variable development and function of collaterals and of CBF. Systemic nitroglycerin (TNG) increases the ratio appreciably in only a few patients. (Modified from ref. 31.)

territories supplied by angiographically normal arteries (see Fig. 10.4), but average flow to the cardiac wall perfused by collaterals did not decrease compared with resting levels, and actually increased in all cases.

Dipyridamole, therefore, caused myocardial ischemia in the collateralized territory, but not through an actual decrease of collateral blood flow occurring as a consequence of lateral steal: the dipyridamole-induced arteriolar dilation actually increased the driving pressure and flow across the collaterals, but the increased collateral flow was insufficient to prevent a drop in perfusion pressure in the collateralized vascular bed. In the absence of detectable lateral steal, myocardial ischemia in the collateralized cardiac wall, which was detected by ^{18}F-labeled-deoxyglucose uptake (and also by ECG changes and angina in three patients and by angina alone in the other three), must have been caused by transmural blood flow steal. As arteriolar vessels in the subepicardial regions became dilated by the drug, the poststenotic perfusion pressure decreased too much to perfuse subendocardial regions adequately, which then became ischemic. Increased flow through subepicardial layers therefore, caused transmural blood flow steal with subendocardial ischemia.

■ *Thus, vasodilator drugs do not cause lateral blood flow steal through well-developed collaterals, at least in patients with single-vessel disease, but only transmural blood flow steal.* ■

10.1.3 Transient impairment of collateral blood flow

The hemodynamic determinants of coronary collateral blood flow (i.e. driving pressure through collaterals and collateral vessel resistance) can be influenced by transient changes in vasomotor tone.

In patients with chronic stable, predominantly effort-related angina, a possible modulation of collateral blood flow by vasomotor tone is suggested by clinical and pharmacologic studies. The pathologic mechanisms responsible for such modulation may not necessarily be the same in previously healthy animals subjected to gradual coronary occlusion.

Clinical observations

The clinical observation of marked variability in the anginal threshold of patients with a single coronary artery occlusion, coronary collaterals, no previous infarction, and no other coronary stenoses, prompted a study that explored the possible role of transient functional impairment of collateral blood flow. The patients studied had no anatomic substratum for dynamic modulation of coronary stenoses; hence, residual coronary flow reserve could be modulated only by constriction of vessels providing or receiving collateral flow. This possible mechanism of ischemia is indicated by three lines of evidence obtained from a group of patients with this model of human disease:[9]

1. Exercise stress testing, repeated in the presence of coronary constrictor or dilator drugs, proved that a marked variability in the ischemic threshold could be induced pharmacologically (see Fig. 10.5A).
2. Ambulatory monitoring during ordinary daily life proved that most ischemic episodes occurred at heart rates much lower than those attained during exercise at the onset of ischemic changes on the ECG. In addition, some ischemic episodes occurred at heart rates 20 or more beats per minute lower than episodes of prolonged tachycardia that were not associated with signs of ischemia (see Fig. 10.5B).

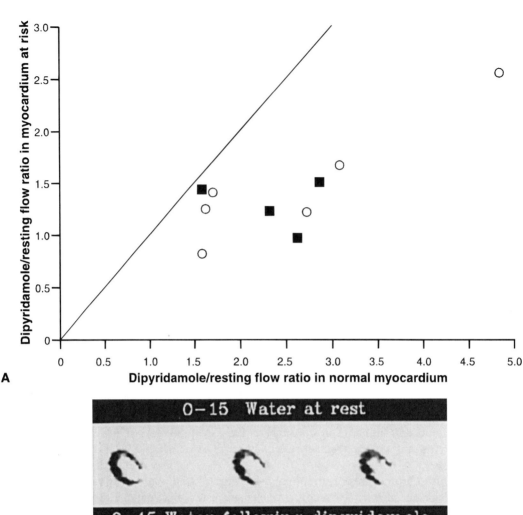

A

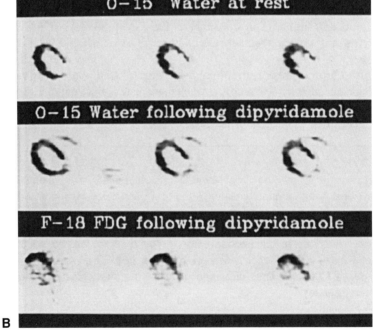

B

Fig. 10.4 Transmural blood flow steal caused by dipyridamole assessed by PET. In patients with single-vessel disease but no previous infarction, the dipyridamole test caused a consistently smaller increase of flow in poststenotic areas than in control areas perfused by nonstenotic arteries (○, with visible collaterals; ■, without visible collaterals). In none of the patients did an important decrease of flow to the collateralized myocardium develop, ruling out the occurrence of dipyridamole-induced lateral steal (**A**). All patients developed regional glucose uptake in the collateralized myocardium after the test, indicative of myocardial ischemia due to transmural blood flow steal (**B**). Ischemia had, most likely, a subendocardial distribution, although this cannot be proved because of the limited spatial resolution of the PET technique. (Modified from ref. 33.)

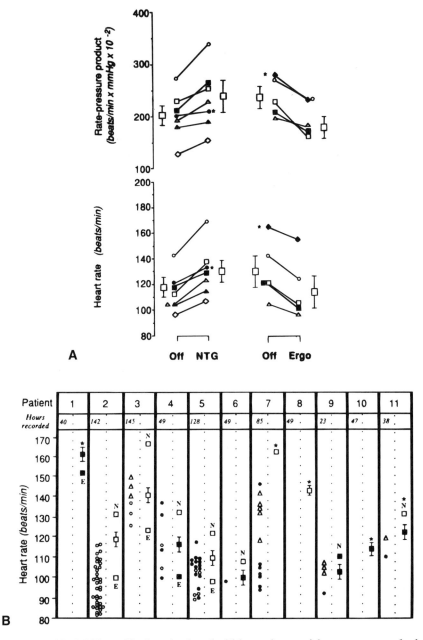

Fig. 10.5 Variability of ischemic threshold in patients with coronary occlusion, no previous infarction, and no substrate for dynamic coronary stenosis. During standardized exercise stress testing the ischemic threshold increased following nitroglycerin (NTG) and decreased following ergonovine (Ergo) (**A**). The variability in the ischemic threshold during Holter monitoring, as assessed by heart rate at the onset of ST-segment depression, was large. In some patients, the heart rate at which many episodes occur during daily life (circles) was 20 beats or more lower than that attained at the onset of ischemia during exercise testing (squares) performed after nitrates (N) or ergonovine (E). Triangles indicate episodes of tachycardia not associated with ST-segment depression during Holter monitoring (**B**). This large variability in the ischemic threshold indicates that residual coronary flow reserve may be modulated to a considerable extent by distal coronary vessel constriction influencing collateral perfusion. (Modified from ref. 9.)

3. Administration of ergonovine during angiography caused marked reduction in collateral filling, with no evidence of epicardial coronary artery spasm, suggesting that collateral blood flow can be impaired by constrictor stimuli that do not cause substantial constriction of large epicardial coronary arteries.

Pharmacologic studies

Intracoronary infusion of serotonin (5-HT) in patients with chronic stable angina caused myocardial ischemia with diffuse constriction of angiographically visible distal vessels and a marked decrease in collateral vessel filling (see 9.2.1). In patients with atypical chest pain, doses of the drug 10 times higher had systemic effects, but failed to cause signs of ischemia. Thus, in patients with a chronic form of ischemic heart disease, 5-HT (at doses in the range that can be produced in the coronary arteries by platelet aggregation) can also impair collateral blood flow, in the absence of appreciable constriction of proximal coronary artery stenoses.[34]

The results of the clinical studies reported above do not allow any conclusions to be drawn as to whether the vasoconstriction occurred selectively in collateral vessels or at proximal and distal sites, because a transient reduction in collateral blood flow can be caused by a reduction in the driving pressure between the origin and the termination of collaterals, by increased resistance across the collaterals themselves, due to selective vasoconstriction, or by a combination of both. In turn, a reduction in collateral driving pressure can be caused by a drop in pressure at the origin of collaterals, due to significant resistance of upstream vessels, by an increase in pressure at the termination of collaterals due to a significant increase in coronary vascular or extravascular resistance in the collateralized territory, or by a combination of both.

Defective endothelial production of either nitric oxide or endothelial-derived hyperpolarizing factor, and hyperreactivity of smooth muscle to constrictor and abnormal neural stimuli, can be responsible for a transient impairment of blood flow at the site of pre- or post-collateral vessels or in the collaterals themselves.

The alterations causing ischemia by transient impairment of collateral blood flow are not necessarily the same in all patients, and may not exist or be the same in experimental animals.

10.2 VARIABLE MYOCARDIAL RESPONSE TO ISCHEMIC INSULTS

The variability in the myocardial response to transient ischemia and necrosis may be due to specific differences in the way that individuals respond. In different groups of patients, the detection of systematic differences in the arrhythmic response to ischemia and infarction and in the mortality rate from infarction could provide valuable indications for individually targeted therapy.

10.2.1 Arrhythmic response to transient myocardial ischemia and MI

Acute myocardial ischemia often causes a broad range of ventricular arrhythmias, but the relationship between ventricular extrasystoles and fatal ventricular tachyarrhythmias (i.e. ventricular tachycardia [VT] and ventricular fibrillation [VF]) in patients is not sufficiently well defined. Arrhythmias should not be grouped indiscriminately together, as some patients may continue to exhibit ventricular extrasystoles for months or years, whereas others without ventricular arrhythmias may develop VF. A reduction in the number of less severe arrhythmias, but an increase in mortality, may be produced by some antiarrhythmic drugs.[35]

In order to cause potentially fatal arrhythmias, ischemia must be severe and, usually, transmural. Fatal ventricular arrhythmias are exceptional in patients with chronic stable angina; they are rare also in patients with unstable angina, but can be observed recurrently in some patients with variant angina, while being notably absent in others. Sustained ventricular tachyarrhythmias are the most frequent cause of SICD in acute MI.

Potentially fatal arrhythmias in transient subendocardial ischemia

In patients who have a normal resting ECG, VT and VF occurring during exercise stress testing are observed exclusively in those cases in which the test is continued in spite of severe ST-segment depression, because the patient does not complain of anginal pain.[36] They are also exceptional during Holter monitoring.[37,38] VF or sustained VT are also infrequent in patients admitted to coronary care units (CCUs) with unstable angina de novo. This suggests that embolization of small coronary vessels by fragments of platelet thrombi, which was shown to be common in unstable patients, is unlikely in itself to be sufficiently arrhythmogenic. Ventricular extrasystoles and runs of unsustained tachycardia can occasionally be observed during transient ST-segment depression in stable and unstable patients, but it is not clear when they are harbingers of VT and VF.

Ischemia-associated arrhythmias are more common in the presence of postinfarction scarring and left ventricular hypertrophy, which indicates an important contributory role of a predisposing anatomic background in ischemia-induced fatal arrhythmias.

SICD is more common during the first few days or weeks after the appearance of unstable angina, but the frequency with which the fatal event occurs as a complication of potentially reversible ischemic episodes, hyperacute infarction, and arrhythmias, not caused by acute ischemia, is not known: a similar question mark lies over the few patients with chronic stable angina who die suddenly.

Fatal arrhythmias in transient transmural myocardial ischemia

Transient transmural myocardial ischemia caused by occlusive coronary artery spasm in patients with variant angina represents a useful human model of ischemia-induced arrhythmogenesis. Ischemia-induced arrhythmias occur in about one-third of patients with variant angina but are consistently absent in the others, in spite of similarities between the number of episodes and the severity and duration of spasm. This is a further indication that the development of ischemia-induced arrhythmias may not merely be a random event, as some patients seem to be persistently more susceptible, and others seem to be consistently protected. In addition, in susceptible patients, arrhythmias occur during a minority of episodes and not necessarily the longest or the most severe. They are equally frequent during the intensification of ST-segment elevation and in the 5 min after the episode has subsided, and occur in both painful and painless episodes. Thus, in this human model, reperfusion arrhythmias are much less common than in animals.

During in-hospital and long-term follow-up studies in a group of 187 consecutive patients with documented variant angina, 32 presented on one or more occasions with episodes of ventricular tachycardia, VF, or severe arrhythmias (group 1) during hospitalization; the remaining 155 patients (group 2) did not.[39] Mean age was not statistically different (53 and 52 years, respectively). The history of old MI was similar (37% and 34%, respectively) and coronary arteriographic findings were not statistically different (for 0-, single-, double- and triple-vessel disease the percentages were 17, 43, 13, and 27, respectively, in group 1, and 9, 33, 34, and 24, respectively, in group 2). ST-segment elevation was predominantly anterior in 60% and inferior in 40% in group 1 and predominantly anterior in 70% and inferior in 30% in group 2.

Group 1. In the past, five patients had reported syncope (preceded by angina in three), and in eight VT, VF, and complete atrioventricular block had been documented in other hospitals. Patients were each monitored for an average period of 28 days (range 7–196 days per patient). A total of 2490 transient episodes of acute myocardial ischemia (documented by typical transient ECG changes) were observed (from 1 to 376 episodes per patient).

During transient ischemic episodes, single ectopic beats and bigeminy were quite frequent and 92 episodes (3.7% of the total) were accompanied by severe rhythm disturbances—66 by VT (22 during asymptomatic episodes), nine by VF, eight by complete atrioventricular block (two followed by cardiac arrest), six by sinus block with severe bradycardia and three by fatal arrhythmias (see below).

In 17 patients there was more than one arrhythmic episode and six had more than one type of arrhythmia. In the 46 episodes in which recording of the entire episode was obtained, severe bradyarrhythmias always occurred during the episode, whereas VT occurred during the episode in 15 and at the moment of its resolution (reperfusion phase) in 21.

Most arrhythmic episodes, including VF, resolved spontaneously (see Fig. 10.6). Three of the 92 episodes of arrhythmias were fatal: one patient had unexpected syncope while in the lavatory during a quiescent phase of his disease (terminal irreversible VF was documented); the other two patients developed cardiac standstill that was followed by complete atrioventricular block and electromechanical dissociation. One additional patient died of pump failure after acute MI. All four patients had triple-vessel disease, confirming the importance of the predisposing abnormal anatomic background.

During follow-up, two of the 28 surviving patients died during the first year: one died suddenly 8 months after a successful bypass operation for an isolated LAD lesion and the other died during an episode of chest pain. A third patient died in the third year of follow-up study soon after the onset of chest pain (he had only minimal irregularities in his coronary arteries

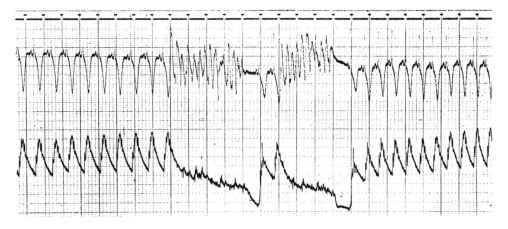

Fig. 10.6 Ventricular fibrillation may be spontaneously reversible. In a patient with a normal coronary angiogram, variant angina, and a history of fainting episodes and documented VT and VF, two episodes of VF, occurring at the end of a painless episode caused by right coronary artery spasm, revert spontaneously to sinus rhythm. These episodes were characterized by the transition from ST-segment elevation to the transient appearance of deep negative T waves. The mechanisms of spontaneous termination of VF are unknown.

and documented spasm of the right coronary artery). No patients died in the second and fourth years of follow-up study.

Group 2. In the past, only six patients had reported syncope, and three episodes of VT or VF had been documented in other hospitals. Patients were each monitored for average periods of 14 days (range 1–80 days per patient). A total of 5109 episodes of acute transient myocardial ischemia were observed (from 1 to 290 episodes per patient). Three patients died after acute MI. During follow-up, two of the 152 surviving patients died of noncardiac causes (neoplasm, hepatitis); two others died in the first year (one suddenly and the other after acute MI); three died during the second year (two during prolonged episodes of chest pain and one during an attack of acute pulmonary edema); two died during the third year (during prolonged episodes of chest pain) and one died during the fifth year (suddenly). Five of the eight patients had a history of MI; coronary arteriography had been performed in five of them, showing single-vessel disease in one patient and double- or triple-vessel disease in the other four.

In patients with variant angina, therefore, fatal arrhythmias tend to recur in the same patients and to be absent in others; thus, they may not occur at random. The reasons why VT and VF occur during only a minority of ischemic episodes, and why they are often self-terminating and tend to recur only in some patients, are not known and should be investigated.

Potentially fatal arrhythmias in acute MI

Fatal arrhythmias are common in acute MI, and SICD is a frequent occurrence in post-MI patients. In acute MI about 50% of patients who die, do so in the first 2 h (usually before admission), most because of VF (see Fig. 10.7).[40] Ventricular fibrillation occurs irrespective of the size of infarction and seems to be more common in patients with increased adrenergic stimulation. A minority of patients die as a result of primary asystole, usually those with a history of severe impairment of cardiac contractility. It is not precisely known why some patients with small infarctions develop fatal arrhythmias whereas others with large infarctions do not.

Monitoring of patients in the early phases of infarction during thrombolysis has proved that reperfusion arrhythmias induced by thrombolysis are quite rare in humans compared with experimental animals. Most arrhythmias occur during persistent elevation of the ST segment rather than immediately after its return to baseline following reperfusion (see Fig. 10.8).[41] Thus, as in transient transmural ischemia, and also during acute infarction and reperfusion, ventricular arrhythmias occur much less frequently than in animal models. After patients have been admitted to a CCU, secondary VF occurs more frequently in patients with the most extensive infarctions and with low levels of serum potassium. Its influence on prognosis is much greater than that of primary VF, which does not seem to have adverse long-term prognostic effects.[42,43]

SICD in post-MI patients. In post-MI patients, SICD is the most common form of death. In one study it represented 72% of cases (29% instantaneous).[44] This high percentage is in sharp contrast with the low frequency of this presenting event in patients with positive exercise tests.[8,45] In about two-thirds of cases of SICD, this was preceded by chest pain, suggesting an ischemic trigger of the fatal arrhythmia; however, with the exception of premature ventricular complexes, no obvious predictor could be identified.

Possible predisposing factors. Secondary VT and VF, occurring after the first 24 h, tend to recur also after discharge, suggesting an important role of the anatomic background

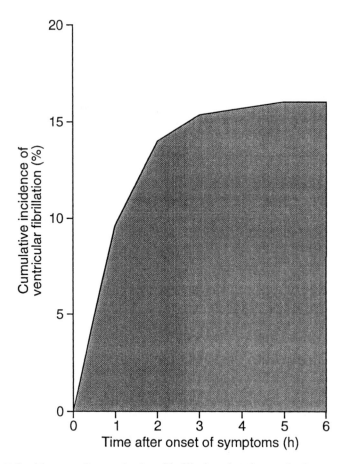

Fig. 10.7 Incidence of ventricular fibrillation in the early hours after the onset of symptoms in acute MI. Two-thirds of patients who develop VF in the first 6 h, do so during the first hour. (Modified from ref. 40.)

favoring reentry circuits and of neurohumoral imbalance, and patients who suffered a cardiac arrest at the onset of a first MI often do so again at the onset of a second. Reentry circuits are likely to have a major role in those patients with previous infarction who continue to develop recurrent arrhythmias. In these patients, SICD may be caused by primary arrhythmias unrelated to acute ischemia (see Ch. 24).

As has been suggested by animal experiments, autonomic nervous imbalance may have an important modulatory role in the genesis of ventricular arrhythmias and/or in their spontaneous reversibility or fatal outcome. A reduced variability of the heart rate[46] represents a useful marker of an autonomic nervous imbalance and has been found to be associated with increased mortality after acute MI.[47,48] The presence of late potentials on the resting ECG tracing[49] represents a marker of an arrhythmogenic background that can favor the development of VT and VF. The short- versus the long-term predictiveness of these parameters, alone and in combination, in different types of patient (anterior versus inferior infarctions, large versus small infarctions, young versus old age) remains to be established.

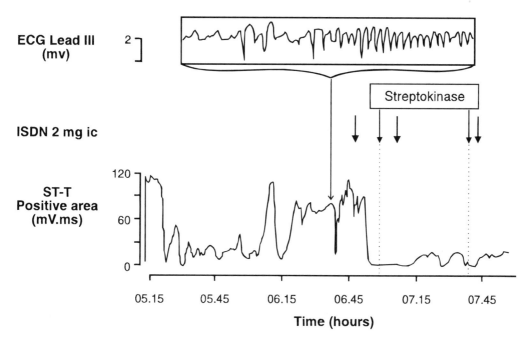

Fig. 10.8 Development of ventricular tachycardia during the first few hours of acute MI. The Holter recording reveals an intermittent return to baseline of ST-segment elevation. VT develops during ST-segment elevation, rather than during one of the multiple episodes of spontaneous reperfusion, indicated by the return to baseline of the ST segment. This was the most common finding in the study. Thus, the relevance of some animal models of reperfusion-induced arrhythmias to human disease may be limited. (Modified from ref. 41.)

■ *In patients with previous infarction, SICD may develop as a result of VT or VF occurring in the absence of an ischemic episode, or may be triggered by a new episode of ischemia or necrosis. The role of random coincidence and of specific predisposing factors for ischemia-induced and nonischemia-related VT and VF has not yet been investigated sufficiently.* ■

10.2.2 Age- and gender-related cardiac response to acute MI

Little is known about the factors that influence the coronary and myocardial response to persistent ischemia, but the variable activation of the endothelium and of cytokine and free-radical generation can contribute to determine the fraction of the area at risk that becomes infarcted and to the development of VT and VF. The coronary and myocardial response to ischemia may be influenced also by the actual causes of ischemia.

The most obvious sources of variability in the cardiac response to persistent ischemia are represented by age and gender. The findings of large multicenter trials on thrombolysis in acute MI show a considerably higher rate of in-hospital mortality in patients over the age of 70. This increased vulnerability to myocardial necrosis with age may not be due to accumulated IHD, as the increased rate of mortality is not related to previous infarction or to a

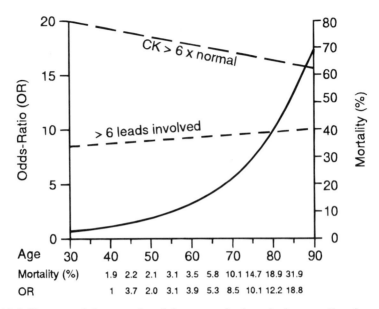

Fig. 10.9 Exponential age-related increase in hospital mortality for acute MI. In patients with their first MI, hospital mortality increased exponentially with age, which was considered as a continuous variable, assuming 40 years as the reference point. The indicators of MI size showed no significant rise with increasing age, as indicated by the percentage of patients with the involvement of more than six ECG leads at entry and with peak CK ratio over six times the upper normal value. The odds-ratio (OR) of death during the hospital phase by age is reported at the bottom. The increase in infarct-related mortality becomes progressively steeper past the age of 65, which can, therefore, be considered a cutoff point in prognostic assessment. The independent predictive value of age was also highly significant in multivariate analysis. The mechanisms of the increasing vulnerability to MI with age, unrelated to detectable differences in the severity of coronary atherosclerosis and to previous ischemic myocardial damage, are not precisely known. (Modified from ref. 50.)

previous history of angina. The incidence of in-hospital mortality was found to increase exponentially with age among 9720 patients with a first infarction, enrolled in the Gruppo Italiano per lo Studio della Sopravvivenza nell'Infarto Miocardico 2 (GISSI-2) study (see Fig. 10.9).[50] Patients with their first MI represented 78.5% of the total number of randomized patients. The age-related increase occurred in both men and women, being higher in women in any age group (see Fig. 10.10). The mortality rate was about 18-fold greater in patients above the age of 80 (31.8%) than in those younger than 40 years (1.9%). Postdischarge (6 months) mortality was about 15-fold higher in patients over the age of 80 (11.3%) than in those younger than 40 years (0.8%): therefore, older patients (i.e. over 80 years of age) with an acute MI who reach hospital have a 30-fold greater incidence of mortality within 6 months than do those younger than 40 years.

The causes of this very large progressive increase in mortality with age, and of the higher rate of mortality in hospital in women, are not precisely known. The incidence of angina was

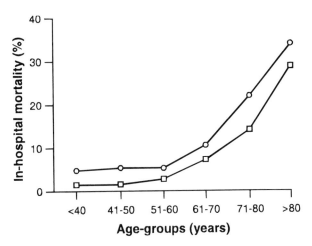

Fig. 10.10 Gender-related increase with age in hospital mortality for acute infarction. The mortality curve for women (○) is parallel to that for men (□), which implies that mortality is about threefold greater than that of men up to the age of 50 and only slightly higher at the age of 80. In studies of mortality from acute MI, therefore, men and women should be grouped separately. The causes of the higher rate of hospital mortality from acute MI in women are not precisely known. (Obtained from data presented in the study in ref. 50.)

low (35%) and was similar in all age groups. Thus, in 65% of patients, MI apparently occurred unheralded as the very first clinically detected manifestation of IHD. Patients with their first unheralded MI may have less severe and less extensive coronary atherosclerosis than patients with chronic stable angina.[13] The size of infarction, as estimated from peak CK and QRS alterations, was similar in all age groups and, if anything, it decreased slightly with age. Available data indicate that, in older patients, in-hospital death was due predominantly to cardiac rupture, but the percentage of patients who had more than two arteries with critical stenoses did not increase with age (see Table 10.1). At predischarge evaluation, patients aged over 70 years also had lower EFs than patients younger than 60 years (47 versus 51%), but age remained the strongest predictor of mortality in multivariate analyses, conferring an average eightfold risk. One of the causes of the progressive increase of myocardial vulnerability to the necrotic insult with age could be a progressive loss of myocytes and their replacement with fibrous tissue.[51] The causes of the greater mortality from acute MI in women (which is about threefold higher below the age of 50) are also unknown.

■ *Thus, the estimated size of the infarct appears to be the most obvious determinant of mortality in patients younger than 65 years, because the age-related vulnerability to myocardial necrosis begins to increase very steeply only after this age.*

Rates of mortality from IHD and the incidence of infarction should be considered separately in epidemiologic studies, as they reflect different pathogenetic and, possibly, different etiological components of IHD, which may be influenced by different types of risk factors and which may benefit from specific therapeutic and preventive strategies. ■

Table 10.1 Cause of in-hospital death in patients receiving thrombolytic therapy*

Age (years)	Death (no. of patients)	Death at time of admission (days 0–1)	Electro-mechanical dissociation	Ventricular fibrillation	Autopsy performed†	Cardiac rupture‡ (no. of patients/ total no. of autopsies)	More than two coronary arteries with critical stenoses§
<60	125/4436	56	13	15	25	6/31 (19)	40
61–70	244/3167	46	20	10	18	25/43 (58)	35
>70	403/2117	52	25	6	21	72/84 (86)	32

* From ref. 50, values are percentages of patients, unless otherwise stated
† Autopsy findings in about 20% of patients enrolled in the GISSI-2 study who died in hospital
‡ Cardiac rupture was the cause of death in 86% of patients above the age of 70 (72/84)
§ The number of patients with more than two coronary stenosed arteries is similar in all age groups

REFERENCES

1. Lee JT, Ideker RY, Reimer KA. Myocardial infarct size and location in relation to the coronary vascular bed at risk in man. Circulation 1981;*64:*526.
2. Helfant RH, Vokonas PS, Gorlin R. Functional importance of the human coronary collateral circulation. N Engl J Med 1971;*284:*1277.
3. Gregg DE, Patterson RE. Functional importance of the coronary collaterals. N Engl J Med 1980;*303:*1404.
4. Gottwik M. Stämmler G, Schaper W, Schlepper M. Collateral development and function in jeopardized human myocardium. Circulation 1984;*70(Suppl.II):*94.
5. Cohen M, Rentrop KP. Limitation of myocardial ischemia by collateral circulation during sudden controlled coronary artery occlusion in human subjects: a prospective study. Circulation 1986;*74:*469.
6. Hansen JF. Coronary collateral circulation: clinical significance and influence on survival in patients with coronary artery occlusion. Am Heart J 1989;*117:*290.
7. Habib GB, Heibig J, Forman SA et al. Influence of coronary collateral vessels on myocardial infarct size in humans. Results of Phase I. Thrombolysis in Myocardial Infarction (TIMI) Trial. Circulation 1991;*83:*739.
8. Epstein SE, Quyyumi AA, Bonow RO. Sudden cardiac death without warning. Possible mechanisms and implications for screening asymptomatic populations. New Engl J Med 1989;*321:*320.
9. Pupita G, Maseri A, Kaski JC et al. Myocardial ischemia caused by distal coronary artery constriction in stable angina pectoris. N Engl J Med 1990;*323:*514.
10. Blumgart HL, Schlesinger MG, Davis D. Studies on the relation of the clinical manifestations of angina pectoris, coronary thrombosis and myocardial infarction to the pathological findings, with particular reference to the significance of the collateral circulation. Am Heart J 1940;*19:*1.
11. Baroldi G, Mantero O, Scomazzoni G. The collaterals of the coronary arteries in normal and pathologic hearts. Circ Res 1956;*4:*223.
12. Watt AH, Penny WJ, Ruttley MST. Left main coronary artery occlusion with preserved left ventricular function: a report of three cases. Br Heart J 1987;*45:*344.
13. Hangartner JRW, Charleston AJ, Davies MJ, Thomas AC. Morphological characteristics of clinically significant coronary artery stenosis in stable angina. Br Heart J 1986;*56:*501.
14. Bogaty P, Brecker SJ, White SE et al. Comparison of coronary angiographic findings in acute and chronic first presentation of ischemic heart disease. Circulation 1993;*87:*1038.
15. Grollier G, Commaneau P, Foucault JP, Potier J. Angioplasty of chronic totally occluded coronary arteries: usefulness of retrograde opacification of the distal part of the occluded vessel via the contralateral coronary artery. Am Heart J 1987;*144:*1324.

16. Cohen M, Sherman W, Rentrop KP, Gorlin R. Determinants of collateral filling observed during sudden controlled coronary artery occlusion in human subjects. J Am Coll Cardiol 1989;*13:*297.
17. Tada M, Yamagishi M, Kodama K et al. Transient collateral augmentation during coronary artery spasm associated with ST-segment depression. Circulation 1983;*67:*693.
18. Piek JJ, Koolen JJ, Hoedemaker G, David GK, Visser CA, Dunning AJ. Severity of single-vessel coronary arterial stenosis and duration of angina as determinants of recruitable collateral vessels during balloon angioplasty occlusion. Am J Cardiol 1991;*67:*13.
19. Maseri A, L'Abbate A, Pesola A et al. Coronary vasospasm in angina pectoris. Lancet 1977;*1:*713.
20. Maseri A, Severi S, De Nes DM et al. Variant angina: one aspect of a continuous spectrum of vasospastic myocardial ischemia. Am J Cardiol 1978;*42:*1019.
21. Yasue H, Omote S, Takizawa A et al. Comparison of coronary arteriographic findings during angina pectoris associated with S-T elevation or depression. Am J Cardiol 1981;*47:*539.
22. Piek JJ. Becker AE. Collateral blood supply to the myocardium at risk in human myocardial infarction: a quantitative post-mortem assessment. J Am Coll Cardiol 1988;*11:*1290.
23. Hirai T, Fujita M, Jakajima H et al. Importance of collateral circulation for prevention of left ventricular aneurysm formation in acute myocardial infarction. Circulation 1989;*79:*791.
24. Forman MB, Collins HW, Kopelman HA et al. Determinants of left ventricular aneurysm formation after anterior myocardial infarction: a clinical and angiographic study. J Am Coll Cardiol 1986;*8:*1256.
25. Saito Y, Yasuno M, Ishida M et al. Importance of coronary collaterals for restoration of left ventricular function after intracoronary thrombolysis. Am J Cardiol 1985;*55:*1259.
26. Schwartz H, Leiboff RL Katz RK et al. Arteriographic predictors of spontaneous improvement in left ventricular function after myocardial infarction. Circulation 1985;*71:*693.
27. Rentrop KP, Feit F, Thornton JC and the Mount Sinai–New York Reperfusion Study Group. The protective potential of collaterals depends on the time of their development. J Am Coll Cardiol 1990;*15:*202A.
28. Ambrose JA, Tannenbaum MA, Alexopoulos D et al. Angiographic progression of coronary artery disease and the development of myocardial infarction. J Am Coll Cardiol 1988;*12:*56.
29. Norell MS, Lyons JP, Gardener JE, Layton CA, Balcon R. Protective effect of collateral vessels during coronary angioplasty. Br Heart J 1989;*62:*241.
30. Flameng W, Schwartz F, Hehrlein F. Intraoperative evaluation of the functional significance of coronary collateral vessels in patients with coronary artery disease. Am J Cardiol 1978;*42:*187.
31. Goldstein RE, Stinson EB, Scherer JL, Seningen RP, Grehl TM, Epstein SE. Intraoperative coronary collateral function in patients with coronary occlusive disease. Circulation 1974;*69:*298.
32. Fam WM, McGregor M. Effect of coronary vasodilator drugs on retrograde flow in areas of chronic myocardial ischemia. Circ Res 1964;*15:*355.
33. Araujo LI, Maseri A, McFalls EO, Galassi A, Lammertsma AA, Jones T. Dipyridamole-induced transmural coronary blood flow steal and ischemia detected by positron emission tomography. 1995. Submitted for publication.
34. McFadden EP, Clarke JG, Davies GJ, Kaski JC, Haider AW, Maseri A. Effect of intracoronary serotonin on coronary vessels in patients with stable angina and patients with variant angina. N Engl J Med 1991;*324:*648.
35. The Cardiac Arrhythmia Suppression Trial (CAST) Investigators. Preliminary report. Effect of encainide and flecainide on mortality in a randomized trial of arrhythmia suppression after myocardial infarction. N Engl J Med 1989;*321:*406.
36. Irving JB, Bruce RA. Exertional hypotension and postexertional ventricular fibrillation in stress testing. Am J Cardiol 1977;*39:*849.
37. Stern S, Banai S, Keren A et al. Ventricular ectopic activity during myocardial ischemic episodes in ambulatory patients. Am J Cardiol 1990;*65:*412.
38. Hausmann D, Nikutta P, Trappe H-J et al. Incidence of ventricular arrhythmias during transient

myocardial ischemia in patients with stable coronary artery disease. J Am Coll Cardiol 1990;*16*:49.

39. Maseri A, Severi S, Marzullo P. Role of coronary arterial spasm in sudden coronary ischemic death. Ann NY Acad Sci 1982;*382*:204.

40. Schomig A, Richardt G. Cardiac sympathetic activity in myocardial ischemia: release and effects of noradrenaline. Basic Res in Cardiol 1990;*85(Suppl.I)*:9.

41. Hackett D, McKenna W, Davies G, Maseri A. Reperfusion arrhythmias are rare during acute myocardial infarction and thrombolysis in man. Int J Cardiol 1990;*29*:205.

42. Toffler GH, Stone PH, Muller JE et al. Prognosis after myocardial infarction complicated by ventricular fibrillation. Circulation 1986;*74(Suppl.II)*:304.

43. Volpi A, Cavalli A, Franzosi MG et al. One-year prognosis of primary ventricular fibrillation complicating acute myocardial infarction. Am J Cardiol 1989;*63*:1174.

44. Goldstein S, Friedman L, Hutchinson R et al. Timing, mechanism and clinical setting of witnessed deaths in postmyocardial infarction patients. J Am Coll Cardiol 1984;*3*:1111.

45. McHenry PL, O'Donnell J, Morris SN, Jordan JJ. The abnormal exercise electrocardiogram in apparently healthy men: a predictor of angina pectoris as an initial coronary event during long-term follow-up. Circulation 1984;*70*:547.

46. Lombardi F, Sandrone G, Pernpruner S et al. Heart rate variability as an index of sympathovagal interaction after acute myocardial infarction. Am J Cardiol 1987;*60*:1239.

47. Kleiger RE, Miller JP, Bigger JT, Moss AJ and the Multicenter Post-Infarction Research Group. Decreased heart rate variability and its association with increased mortality after acute myocardial infarction. Am J Cardiol 1987;*59*:256.

48. Bigger JT, Fleiss JL, Rolnitzky LM, Steinman RC. The ability of several short-term measures of RR variability to predict mortality after myocardial infarction. Circulation 1993;*88*:927.

49. Simson MB. Noninvasive identification of patients at high risk for sudden cardiac death. Signal-averaged electrocardiography. Circulation 1992;*85(Suppl I)*:I-145.

50. Maggioni AP, Maseri A, Fresco C et al on behalf of GISSI-2 investigators. Age-related increase in mortality of patients with first myocardial infarction treated with thrombolysis. New Engl J Med 1993;*329*:1442.

51. Olivetti G, Melissari M, Capasso JM, Anversa P. Cardiomyopathy of the ageing human heart. Myocyte loss and reactive cellular hypertrophy. Circ Res 1991;*68*:1560.

Mode of first presentation: acute, chronic, and quiescent phases of IHD

INTRODUCTION

Ischemic heart disease (IHD) is traditionally considered in a cross-sectional way, attention being focused on each presenting syndrome according to the angle from which it is viewed by pathologists, epidemiologists, physicians, and cardiologists.

Pathologists consider patients according to the syndrome that brought them to autopsy (although often such patients had suffered a composite sequence of multiple ischemic syndromes). They traditionally assume that the different ischemic syndromes are the random expression of the same basic pathologic process, i.e. the progressive development of coronary atherosclerosis.

Epidemiologists have observed that the mode of first presentation of IHD is usually unheralded and dramatic, with the occurrence of myocardial infarction (MI) or sudden ischemic cardiac death (SICD), rather than gradual, with progressive worsening of effort-induced angina. They have also observed that the incidence of angina differs in men and women and that it reaches a plateau in men after the age of 60, whereas the incidence of infarction continues to increase linearly with age in both men and women (at least up to the age of 75), remaining about threefold higher in men. The plateau in the incidence of angina and the linear increase of infarction are in sharp contrast with the exponential increase in the rate of mortality from IHD with age in both sexes.

Physicians and cardiologists are often concerned with the ischemic manifestations in a longitudinal view of IHD, and those who follow patients over the years are impressed, not only by the frequent sudden and unpredictable onset of major ischemic events, but also by both the common waning of symptoms and the alternance or recurrence of ischemic syndromes in the same patient. Some patients who first present with chronic stable angina go on to develop unstable angina or infarction; others who first present with acute MI go on to develop unstable or chronic stable angina; many patients with recent-onset chronic stable angina or acute MI may enter quiescent and totally asymptomatic phases that last for months or years, only to present again, unpredictably, with chronic stable or unstable angina or with unheralded MI or SICD.

As discussed in Chapter 8, the relationship between the severity of coronary atherosclerosis and the severity of ischemic manifestations is extremely variable. This variability, which is most obvious among patients at the time of their first presentation with IHD, should not be surprising because the data reviewed in the last three chapters indicate five major sources of variability:

1. The vast majority of individuals have coronary atherosclerosis, but only a few have symptoms or signs of myocardial ischemia or necrosis.
2. Angina pectoris, the most common sign of recurrent ischemia, has multiple causes and is associated with a very variable course and outcome, largely dependent on whether its causes are stable or unstable.
3. For reasons that are not yet clear, infarction is caused by acute coronary lesions that develop suddenly and unpredictably on a very variable atherosclerotic background, whereas, in chronic stable patients, severe stenoses can remain stable for years and complete occlusion may not be associated with any signs of infarction.
4. In some patients, fatal arrhythmias develop unpredictably, not only in the very early hours of acute infarction, irrespective of its extent, but also during episodes of transient ischemia caused by occlusive coronary artery spasm, and even in the absence of acute necrosis or ischemia in some patients with postinfarction scarring.
5. Progression of coronary atherosclerosis appears to reach a plateau at about the sixth decade, whereas the rate of mortality from IHD continues to increase exponentially with age.

Thus, a common predisposing atherosclerotic background cannot be considered in itself to be a sufficient explanation for the following:

a. the mode of first presentation of IHD
b. the variable occurrence, recurrence, and alternation of acute phases of IHD (characterized by unstable angina and acute MI), chronic phases (characterized by occasional ischemic episodes recurring with a stable pattern), and quiescent phases (characterized by the absence of spontaneous or inducible ischemic episodes after the initial presentation of IHD)
c. the age- and gender-related incidence and prevalence of angina, infarction and mortality from IHD.

The waxing and waning of different ischemic stimuli, rather than the gradual progressive increase of atherosclerotic stenoses, must represent the most common explanation for the sudden onset of IHD and its variable course. As discussed in Chapter 9, ischemic stimuli have no evolutive tendency in chronic stable angina, but may cause sudden interruption of myocardial blood flow in unstable angina and acute MI. The causes of ischemic episodes in stable and unstable phases are different, although some types of coronary lesions at least may be common predisposing factors to both.

11.1 MODE OF FIRST PRESENTATION OF IHD

The frequently unexpected and dramatic first presentation of IHD has been documented in the prospective follow-up of previously healthy individuals in community studies and in the clinical histories of patients presenting with acute MI. The most thorough and representative community longitudinal study of healthy individuals at entry took place in Framingham (Massachusetts, USA) and a representative cross-sectional observation is provided by the clinical data collected prospectively in the large multicenter Gruppo Italiano per lo Studio della Sopravvivenza nell'Infarto Miocardico-2 (GISSI-2) study.

11.1.1 Mode of first presentation of IHD in the community

In the Framingham study,[1,2] a total of 5127 individuals (aged from 30 to 62 years), who were followed up on a biennial basis over a period of 14 years, were found to have no manifestations of IHD at the time of initial examination. The incidence of IHD was distinctly higher in men than in women, who lagged behind by about 20 years in both the incidence of MI and the rate of mortality from IHD, and by about 10 years in the incidence of angina pectoris.

The mode of first presentation of IHD was similar in individuals aged between 30 and 49 years and between 50 and 62 years at entry; irrespective of age, the mode was predominantly infarction (45%) in men and predominantly angina (56%) in women—severe unstable angina in 9 and 11% and SICD in 14 and 10%, respectively (see Fig. 11.1). Approximately one-quarter of all MIs were detected only by the routine biennial examination and, hence, were not recognized clinically; an estimated 15% were totally asymptomatic. More than one-half of the deaths due to IHD were sudden and unexpected and two-thirds of deaths occurred outside hospital.

The unexpected, dramatic common first presentation of IHD with MI, rather than with gradually worsening effort-related angina, is consistent with the observation presented in Chapters 8 and 9, that acute coronary occlusion usually occurs suddenly at the site of non-flow-limiting stenoses.

In the Framingham study, 45% of cases of angina occurred subsequent to MI in men, but only 15% of cases in women. This observation, together with the higher frequency of chronic stable angina presenting as the first manifestation of IHD in women (in whom the occurrence of flow-limiting stenoses is delayed by over a decade compared with men) (see Fig. 8.6), is suggestive of a different prevalence of pathogenetic mechanisms of angina in the two sexes.

11.1.2 Mode of first presentation of IHD in cardiological practise

The frequent occurrence of MI as the first manifestation of IHD documented in the Framingham study is confirmed by the information collected prospectively in the GISSI-2

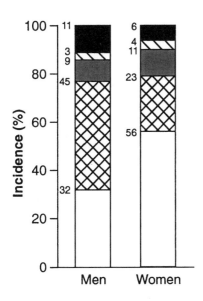

Fig. 11.1 Mode of first presentation of IHD in the Framingham study. Chronic angina pectoris (□) was the first manifestation of IHD in only 32% of men and in 56% of women. The common first presentation with MI (▨), sudden death (■), coronary death (▧), or acute coronary insufficiency (■), rather than with gradual worsening of chronic stable angina, suggests that these sudden, dramatic events are not the result of gradual progression of coronary stenoses. (Modified from ref. 2.)

study.[3] Of a total of 12 381 patients who were randomized to receive thrombolytic therapy, 9720 were cases of first confirmed MI. About 65% had no previous history of IHD; of the remaining 35% with a history of angina, about one-half had recent-onset angina (less than 1 month) and the other one-half chronic stable angina. These proportions were similar in men and women and also in different age-groups. Thus, in this large series of patients also, infarction was the very first manifestation of IHD and was preceded by chronic stable angina in only a minority of cases. The low frequency of preinfarction angina may be due to a limited degree of diagnostic recall by patients with IHD, such as that observed in the British Heart Study.[4] The possibility of a poor diagnostic recall is less likely in Italian patients, who are, in general, more health conscious than British patients; similarly, a recent Swedish study reported a very high degree of diagnostic recall in Swedish patients.[5] The recall of symptoms was, however, good in the British Heart Study. The data from this large cross-sectional study of patients presenting with their first MI are, therefore, consistent with the findings obtained in the longitudinal community follow-up study in Framingham, which showed that in only 23% of cases was acute MI preceded by a history of chronic stable angina.

11.2 ACUTE, CHRONIC, AND QUIESCENT PHASES OF IHD

Following the first presentation of IHD, its evolution is variable (see Fig. 11.2). Survivors of acute MI may develop chronic ischemic cardiac failure when infarction causes a severe impairment of ventricular function, chronic stable angina when thrombus organization causes flow-limiting stenoses in nonnecrosed segments of the wall, or enter into a quiescent phase. In patients presenting with unstable angina, IHD may evolve into acute MI, SICD, chronic stable angina, or a quiescent phase and in patients presenting with uncomplicated stable angina it may evolve into unstable angina, acute MI, SICD, or a quiescent phase.

Although acute, chronic, and quiescent phases may alternate in the same patients, the etiological components of acute and chronic phases may possibly differ substantially.

Acute phases include acute MI and unstable angina. They are most likely caused by unstable coronary lesions.

Chronic phases include chronic stable angina and chronic postischemic cardiac failure.

Quiescent phases are characterized by the absence of symptoms and signs of myocardial ischemia (spontaneous or stress induced).

11.2.1 Acute phases

As previously described, acute phases, represented by unstable angina and acute MI, can be the very first manifestations of IHD in about 60% of patients. In the remaining 40%, acute phases can develop in patients with previous infarction, in patients in a quiescent phase (about 25%), or in patients with chronic stable angina (about 15%). Acute phases are caused by the sudden development of unstable coronary lesions that can increase over a period of weeks, days, or only hours and cause either unstable angina or MI. Such lesions can leave organized mural thrombi, causing flow-limiting stenoses and chronic stable angina, or cause no detectable progression of stenoses and subside into a quiescent phase.

In patients with no previous history of MI, the prognosis of acute phases is related to the following:

a.   the severity of the atherosclerotic background (the more proximal, numerous and severe the flow-limiting coronary stenoses, the larger the area of myocardium at risk)

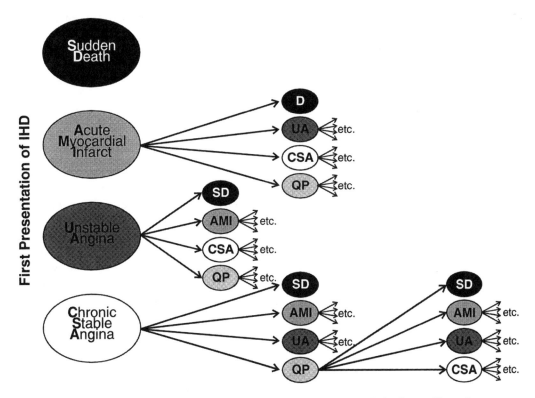

Fig. 11.2 Possible evolution of IHD following its first clinical manifestation.
The time interval between the different manifestations (SD, sudden death; D, death;
AMI, acute myocardial infarction; UA, unstable angina; CSA, chronic stable angina;
QP, quiescent phase) may vary considerably. The extent to which the first manifesta-
tion conditions those subsequent to it is still far from clear.

b. the intensity of ischemic stimuli (thrombotic and vasoconstrictor and their positive
feedback mechanisms) (as discussed in Ch. 9)

c. the response of the myocardium to the ischemic insult (collateral vessel development and function, age and vulnerability to ischemia-induced necrosis and fatal
arrhythmias) (as discussed in Ch. 10).

In patients with previous MI, the prognosis of acute phases is also influenced considerably
by preexisting ventricular dysfunction due to scar tissue, which favors the development of
ventricular failure and fatal arrhythmias and makes the heart more vulnerable to further
losses of myocardium and ischemic insults.

Thus, patients in whom acute MI and unstable angina appear as the first manifestations
of IHD have, in general, a better prognosis than those in whom acute phases develop in the
presence of preexisting impairment of left ventricular function due to previous MI.

In post-MI patients, SICD represents about 65% of the causes of cardiac death.[6–8]

Unless specific markers of an individual's susceptibility to develop acute phases of IHD
can be identified, only the sudden appearance of spontaneous angina and/or an unexplained
waxing of symptoms and signs of ischemia can indicate the onset of an unstable phase or its
transition from a stable phase; similarly, only the absence of symptoms and signs of ischemia
or their stability over a period can indicate the conversion of an acute unstable phase into a

chronic stable phase. The recognition of the transition between acute unstable phases and chronic stable phases, and vice versa, is made difficult by:

a.   the similar features of anginal pain in stable and unstable angina
b.   the inability of a positive exercise stress test (or Holter recording) to differentiate between stable and unstable phases of ischemia
c.   the inability of coronary angiography to differentiate accurately between stable and unstable lesions as stenoses may be smooth yet unstable, or irregular yet (now) stable.

Like volcanoes, plaques can be formed by an eruption; like smokeless volcanoes, plaques that cause no symptoms may, nevertheless, still be active and about to erupt, or be quiescent and remain so. In some patients, the severity of a culprit stenosis may not change with the development of unstable angina or MI, like some volcanoes exhibiting devastating eruptions without major changes occurring in their morphology. Other plaques may form like mountains, rather than like volcanoes, having no eruptive potential and, therefore, being indistinguishable from inactive volcanoes. The greater the number of vessels with plaques, the greater the probability that the patient has the predisposition to develop "volcano-like" plaques that may produce acute coronary syndromes in the presence of unfavorable local and systemic circumstances.

11.2.2 Chronic phases

IHD may cause chronic persistent symptoms in the absence of (or even in the presence of) continuous therapy, because of either chronic stable angina or chronic postischemic cardiac failure. Chronic ischemic manifestations may occur in patients with a history of previous MI and in those without; the two groups should be kept separate because of differing prognoses.

Uncomplicated chronic stable angina

Uncomplicated chronic stable angina can be defined as angina with documented myocardial ischemia, with no evidence of either previous infarction or phases of instability and with normal ventricular function.[9] As discussed in Chapter 9, the chronic causes of ischemia can be multiple and include:

a.   severe fixed flow-limiting stenoses in proximal coronary arteries (one or several)
b.   a stenosis with an important dynamic component
c.   distal coronary vessel constriction in the presence of angiographically normal vessels and non-flow-limiting stenoses.

Although all examples described above can be defined as chronic stable angina, the susceptibility of each patient to acute unstable phases of IHD differs: in general, it is highest in patients with multivessel coronary stenoses; it is also high in patients with a very reduced ischemic threshold; it is lower in those with a high ischemic threshold, and lowest in those with angiographically normal arteries. Effort tolerance is usually most severely reduced in patients with the severest proximal coronary stenoses, who also have more frequent ischemic episodes, with and without pain on ambulatory Holter recordings. In such stable patients, it is not clear whether the predisposition to develop acute, unstable phases is indicated more by the frequency of ischemic episodes or by the severity of the underlying coronary atherosclerosis. The stability of ischemic manifestations is not necessarily indicative of the lack of progression of flow-limiting stenoses, as collateral development may prevent a reduction of effort tolerance.[10] The observation that, in patients with a positive exercise test, SICD occurs much less frequently than in those with a negative test, suggests a possible protective role of collateral development due to flow-limiting stenoses.[11]

■ *Knowledge of the origin of flow-limiting stenoses ("volcano-like" or "mountain-like") would be helpful in predicting the susceptibility to acute ischemic phases of patients with chronic stable angina.* ■

Complicated chronic stable angina

Complicated chronic stable angina can be defined as angina in patients with a previous acute MI. In the Framingham study[1] it represented 45% of cases in men and 15% of cases in women. Postinfarction angina was reported at 6 months in 17% of cases of non-Q-wave infarction and in 15% of Q-wave thrombolyzed infarctions in the GISSI-2 study.[12] Patients with postinfarction chronic stable angina are much less likely to have angiographically normal coronary arteries than patients with uncomplicated chronic stable angina. The factors that determine their prognosis are the same as those in uncomplicated patients, but with the important additional components related to the impairment of ventricular function and the increased vulnerability to ischemia-induced arrhythmias caused by the previous MI. In addition, such patients should be separated from those with uncomplicated chronic stable angina because their susceptibility to MI is proven and because some plaques at least are likely to have originated from "volcano-like" eruptions.

Chronic postischemic cardiac failure

Chronic postischemic cardiac failure is mainly determined by the amount of myocardium that has been lost and the consequent remodeling of the ventricle which, without antifailure treatment, prevent the heart from maintaining an adequate function. It is a frequent complication of infarction, particularly in elderly patients. In the GISSI-2 study, signs of cardiac failure were present at 6 months post-MI in 9% of 9860 patients who received thrombolytic therapy but, as 19% were treated with diuretics the actual prevalence could have been higher.[13]

Patients with postischemic cardiac failure are much more vulnerable to new acute ischemic insults because of their reduced residual contractile reserve and their increased vulnerability to ischemia-induced arrhythmias.

11.2.3 Quiescent phases

Totally asymptomatic periods lasting many months or even years are frequently observed after acute MI, recent-onset angina, or periods of chronic stable angina. If, during such asymptomatic periods, no signs of silent ischemia can either be induced by exercise testing or other provocative tests, or observed during ambulatory Holter recordings, patients are classified as being in a quiescent phase of IHD. The prognosis of patients in a quiescent phase differs according to the original presenting ischemic syndrome.

In the Framingham study, remissions of at least 2 years were observed in 32% of men and in 44% of women who presented with recent-onset angina, and in 14% of men and in 19% of women with a history of chronic stable angina. Asymptomatic phases are common also after MI. About 89% of patients discharged from hospital in the GISSI-2 trial were free from angina at 6 months, about 80% were receiving neither diuretics nor digitalis, and less than 20% had positive ECG exercise stress tests.

Quiescent phases can last for months or even decades in the absence of anti-ischemic treatment. Alternatively, after variable periods of time, they can be interrupted by either acute phases (unstable angina, unheralded MI, or SICD) or by the appearance of chronic stable angina. The known prognostic indicators are represented by the history of previous infarction, by its extension, by the number of coronary arteries with flow-limiting stenoses, and by the patient's susceptibility to potentially fatal arrhythmias, but prognosis is better than when ischemia is present or inducible. As discussed in Chapter 13, patients with chronic stable angina or post-acute MI with inducible ischemia at low work loads, have a worse prognosis than those in whom ischemia is inducible only at high work loads or is not inducible at all.

The mode of recurrence of active ischemic phases is unpredictable, although the clinical impression is as follows:

1. A recurrence of infarction, without warning symptoms, is more commonly found in patients first presenting with an unheralded infarction.
2. A recurrence of chronic stable angina is more frequent in those first presenting with uncomplicated chronic stable angina.
3. SICD is the most common cause of death in post-MI patients.

Thus, when patients enter an asymptomatic, quiescent phase after either acute MI or unstable angina, they seem to remain at a higher risk than those who are in a quiescent phase after uncomplicated chronic stable angina.

■ *The prognosis of patients with IHD in a quiescent phase should be assessed accurately in order to judge the risk, as well as the inconvenience and cost–benefit ratio, of treatment intended to increase both the expectancy of life free from ischemic events and also total life expectancy.* ■

11.3 AGE- AND GENDER-RELATED MORTALITY: INCIDENCE AND PREVALENCE

Mortality rates of IHD are influenced considerably by age and by gender; similarly, the incidence and prevalence also vary with age and gender. The reasons for the variable age- and gender-related rates of IHD mortality and the incidence of ischemic syndromes are not precisely known (see Ch. 12).

11.3.1 Age- and gender-related mortality from IHD

Mortality from IHD increases exponentially with age in both men and women, doubling approximately every 10 years, but mortality rates are much lower in younger women and the two gradually converge at about 90 years of age. Furthermore, mortality from acute MI shows an exponential increase in both men and women, with no detectable breakpoint being associated with the time of the menopause (see Fig. 11.3A,B).[14]

The lower mortality from IHD in younger women is associated with a lower incidence of coronary stenoses, compared with men, before the seventh decade of life (see Fig. 8.6).

The fraction of total mortality caused by IHD also varies with age in men and women. In men, it increases steeply up to the age of 40 and then more gradually up to the age of 60, reaching a maximum of 16% in Italy and 34% in the USA. In women, it increases progressively with age, reaching a maximum of 13% in Italy and 34% in the USA.[15] Above the age of 74, mortality from IHD is similar in men and women, in both Italy and the USA (see Fig. 11.4). SICD accounts for about 50% of fatal cases in patients with known IHD, regardless

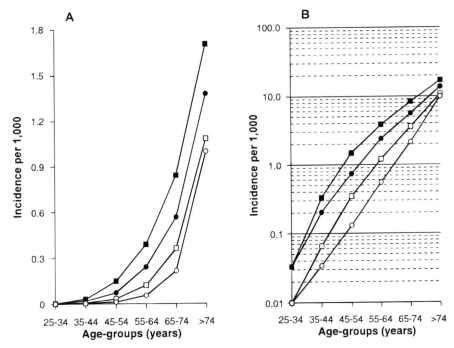

Fig. 11.3 Age- and gender-related incidence of mortality for acute MI. In the USA and in Italy the incidence is higher in men (●, Italy; ■, USA) than in women (○, Italy; □, USA) and increases markedly with age (**A**). Although the incidence is higher in the USA than in Italy, in both countries mortality is substantially lower in women. The semilogarithmic plot of the same data shows that male and female rates of mortality tend to converge in old age and that no change in the slope of the curve is detectable in women in association with the menopausal years (**B**). (Based on data from ref. 14.)

of their New York Heart Association functional classification (NYHA Classes I–IV). It is not known how many cases of SICD are caused by primary arrhythmias, by arrhythmias induced by a new ischemic episode, by acute cardiac failure, or by infarct-related cardiac rupture, which is particularly common in the elderly (see Ch. 10). In-hospital mortality from acute MI is about threefold higher in young women than in men, but is only 20% higher in older women (see Ch. 10). The causes of the increased vulnerability of women to infarction are not precisely known.

■ *Prospective studies are needed to ascertain the frequency of individual causes of death in relation to age and gender. Appropriate studies are needed also to assess the causes of the increasing incidence of infarction—as well as the increasing vulnerability to necrotic insults—with age and gender, and to understand the mechanisms that provide protection from infarction in younger women.* ■

11.3.2 Incidence and prevalence of ischemic syndromes

The incidence rates of IHD define the number of new cases that occur in the population each year. The prevalence rates of IHD define the number of individuals with the disease at a given point in time, hence reflecting the difference between the incidence of new cases and

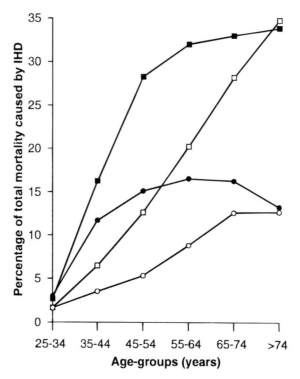

Fig. 11.4 Age- and gender-related percentage of total mortality caused by IHD in the USA and Italy. The percentage total mortality caused by IHD increases rapidly up to the fifth decade of life in men and progressively up to the seventh decade in women in both countries (symbols as in Fig. 11.3). Mortality from IHD is a much smaller fraction of total mortality in Italy than in the USA. The difference between the two countries is larger than expected on the basis of mortality due to MI (see Fig. 11.3). The causes of this difference are unknown. (Data obtained for the year 1987 from ref. 14.)

the deaths of patients with the syndrome (or, in the case of angina, the disappearance of symptoms). The incidence and prevalence of MI and angina increase with age in both men and women, but the intergender differences are much wider for infarction than for angina.

In the text, prevalence and incidence are expressed per 100 individuals, a dimension more familiar to physicians, who are used to dealing with a limited number of patients with a high incidence of events. In the figures, they are expressed per 1000, a figure more familiar to epidemiologists, who are used to dealing with large population samples with a low incidence of events.

Incidence

In the Framingham Heart Study, the incidence of infarction was found to increase with age in both men and women, reaching about 1.2 and 0.3% per year, respectively, at the age of 70 (see Fig. 11.5A).[15] The incidence of SICD at age 60 was about 0.27% in men and about 0.04% in women. Furthermore, the annual incidence of angina was found to increase progressively with age up to about 0.7% per year at the age of 60 in both men and women, and then to remain stable up to 70 (see Fig. 11.5B).[15] Similar figures have been reported in other studies.[16]

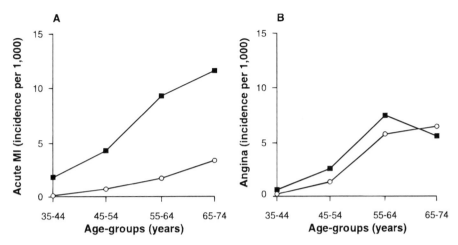

Fig. 11.5 Age- and gender-related incidence of acute MI and angina in the Framingham Heart Study. The incidence of infarction is about 3.5 times greater in men up to the seventh decade of life (**A**), whereas that of angina is similar for men (■) and women (○) (**B**). The large difference between the incidence of MI and that of angina suggest different gender-related pathogenetic mechanisms. The discrepancy between the large intergender difference in the incidence of MI and the relatively small difference in MI-related mortality in the seventh decade may be explained by the greater mortality from infarction in women, reported in Chapter 10. (From data in ref. 15.)

Prevalence

The prevalence of angina and infarction depends on the balance between the incidence of new cases, mortality in old cases, and on the waning of angina. In a study of over 2000 residents of Rochester, Minnesota,[17] the prevalence rates of infarction in men increased progressively with age and were much higher than in women throughout life (still about threefold higher above the age of 74) (see Fig. 11.6A). Conversely, the prevalence rates of angina were about double in men compared with women up to the age of 60, but became similar at the age of 75 (see Fig. 11.6B). In the British Cardiovascular Health study[18] the prevalence rates of definite MI and angina were 11 and 15%, respectively, among men aged 65–69 years and 16 and 18%, respectively, among men aged 75–79 years. The comparable rates for women were 4 and 8%, and 7 and 12%, respectively.

■ *The variability in the age-related incidence and prevalence of angina and infarction and in mortality from IHD between men and women is a further indication of the inadequacy of the epidemiologic correlation of risk factors with combined IHD events, and of the need for ischemic stimuli and the cardiac response to ischemic insults in relation to gender and age to be considered separately.* ■

Pathophysiologic implications

The differences in the age-related incidence and prevalence of angina and in mortality rates from IHD among men and women suggest major differences in the susceptibility of different individuals to the disease, in the pathogenetic mechanisms, and in the vulnerability to ischemic insult. The small difference between men and women in the age-related incidence and prevalence of angina is in sharp contrast to the large difference in the age-related inci-

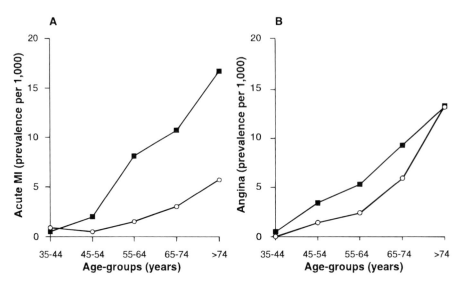

Fig. 11.6 Age- and gender-related prevalence of MI and angina in Rochester, Minnesota, USA. The prevalence of MI (**A**) and angina (**B**) increases with age. The intergender difference is much smaller for angina than for MI. Over the age of 75 there is still a threefold higher prevalence of MI in men (■) than in women (○), but a similar prevalence of angina. (Modified from ref. 17.)

dence and prevalence of infarction. The threefold difference between men and women above the age of 75 in the incidence and prevalence of infarction is also a sharp contrast to the minor difference in mortality rates for acute MI and for total IHD mortality at the same age. The contrast between the age-related exponential increase in mortality rates for acute MI and the linear increase in the incidence of infarction can be explained by the exponential age-related increase in mortality from acute MI observed in patients receiving thrombolytic therapy (see Ch. 10).[3] Finally, the age-related increase in flow-limiting coronary stenoses (see Fig. 8.6) appears to be similar only to the age-related incidence of angina in men. The contrast between the similar age-related incidence and prevalence of angina in men and women and the large difference in the age-related increase in flow-limiting coronary stenoses in the two sexes up to the age of 70, suggests a different prevalence of pathogenetic mechanisms of angina pectoris. Accordingly, these major differences in the heart's response to ischemic insults are supported, not only by the threefold higher rate of in-hospital mortality for acute MI in young women compared with young men but also the threefold higher incidence and prevalence of infarction in men, compared with women, up to the age of 75, in the presence of a nearly similar incidence of total IHD mortality. The large gender- and age-related epidemiologic differences in the incidence and prevalence of angina and infarction, in the prevalence of flow-limiting coronary stenoses, and in the rates of IHD mortality, are further indications that epidemiologic studies cannot provide clinically useful data and may lead to misleading conclusions when inhomogeneous individuals and events are grouped together in order to obtain statistically significant information within a short period of time.

■ *These conclusions suggest the urgent need for a gender- and age-specific analysis of each ischemic syndrome according to incidence, clinical presentations, fatal or non-fatal outcome, and specific risk factors.* ■

REFERENCES

1. Kannel WB, Feinleib M. Natural history of angina pectoris in the Framingham study. Am J Cardiol 1972;29:154.
2. Kannel WB. Some lessons in cardiovascular epidemiology from Framingham. Am J Cardiol 1976;37:269.
3. Maggioni AP, Maseri A, Fresco C et al on behalf of GISSI-2 Investigators. Age-related increase in mortality in patients with first myocardial infarction treated with thrombolysis. N Engl J Med 1993;329:1442.
4. Shaper AG, Cook DG, Walker M, MacFarlane PW. Recall of diagnosis by men with ischaemic heart disease. Br Heart J 1984;51:606.
5. Olsson L, Svärdsudd K, Nilsson G, Ringqvist I, Tibblin G. Validity of a postal questionnaire with regard to the prevalence of myocardial infarction in a general population sample. Eur Heart J 1989;10:1011.
6. Goldstein S, Friedman L, Hutchinson R et al. Timing, mechanism and clinical setting of witnessed deaths in postmyocardial infarction patients. J Am Coll Cardiol 1984;3:1111.
7. Marcus FI, Cobb LA, Edwards JE et al. Mechanisms of death and prevalence of myocardial ischemic symptoms in the terminal event after acute myocardial infarction. Am J Cardiol 1988;61:8.
8. Wilcox RG, Von der Lippe G, Olsson CG, Jensen G, Skene AM, Hampton JR. Effects of alteplase in acute myocardial infarction: 6-month results from the ASSET study. Lancet 1990;335:1175.
9. Bogaty P, Brecker SJ, White SE et al. Comparison of coronary angiographic findings in acute and chronic first presentation of ischemic heart disease. Circulation 1993;87:1938.
10. Crake T, Tousoulis D, Kaski JC, Maseri A. Stability of symptoms in chronic angina pectoris in spite of severe coronary stenosis progression. 1995. Submitted for publication.
11. Epstein SE, Quyyumi AA, Bonow RO. Sudden cardiac death without warning. Possible mechanisms and implications for screening asymptomatic populations. New Engl J Med 1989;321:320.
12. Maggioni AP, Gardinale E, Mauri F, Mafrici A, Santoro E, De Vita C a nome dei ricercatori degli studi GISSI. Decorso dell'infarto miocardico acuto non Q nelle diverse presentazioni In: Rovelli F, De Vita C, Moreo A (eds). Cardiologia 1993. Librex Spa, Milano, p. 326.
13. Volpi A, De Vita C, Franzosi MG et al. Determinants of 6-month mortality in survivors of myocardial infarction after thrombolysis. Results of the GISSI-2 data base. Circulation 1993;88:416.
14. World Health Organization: World Health Statistics Annual 1990. WHO, Geneva.
15. Margolis JR, Gillum RF, Feinleib M, Brasch R, Fabsitz R. Community Surveillance for Coronary Heart Disease: The Framingham Cardiovascular Disease Survey. Comparison with the Framingham Heart Study and previous short-term studies. Am J Cardiol 1976;37:61.
16. Jensen G. Epidemiology of chest pain and angina pectoris. Acta Med Scand 1982;Suppl.682:1.
17. Phillips SJ, Whisnant JP, O'Fallon WM, Frye RL. Prevalence of cardiovascular disease and diabetes mellitus in residents of Rochester, Minnesota. Mayo Clin Proc 1990;65:344.
18. Mittelmark MB, Psaty B, Rautaharju PM. Prevalence of cardiovascular diseases among older adults. Am J Epidemiol 1993;137:311.

12 | Risk factors and etiologic components of IHD

INTRODUCTION

The development of specific therapeutic and preventive strategies for ischemic heart disease (IHD) depends on a precise understanding of the etiologic factors that lead to the development of ischemic syndromes. As the pathogenetic components of IHD discussed in Chapters 8, 9, and 10 are multiple and varied, the etiologic factors of IHD must also be multiple and varied. They have not yet been completely elucidated and are of variable importance in different ischemic syndromes and in different individuals.

In their craving for a simple, unifying solution to this problem, researchers have focused on the most obvious features of the disease.[1] These features vary, depending on the angle from which they are viewed; average differences between patients and controls are emphasized and accepted as plausible explanations without sufficient consideration being given either to the frequently broad overlap between findings in patients and in controls, who have no signs of disease, or to the possibility that other, as yet unexplored, causes may have important contributory roles.

Thus, *epidemiologic studies* of IHD focus on variables suggested by prevailing hypotheses that are easily measurable and correlated with total IHD mortality figures. An observed association is frequently accepted as having a cause–effect relationship when it agrees with the hypothesis under consideration. *Pathologic studies* are based on those patients who have succumbed to the disease; they have focused on the most readily available explanations, such as the chronic atherosclerotic background, coronary thrombosis, and plaque fissure, as plausible triggers of ischemic events. *Experimental pathogenetic studies* focus more on the development of the chronic atherosclerotic background (which is easily quantifiable) than on the development of ischemic events and their consequences (which are much more difficult to assess). *Physicians* are often puzzled by the discrepancies that exist between ischemic manifestations, severity of coronary atherosclerosis, and risk factors.

Because of the unpredictable onset, course, and outcome of the various ischemic syndromes in individual patients, a common single etiology has been sought by examining the variables that are associated with its most easily detectable manifestations in the population at large, i.e. IHD-associated mortality and infarction. This generalization, which is certainly valid as a first-generation hypothesis, may prevent our understanding of the precise etiologic components of the various ischemic syndromes.

For such a heterogeneous disease as IHD, epidemiologic information highlights those associations that are more prevalent in the population. Studies have been based on the following assumptions:

a. that IHD in general can be equated with coronary atherosclerosis
b. that atherosclerosis is, in general, a single disease entity
c. that angina pectoris, myocardial infarction (MI) and sudden ischemic cardiac death (SICD) can be taken, in general, as endpoints of the same gradual disease process, which occur largely at random when a gradual progression of coronary atherosclerosis, began in childhood, reaches a critical threshold.

The common acceptance of this view is illustrated by the widespread use of the term "coronary artery disease" rather than "ischemic heart disease" (see Introductory Chapter). This unifying view does not take into consideration the very high prevalence in the population of individuals with extensive coronary artery atherosclerosis (but no symptoms or signs of myocardial ischemia), the various possible causes of atherosclerosis, and the frequently small degree of coronary atherosclerosis observed in many patients with MI or SICD occurring as the very first manifestation of IHD.

Angina pectoris, MI, and SICD can each be caused by several different mechanisms: thus, the causes of IHD mortality can be multiple. About three-quarters of IHD-related deaths occur in individuals over the age of 65, and the increase in mortality from IHD with age is related not only to an increased incidence of IHD but also to a greater cardiac vulnerability to ischemic insults in old age. When the causes of a syndrome are multiple, the search for common risk factors is influenced by the prevalence of the type of patients included in the study group. For example, an analogy would be the search for a single common cause of anemia, which would be affected by the prevalence in the group studied of individuals with iron, vitamin B_{12}, or folic acid deficiencies and of hemoglobin or enzymatic defects; in turn, the prevalence of the cause among the population studied may vary according to living standards, ethnic grouping, and geographic location.

Past studies have established convincingly that individuals with severe coronary atherosclerosis have, in general, a much greater incidence of all ischemic syndromes. They have also established that individuals with high levels of known risk factors have significantly higher rates of mortality from IHD. However, although the predictive value of combined multiple risk factors is high, it identifies only some of the patients who die from IHD, as most of them have average levels of risk factors: conversely, some with high levels of risk factors may not develop IHD and may die from noncardiac causes in old age.

Future studies, therefore, should consider specifically two aspects of the disease:

1. Whether or not the three pathogenetic components of IHD outlined in the previous chapters, are associated individually with specific etiologic risk factors (known or as yet unknown) contributing to the development and outcome of the various ischemic syndromes.

It would be important to ascertain whether there are particular risk factors that favor the development of chronic stable angina and that are separate from other factors that favor the development of unstable angina and MI and also separate from yet others that favor the extension of MI, cardiac rupture, fatal arrhythmias, and SICD. For example, it is not known to what extent the reduction in the mortality rate from IHD consistently observed during the last few years in most industrialized countries, is attributable to a decreased incidence of coronary atherosclerosis, MI, mortality from MI, or SICD.

2. Whether all individuals (or only some) are susceptible to a given risk factor, so that screening and prevention could be targeted more specifically.

This chapter does not offer definite solutions to these complex problems, but analyses the data available in order to set the stage for the development of additional, more specific, preventive strategies, with special emphasis given to those aspects not currently receiving as much attention as already proven causal risk factors such as lipids, smoking, and hypertension.

12.1 RISK FACTORS AND IHD

Epidemiologic studies in different populations have shown that the rate of IHD-associated mortality is more obviously correlated with environmental factors than with race. Although reliable data are lacking for most Asian, African, and Latin American countries, it is believed that IHD is uncommon in nonindustrialized countries. There is at least a 10-fold variation in international rates of mortality from IHD. The higher rates appear to be broadly associated with the process of industrialization, with the notable exception of Japan. The variable incidence of IHD is commonly attributed to different dietary habits, but genetic, lifestyle, and cultural differences in low-risk populations such as the Japanese and French, and in high-risk populations such as the Finnish and Scottish, may also have important protective or causative roles.

Within the same country, the disease appears to be more prevalent in urban than in rural areas. For example, mortality rates in the industrialized states of the mid-West and Atlantic coast of the USA are higher than those in the rural areas of the Great Plains and mountain states. On the basis of differences in traditional risk factors, there is not always a satisfactory explanation for the fact that mortality from IHD varies from region to region in the same country, an example being the two- to threefold higher rate of mortality from IHD in the west of Scotland than in the densely populated south-east of England.

Observations on migrant populations provide further interesting material for speculation about racial, genetic, and environmental components. In the USA, the mortality rate from IHD in black Americans is similar to that of Caucasians and is many times higher than that of Negroes in Africa. Japanese who migrated to Hawaii and California have about twice the rate of IHD compared with those in Japan, but this is still less than one-half that of Caucasians. Migrants are not only exposed to different diets (a commonly invoked explanation), but also to different lifestyles and to the distress caused by cultural dysadaptation (see below).

Family clustering of IHD (suggestive of a genetic influence) has been observed when IHD brings about premature infarction, but this clustering cannot be clearly detected in subjects who develop MI past the age of 60. The mechanisms by which causative and protective environmental and genetic factors influence racial and individual vulnerability to the disease are still unknown. Some of these mechanisms may initiate, potentiate, or protect an individual from "atherosclerosis;" others may predispose to the development of, or provide protection from, MI and its fatal consequences (see below).

Correlations have been sought between statistical predictors of IHD (risk factors) and IHD mortality, as well as between risk factors and atherosclerosis.

The risk factors that have been explored so far have been selected from variables suggested by prevailing pathogenetic theories and by the ease with which they could be measured in population studies. Thus, for example, lipid risk factors began to be studied actively in the 1950s and have been pursued with much greater vigor and investment of resources than have coagulation, psychological, and inflammatory risk factors.

Risk factors can be causally related to IHD or may represent markers associated only indirectly with the disease through other variables. The final proof of causality is provided only by the reduction of the incidence of IHD after elimination or reduction of the risk factor.

■ *Proof that a risk factor is causally related to the development of IHD does not imply that it is causal in all individuals; it merely indicates that it is a determinant of the disease in a sufficiently large number of individuals in the population studied.* ■

12.1.1 Relative risk versus absolute risk

The impact of a risk factor in a population derives from the combination of two elements:

a. the relative risk that it confers on susceptible individuals above their baseline risk
b. the prevalence in the population of individuals susceptible to the risk factor (see Fig. 12.1).[2]

For any given level of risk factor, low-risk populations may lack hidden, associated risk factors that are present in the population at higher risk, may have protective factors that are lacking in the higher-risk population, or may have a lower prevalence of susceptible individuals. The explanation for the differences in the incidence of IHD among different populations on the basis of a single correlation that fits into a prevailing hypothesis (such as mean serum cholesterol levels or dietary habits), neglects other possible genetic, environmental, or cultural etiologic components.

The average importance of a risk factor in any community can be evaluated from the *relative risk* conferred by its presence (or a certain level of risk factor) compared with its absence (or a lower level). The most direct means of identifying the relative risk conferred by any given factor is represented by prospective population studies in healthy individuals categorized by risk factor levels. The number of new cases of IHD in individuals exposed to risk versus the number of cases in nonexposed individuals gives the relative risk conferred by the factor in that population.

Thus, risk factors can be broadly considered as multipliers of the *baseline risk* of the disease, which varies considerably with age and gender and among different populations because of the prevalence of genetic factors and other, as yet unidentified, environmental factors (see Table 12.1). Hence, the *absolute risk* is the product of the *relative risk* and the *baseline risk*.

A relative risk of 4, for example, indicates that individuals with that risk factor, or with that level of risk factor, have, on average, a fourfold probability of dying from IHD, compared with individuals with the baseline risk. Thus, a relative risk of 4 will result in an expected average absolute risk of IHD mortality of 0.2% per year in a group with an average baseline IHD mor-

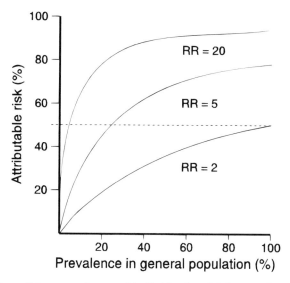

Fig. 12.1 Effect of the prevalence of individuals with increasing susceptibility to IHD on the average risk in the population. In general, for any given risk factor the average risk attributable to the total population increases progressively with the prevalence in the population of individuals susceptible to it. The practical implications of this concept are considerable: for example, for a given risk factor a 50% attributable risk to the total population can result from (a) a 100% prevalence of individuals with a risk ratio (RR) of 2, (b) a 25% prevalence of individuals with an RR of 5 or (c) a 5% prevalence of individuals with a RR of 20. For a given risk factor, only susceptible individuals require reduction of the risk; therefore, the reduction of the population attributable risk would be best achieved by identifying and treating highly susceptible individuals. (Modified from ref. 2.)

Table 12.1 Variables associated with IHD mortality: ratio of mortality rates. (Mortality rates for IHD are influenced to varying degrees by several modifiable variables. These are often present in the same individual, further increasing the risk.)

Variable	Comparison	Increase in mortality rate
Age (years)	80 vs 40	>100-fold
Population	East Finland vs Japan	>10-fold
Sex	Age-matched men vs premenopausal women	>6–8 fold
Family history*		>4–8 fold
Weight at birth (kg)	<2.5 vs >3.5	>2-fold
Total serum cholesterol (mg)	<165 vs >265	>4-fold (MRFIT)†
Systolic blood pressure (mmHg)	>150 vs random value <110	>3-fold
Smoking (no. of cigarettes/day)	>10 vs 0	>2-fold
Multiple risks	Upper‡ vs lower decile	>5-fold

* History of a first-degree relative with a history of myocardial infarction before the age of 60
† Multiple Risk Factor Intervention Trial (MRFIT)
‡ Smokers with cholesterol levels >285 mg, systolic blood pressure >150 mmHg (MRFIT)

tality of 0.05%, but in an absolute risk of 0.02% in a group with an average baseline risk of 0.005%.

The baseline risk varies considerably among different populations and with age within the same population. Age-adjusted IHD mortality rates can vary by a factor of about 10 in different countries and by a factor of at least three within the same country. Thus, for example, the relative risk conferred by increased cholesterol levels in the Framingham Study correctly predicted the risk ratio between lower and upper quintiles, but overestimated by 200% the rate of mortality from IHD actually observed in southern Europe.

The extent to which the differences in the incidence of IHD among populations are related to modifiable and nonmodifiable environmental or genetic risk factors is unknown. Differences in risk between populations have mainly been considered in terms of diet and its effect on serum cholesterol levels. Insufficient information is available about the following:

a. other dietary factors (such as fiber intake, types of fatty and amino acids, carbohydrate intake, and other components that could influence, for example, antioxidant levels in blood and tissues, as well as the procoagulant and anticoagulant activity of the blood)
b. cultural and psychosocial factors
c. nutritional state in the uterus and in infancy, and genetic predisposing or protective factors
d. the prevalence of subclinical infectious disease, viral or bacterial (see below).

The low incidence of IHD in Eskimos that is associated with their fish oil diet, received attention with respect to the potentially antithrombotic effects of the latter, but environmental, cultural, and genetic differences could also contribute to their low incidence of IHD. Within populations, the baseline risk varies with age, gender, family history, and regional environmental risk factors.

■ *The concept of absolute risk is as important as that of relative risk because, for the same variation in the relative risk, the change in the total number of cases affected is large only when the baseline risk is high.* ■

12.1.2 Quantitation of IHD risk

Population studies have assessed the importance of a number of nonmodifiable and modifiable risk factors for IHD-associated mortality.

Major *nonmodifiable* risk factors considered so far include age, gender, belonging to certain racial groups, and a family history of premature MI in first-degree relatives. They determine the baseline risk. Major *modifiable* risk factors considered so far include hypercholesterolemia, diastolic and systolic hypertension, smoking, and blood levels of fibrinogen.

By far the greatest risk of mortality from IHD is conferred by nonmodifiable risk factors. The baseline risk thus conferred is modulated by modifiable risk factors such as cigarette smoking, hypertension, and hypercholesterolemia. Modifiable risk factors account for about 50% of cases of IHD-related mortality;[3] conversely, in the Framingham study, 85% of individuals in the top quintile of risk remained free from IHD during 20 years of follow-up.[4] The conclusions of the Western Collaborative Study, after an 8½ year follow-up of 3154 employed men aged 39–59 years, can be taken as fair and representative of similar prospective studies. Three-quarters of men in the highest risk decile remained free from IHD over the period of follow-up and "even the combination of many known risk factors still falls significantly short of error-free prediction of coronary heart disease in middle aged males. . . . It appears, therefore, that other factors play an important pathogenetic role in the incidence of the disease."[5]

Major nonmodifiable risk factors

Age. Age is by far the *major* risk factor as the risk of death from IHD increases exponentially and is about 100-fold greater for an 80-year-old man than for a 40-year-old man (see Fig. 11.3). The higher risk of mortality from IHD with age is due not only to a higher incidence of MI but also to an exponential increase in mortality within 6 months of an acute MI, which results in an approximately 30-fold increase in mortality in 80-year-old compared with 40-year-old patients (see Ch. 10). Thus, age becomes the major determinant of mortality from MI in multivariate statistical analysis only when many individuals included in the study group are over the age of 65.

Gender. Gender is another major independent determinant of IHD mortality: for a 40-year-old man the risk of IHD-related mortality is 6–8 times greater than for a 40-year-old woman, but for a 65-year-old man the risk is reduced to about twice that for a woman of the same age. Women, however, appear more vulnerable to myocardial necrosis as the percentage of in-hospital mortality for acute MI in young and middle-aged women is about threefold greater than in young and middle-aged men (see Fig. 10.11). Mortality from IHD in women converges gradually with that of men at about the age of 90 and the percentage of mortality for hospitalized patients becomes nearly the same. There are no detectable discontinuities in the increase of mortality rates for IHD associated with the period of the menopause (see Fig. 11.3B).

Weight at birth. Weight at birth, at 3 months, and at 1 year is correlated inversely with the rate of IHD-associated mortality (see Fig. 12.2).[6] This correlation, observed also for other diseases such as chronic bronchitis, may be a marker of poor socio-economic conditions. This possibility is suggested by the correlations between the geographic distribution of IHD mortality and poor child health indicators, neonatal and postneonatal mortality rates between 1921 and 1925, and standardized mortality ratios in adults for IHD between 1968 and 1978 within the same geographic regions in England and Wales (see Fig. 12.3).[7] These correlations were attributed to an inverse relation between fetal growth and blood pressure during life and also to the long-term "programing" of metabolism during infancy in response to infant feeding.[8]

Genetic predisposition. The genetic differences that may predispose to IHD can be multiple and may have variable penetrance, depending on both their association in the same individual and the exposure to environmental factors. There is evidence of familial aggregation according to the type of IHD manifestation—fatal or non-fatal MI or angina (see below).[9,10] A genetic predisposition to IHD can derive from point mutations causing important dysfunctions of the low-density lipoprotein (LDL) pathway such as those described by Brown and Goldstein in their classic studies of familial hypercholesterolemia, and from point mutations in apoprotein genes (see Fig. 12.4).[11] Twin studies by Berg[12] suggest the importance of genetic factors controlling lipid metabolism at various levels, unrelated to the LDL pathway outlined in Fig. 12.4, including effects on lipoprotein (a) apoproteins, high-density lipoproteins (HDL), apoproteins and apoprotein E variations. In addition, genes

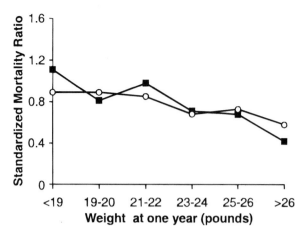

Fig. 12.2 Weight at 1 year is inversely correlated to IHD mortality. The lower the weight at 1 year, the higher the rate of mortality from IHD (■) later in life (○, all causes). On the abscissa, 1.0 refers to the average mortality rate in the population studied. The correlation is statistically significant. Low weight at 1 year is attributed to poor child health, which may influence the setting of blood pressure levels and metabolism and reduce body defenses in general. (From data in ref. 6.)

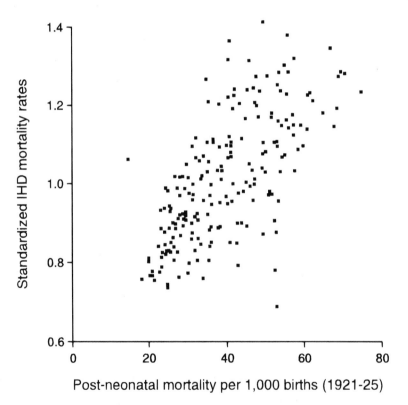

Fig. 12.3 The geographic distribution of standardized IHD mortality is correlated with infant mortality 50 years previously. In England and Wales, mortality rates for IHD between 1968 and 1978 are positively correlated with neonatal and postneonatal mortality rates in the same geographic regions in the years 1921–1925 ($r = 0.68$). On the abscissa 1.0 refers to the average mortality rate in the population studied. This correlation is similar to that found in mortality for chronic obstructive lung disease and was also attributed to the effects of poor child health later in life, as these geographic differences cannot be explained on the basis of known risk factors. (Modified from ref. 7.)

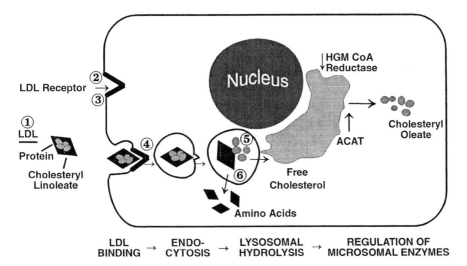

LDL → ENDO- → LYSOSOMAL → REGULATION OF
BINDING   CYTOSIS   HYDROLYSIS   MICROSOMAL ENZYMES

Fig. 12.4 Point mutations can alter sequential steps in the LDL pathway. The sites at which mutations have been found are identified by numbers: 1, abetalipoproteinemia; 2, familial hypercholesterolemia, receptor negative; 3, familial hypercholesterolemia, receptor defective; 4, familial hypercholesterolemia, internalization defect; 5, Wolman syndrome; 6, cholesteryl ester storage disease. HMG-CoA reductase denotes 3-hydroxy-3-methylglutaryl coenzyme-A reductase and ACAT denotes acyl-coenzyme A: cholesterol acyltransferase. Multiple genetic defects can also cause similar phenotypic alterations. (Modified from ref. 11.)

belonging to the low risk polymorphisms can influence blood lipid composition[13] and be associated with IHD.[14]

A genetic component of IHD, unrelated to known risk factors, is suggested by family clustering of MI in patients below the age of 60 (and especially below the age of 50), even after excluding cases with genetically determined dyslipidemias. The inheritability of MI in young individuals (after excluding cases related to lipid abnormalities) was estimated as 0.56,[15] which compares with the figure of 0.66 in monozygotic twin pairs (0.25 in dizygotic twin pairs).[12] In patients who develop MI before the age of 60, the number of first-degree relatives with infarction is significantly higher than that of matched controls, and patients with two first-degree relatives who developed infarction before the age of 60 may have a 20-fold risk of developing infarction.[16]

A deletion polymorphism in the gene for the angiotensin-converting enzyme (ACE) was found to be a potent risk factor for MI.[17] The association was especially strong in individuals with a low body-mass index and low plasma levels of ApoB. The risk may be associated with the presence of the DD genotype, which is associated with higher levels of circulating ACE than the ID and II genotypes. This enzyme has key roles in the production of angiotensin II and in the catabolism of bradykinin, two peptides involved in the control of vasomotor tone and in the proliferation of vascular smooth muscle cells. Insulin resistance-related increased risk of IHD may also be genetically determined (see below).

The penetrance of genetic defects. The penetrance of genetic defects favoring the development of IHD is variable, as infarction among monozygotic twins does not necessarily occur at a similar age. IHD may also develop at very different ages in patients with both homozygous and heterozygous familial hypercholesterolemia due to LDL-receptor defects,

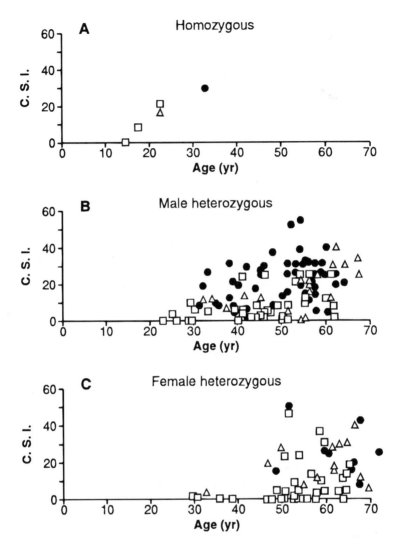

Fig. 12.5 Coronary stenoses and ischemic manifestations in patients with familial hypercholesterolemia. Homozygous patients had mean serum cholesterol levels of 592 ± 84 mg% and heterozygous men and women had levels of 322 ± 63 and 346 ± 68 mg%, respectively. Three homozygous patients (□) had no symptoms or signs of IHD, one had MI (●), one had angina (△) (**A**). In heterozygous men (**B**) and women (**C**) a very variable relationship between age, coronary stenosis index (CSI), and ischemic manifestations is apparent. The absence of IHD in some of these patients with very elevated serum cholesterol levels, in spite of advanced age, is in sharp contrast with the observation that 30% of patients with their first MI enrolled in the GISSI-2 study had cholesterol values below 190 mg%. (Modified from ref. 19.)

in spite of similar levels of serum cholesterol (see Fig. 12.5).[18] Among affected patients with homo- and heterozygous familial hypercholesterolemia, a large variability was observed between serum cholesterol levels and ischemic manifestations and coronary angiography stenosis score (see Fig. 12.5).[18] One-half of male patients younger than 50 years and one-quarter of those over 50 with mean serum cholesterol levels above 280 mg% had no symptoms or signs of IHD; the percentages for women were 60 and 50% respectively. These figures contrast sharply with the development of infarction in a substantial number of patients with serum cholesterol levels below 200 mg% (see below).

The prevalence of causative or protective genetic components of IHD is likely to vary in different populations and the effects may be age related.

■ *The study of the genetically determined components of IHD is made difficult by the variable penetrance of the genetic defects, by their variable prevalence in different populations and age groups, by the considerable interaction of environmental risk factors, and by the frequent unexpected death of many affected individuals, either at the time of first manifestation or soon after they manifest the disease, which prevents collection of their genomic DNA.* ■

Major modifiable risk factors

Total cholesterol. In middle-aged men, mortality from IHD is about four times higher in those with values of total cholesterol in the higher decile than in those with values in the lower decile: the gradient of risk increases continuously in a log-linear fashion for cholesterol levels in the same way that it does for values of diastolic and systolic arterial blood pressure (see Figs 12.6A,B).[19,20] However, 70% of mortality from IHD occurs in individuals with cholesterol levels below the upper quintile of risk. In the Framingham Study, the cholesterol-related gradient of risk of IHD in women was detectable only in the 40–50 age-group, and was not detectable in men over the age of 56. Furthermore, a 30-year follow-up of total and cardiovascular mortality was significantly related to serum cholesterol levels in men aged 31–39 years and, to a lesser extent, in those aged 40–55, but not in those aged between 56 and 65 years or in women of any age (see Fig. 12.7A–D).[21] In the same study, falling cholesterol levels over the first 14 years of follow-up were associated with increased cardiovascular mortality rates over the next 16 years.

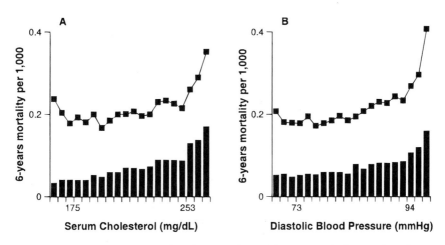

Fig. 12.6 Increase in IHD-related mortality with serum cholesterol and arterial blood pressure levels. Both mortality from IHD (black bars) and total mortality (squares) increase continuously as a function of total serum cholesterol levels (**A**) and diastolic arterial blood pressure (**B**). As the increase is markedly curvilinear for both variables, over two-thirds of fatal cases occur in individuals with risk levels below the upper quintile. Total mortality increases steeply only above the upper quintile. (Modified from ref. 19.)

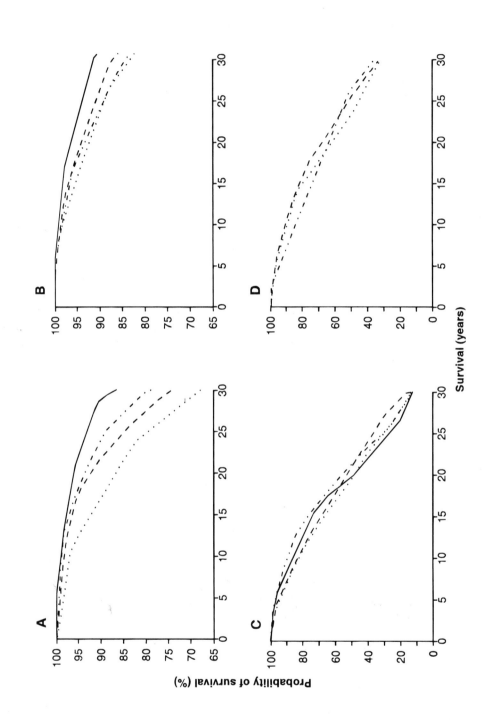

The average values of total serum cholesterol in population samples from different countries were found to be correlated with average IHD mortality in the whole country in men
(see Fig. 12.8),[22] but not in women; however, even in men, life expectancy was not related
to serum cholesterol values (see Fig. 12.9).[22,23] Moreover, gradients ranking populations in
approximately the same order as those in which average cholesterol levels rank IHD mor-

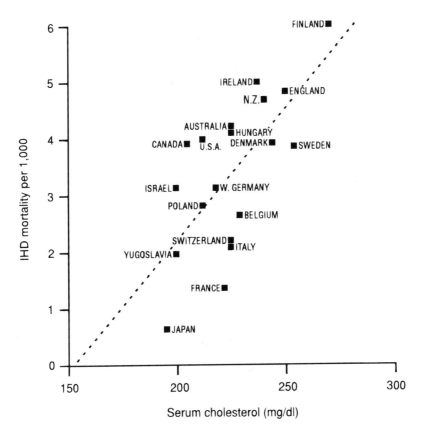

Serum cholesterol (mg/dl)

**Fig. 12.8 Relationships between IHD-related mortality rates and average val-
ues of serum cholesterol in different countries.** Mortality rates for IHD in men
vary over a nearly 10-fold range in different countries and were found to be correlated with average values of serum cholesterol assessed in population samples. This significant correlation is commonly taken as evidence of the causal relation between
serum cholesterol levels and IHD mortality, but this extrapolation does not appear to
be justified (see Figs 12.9–12.12). (Modified from ref. 22.)

Fig. 12.7 30-year mortality predicted by serum cholesterol levels. In the
Framingham study, survival over 30 years was influenced by the values of serum cholesterol (A–C: –, <181; ••–, 181–220; – –, 221–260, and •••, >260 mg cholesterol/dl;
D: ••–, <221; – –, 221–260, and •••, >260) only in young individuals. Life expectancy was influenced by cholesterol levels in men aged between 31 and 39 years (**A**) and,
to a lesser extent, in women in the same age range (**B**). Cholesterol levels had a smaller influence on individuals aged 40–47 and failed to influence mortality in men and
women aged 48–55 years at entry (**C, D**). A reduction of cholesterol during the first
14 years of follow-up was associated with an increased rate of cardiovascular mortality over the following 16 years. (Modified from ref. 21.)

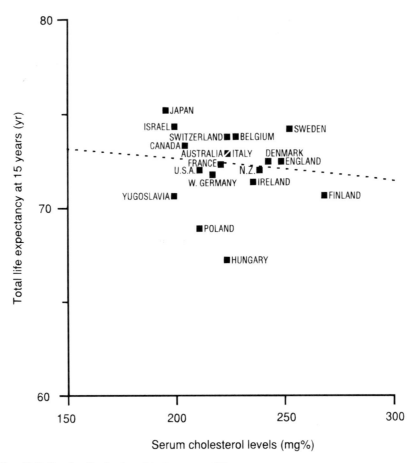

Fig. 12.9 Lack of relationship between life expectancy and serum cholesterol levels in the same countries depicted in Figure 12.8. Life expectancy for living male adolescents at age 15 is not correlated with the same average serum cholesterol levels that correlated with IHD death rates in Figure 12.8. (From data presented in refs 22 and 23.)

tality have been found for wine consumption (see Fig. 12.10)[24] and also for incidence of juvenile diabetes and mean yearly temperature (see Fig. 12.11).[25] These observations suggest that correlations between variables measured in samples of individuals and events in average populations should be considered with caution before interpreting the association as causal. The results of the prospective MONICA study[26] organized by the World Health Organization failed to confirm the close correlation observed in previous studies between median cholesterol levels and IHD mortality in different countries (see Fig. 12.12).

In the classic study by Goldstein et al[27] on 500 3-month survivors of MI under 60 years of age, 31% had hyperlipidemia, more commonly men under the age of 40 (60% frequency) and women under the age of 50 (60% frequency). Elevation of serum cholesterol values alone was found in 7.6% of cases. The prevalence of individuals with genetic forms of hypercholesterolemia is low: cases of heterozygous familial hypercholesterolemia are estimated as 1 in 500, cases of familial combined hyperlipidemia are estimated as 1 in 300, and cases of familial dysbetalipoproteinemia are estimated as 1 in 10 000 subjects.

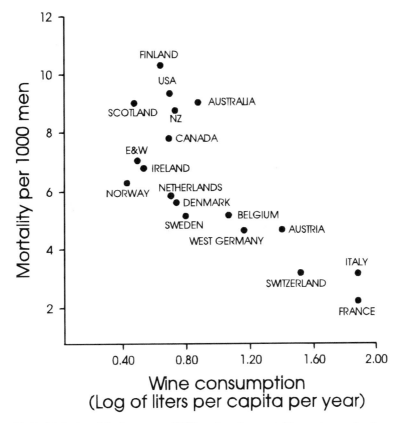

Fig. 12.10 Relationship between IHD-related mortality rates and wine consumption in different countries. A strong negative association between deaths from IHD in men aged 55–64 years and wine consumption was interpreted as a possible protective effect of alcohol. The observed relation is similar to that observed in Figure 12.8 for serum cholesterol levels and mortality. Data for Japan and China, however, where both wine consumption and IHD-related mortality are very low, are not included in the figure or in the calculation. The interpretation as causal of an association between variables observed in different countries must be very guarded. (Modified from ref. 24.)

Among the 9720 patients with their first infarction enrolled in the Gruppo Italiano per lo Studio della Sopravvivenza nell'Infarto Miocardio-2 (GISSI-2) study, 30% had serum cholesterol values on admission less than 190 mg% and 10% less than 170 mg%.[28] In contrast, only 10.3% of 2789 men with MI in the Coronary Drug Project placebo group[29] had cholesterol values below 200 mg%, suggesting that important unknown pathogenetic factors are superimposed over a variable distribution of cholesterol levels in different populations, consistent with findings in population studies. IHD is lower than would be expected in southern France despite high serum cholesterol levels and widespread cigarette smoking.[30,31] The results of the Russian Lipid Research Clinics Program showed a J-shaped cholesterol/IHD relationship for both total and LDL-cholesterol in the two lowest quintiles and no relation with HDL-cholesterol.[32]

The increased risk conferred by raised total serum cholesterol levels seems to be related to elevated levels of LDL-cholesterol, but the individual susceptibility to LDL-cholesterol may be

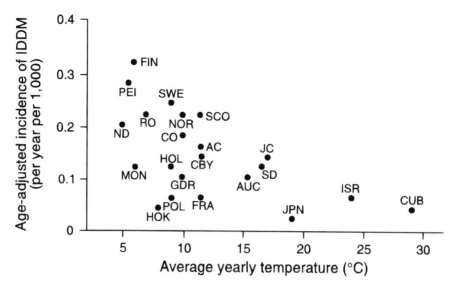

Fig. 12.11 Relationship between the incidence of juvenile diabetes (IDDM) and average yearly temperatures in different countries. The relationship between the incidence of juvenile diabetes and average yearly temperatures ranks countries in an order similar to that in which average cholesterol levels rank IHD mortality rates. (Modified from ref. 25.)

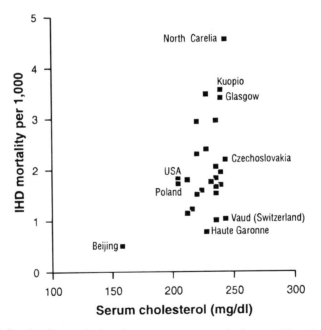

Fig. 12.12 Lack of correlation between average cholesterol levels and IHD-related annual mortality rates in the MONICA project. The findings of the WHO-organized MONICA project, in which risk factors and the development of IHD were correlated in selected areas of different countries, showed no relation between serum cholesterol levels and rates of annual IHD-related mortality. These carefully collected data raise further questions about the common interpretation of the correlation reported in Figure 12.8. (Based on data from ref. 26.)

modulated by factors that influence its oxidation (see below). Information currently available on reduced levels of HDL-cholesterol is less conclusive: some studies have indicated that it is inversely associated with an increased risk of IHD; however, in six prospective studies in which it was measured at initial examination, the differences in the concentrations of HDL-cholesterol between individuals who developed MI and those who did not was of the order of only 0.1 mм/l. In only some studies does HDL-cholesterol remain a significant factor in multivariate regression analysis. In one study,[33] low values of HDL-cholesterol alone was found to be the most common type of dyslipidemia in patients with premature IHD (19.3% versus 4.4% in controls). So far, the proof of causality for HDL-cholesterol (i.e. a reduction of risk by elevation of HDL-cholesterol) is lacking.

Although the elevated concentration of serum triglycerides has emerged as a positive risk factor for IHD in univariate analysis, it does not retain an independent relationship with major IHD events in multivariate analysis.[34] Indeed, serum triglycerides are significantly positively correlated with total body-mass index, total and LDL-cholesterol, insulin resistance, and the presence of diabetes and are marginally correlated with HDL-cholesterol.

A markedly elevated level of serum cholesterol is a proven causal factor for IHD in middle-aged men because its reduction lowers cardiovascular mortality and nonfatal ischemic events. This proof is not yet available for women, for elderly individuals, and for moderately elevated values of serum cholesterol. No definite proof of causality is yet available for the other lipid abnormalities mentioned above; as they are so numerous and so prevalent, it is possible that at least one may be found in most individuals with IHD, but, however plausible they might appear, they cannot be considered causal until proven so.

It is worth noting that many patients with heterozygous familial hypercholesterolemia die in their sixties or even later, whereas many patients who die in their forties or fifties have cholesterol levels below 200 mg%, suggesting either a major role of a very variable individual susceptibility to this risk factor or that other risk factors are of major importance.

Cigarette smoking. For subjects smoking more than 10 cigarettes a day, the risk is at least double that of nonsmokers; heavy smokers have a higher risk than moderate smokers. Cessation of smoking abolishes the increased risk within 1 year, thus proving its causal role.[35]

Blood pressure. For subjects with a random reading of systolic blood pressure levels greater than 150 mmHg, the risk is three times that of subjects with systolic blood pressure levels less than 110 mmHg. In the Multiple Risk Factor Intervention (MRFIT) study, IHD mortality in subjects with diastolic blood pressure levels of 100 mmHg was three times that of those with diastolic blood pressure levels of 70 mmHg. In addition, systolic blood pressure levels are linearly related to IHD mortality, with a continuous gradient of risk from 100 mmHg upwards (see Fig. 13.3) and, in the elderly, systolic blood pressure is a better predictor of IHD risk than diastolic blood pressure.[20]

Control of hypertension is associated with a reduction of IHD risk, indicating a causal role for clearly hypertensive levels, but a causal relationship is not clearly proven for moderate elevation of diastolic blood pressure or for systolic blood pressure levels (see below).

Fibrinogen. The difference in the relative risk between subjects with fibrinogen levels in the higher or lower tertiles was about twofold in the Framingham Study and, in men, the risk increased linearly. The gradient of risk was highest in 50-year-old women and was absent in 70-year-old men.[36] The relative risk was about fourfold in the Northwick Park study.[37] Blood levels of fibrinogen were better predictors of major IHD events than serum cholesterol levels in a British study[38] and they also have synergistic effects with cholesterol and blood pressure levels, which lose considerable prognostic value with the presence of low levels of fibrinogen.[39,40] It is not clear whether the association is causal, as an elevated level of fibrinogen is associated with smoking, increased blood viscosity, platelet aggregation,[41] white cell count[38] and with job stress[42] and may also be a marker of an enhanced acute phase reaction (see below).

Psychosocial factors and stress. Although these are often not considered to be major risk factors, inquiring physicians cannot help being impressed by the very frequent reports (particularly among young and middle-aged patients) of the occurrence of distressing emotional situations, which the patient found difficult to overcome, before the onset of acute MI.

As discussed in Chapter 9, this emotional distress results from a combination of the intensity and duration of the stress and on the patient's sensitivity to it, which, in turn, is influenced not only by personality, but also by cultural background, psychological stability, and levels of social support. The difficulty in assessing accurately the complex balance between distressing events and emotional reactions has led to approaches that have considered either personality as a factor separate from socioenvironmental distress, or stressful events separate from personality, social support, and the cultural ability to cope. On the one hand, the consideration of personality type alone does not take into account whether types A and B individuals are fulfilled or frustrated by their lives, have social support or lack it, and whether they are able or unable to cope with their problems. On the other hand, studies that focus on life events and occupational stress consider neither an individual's personality, cultural ability to cope, levels of social support, nor levels of fulfilment or frustration. Thus, neither approach considers adequately the relationship between the intensity of stress and the ability to cope resulting in distress and frustration. Chronic dysadaptation, inability to cope, distress, frustration, and dissatisfaction can predispose indirectly to IHD by favoring the clustering of risk factors (see below), and acute distress may directly favor the development of acute ischemic events.

According to these considerations, it may not be surprising that the predictive value of a type A personality reported in the Western Collaborative study[5] was not confirmed in the MRFIT study.[43] However, the Civil Servant Study[44,45] indicated that the mortality rate for IHD (as well as the rate of total mortality) is significantly higher for the lower employment grades than for executives. Within each employment grade, mortality was correlated with cholesterol levels, thus indicating a strong synergistic prognostic effect between these two risk factors. The mechanisms through which socioeconomic risk factors contribute to IHD mortality, independent of other risk factors such as serum cholesterol levels, may also be related to poor living standards at birth and thereafter.[8]

Minor modifiable risk factors

For minor modifiable risk factors, the association with IHD mortality is even less obvious. Each factor may be casual, resulting from its association with known major risk factors or other unidentified mechanisms, or may be a marker of dysadaptation.

Obesity. This is an independent risk factor when an individual is 30% or more overweight. The independent role of lower levels of obesity (a fairly common tendency as about 20% of individuals in the USA are 20% over their ideal weight) is uncertain because of its frequent association with other major risk factors and the variability of criteria used to define obesity. In the Framingham Study it is interesting to note that an individual's recollection of being over-weight at the age of 25 was the strongest indicator of the development of IHD in the following 30 years.

Diet. Patients who developed IHD were consistently found to have, on average, a lower calorific intake than unaffected individuals. As the inverse correlation between energy intake and IHD is even stronger when related to body weight, it was interpreted as an indication that the individuals who developed IHD had, on average, a lower level of physical activity.

The percentage of calories derived from saturated fatty acids and a low ratio of polyunsaturated to saturated fatty acids (P/S ratio) was found to be highly correlated with total serum cholesterol levels and the incidence of IHD among different populations, but not within single countries and cultures. This certainly does not explain, for example, the doubled rate of incidence of mortality from IHD in Scotland compared with the south-east of England.

The intake of dietary cholesterol usually contributes only about 10% to serum cholesterol levels, which are mainly determined by LDL receptors, regulation of endogenous cholesterol synthesis, lipoprotein kinetics, and intestinal reabsorption of bile acids. A Mediterranean diet is commonly thought to be associated with a lower incidence of mortality from IHD, but the mortality rates from MI in Italy (which has a Mediterranean diet) are the same as those in Switzerland and Austria (which do not).[23]

Alcohol. Although heavy drinking is associated with an increased mortality from IHD, individuals who consume moderate amounts of alcohol have about a 30% lower incidence of IHD than teetotalers.

Physical activity. Sedentary individuals present a somewhat higher (about double) incidence of IHD than individuals engaged in regular physical activity. However, there is no hard evidence that more intense physical activity may further reduce the risk of IHD.

Diabetes. Diabetes increases the risk of IHD, independent of associated risk factors such as hypertension, obesity, and serum lipid alterations. Notably, premenopausal women with type 1 diabetes have the same incidence of IHD as men in the same age group. The risk of IHD in individuals with insulin resistance is discussed in 12.1.3.

Hyperuricemia. Although this is associated with IHD, it appears to be an indirect indicator of the metabolic abnormalities associated with IHD, as elevated concentrations of serum uric acid were not found to be independent predictors of IHD.

Estrogens. The reason for the sixfold lower incidence of IHD in women than in men under 45 is not known. The beneficial effects of estrogen on IHD mortality in postmenopausal women are reasonably well established, but administration of estrogen in men appears to *increase* IHD mortality. Oral contraceptives increase the risk of infarction by two- to fourfold, and up to 20-fold in heavy smokers over the age of 35. The mechanisms of this deleterious effect are not known but are not related to the more obvious development of angiographically detectable coronary atherosclerosis.

Blood viscosity. Blood viscosity, which is closely correlated with fibrinogen blood levels, may also play a part in occlusive coronary thrombosis, but this risk factor has received little attention.

Because of the multiplicity of putative risk factors, the development of IHD in almost all patients may be blamed on the risk factor present, without due consideration being given to the fact that virtually everyone has at least one major or minor risk factor. Blind acceptance of readily available plausible explanations hinders the search for the precise causes of the disease.

12.1.3 Clustering of modifiable, causal risk factors

Major causal modifiable risk factors tend to cluster in individuals and populations, and this clustering often represents a consequence of social, cultural, and personal dysadaptation and/or of a genetic predisposition. Lipid and coagulation abnormalities often coexist and may be interrelated.[46] Smoking is correlated with distress and coagulation abnormalities. Insulin resistance is correlated with hypertension, lipid abnormalities, and elevated levels of acute-phase proteins (see below). Heart rate is correlated with atherogenic blood lipid fractions.[47] Obesity during adolescence is correlated with subsequent IHD events in adulthood and old age independent of adult weight.[48] The importance of a single putative risk factor may, therefore, be indirect and influenced by its prevalence compared with other risk factors in the group studied. Environmental and genetic risk factors seem to have multiplicative effects when they are combined.

Dysadaptation

The role of cultural dysadaptation can be inferred from the differences in IHD mortality rates in various countries, among rural, urban, and migrant populations. The much higher population density and faster pace of life, together with the much lower levels of social support in urban than in rural areas (which applies also to migrant populations), can favor dysadaptation. Social dysadaptation can cause clustering of risk factors in two ways:

a. by favoring the development of established risk factors such as hypertension, hypercholesterolemia, smoking, obesity, physical inactivity, and diabetes (all of which tend to cluster in most populations with a high rate of mortality from IHD)
b. by contributing to psychological distress and inability to cope.

Assortative mating for lifestyle and risk factors was proposed in order to explain the increased occurrence of MI in the relatives or wives of survivors of MI.[49]

Genetic predisposition

Clustering of hypertension, hypertriglyceridemia, low plasma levels of HDL-cholesterol, and insulin resistance have been observed in patients with IHD as part of a metabolic disorder defined as metabolic syndrome X, possibly genetically determined.[50-52] Resistance to insulin-stimulated glucose uptake and hyperinsulinemia can be associated with IHD, not only through the associated known risk factors but also directly, as insulin is known to be directly atherogenic and an impaired glucose tolerance can be an independent risk factor for IHD. Endogenous hyperinsulinemia is associated with an increased risk of IHD in immigrants from the Indian subcontinent in London, although they have low plasma levels of LDL-cholesterol, and elevated levels of plasminogen activator inhibitor-1 (PAI-1) and acute-phase reactants (C-reactive protein and fibrinogen) in angina pectoris.[53]

Interaction of environmental and genetic factors

Interaction of genetic and environmental risk factors may, for example, influence blood lipid levels[9,10] and may have a combined effect on the development of IHD. Hypercholesterolemia and smoking have been found to be multiplicative, rather than additive, risk factors for MI in patients with a family history of MI in first-degree relatives below the age of 60.[16] Environmental or genetic protective factors may account for the variable penetrance of genetic defects associated with IHD.

Practical implications of risk factor clustering

The first implication is that the clustering of risk factors can identify patients at high risk of developing IHD; however, as previously indicated, the greater the specificity of multiple combined predictors, the lower the sensitivity, as most patients with IHD are those without such high levels of risk factor clustering. In population screening, the overall quantitative predictive power of major known combined modifiable risk factors is exemplified by the results of a major study. The MRFIT study[19] demonstrates that, of 361 662 men aged between 37 and 57 years who were screened in lipid clinics in the USA, 12 866 (3.6%) were identified as being in the top 10% at risk of developing IHD, as estimated from the Framingham data. During the 6-year follow-up, the rate of mortality from IHD among that highly selected group was about 0.25% a year—about four times that of individuals in the lower 10% of risk, who had a mortality rate of about 0.06% per year.

This relatively low gradient of risk implies that not only the vast majority of deaths from IHD occurred in the 358 796 individuals who were in the group with risk factors below the top 10%, but also that only a small minority of those in the top decile of risk died.

■ *Thus, although they are significant indications of risk for the population at large, even combined risk factors have a rather low sensitivity and specificity in clinical practise.* ■

The second implication is that intervention against one risk factor in individuals who also have others (and, hence, a higher baseline risk) may produce a larger reduction in the total number of cases of IHD for the same reduction in relative risk. Concentrating on the reduction of a single risk factor alone, however, may give the false impression that the total risk is being dealt with (see Ch. 13).

■ *Thus, when the population attributable risk is considered, it is possible only to adopt an approach of global risk factor reduction until more specific risk factors and vulnerable individuals are identified (see Ch. 13).* ■

12.1.4 Major risk factors and coronary atherosclerosis

In postmortem studies the relationship of coronary atherosclerosis with major risk factors has been assessed in different populations. The major finding of the International Atherosclerosis Project[54] was that "many (almost all) people have atherosclerosis, while relatively few have clinical disease due to atherosclerosis." "Atherosclerosis" included gross lesions (not fatty streaks) manifested by fibrous plaques, calcified lesions, and lesions complicated by hemorrhage, ulceration, and thrombosis. On a group basis, the severity of mural atherosclerosis in different populations was found to be closely associated with the incidence of IHD. The severity of mural atherosclerosis could not, however, be considered to be "the only condition determining risk of clinical disease due to atherosclerosis." This conclusion was supported by the "wide variety in the extent of lesions among patients who have died of IHD" and also by the "failure to detect stenosis (greater than 40% reduction of luminal diameter) in approximately one-third of the persons who had myocardial scarring." A striking variability in the severity of atherosclerosis was observed even in the most homogeneous groups. This was the major common finding of all the centers participating in the study.

As reported in Chapter 8, the percentage of the surface of epicardial coronary arteries covered by raised plaque is very large in many individuals without IHD and, in general, it ranks the geographic and ethnic groups in the same order as their average incidence of mortality from IHD. The severity of age-related atherosclerosis in the various geographic locations and racial groups suggests that etiologic environmental agents do not initiate a detectably different process in high-risk populations, but, in general, enhance a process that occurs to some degree in most human beings. However, even in populations with the highest average severity of atherosclerosis, some individuals have only minimal atherosclerosis, even in old age, thus providing evidence that the process cannot simply be related to aging.

The extent of raised lesions and the presence of coronary artery stenoses are both fairly weakly correlated with total serum cholesterol levels[55] (see Fig. 12.13), with a large scatter of values about the average relationship, but neither are correlated with systolic blood pressure levels[56] or smoking[57] (see Figs 12.14 and 12.15). In the Oslo Study, HDL-cholesterol was found to be correlated inversely with the extent of coronary atherosclerosis. Correlations between total and HDL-cholesterol levels and raised lesions are much weaker than those between the extent of raised lesions and the presence of coronary stenoses. The correlation coefficient between total serum cholesterol and raised lesions was 0.38 and was slightly lower with stenoses reducing the diameter more than 40% in one, two, or three coronary arteries. Conversely, the correlation coefficients between raised lesions and critical stenoses of one, two, or three coronary arteries ranged between 0.68 and 0.76.[58] In addition, an association between severity of coronary artery obstructions (assessed by angiography) and major risk factors can be observed in vivo, but it is fairly weak.

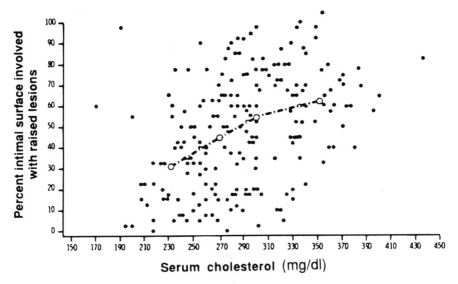

Fig. 12.13 Weak correlation between serum cholesterol levels and coronary atherosclerosis. The percentage of the intima of the main epicardial coronary arteries covered by raised fibrous plaque is weakly correlated to cholesterol levels. The average correlation indicated by the circles joined by the dashed line is often presented as an illustrative example of the relation of baseline serum cholesterol levels and coronary atherosclerosis. The very large dispersion of individual data points about the average values indicates that some individuals have a remarkable degree of protection against the adverse effects of cholesterol, whereas others are very susceptible or have other important causal factors. (Modified from ref. 55.)

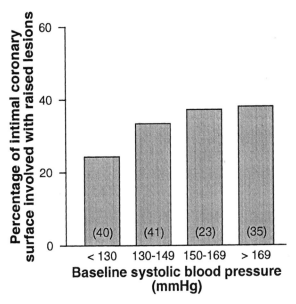

Fig. 12.14 Lack of relationship between values of systolic blood pressure and coronary atherosclerosis. The percentage of the intima of the main epicardial coronary arteries covered by raised fibrous plaques is not related to the values of systolic blood pressure. The linear relationship between IHD mortality and systolic blood pressure values presented in Figure 12.6 does not, therefore, appear to be mediated by the development of coronary atherosclerosis. (Modified from ref. 56.)

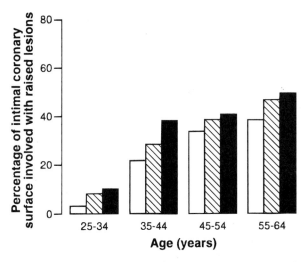

Fig. 12.15 Lack of relationship between cigarette smoking and coronary atherosclerosis. The percentage of the intima of the main epicardial coronary arteries covered by raised fibrous plaque is not related to cigarette smoking (□, non-smokers; ▨, 1–24; ■, ⩾25 cigarettes/day). The increased risk of IHD conferred by smoking does not, therefore, appear to be mediated by the development of coronary atherosclerosis. (Modified from ref. 57.)

In a subgroup of 8807 patients registered in the Coronary Artery Surgery Study (CASS),[59] 6688 had stenoses that reduced the diameter by more than 50%, 417 had stenoses with less than 50% diameter reduction and 1702 had no angiographic evidence of coronary athero- sclerotic stenosis. In this large subgroup, age, gender, cigarette smoking, and serum choles- terol levels best distinguished the groups with and without evidence of coronary stenoses. In male patients 36–55 years of age, total serum cholesterol levels were 218 mg in those with- out, and 239 mg in those with, angiographic evidence of the disease. The difference was smaller in those aged 56–65 years—214 mg in those without stenoses versus 228 mg in those with stenoses. At all ages, the variability in the relation between blood cholesterol levels and severity of coronary atherosclerosis was very wide.

The weak association, observed in postmortem and angiographic studies, between coro- nary atherosclerosis and major risk factors indicates that major known risk factors are of limited value in predicting which individuals would have extensive coronary atherosclerosis at postmortem or flow-limiting stenoses on angiography.

■ *The causal relationship of risk factors with IHD mortality is not mediated, therefore, merely by the formation of the chronic atherosclerotic background.* ■

12.1.5 Risk factors and individual ischemic syndromes

The association of major known risk factors with angina, non-fatal MI, and SICD is less clear than that with IHD mortality, not only because angina is a soft endpoint in epidemi- ologic studies, but also because the incidence of non-fatal MI cannot be assessed accurate- ly in epidemiologic studies, and cases of SICD include very heterogeneous groups of patients in various stages of IHD, with or without hyperacute MI. Although the relationship is consistent with that observed for IHD mortality, suggesting that in many patients these syndromes may have common underlying risk factors, the association with major known risk factors is not exactly the same in the various ischemic syndromes.

Studies of family clustering of MI demonstrate a strong association with premature MI, but not with angina or SICD in first-degree relatives. Uncomplicated angina pectoris was found to be associated with lipid abnormalities that differed from those associated with MI in school children with a family history of unheralded MI or uncomplicated chronic stable angina.

Rissanen and Nikkilä[9,10] found that levels of serum triglycerides were higher in the relatives of patients with chronic stable angina than in controls, whereas levels of total cholesterol were similar. Conversely, levels of serum cholesterol were higher in the relatives of patients with MI than in controls, whereas levels of triglycerides were similar to those of controls. Crea et al[60] found that, among 1000 schoolchildren, those with family histories of MI had an LDL/HDL-cho- lesterol ratio significantly higher than that found in controls. In children with family histories of uncomplicated chronic stable angina, the ratio was lower than in controls. Conversely, levels of serum HDL-cholesterol and apolipoprotein A_1 were higher in children with family histories of stable angina than in either children with family histories of MI or controls.

12.1.6 Atherosclerosis and risk factors in cardiac, cerebral, and peripheral ischemic syndromes

The widespread notion of a common atherosclerotic background and common risk factors for cardiac, cerebral, and peripheral vascular ischemic syndromes is suggested by the common development of infarction, stroke, and peripheral vascular disease in the same patient. This association suits the inclination to attribute all ischemic syndromes to a common atherosclerotic process, generally related to known established risk factors. However, this association is found much more frequently in older and diabetic patients than in individuals below the age of 60. The involvement of the intima of epicardial coronary arteries by raised fibrous plaques was found to be higher in patients who died of IHD than in those who died of other vascular diseases or of other causes (see Fig. 12.16).[56]

The first most notable discrepancy is observed in patients with familial hypercholesterolemia. In homozygous patients, cholesterol accumulation at the level of the aortic valve can be sufficient to cause severe aortic stenosis, with extensive coronary artery obstructions and IHD; nevertheless, cerebral and peripheral vascular diseases are extremely rare in such patients. Heterozygous patients also have a much higher incidence of IHD than of cerebral and periph-

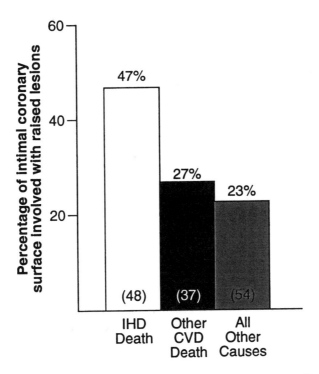

Fig. 12.16 Coronary atherosclerosis in patients who died of IHD and other cardiovascular causes. The percentage of the coronary intimal surface covered by raised fibrous plaque is greater in patients who died of IHD (□) than in patients who died of other vascular diseases (■) or from all other causes (■). This finding suggests a differential involvement of different vascular beds by atheroma in cardiac and peripheral or cerebral vascular syndromes. (Modified from ref. 56.)

eral vascular disease. The second discrepancy is that patients with genetically determined familial dysbetalipoproteinemia are much more prone to peripheral vascular disease than to IHD.[61] Lastly, patients without genetically determined familial dyslipidemias, who develop cerebral or peripheral vascular diseases below the age of 60, have a different lipoprotein risk factor profile than those who develop IHD below the age of 60.[62] They also have a more frequent family history of stroke or peripheral vascular disease than of MI, suggesting that, in younger individuals, family clustering may be specific for cerebral or peripheral vascular disease or IHD. Unselected patients with peripheral vascular disease were found to have a higher incidence of smoking and a higher frequency of specific fibrinogen genotype than patients with IHD, but a lower incidence of elevated apolipoprotein A.[63–65]

In elderly individuals and diabetic patients, the severity and extent of vascular damage are likely to progress and spread to various vascular beds, whatever their predisposing or precipitating mechanisms. When the vascular damage is extensive and severe, the probability of ischemic manifestations developing in multiple districts becomes higher, because even minor ischemic stimuli can cause gross damage and also because a prothrombotic state may develop as a result of the extent of the chronic vascular damage.

Analysis of risk factors in patients presenting with their first cardiac, cerebral, or peripheral vascular ischemic syndrome, would allow the investigation of the individual association of each ischemic syndrome with risk factors.

■ *The differences between the prevalence of a disease-specific family history and of risk factors among cardiac, cerebral, and peripheral vascular ischemic syndromes, indicate that they may not always be the expression of a random occurrence of ischemic manifestations in different vascular beds on the same common type of atherosclerotic background.* ■

12.1.7 Risk factors for IHD and life expectancy

As over three-quarters of the incidence of mortality from IHD occurs in individuals above the age of 65, it is interesting to examine the effects of risk factors on life expectancy in different populations. As illustrated in Figures 12.8 and 12.9, the wide differences in IHD mortality rates from country to country, associated with mean levels of serum cholesterol, are not accompanied proportionately by differences in mean life expectancy. These findings are consistent with those of the Framingham Heart study (see Fig. 12.17). This observation suggests that, within a given population, individuals above a certain age who do not die of IHD are exposed to other causes of death that contribute importantly to determine their life span. If mortality from cardiac causes were eliminated, the calculated increase in life expectancy would be about 5.8 years (see Fig. 12.17) if the age-specific rate of mortality from each of the other causes remained constant. Individuals spared from cardiac death, however, become exposed to other causes of death and the anticipated prolongation of life would thus be about 2.5 years.[66]

The risk factors that mostly reduce life expectancy, therefore, are those associated with premature IHD mortality and with other causes of mortality. The most typical example of premature IHD mortality is homozygous familial hypercholesterolemia, but the general relationship between serum cholesterol levels and ischemic manifestations is very variable and only weakly related to age (see Fig. 12.5). Typical examples of risk factors for IHD that are also associated with other diseases are cigarette smoking (strongly associated with the development of lung and other forms of cancer, as well as with chronic, obstructive lung disease) and systolic and diastolic hypertension (strongly associated with cerebrovascular dis-

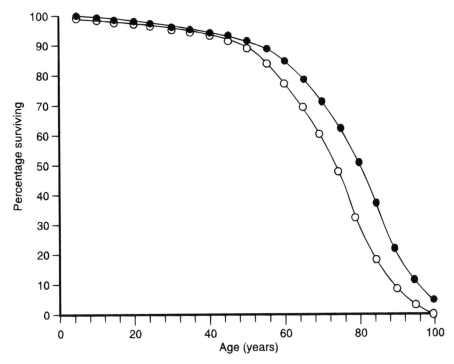

Fig. 12.17 Effect of theoretical elimination of all cardiac causes of death on life expectancy in the population. The prolongation of life expectancy calculated assuming the elimination of all cardiac causes of death (●) in white males in the USA (based on 1980 estimates) is of about 5 years, assuming that the age-specific mortality from each of the other causes (○) remains unchanged. However, as individuals spared from death from IHD are at risk of other causes of death, elimination of cardiac mortality would extend life expectancy by about 2.5 years. (Modified from ref. 66.)

ease). Additionally, although levels of serum cholesterol in young men are predictive of the subsequent development of cardiovascular disease, they do not predict the overall risk of death.

■ *Correction of risk factors that are not associated with premature IHD mortality or with other causes of mortality, may not result in a significant increase in life expectancy or even in a detectable reduction of total mortality* ■.

Decreasing rates of mortality from IHD

Mortality rates for IHD are declining progressively in most industrialized countries and increasing progressively in eastern European countries. In the USA, the total number of deaths from all causes was 1 930 082 among an estimated midyear population of 198 million in 1968 and 1 924 000 among an estimated population of 218 million in 1978. Over this period, mortality from IHD declined from 674 747 to 641 140.[67]

The reduction in IHD mortality rates is similar in all age groups and also in men and women, but its time course differs from that of all other causes of death and of stroke (see Fig. 12.18).[68] The decline in IHD mortality may result not only from a decrease in the num-

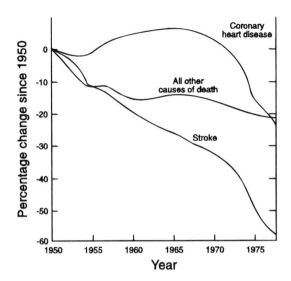

Fig. 12.18 Changes in IHD-related mortality rates from 1950 to 1978 in the USA. This figure exemplifies the difficulties encountered in establishing the reasons for the recent decrease in mortality from IHD in most industrialized countries. The decrease follows an increase up to 1965 when the decline began, too early to be accounted for by the effects of the campaign for the control of risk factors or the introduction of coronary care units or bypass surgery. The decline in IHD mortality followed that for stroke, which occurred despite the increasing longevity of the population and began before antihypertensive therapy was widely adopted. Thus, opportunistic interpretations of mortality trends should be considered with great caution. (Modified from ref. 69.)

ber of cases of IHD but also from an enhanced resistance to ischemic insults and a consequent reduction in the number of fatalities. This latter possibility is suggested by the lack of any consistent downward trend in hospital discharge rates for acute MI in the USA.[69] The possibility of a decline in the number of fatalities from IHD, rather than in the incidence of MI, is also suggested by the lack of change in the incidence and mode of first presentation of IHD in the Rochester Heart study over the years 1954–1982 (see Fig. 12.19A,B).[70]

This progressive reduction of IHD mortality is generally attributed to improved cardiac care by cardiologists and to the improved control of risk factors by community health experts, but the precise causes are not known. It should be stressed that the decline began in 1965 in the USA (i.e. before the campaign for risk reduction) and 10 years later in England and Wales, and in all it was preceded by a progressive increase that still persists in some eastern European countries (see Fig. 12.20).[71] The causes of this rise and fall are complex,[8] and may include improved living standards and infant nutrition and other environmental causes responsible for changes occurring in other diseases. No substantial changes in the estimated total and fat-attributable calorie intake was observed in the USA and Italy over the years 1955–1980 (see Fig. 12.21).[72] In addition, the decline in cigarette smoking does not appear sufficient to account for the decrease.[72]

First presentation of IHD

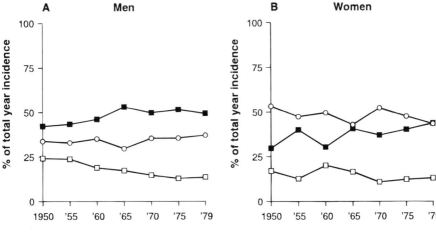

Fig. 12.19 Changes in the mode of first presentation of IHD. The mode of first presentation of IHD in the Rochester Heart Study for men (**A**) and women (**B**) from 1954 to 1987 shows a trend for a large percentage decrease in SICD (□), a small percentage increase of MI (■) in men and a small percentage decrease of angina (○) in women. (Modified from ref. 71.)

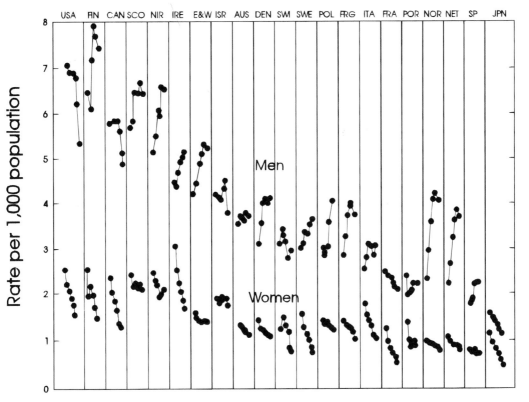

Fig. 12.20 Trends in mortality from heart disease in different countries from 1950 to 1976. Large changes in IHD mortality rates in men (upper waves) and women (lower waves), often in opposite directions, were observed in different countries over the years. When globally considered, these variations cannot be easily related to any known plausible cause and exemplify the complexity of the epidemiology of IHD. Each column represents the period 1950–76 for each country. (Modified from ref. 71.)

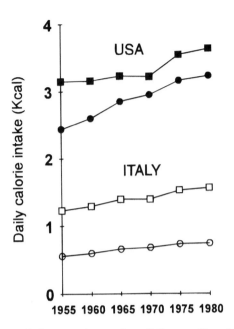

Fig. 12.21 Estimated changes in total and fat-attributable caloric intake in Italy and USA. Both total (filled symbols) and fat-attributable (open symbols) caloric intake are much higher in the USA (squares) than in Italy (circles). This difference would be compatible with the high incidence of IHD in the USA, but cannot be taken as an explanation for the decline in IHD-related mortality observed in both countries, as both total and fat-attributable caloric intake have increased rather than decreased. (From data in ref. 71.)

12.2 ETIOLOGIC COMPONENTS OF IHD

Of all the putative risk factors for IHD considered so far, proof of a causal role is available only for smoking, severe hypertension, and very high levels of serum cholesterol, because their reduction decreases the risk of IHD in middle-aged men. No such conclusive evidence for older men and women is yet available, nor regarding mild hypertension and moderately elevated cholesterol levels.

The pathogenetic mechanisms through which proven etiologic factors influence the risk of IHD are not precisely known; another unknown factor is whether the observed reduction of risk associated with the control of these risk factors is uniform in all individuals exposed to the risk, or whether it occurs only in susceptible individuals.

As currently known risk factors for IHD can explain only about 50% of the rate of IHD mortality,[3-5] other important, but as yet unconsidered, etiologic factors that influence the formation of the atherosclerotic background, the type of atherosclerotic lesions, the development of ischemic stimuli, or the response of the heart to ischemic insults need to be identified.

12.2.1 Proven etiologic factors

Conclusive evidence of a causal role is provided by the reduction of ischemic events and mortality following the cessation of cigarette smoking, the control of severe hypertension, and the reduction of high levels of serum cholesterol in hypercholesterolemic middle-aged men. The effects of smoking, severe hypertension and very high levels of serum cholesterol on ischemic events and mortality are, therefore, strong enough to be detectable in primary prevention studies and prove that these high levels of risk factors are causal factors of IHD. The absence of definite evidence that the risk of IHD is reduced by treatment of mild hypertension and mild hypercholesterolemia may be due, in part, to the lack of sufficiently powerful studies, because in individuals without very elevated levels of risk factors the incidence of fatal and nonfatal cardiac ischemic events is relatively low. When very large numbers of individuals and very long follow-up periods are required in order to prove a reduction of relative IHD risk, the number of events prevented per 1000 patients treated per year of treatment is low. An alternative reason for the lack of direct evidence is the possibility that the relationship becomes causal only for high levels of hypertension and serum cholesterol, but it is predominantly mediated by other associated causal risk factors for lower levels of blood pressure and cholesterol, for example the increase of serum cholesterol and blood pressure levels with age.

12.2.2 Mechanisms of action of proven causal risk factors

The lack of correlation between the extent or severity of coronary atherosclerosis with smoking and with arterial blood pressure levels, and the weak correlation with cholesterol levels, suggests that these risk factors may act predominantly by influencing the other major pathogenetic components of IHD, i.e. the development of ischemic stimuli and the response of the heart to ischemic insults. Alternatively, the poor correlation between these risk factors and coronary atherosclerosis may be due to the confounding effects of other factors that independently produce atherosclerosis in some individuals.

Smoking may favor the development of ischemic stimuli and the response of the heart to ischemic insults by influencing the hemostatic, vasomotor and neurohumoral equilibrium and, hence, the development of ischemia, necrosis, and fatal arrhythmias.

Severe hypertension may favor the development of ischemic stimuli by increasing both the coronary vascular reactivity to vasoconstrictor stimuli and the vulnerability of the heart to ischemic insults as a consequence of left ventricular hypertrophy, an important risk factor for IHD mortality which seems also to have a prognostic value independent of blood pressure levels.[73] Mild hypertension may also be a marker of IHD susceptibility because of its association with age and with the clustering of other risk factors.

Hypercholesterolemia is commonly thought to be a causal mechanism of IHD because it produces atherosclerotic plaques in the coronary arteries. This hypothesis is suggested because cholesterol is found in many large coronary plaques, and plaque fissures are also found in cholesterol-rich plaques. However, as in animals, an individual's susceptibility to the development of atherosclerotic plaques in response to hypercholesterolemia is extremely variable and may be related to several other factors such as:

a. different lipoprotein patterns, such as low levels of apolipoprotein A_1, high levels of apolipoprotein B and lipoprotein(a)
b. certain polymorphisms of the apolipoprotein A_1 and B genes
c. different rates of oxidation of LDL, which represents a potential immunogenic or inflammatory stimulus related to genetic or environmental factors.

However, the weak correlation between extent of coronary atherosclerosis and IHD suggests that hypercholesterolemia may be related to IHD mortality through a complex chain of events that includes the development of ischemic stimuli and the response of the heart to ischemic insults. This possibility is supported by the discrepancy, observed in recent studies, between the significant reduction of ischemic events and the limited regression or lack of progression of coronary atherosclerotic lesions (see Ch. 13), but so far has not received appropriate attention.

12.2.3 Other possible specific causal risk factors

A rational search for specific causal risk factors for IHD should focus on each individual major pathogenetic component of IHD. The first priority should be the risk factors for the acute coronary ischemic stimuli responsible for unstable angina and MI; the second priority is the atherogenic risk factors specifically predisposing to acute coronary stimuli, and the third priority is the risk factors that influence unfavorably the heart's response to ischemic insults. The search should consider the age- and gender-related importance of risk factors and their prevalence in different populations.

Risk factors for acute coronary ischemic stimuli

A fundamental observation that must receive appropriate consideration is the minimal predictive value of classic coronary risk factors for identifying unstable angina or acute MI among patients presenting to the emergency department with chest pain.[74] As discussed in Chapter 9, the high prevalence of acute coronary thrombosis in unstable angina, MI, and SICD suggests a possible causal role of thrombotic risk factors, which began to receive attention in the 1980s (whereas research into lipid risk factors began in the 1950s). Thrombosis, however, occurs in response to acute coronary intimal damage, due either to primary mechanical rupture of a plaque occurring as a random process or to specific local acute thrombogenic stimuli. Thus, risk factors for thrombogenic stimuli should also receive appropriate attention and, among these, inflammatory risk factors are worthy candidates in view of the growing histologic and humoral evidence of an inflammatory component in unstable angina.

Thrombotic risk factors. The search for thrombotic risk factors is based on the hypothesis that a "prothrombotic state," resulting from the presence of such risk factors, could cause the process of repair of intimal injury to evolve more unfavorably than in their absence. This hypothesis implies that a subliminal thrombogenic stimulus would cause coronary occlusion only in the presence of the thrombogenic risk factor (whereas a supraliminal stimulus would cause thrombosis even in its absence). Suggestive evidence about the existence of a potential prothrombotic state in IHD is available from cross-sectional studies in patients with IHD and from prospective epidemiologic studies. Proof of causality will be difficult to obtain: this is because, first, the observed association between the potential elements of a prothrombotic state and IHD may be a consequence of the disease in patients with IHD, and a marker of other associated causal factors in individuals included in prospective epidemiologic studies; second, pharmacologic control of the prothrombotic state may reduce not only the pathologic response to subliminal but also the physiologic response to supraliminal thrombogenic stimuli.

Fibrinogen and factor VII$_c$ plasma levels were found to correlate with both nonfatal MI and total IHD mortality in the Northwick Park Heart study[37] and in four other studies.[36,38,39,42] The relationship may be a causal one, as fibrinogen increases platelet aggregation, fibrin formation, atheroma, and plasma viscosity,[38] but the moderate preventive effects of antivitamin K in MI suggests that a direct role on coagulation may not be a major one, as has been argued in a review on the subject.[75] Elevated levels of fibrinogen may be genetically determined,[76] or could be markers of an unfavorable pattern of acute-phase response (of which fibrinogen is part), together with von Willebrand's factor, sialic acid, and acute-phase proteins (see below).

A prothrombotic state in the elderly was detected by measuring the plasma levels of activation peptides of proenzymes of the coagulation chain, which increase gradually with age in apparently healthy individuals. This is indicative of procoagulatory mechanisms having prevalence over natural anticoagulatory mechanisms,[77] but the age-related increase may also reflect a greater rate of repair of vascular damage due to greater wear and tear of the vascular bed in old age. Decreased fibrinolysis observed in patients with IHD[78] may be an additional component of a prothrombotic state.

Increased platelet volume was also found to be correlated with IHD mortality,[79] but it is not clear whether the relationship is causal or is mediated by hidden factors.

Elevated levels of PAI-1 were found to be predictive of reinfarction,[80] but it is not clear whether the effect was causal or was a marker of an unfavorable pattern of acute-phase response.

Risk factors for thrombogenic stimuli. Rupture of a coronary atherosclerotic plaque occurring at random as a result of purely mechanical forces at weak points in lipid-rich plaques should, in general, be proportional to the extent and severity of coronary atherosclerosis. As this is not the case, other factors not randomly associated with the severity of stenoses or to the extent of the atherosclerotic background should be postulated. Inflammatory risk factors represent a novel avenue of research, as recent observations have shown an inflammatory component in the intima and adventitia of plaques and evidence of systemic inflammation in unstable angina. The inflammatory component could be due to several stimuli, such as oxidized LDL, local immunologic stimuli,[81] reactivation of dormant cytomegalovirus or herpesvirus or of *Chlamydia pneumoniae*. In turn, the "gain" of the inflammatory process could be increased by an enhanced acute-phase response. The inflammatory stimulus may be localized to a single plaque, or may be generalized and become more obvious at the site of plaques because of favorable localizing conditions, in the same way that infective endocarditis represents the localization of a systemic infection on one valve (see Ch. 9).

Elevated plasma levels of acute-phase reactants. Elevated plasma levels of acute-phase reactants were found to be predictive of IHD events and mortality. Plasma levels of sialic acid were found to be correlated with IHD mortality over a 20-year follow-up period.[82] In addition, plasma levels of C-reactive protein (CRP), although often within the normal range, were found to be independent strong predictors of MI in a recent European prospective study that included 3000 patients with angina pectoris.[83] As discussed in Chapter 9, the elevation of acute-phase proteins is strongly predictive of an unfavorable evolution in unstable angina. Plasma levels of protein C were found to be correlated with both plasma levels of insulin and PAI-1 levels in patients with angina pectoris undergoing cardiac catheterization.[53] Thus, elevated values of acute-phase reactants may not only be causal factors but also markers of an enhanced response to inflammatory stimuli that adversely influence coronary and myocardial susceptibility and the response to ischemic stimuli. This possibility is suggested by the correlation between elevated CRP values and seasonal peaks of acute IHD events.[84]

Atherogenic risk factors specifically predisposing to acute coronary stimuli

As the development of acute ischemic events is only weakly correlated to the severity and extent of coronary atherosclerosis, only some specific types of plaques may favor the development of thrombogenic stimuli. At present, the existence of such risk factors (which, besides causing the formation of chronic atherosclerotic plaques, have in themselves the potential to favor specifically the development of coronary thrombogenic stimuli) is mere speculation, but they are outlined here only to stimulate research into this potentially critical area. Risk factors that allow or stimulate the oxidation of LDL-cholesterol (i.e. lack of antioxidants and/or oxidants), endothelial viral and *C. pneumoniae* infections, immune complex deposition, and antibodies or autoantibodies against plaque constituents can all cause a local inflammatory response. The prevalence of cytomegalovirus antibodies in the adult population in various parts of the world is very high.[85] Its ability (shared with other herpesviruses) to remain latent after occasioning an acute infection in the host, and its demonstration in atherosclerotic plaques, makes it a plausible candidate. Dormant viruses in coronary plaques may be reactivated in analogy to the episodic reactivation of herpes simplex, in response to physical stimuli such as intense exposure to the sun, to infections, or to intense psychological stress. *C. pneumoniae*,[86] which is also commonly found in endothelial cells and atherosclerotic plaques together with immunocomplexes (see Ch. 9), may also be a possible atherogenic stimulus.

Risk factors influencing unfavorably the cardiac response to ischemic insults

The existence of such risk factors is also speculative, but is suggested by the association of psychological distress and vital exhaustion with MI (reported in Ch. 9) and SICD. This association may be mediated by an increased vulnerability to inflammatory stimuli, by an enhanced acute-phase response and by a neurally mediated predisposition to ischemia-related fatal arrhythmias. The assessment of risk factors influencing the cardiac response to ischemic insults, such as the preexistence of intercoronary anastomoses (which influence the severity of ischemia), an autonomic nervous imbalance, or an abnormal cytokine response (which may influence the development of myocardial necrosis and fatal arrhythmias), is difficult because they become important only in the presence of coronary ischemic stimuli, which, in turn, are more likely to develop on a predisposing chronic atherosclerotic background.

12.3 THE WAY FORWARD

Precise understanding of the nature and role of the etiologic components of IHD is not yet possible for the following reasons:

1. The atherogenic stimuli, which may initiate the cascade of events that leads to plaque formation and growth, are multiple, may have a different prevalence in different age-groups, populations and communities and may cause a variable predisposition to chronic or to acute ischemic stimuli.
2. Not only are the pathogenetic mechanisms that cause angina multiple, but those that may cause MI are also multiple and may have a variable prevalence in different groups of patients.
3. The response of the heart to ischemic insults, which is a major determinant of prognosis, is also variable with gender and age.

The proof of the causal roles of smoking, hypercholesterolemia, and hypertension, together with the efforts to control them, have so far largely monopolized etiologic research into IHD, although they can explain only about 50% of cases of mortality from IHD. In addition, two facts are clearly established. First, some individuals with elevated levels of these risk factors do not develop IHD either because they may lack other unknown risk factors that are necessary for the development of the disease, or because they are protected against them. Both favoring and protective factors can be environmentally or genetically determined. Second, many subjects develop IHD in spite of low (or very low) levels of these risk factors. They may lack protective factors, have an enhanced susceptibility to known risk factors, or have other causal mechanisms, independent of known risk factors.

These complexities can no longer be ignored, and two general approaches, not mutually exclusive, are available in order to overcome this long-lasting impasse:

1. The first approach is to search for a more precise definition of the mechanisms through which genetic and environmental factors determine the variable individual response to proven risk factors, so that it will, for example, become possible to explain the paradox of patients with familial hypercholesterolemia developing IHD in their sixties (or not at all) and that of patients with premature IHD often having cholesterol values below 200 mg%.
2. The second approach is to search for other causal risk factors distinct from those already proven.

With both approaches it would be necessary not only to prove a causal role of established and newly identified putative risk factors but also to define both their gender-, age- and population-related prevalence and the individual susceptibility and protection to each of them.

12.3.1 Research on the lipid hypothesis

The lipid hypothesis began to be tested in the 1950s and stimulated research that led to the identification of a large number of lipid- and lipoprotein-related abnormalities associated with IHD in some groups of individuals. It is possible that a better understanding of the role of newly identified lipid atherogenic mechanisms may explain the cases of MI or SICD that occur in the absence of elevated levels of total and/or LDL-cholesterol, as well as the reasons why some individuals fail to develop IHD in spite of elevated levels of total and/or LDL-cholesterol. As there are many lipid and apolipoprotein abnormalities, and as their prevalence in the population is high, a comprehensive investigation is likely to identify at least one such individual abnormality in nearly all patients with IHD and low levels of total and/or LDL-cholesterol, and at least one combined abnormality that could explain the protective factors in nearly all individuals with high levels of total and/or LDL-cholesterol but not IHD. These associations, though plausible, cannot be accepted as causal without independent proof of IHD fatal and nonfatal events merely because they are so numerous and common in the general population. It is also imperative to investigate the extent to which lipid risk factors influence not only the formation of the chronic coronary atherosclerotic background, but also the development of acute ischemic stimuli, and the response of the heart to the ischemic insult.

12.3.2 Research on other causal risk factors

As discussed in Chapters 8–10 and in 12.2.3, there is compelling evidence that the chronic atherosclerotic background can also be caused by nonlipid abnormalities, such as inflammatory and thrombogenic ischemic stimuli, and that although the end product of these varied stimuli, (i.e. coronary atherosclerosis) is an extremely common denominator of IHD, it is neither a sufficient nor a necessary element for the development of myocardial ischemic events. Thus, it is imperative to pursue more vigorously (along the lines outlined in 12.2.3) the search not only for risk factors that cause coronary lesions with the potential to trigger coronary ischemic stimuli, and genetic and environmental protective factors, but also the factors that can influence unfavorably the response of the heart to ischemic insults or can protect it.

12.3.3 Identification of susceptible and protected individuals

The results of reducing a particular risk factor in a population or group of patients proves its causal role, independent of the prevalence of susceptible individuals (see Fig. 12.1); however, if the number of individuals who are potentially susceptible to that risk factor is low, a large number will be worried and treated unnecessarily for a lifetime. In the future, predisposing or protective roles of genetic, environmental, gender- and age-related factors (such as neonatal growth, dysadaptation, distress, antioxidants in the diet, and genetic polymorphism) need to be considered specifically for ischemic stimuli and for the cardiac response to ischemic insults.

REFERENCES

1. James TN. Presidential Address AHA 53rd Scientific Session. Sure Cures, Quick Fixes and Easy Answers. A Cautionary Tale About Coronary Disease. Circulation 1981;63:1199A.
2. Hopkins PN, Williams RR. Identification and relative weight of cardiovascular risk factors. Cardiol Clin 1986;4:3.
3. Oliver MF. Prevention of coronary heart disease—propaganda, promises, problems and prospects. Circulation 1986;73:1.
4. Kannel WB. Metabolic risk factors for coronary heart disease in women: perspective from the Framingham study. Am Heart J 1987;114:413.
5. Rosenman RH, Brand, RJ, Sholtz RI, Friedman M. Multivariate prediction of coronary heart disease during 8.5 year follow-up in the Western Collaborative Study Group. Am J Cardiol 1976;37:903.
6. Barker DJP, Osmond C, Golding J, Kua D, Wadsworth MEJ. Growth in utero, blood pressure in childhood and adult life, and mortality from cardiovascular disease. Br Med J 1989;298:564.
7. Barker DJP, Osmond C. Infant mortality, childhood nutrition, and ischaemic heart disease in England and Wales. Lancet 1986;1:1077.
8. Barker DJP. Rise and fall of Western diseases. Nature 1989;338:371.
9. Rissanen AM, Nikkilä EA. Coronary artery disease and its risk factors in families of young men with angina pectoris and in controls. Br Heart J 1977;39:875.
10. Rissanen AM, Nikkilä EA. Aggregation of coronary risk factors in families of young men with fatal and non-fatal coronary heart disease. Br Heart J 1979;42:373.
11. Goldstein JL, Brown MS. The low-density lipoprotein pathway and its relation to atherosclerosis. Ann Rev Biochem 1977;46:897.
12. Berg K. The genetics of the hyperlipidemias and coronary artery disease. In: Bonne-Tamir B (ed.), Cohen T, Goodman RM (assoc eds) Human Genetics, Part B: Medical Aspects. Alan R. Liss Inc, New York 1982, p. 111.
13. Shoulders CC, Ball MJ, Baralle FE. Variation in the apo AI/CIII/AIV gene complex: its association with hyperlipidemia. Atherosclerosis 1989;80:111.
14. Price WH, Kitchin AH, Burgon PRS, Morris SW, Wenham PR, Donald PM. DNA restriction fragment length polymorphisms as markers of familial coronary heart disease. Lancet 1989;1:1407.
15. Nora JJ, Lortsher RH, Spangler RD, Nora AH, Kimberling WJ. Genetic epidemiologic study of early onset ischemic heart disease. Circulation 1980;61:503.
16. Roncaglioni MC, Santoro L, D'Avanzo B et al. The role of family history in patients with myocardial infarction: an Italian case–control study. Circulation 1992;85:2065.
17. Cambien F, Poirier O, Lecerf L et al. Deletion polymorphism in the gene for angiotensin-converting enzyme is a potent risk factor for myocardial infarction. Nature 1992;359:641.

18. Mabuchi H, Koizumi J, Shimizu M, Takeda R and the Hokuriki FH-CHD Study Group. Development of coronary heart disease in familial hypercholesterolemia. Circulation 1989;*79*:225.
19. Martin MJ, Browner WS, Hulley SB, Kuller LH, Wentworth D. Serum cholesterol, blood pressure, and mortality: implications from a cohort of 361 662 men. Lancet 1986;*2*:933.
20. Neaton JD, Wentworth D for the Multiple Risk Factor Intervention Trial Research Group. Serum cholesterol, blood pressure, cigarette smoking, and death from coronary heart disease. Overall findings and differences by age for 316 099 white men. Arch Intern Med 1992;*152*:56.
21. Anderson KM, Castelli WP, Levy D. Cholesterol and mortality. 30 years of follow-up from the Framingham Study. J Am Med Ass 1987;*257*:2176.
22. Simons LA. Interrelations of lipids and lipoproteins with coronary artery disease mortality in 19 countries. Am J Cardiol 1986;*57*:5G.
23. World Health Organization: World Health Statistics Annual 1990. WHO, Geneva.
24. St. Leger AS, Cochrane AL, Moore F. Factors associated with cardiac mortality in developed countries with particular reference to the consumption of wine. Lancet 1979;*1*:1017.
25. Diabetes Epidemiology Research International Group. Geographic patterns of childhood insulin-dependent diabetes mellitus. Diabetes 1988;*37*:1113.
26. World Health Organization: MONICA Project. Geographical variation: the major risk factors of coronary heart disease in men and women aged 35–66 years. World Health Statistics Quarterly 1988;*41*:115.
27. Goldstein JL, Hazzard WR. Schrott HG et al. Hyperlipidemia in coronary heart disease. 1. Lipid levels in 500 survivors of myocardial infarction. J Clin Invest 1973;*52*:1533.
28. Maggioni AP, Maseri A, Fresco C et al on behalf of GISSI-2 Investigators. Age-related increase in mortality in patients with first myocardial infarction treated with thrombolysis. N Engl J Med 1993;*329*:1442.
29. Coronary Drug Project Research Group. Natural history of myocardial infarction in the coronary drug project: long-term prognostic importance of serum lipid levels. Am J Cardiol 1978;*42*:489.
30. Richard JL. Les facteurs de risque coronarien. Le paradoxe français. Arch Mal Coeur 1987;*80*:17.
31. Tunstall-Pedoe H. Autre pays, autres moeurs. Br Med J 1988:*297*:1559.
32. Shestov DB, Deev AD, Klimov AN, Davis CE, Tyroler HA. Increased risk of coronary heart disease death in men with low total and low-density lipoprotein cholesterol in the Russian lipid research clinics prevalence follow-up study. Circulation 1993;*88*:846.
33. Genest J Jr, McNamara JR, Ordovas JM et al. Lipoprotein cholesterol, apolipoprotein A-I and B and lipoprotein(a) abnormalities in men with premature coronary artery disease. J Am Coll Cardiol 1992;*19*:792.
34. Criqui MH, Heiss G, Cohn R, Cowan LD, Suchindran CM, Bangdiwala S. Plasma triglyceride level and mortality from coronary heart disease. N Engl J Med 1993;*328*:1220.
35. Department of Health and Human Services. Reducing the health consequences of smoking: 25 years of progress: A Report of the Surgeon General. Government Printing Office, Washington DC 1989 (DHHS publication no. (CDC) 89-8411).
36. Kannel WB, Wolf PA, Castelli WP, D'Agostino RB. Fibrinogen and risk of cardiovascular disease. J Am Med Ass 1987;*258*:1183.
37. Meade TW, Mellows S, Brozovic M et al. Haemostatic function and ischaemic heart disease: principal results of the Northwick Park Heart Study. Lancet 1980;*2*:533.
38. Yarnell JWG, Baker IA, Sweetnam PM et al. Fibrinogen, viscosity, and white blood cell count are major risk factors for ischemic heart disease. Circulation 1991;*83*:836.
39. Wilhelmsen L, Svärdsudd K, Korsan-Bengtsen K et al. Fibrinogen as a risk factor for stroke and myocardial infarction. N Engl J Med 1984;*311*:501.
40. Assmann G, Schulte H. Results and Conclusions of the Prospective Cardiovascular Münster (PROCAM) Study. In: Assmann G (ed). Lipid Metabolism Disorders and Coronary Heart Disease, 2nd edition. MMV Medizin Verlag, Munich, 1993, p. 19.
41. Landolfi R, De Cristofaro R, De Candia E, Rocca B, Bizzi B. Effect of fibrinogen concentration on the velocity of platelet aggregation. Blood 1991;*78*:377.
42. Markowe HLJ, Marmot MG, Shipley MJ et al. Fibrinogen: a possible link between social class and coronary heart disease. Br Med J 1985;*291*:1312.

43. Ragland DR, Brand RJ. Type A behavior and mortality from coronary heart disease. N Engl J Med 1988;*318*:65.
44. Marmot M, Theorell T. Social class and cardiovascular disease: the contribution of work. Int J Health Serv; 1988;*18*:659.
45. Davey Smith G, Shipley MJ, Marmot MG, Rose G. Plasma cholesterol concentration and mortality. The Whitehall Study. J Am Med Ass 1992;*267*:70.
46. Cortellaro M, Boschetti C, Cofrancesco E et al and the PLAT Study Group. The PLAT Study: a multidisciplinary study of hemostatic function and conventional risk factors in vascular disease patients. Atherosclerosis 1991;*90*:109.
47. Bønaa KH, Arnesen E. Association between heart rate and atherogenic blood lipid fractions in a population. The Tromsø Study. Circulation 1992;*86*:394.
48. Must A, Jacques PF, Dallal GE, Bajema CJ, Dietz WH. Long-term morbidity and mortality of overweight adolescents. A follow-up of the Harvard Growth Study of 1922 to 1935. N Engl J Med 1992;*327*:1350.
49. Ten Kate LP, Boman H, Daiger SP, Motulsky A. Increased frequency of coronary heart disease in relatives or wives of myocardial infarct survivors: assortative mating for lifestyle and risk factors? Am J Cardiol 1984;*53*:399.
50. Fuller JH. Coronary-heart-disease risk and impaired glucose tolerance. The Whitehall Study. Lancet 1980;*1*:1373.
51. Reaven GM. Insulin resistance and compensatory hyperinsulinemia: role in hypertension, dyslipidemia, and coronary heart disease. Am Heart J 1991;*121*:1283.
52. De Fronzo RA, Ferranini E. Insulin Resistance. A multifaceted syndrome responsible for NIDDM, obesity, hypertension, dyslipidemia, and atherosclerotic cardiovascular disease. Diabetes Care 1991;*14*:173.
53. Juhan-Vague I, Alessi MC, Joly P et al. Plasma plasminogen activator inhibitor-1 in angina pectoris. Influence of plasma insulin and acute-phase response. Arterosclerosis 1989;*9*:362.
54. McGill HC, Arias-Stella J, Carbonell LM. General findings of the International Atherosclerosis Project. Lab Invest 1968;*18*:38.
55. Solberg LA, Strong JP. Risk factors and atherosclerotic lesions. A review of autopsy studies. Arteriosclerosis 1983;*3*:187.
56. Sorlie PD, Garcia-Palmieri MR, Castillo-Staab MI, Costas R Jr, Oalmann MC, Havlik R. The relation of antemortem factors to atherosclerosis at autopsy. Am J Pathol 1981;*103*:345.
57. McGill H. The cardiovascular pathology of smoking. Am Heart J 1988;*115*:250.
58. Holme I, Solberg LA, Weissfeld L. Coronary risk factors and their pathway of action through coronary raised lesions, coronary stenoses and coronary death. Am J Cardiol 1985;*55*:40.
59. Vlietstra RE, Frye RL, Kronmal RA et al and Participants in the Coronary Artery Surgery Study. Risk factors and angiographic coronary artery disease: a Report from the Coronary Artery Surgery Study (CASS Study). Circulation 1980;*62*:254.
60. Crea F, Gaspardone A, Tomai F et al. Risk factors in school children associated with a family history of specific coronary syndromes in adult relatives. J Am Coll Cardiol 1994;*23*:1472.
61. Austin MA, Breslow JL, Hennekens CH et al. Low-density lipoprotein subclass patterns and risk of myocardial infarction. J Am Med Ass 1988;*260*:1917.
62. Wiseman SA, Powell JT, Barber N, Humphries SE, Greenhalgh RM. Influence of apolipoproteins on the anatomical distribution of arterial disease. Atherosclerosis 1991;*89*:231.
63. Fowkes FG, Housley E, Riemersma RA et al. Smoking, lipids, glucose intolerance, and blood pressure as risk factors for peripheral atherosclerosis compared with ischemic heart disease in the Edinburgh Artery Study. Am J Epidemiol 1992;*135*:331.
64. Fowkes FGR, Connor JM, Smith FB. Fibrinogen genotype and risk of peripheral atherosclerosis. Lancet 1992;*339*:693.
65. Groves P, Rees A, Bishop A et al. Apolipoprotein (a) concentrations and susceptibility to coronary artery disease in patients with peripheral vascular disease. Br Heart J 1993;*69*:26.
66. Curtin LR, Armstrong RJ (NCHS). United States life tables eliminating certain causes of death. US Decennial Life Tables for 1979–82. DHHS Publ No. (PHS) 1988;*88*:1150.
67. Feinleib M, Rifkind BM. Changing patterns of cardiovascular disease mortality in the United States. Isr J Med Sci 1982;*18*:1098.

68. Levy RI. Declining mortality in coronary heart disease. Arteriosclerosis 1981;*1:*312.
69. Gillum RF. Acute myocardial infarction in the United States, 1970–1983. Am Heart J 1987;*113:*804.
70. Elveback LR, Connolly DC, Melton JL III. Coronary heart disease in residents of Rochester, Minnesota. VII. Incidence, 1950 through 1982. Mayo Clin Proc 1986;*61:*896.
71. Thom TJ, Epstein FH, Feldman JJ, Leaverton PE. Trends in total mortality and mortality from heart disease in 26 countries from 1950 to 1978. Int J Epidemiol 1985;*14:*510.
72. La Vecchia C, Harris RE, Wynder EL. Comparative epidemiology of cancer between the United States and Italy. Cancer Res 1988;*48:*7285.
73. Frohilich ED, Tarazi RC. Is arterial pressure the sole factor responsible for hypertensive cardiac hypertrophy? Am J Cardiol 1979;*44:*959.
74. Jayes RL Jr, Beshansky JR, D'Agostino RB, Selker HP. Do patients' coronary risk factor reports predict acute cardiac ischemia in the emergency department? A multicenter study. J Clin Epidemiol 1992;*45:*621.
75. Hirsh J. Hypercoagulability. Semin Hematol 1977;*14:*409.
76. Humphries SE, Cook M, Dubowitz M, Stirling Y, Meade TW. Role of genetic variation at the fibrinogen locus in determination of plasma fibrinogen concentrations. Lancet 1987;*1:*1452.
77. Bauer KA, Weiss LM, Sparrow D, Vokonas PS, Rosenberg RD. Aging associated changes in indices of thrombin generation and protein C activation in humans. J Clin Invest 1987;*80:*1527.
78. Francis RB, Kawanishi D, Baruch T, Mahrer P, Rahimtoola S, Feinstein DI. Impaired fibrinolysis in coronary artery disease. Am Heart J 1988;*115:*776.
79. Martin JF, Rath PMW, Burr ML. Influence of platelet size on outcome after myocardial infarction. Lancet 1991;*II:*1409.
80. Hamsten A, De Faire U, Walldius G et al. Plasminogen activator inhibitor in plasma: risk factor for recurrent myocardial infarction. Lancet 1987;*II:*3.
81. Libby P, Hansson GK. Biology of disease. Involvement of the immune system in human atherogenesis: current knowledge and unanswered questions. Lab Invest 1991;*64:*5.
82. Lindberg G, Eklund GA, Gullberg B, Rastam L. Serum sialic acid concentration and cardiovascular mortality. Br Med J 1991;*302:*143.
83. Thompson SG, Kienast J, Pyke SDM, Haverkate F, Van de Loo JCW, for the European Concerted Action on Thrombosis and Disabilities Angina Pectoris Study Group. Hemostatic factors and the risk of myocardial infarction or sudden death in patients with angina pectoris. New Engl J Med 1995;*332:*635.
84. Woodhouse PR, Khaw KT, Foley A, Meade TW. Seasonal variations of plasma fibrinogen and factor VII activity in the elderly: winter infections and death from cardiovascular disease. Lancet 1994;*343:*435.
85. Ho M. Epidemiology of cytomegalovirus infections. Rev Infect Dis 1990;*12:*S701.
86. Linnanmäki E, Leinonen M, Mattila K, Nieminen MS, Valtonen V, Saikku P. Chlamydia pneumoniae-specific circulating immune complexes in patients with chronic coronary heart disease. Circulation 1993;*87:*1130.

13 | Determinants of prognosis: primary and secondary prevention

INTRODUCTION

The uncertainty about prognosis occupies a particularly prominent position in the minds of patients with ischemic heart disease (IHD) and of their physicians, so that diagnostic and therapeutic approaches are often conditioned more by the desire to avoid the possible occurrence of myocardial infarction (MI) and sudden ischemic cardiac death (SICD) than by symptoms. Indeed, with the exception of very severe forms of angina, symptoms may be mild; for most patients anginal pain is not always unbearable, it may last only a few minutes, may not occur every day, and may even be absent altogether for weeks or months. On the other hand, although MI and SICD are very rare events, they may be the first manifestations of IHD or may occur unpredictably during periods free, or relatively free, from symptoms: hence the understandable anxiety and the urge to identify and prevent the occurrence of these baffling events. However, whereas the success of treatment aimed at relieving symptoms can be judged from the degree of symptomatic relief provided, the improvement of prognosis requires some reasonable knowledge of both the reduction of life expectancy and the expectancy of life free from disability resulting from non-fatal IHD in clinically defined groups of patients.

Total life expectancy

The reduction of life expectancy due to IHD mortality can be assessed easily in patients in whom the probability of IHD-related death is high and, hence, becomes the major cause of premature mortality (i.e. patients with previous MI, impaired ventricular function, multivessel coronary disease, and low effort tolerance). In such patients the average survival curve is significantly lower than that defined by life tables for the normal population. The reduction of life expectancy cannot be assessed easily in middle-aged individuals with moderate levels of risk factors for IHD (but with no evidence of its development) because, although they are at a higher risk of death occurring as a result of IHD, mortality from IHD may not represent the major cause of premature deaths. Individuals not dying of IHD, therefore, may die of some other intervening cause and their average survival curves may not differ significantly from those of the normal control population. Hence, very large numbers of individuals are required to be followed for several years in order to detect a statistically significant difference from life table curves for the control population.

In patients in whom IHD is not the major cause of premature mortality and, therefore, in whom the reduction of life expectancy is not immediately apparent, the increased risk of IHD-related mortality is commonly assessed in terms of its occurrence during a follow-up period compared with controls (odds-ratio) (i.e. the ratio of mortality from IHD in the individuals at risk compared with controls during follow-up). However, odds-ratios provide only relative information, because the total number of individuals who will die as a result of the risk under consideration (i.e. the absolute risk) varies in proportion to the baseline IHD mortality rates of the control group; for example, a threefold increase in the odds-ratio implies 15 deaths instead of five when the baseline risk is 5%, but only three deaths instead of one when the baseline risk is 1%. This concept has obvious implications for the number of individuals or patients that could be saved among the total number treated by interventions.

The incidence of IHD in the general adult population as a result of the combination of relative risk in specific subgroups at progressively higher risk was outlined clearly by Myerburg et al for sudden death (see Fig. 13.1)[1] but the same principle may apply to for MI.

The overall incidence of SICD in the adult population in the USA is estimated at about 300 000 (about 0.1% per year). About 100 000 cases occur in individuals who cannot be considered at

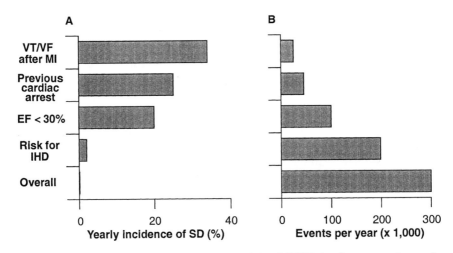

Fig. 13.1 Identification of individuals at risk of SICD in the general population as a function of the size of subgroups at different risk. There is an inverse relation between the predictive power of risk factors and the total number of patients identified. Patients who had experienced ventricular tachycardia (VT) or ventricular fibrillation (VF) in the convalescent phase of MI have an estimated 30% incidence of sudden death (SD) per year (**A**), but they represent only 20000 of the 300000 cases of SD in the population of the USA (**B**). Patients who previously suffered a cardiac arrest and those with a left ventricular EF below 30% have an approximately 20% yearly incidence of SD, but represent only 30 000 and 100 000 cases, respectively, of total cases in the USA. Patients with IHD, or with the highest levels of risk factors for IHD, have a 2% risk of SD (**A**), and represent 200 000 cases of SD in the population. (Some patients belong to more than one category.) Similar principles also apply for the incidence of MI. (Modified from ref. 1.)

high risk for IHD as they have average or low levels of risk factors for IHD. About 200 000 cases occur in individuals with IHD or with high levels of risk factors for IHD with an average risk of about 2% per year. Among this subgroup the risk varies from 0.5% per year in individuals without IHD but with high levels of multiple risk factors (about 50000 cases per year), to 5% per year in patients with previous coronary events (about 150000 cases per year), to 20% in patients with heart failure and ejection fraction (EF) less than 30% (about 100 000 cases per year), to 30% per year in patients in the convalescent phase of acute MI with low EF and malignant ventricular arrhythmias (about 20 000 cases per year).

These considerations indicate that the more predictive the risk factors, the smaller the number of patients identified. Moreover, the same authors indicate that there is a time dependence of risk following the initial major coronary event. The risk decreases progressively following the event and after 6–18 months becomes similar to that of the low-risk group of patients with IHD but no major ischemic event (see Fig. 13.2).[2]

The increase in life expectancy produced by therapeutic or preventive strategies is also, therefore, assessed most easily in those groups of patients with high rates of premature IHD-

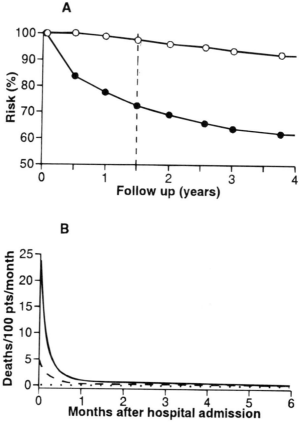

Fig. 13.2 Time dependence of risk after major cardiovascular events. A. The risk of SICD is highest soon after acute MI (●), but after about 1 year the risk becomes similar to that of patients with chronic IHD (○). (Modified from ref. 1.) **B.** The risk of death is highest soon after acute MI (—) than after unstable angina (- - -) and becomes similar to that of chronic stable angina (·····) after about 3 months. (Modified from ref. 2.)

related mortality, causing a large deviation from the survival curve of matched controls. In order to demonstrate an increased life expectancy, both the number of patients that need to be included in controlled trials and the duration of observation are inversely proportional to the mean probability of IHD-related mortality in the group. In groups of patients in whom IHD-related mortality does not cause premature death with a consequent, obvious deviation from the survival curve of controls, the increase in life expectancy may not be demonstrable unless very large numbers of patients are followed for many years, even when the percentage reduction of IHD mortality is as high as 50%; at the same time, the number of patients that could be saved would be a very tiny fraction of those treated.

■ *The reduction of odds-ratios of IHD-related mortality may not be a relevant endpoint unless it is associated with improved life expectancy or with the expectancy of significantly longer periods of life free from IHD events and a better quality of life. For a given reduction of the odds-ratio, the total number of events prevented per patient treated depends on their absolute baseline risk.* ■

Life expectancy free of IHD-related disability

The reduction of IHD-related disability, with the consequent improvement in the quality of life, becomes the most important component of the prognostic assessment in patients in whom the IHD-related reduction in life expectancy is not obvious. The quality of life is influenced not only by the degree of disability resulting from nonfatal IHD but also by two opposing subjective components: these are, on the one hand, the inconvenience of having to take the appropriate medication, to undergo the necessary interventions, and to make lifestyle changes and, on the other hand, the fear of the disease, which causes anxiety about prognosis. The importance of these components of the quality of life varies according to the patient's cultural background, personality, and levels of social support and cannot be assessed easily.

■ *The reduction in the number of nonfatal IHD events, as well as the subjective components of the quality of life, should both be included in the overall evaluation of the cost–benefit ratios of those therapeutic and preventive strategies for which a statistically significant improvement in life expectancy cannot be demonstrated.* ■

13.1 DETERMINANTS OF REDUCED TOTAL AND IHD EVENT-FREE LIFE EXPECTANCY

The determinants of reduced life expectancy and IHD disability-free life expectancy should be considered in terms of nonmodifiable risk factors that contribute to the baseline risk and potentially modifiable determinants of risk. The product of the modifiable risk and the baseline risk determines the absolute risk, as indicated in Chapter 12. The baseline risk conferred by nonmodifiable risk factors determines the total number of patients that can be saved for a given percentage reduction of mortality produced by correction of modifiable risk factors.

13.1.1 Individuals with no evidence of IHD

Most of the information available on the effects of modifiable risk factors on the incidence of ischemic events concerns middle-aged men, but inferences are often made about older men and about women, for whom information is scarce. In individuals with no evidence of IHD, the probability of IHD-related mortality or nonfatal IHD can be predicted on the basis of the baseline risk in relation to nonmodifiable risk factors (i.e. age, gender, family history, diabetes, and glucose intolerance), and also of the additional risk conferred by proven, modifiable risk factors (i.e. high levels of serum cholesterol, cigarette smoking, systemic hypertension) (see Fig. 13.3A–C).[3]

Both the odds-ratio and the absolute risk increase markedly in individuals with clustering of multiple nonmodifiable and modifiable risk factors,[4] particularly when they are associated with ECG abnormalities such as signs of left ventricular hypertrophy (i.e. evidence of a cardiac abnormality rather than a risk factor) (see Fig. 13.4); however, clustering of causal

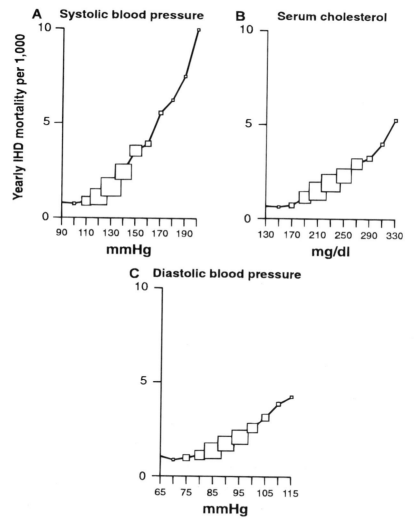

Fig. 13.3 Comparative mortality associated with major risk factors for IHD.
Systolic blood pressure values (**A**) are associated with the highest risk of IHD-related mortality per 1000 individuals per year, followed by serum cholesterol levels (**B**) and by diastolic blood pressure values (**C**). The size of the square indicates the size of the population with the particular level of risk factors. Patients at the highest risk are a tiny minority and hence account for a minimal number of cases occurring in the general population (as illustrated in Fig. 13.1). (Derived from data in ref. 3.)

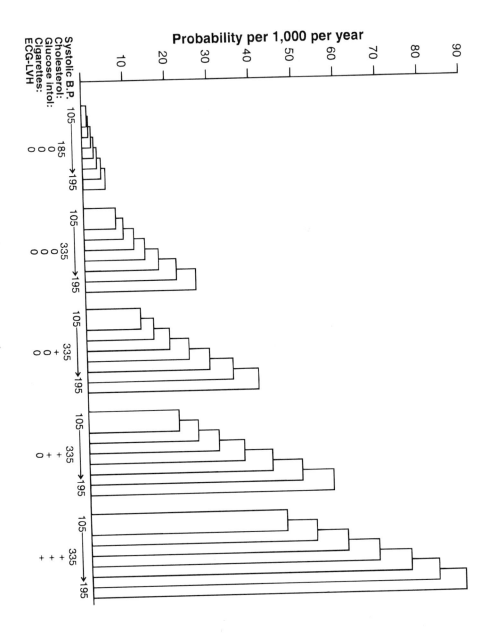

Probability per 1,000 per year

Systolic B.P.
Cholesterol:
Glucose intol:
Cigarettes:
ECG-LVH

risk factors is rare (see Fig. 13.5),[5] and thus it identifies only a minority of those who will develop IHD. In addition, many individuals with multiple risk factors may not develop IHD.

As discussed in Chapter 12, total mortality is increased in only young individuals with very high levels of serum cholesterol that cause premature IHD-related death, in individuals with clustering of high levels of multiple risk factors, and in individuals with risk factors for IHD, such as smoking and hypertension, which also cause non-IHD-related premature mortality; nevertheless, many individuals in these groups will not develop IHD.

■ *Proven risk factors, although useful for assessing population attributable risk, are not sufficiently sensitive or specific to provide an accurate prediction of an individual's prognosis because the determinants of the individual susceptibility to risk factors are largely unknown.* ■

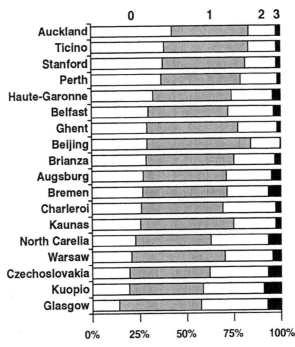

Fig. 13.5 Prevalence of risk factors in selected regions in the MONICA study. Most individuals screened had one or no risk factor: only a minority had three risk factors. Thus, most ischemic events will occur in individuals with one or two risk factors. (Based on data from ref. 5.)

Fig. 13.4 Effect of combined risk factors on the probability of mortality occurring in middle-aged men. The probability of cardiovascular death occurring is correlated linearly with systolic blood pressure in individuals with various combinations of risk factors. This correlation is related partly to the increase in levels of systolic blood pressure with age. The presence of electrocardiographic signs of left ventricular hypertrophy is an indication of increased risk, even when systolic blood pressure is as low as 105 mmHg. Mortality increases from about 1/1000 per year in the lowest-risk group to 90/1000 per year in the highest-risk group. (Modified from ref. 4.)

13.1.2 Patients with evidence of IHD

Patients with evidence of IHD have a reduced ischemic event-free and total life expectancy, even when in a quiescent phase, because their susceptibility to IHD is already proven. On average, they have a relative risk 5–7 times higher than individuals without IHD,[6,7] but their individual prognosis can be extremely variable, depending not only on chronic non-modifiable and modifiable determinants but also on their susceptibility to unstable phases and on their cardiac response to ischemic insults (see Table 13.1). Following acute phases, the time dependency of risk, decreasing progressively after the acute events, should be considered.

In totally asymptomatic individuals, a positive ECG exercise stress test confers an additional risk. In the Multiple Risk Factor Intervention (MRFIT) study, exercise stress testing was positive in about 12% of 12 422 individuals who were selected as being in the top 10% of risk among the 361 662 screened. A positive test conferred a risk ratio of 3.5 (0.7% compared with 0.2% per year) compared with a negative test in individuals who were in the usual care group, but failed to increase the risk in individuals who were in the special intervention group (see Fig. 13.6).[8]

Patients with evidence of stress-induced myocardial ischemia in a stable phase of the disease are much more likely to present with MI than with SICD, in contrast to patients with a negative test who present more often with SICD than with MI. In patients with a positive test, this difference may be due to the presence of flow-limiting coronary stenoses responsible for the development of collaterals, which can reduce the severity of ischemia during sudden coronary occlusion.[9] Conversely, in the Coronary Artery Surgery Study (CASS) registry, SICD could not be identified by any angiographic parameters.[10]

The information available on prognosis is not directly applicable to individual patients because the desire for an objective doctor-independent assessment has often led to patients being classified according to single criteria, either clinical (stable or unstable angina, post-MI), angiographic (single-, double-, or triple-vessel disease or low EF) or ECG, scintigraphic, or echocardiographic exercise stress test results (positive or negative). Moreover, broad inclusion criteria are usually adapted in order to obtain, within a short period, groups large enough for the purposes of statistical analysis. The broader the inclusion criteria, the less meaningful the average values thus obtained for individual patients.

The very variable relationship between coronary anatomy, ventricular function, residual coronary flow reserve, and ischemic manifestations is not given sufficient consideration. On the one hand, it is usually assumed that patients with similar symptoms have similar prog-

Table 13.1 Major determinants of prognosis in patients with known IHD

Type of determinants of prognosis*	Determinants
Chronic, nonmodifiable	Severity of postinfarction left ventricular dysfunction Nonmodifiable risk factors General clinical condition
Chronic, modifiable	Susceptibility to malignant arrhythmias Number of flow-limiting stenoses potentially treatable by revascularization procedures Modifiable, causal risk factors
Acute	Susceptibility to unstable angina and MI Vulnerability of the heart to ischemic insults

*IHD event-free and total life expectancy is determined by a combination of chronic, nonmodifiable and modifiable determinants with acute determinants of prognosis

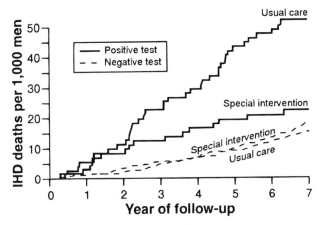

Fig. 13.6 Risk of IHD-related death conferred by a positive exercise stress test in individuals in the top decile of risk. Among the more than 360 000 individuals included in the MRFIT Study, 3% were in the top 10% decile of risk (i.e. about 12 500 patients). The ECG exercise stress test was positive in about 12% of these top-risk individuals. Mortality rates were similar in individuals with positive tests and in those with negative tests in the special intervention group (about 0.2% per year) and was about threefold higher (0.75% per year) in those with positive tests in the usual care group. Thus, even in top-risk individuals, positive exercise stress tests are rare and have a rather limited prognostic value. (Modified from ref. 6.)

noses, independent of the cause of their symptoms, their coronary anatomy, and ventricular function. On the other hand, patients with a similar coronary anatomy are often thought to have a similar prognosis, independent of the causes of ischemia, the severity of symptoms, and the reduction of ventricular function and coronary flow reserve.

Prognostic studies that include patients at very low and very high risk, together with patients at intermediate risk, suffer from the hidden assumption that the risk of intermediate patients is a continuous variable, linearly related to the parameters that separate patients at very high risk from those at very low risk.

Attempts to correlate prognosis with the results of a single test, neglecting readily available information from other sources, are favored by the subdivision of cardiology departments into separate services, such as clinical, ECG, echocardiography, nuclear cardiology, and cardiac catheterization.

The assessment of prognosis should be based on all easily available information, rather than on a single parameter, even if it was obtained using the latest and most sophisticated technique. In clinical practise the combination of available routine data alone allows the stratification of low-, intermediate-, and high-risk patients: for example, the size of the infarct can be inferred from the peak of the enzyme curve together with the number of ECG leads with Q waves and a semiquantitative echocardiographic study at the time of discharge; the severity of impairment of ventricular function can be assessed from a history of MI complicated by cardiac failure, from increased heart size or congested lung fields on standard chest radiographs, and from semiquantitative echocardiographic assessment of ventricular function; the severity of impairment of coronary flow reserve can be judged from the threshold of exertional angina and from the work load at which the exercise stress test becomes positive after sublingual nitrates. The prognostic value of myocardial perfusion studies, quantitative estimates of left ventricular EF and ventricular volumes, and coronary angiography must be assessed in terms of the additional information that they provide over and above generally available baseline determinants in uncertain cases. For example, the prognostic value of EF measurements and of thallium uptake in the lungs may provide no additional information in patients with very large infarctions, enlarged hearts, and histories of cardiac failure or in patients with very small infarctions, normal-sized hearts, no signs of failure, and good effort tolerance.

This section discusses the determinants of prognosis in patients in a quiescent phase of IHD or with stable, mild symptoms, for whom treatment is aimed predominantly at improving prognosis. The chronic determinants of prognosis are separated into nonmodifiable baseline factors (such as the extent of myocardium lost because of MI and age) and potentially modifiable coronary factors (such as flow-limiting coronary stenoses susceptible to revascularization procedures) and proven modifiable risk factors for IHD. It thus becomes possible to define a group of patients with known IHD who are at relatively low risk and in whom, therefore, diagnostic tests have a very low predictive accuracy of ischemic events. The specific prognostic determinants relating to acute MI, unstable and stable angina, chronic postinfarction cardiac failure and the time dependency of risk post-MI are discussed in the pertinent chapters.

Chronic, nonmodifiable baseline determinants of prognosis

The major chronic nonmodifiable baseline determinants of prognosis are the severity of postinfarction ventricular dysfunction and age. Evidence of previous MI (albeit small) is, in itself, indicative of a patient's susceptibility to further MI, but the independent prognostic role of a small, uncomplicated MI is not known. It is also not known whether a history of resolved unstable angina represents an independent indicator of risk.

Left ventricular dysfunction. Left ventricular dysfunction reflects the extent of myocardial necrosis and, hence, an enhanced vulnerability to further losses of myocardium. It is indicated by a history of cardiac failure and by enlargement of the ventricle (increased end-systolic and end-diastolic volumes). A reduced EF is the index of left ventricular dysfunction used most commonly in clinical practise because it can more easily be quantified numerically. The relationship between EF and survival post-MI is exponential: the point of major flex on the curve corresponds to an EF of about 40%, below which it becomes a major determinant of prognosis (see Figs 13.7 and 22.5).[11] The application of the average survival figures related to EF measurements to an individual patient is somewhat limited, because they were collected in unselected patients of different ages, with or without signs of failure, with or without recurrent or inducible myocardial ischemia or ventricular arrhythmias, and with variable levels of modifiable risk factors.

Age. Age is the other most important nonmodifiable prognostic determinant. In-hospital mortality for acute MI and mortality at 6 months after discharge both increase exponentially with age: the point of a major flex on the curve occurs at about 65 years of age, above which it becomes a major determinant of prognosis (see Figs 10.10 and 22.4).

■ *Thus, post-MI patients younger than 65 years and with a left ventricular EF greater than 40% can be grouped together to assess the effects of modifiable determinants of prognosis.* ■

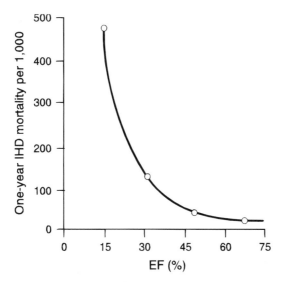

Fig. 13.7 Relationship between left ventricular ejection fraction (EF) and post-MI mortality. One-year mortality post-MI increases exponentially with the reduction of left ventricular EF. The increase becomes very steep below 40%. (Modified from ref. 11.)

Chronic, modifiable determinants of prognosis

Among the chronic, potentially modifiable determinants of prognosis, the most widely considered is the number of coronary arteries with flow-limiting coronary stenoses. In the CASS registry, patients with three-vessel disease had worse survival curves than those with two- or one-vessel disease. As expected, this angiographic prognostic indicator was influenced strongly by the severity of preexisting left ventricular dysfunction (see Fig. 13.8)[12] and by the results of exercise stress testing (see Fig. 13.9).[13] Although the presence of flow-limiting proximal coronary stenoses is obviously a causal risk, it may also be a marker of susceptibility to the development of new coronary obstructions and of major ischemic events. Patients who exhibited coronary stenosis progression at repeated angiography had a higher incidence of new ischemic events during the subsequent follow-up period than those who did not.[14]

Other chronic, modifiable risk factors include the proven causal risk factors for IHD (i.e. cigarette smoking, hypercholesterolemia, hypertension). For example, high levels of serum cholesterol are associated with a much higher rate of mortality from IHD in patients with the disease than in individuals without it (see Fig. 13.10),[15] because they are multipliers of a high baseline risk and possibly because of a greater prevalence of individuals susceptible to the adverse effects of elevated serum cholesterol levels among patients with known IHD.

Patients with known IHD at low risk

Identification of patients with known IHD who are at low risk is important, first, because it is reassuring for the patient; second, because in such a group the prognostic accuracy of any diagnostic test becomes very low; third, because it is difficult to demonstrate that even the

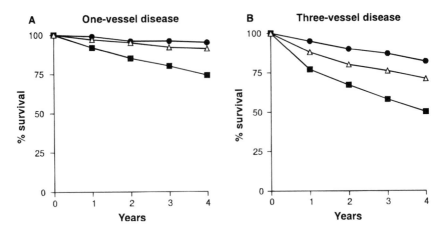

Fig. 13.8 Combined effect of the number of coronary arteries with flow-limiting stenoses and a reduced ejection fraction (EF) on survival. Survival is about 95% in patients with single-vessel disease and an EF greater than 50% (●) (A); it is lowest in those with triple-vessel disease and an EF lower than 35% (■) (B). The survival curves of patients with an EF >50% represent an average of patients with and without a previous MI and with a positive or a negative exercise test. Patients with no previous infarction and with negative exercise stress tests should have a better than average rate of survival. (Modified from ref. 12.)

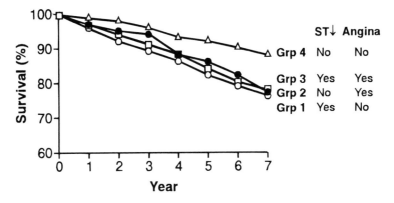

Fig. 13.9 Influence of the results of exercise stress testing on prognosis. Seven-year cumulative survival rates for 1583 patients with coronary artery disease in the CASS registry were significantly greater for patients who had negative exercise stress tests (Grp 4) than for those with angina and ST-segment depression who had positive tests (Grp 3), or only angina (Grp 2) or only ST-segment depression (Grp 1). These results refer to unselected patients. Those without a previous MI or those having had an MI but with good ventricular function can be expected to have a better than average prognosis. (Modified from ref. 13.)

most aggressive treatments can significantly increase life expectancy when the latter is not reduced appreciably.

Clinical and noninvasive information may be sufficient to identify groups of low-risk patients in whom life expectancy cannot be improved significantly by any aggressive or prolonged treatment because it is not significantly reduced compared with life tables.

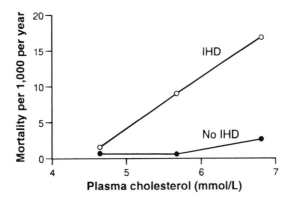

Fig. 13.10 Relationship between serum cholesterol levels and mortality in individuals with and without IHD. Patients with IHD (○) exhibit a much higher mortality than individuals with no evidence of IHD (●) (1.5% versus 0.2% for cholesterol levels of about 7 mmol/L) for the same levels of serum cholesterol, which is a multiplier of the higher baseline risk. (Modified from ref. 15.)

Post-MI patients. Follow-up studies in very large multicentric trials have demonstrated that the average survival of unselected patients discharged from hospital after thrombolysis is much better than that reported in selected groups from individual institutions (as the latter most likely admitted a greater number of severe cases). In the Gruppo Italiano per lo Studio della Streptochinasi nell'Infarto Miocardico-1 (GISSI-1) study, the 1-year survival curve of patients receiving thrombolytic therapy was parallel to that of non-thrombolyzed patients, although the rate of revascularization procedures in thrombolyzed patients was below 2%.[16] Thus, early coronary reperfusion did not appear to involve a subsequent increased risk of death, even in the absence of coronary revascularization (see Ch. 22).

The low rate of mortality post-MI was confirmed in GISSI-3, in which about 60% of patients admitted to coronary care units (CCUs) were enrolled,[17] and hence provides a reliable estimate of the average survival of thrombolyzed patients discharged from hospital, of which less than 2% were subjected to revascularization procedures (see Ch. 22).

A greater than average survival should be expected for patients younger than 65 years, with left ventricular EF greater than 50% and with no angina, no arrhythmias, and a negative exercise stress test. In this group of patients at very low risk, the predictive value of diagnostic tests is very low and the improvement of prognosis produced by treatment is difficult to assess.

Patients with chronic stable angina. Unselected patients with known IHD who can continue to exercise on the Bruce protocol into stage 4, have excellent prognoses even in the presence of ST-segment depression of more than 2 mm[18] and mortality was less than 1% per year also in those with triple-vessel disease.[19,20] In this group, therefore, prognosis should be even better for patients who not only manage to exercise beyond stage 4 but, in addition, have no history of a previous MI, have a normal resting ECG, and have a negative test. In this low-risk group, therefore, the predictive value of tests is very low and coronary arteriography would be unable to exclude the risk of infarction developing in the absence of coronary stenoses or in the presence of nonflow-limiting stenoses (see Chs 8 and 9). A multicenter 5-year prospective study by the Italian National Research Council has shown that, of a total of 1083 patients younger than 65 years who were subjected to coronary angiography because of a history of angina or infarction, only three patients developed MI out of 202 who had normal ECG exercise stress tests and no previous infarction, and these patients were not identifiable on the basis of the angiographic findings.[21]

13.2 PRIMARY AND SECONDARY PREVENTION

Primary prevention, in general, is the concern of community medicine and health authorities. Primary prevention in individuals with high levels of risk factors and secondary prevention in patients with known IHD are mainly the concern of physicians. For both primary and secondary prevention, currently available strategies are limited by our incomplete knowledge not only of the etiologic components that cause coronary atherosclerosis, precipitate MI, and determine an unfavorable cardiac response to ischemic insults but also of the individual genetic or acquired susceptibility to (or protection from) known and unknown risk factors.

For individuals at risk of IHD and for patients with either no or only mild IHD-related symptoms, it would be useful to know by how much life expectancy may be prolonged by lifelong therapeutic regimens, by invasive interventions and by making lifestyle changes. When there is no evidence of a statistically significant prolongation of life expectancy, it would be useful to know by how long a nonfatal IHD event, which could jeopardize the quality of life, could be delayed as a result of a particular treatment. Only accurate information on improved total and event-free life expectancy would allow a rational evaluation of lifelong therapeutic regimens and invasive interventions prescribed in order to improve prognosis, rather than to correct symptoms, signs, and consequences of myocardial ischemia.

◤ *Currently available assessments of risk factors and of determinants of prognosis have a reasonably good predictive value only in groups of patients who are at high risk of IHD-related events.*

The benefits of interventions and of compliance with lifelong preventive strategies are likely to increase in proportion to the estimated risk of a reduced ischemic event-free and total life expectancy. ◼

13.2.1 Primary prevention

A theoretical upper limit to the possible increase of life expectancy that could be expected from a reduction of IHD-related mortality is provided by calculations that assume the total elimination of cardiac mortality: as reported in Chapter 12, average life expectancy would be prolonged by only 2.5 years because individuals spared from cardiac deaths are exposed to other causes of death (see Fig. 12.17).

At present, the reduction of IHD risk in the general population can be based only on a widespread reduction of those modifiable causal risk factors identified so far, but, as discussed in Chapter 12, smoking, blood pressure, and cholesterol levels account for no more than one-half of the cases of IHD. Thus, it is not surprising that the benefits of available primary prevention strategies obtained in randomized trials have, so far, been less than expected, even in individuals considered at high risk on the basis of known risk factors.

Results of randomized trials

The reduction of a single causal risk factor for IHD (i.e. serum cholesterol or arterial blood pressure) and/or the control of multiple, moderately elevated risk factors (i.e. smoking, hypertension, and serum cholesterol) was found to be associated with a variable reduction of fatal and nonfatal ischemic events, but not always with a statistically significant reduction in total mortality. In any case, when causal risk factors and the baseline risk are not markedly elevated, the number of patients saved and also the number of events prevented are very small relative to the number of patients treated (see Table 13.2).

Reduction of total serum cholesterol. A meta-analysis of a large number of trials (which included a total of 103 598 individuals)[22] indicates that the incidence of fatal and nonfatal ischemic events decreased linearly in proportion to the reduction of cholesterol levels by diet or other treatments (see Fig. 13.11A/B). However, total mortality was not reduced significant-

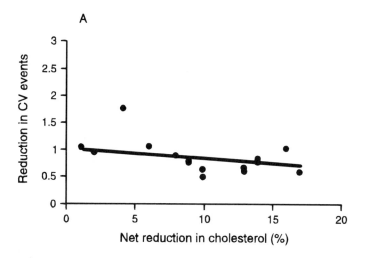

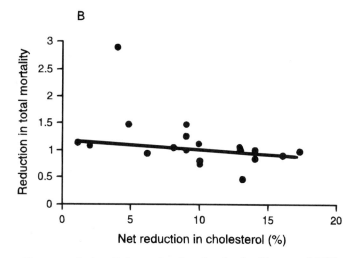

Fig. 13.11 Meta-analysis of the reduction in the incidence of IHD and total mortality in cholesterol reduction trials involving 103598 men. The odds-ratio of the incidence of IHD (**A**) and of total mortality (**B**) are plotted against the net percentage reduction of serum cholesterol levels achieved by various intervention trials. On average, the reduction of the relative risk is linearly related to the decrease of serum cholesterol levels, but the results of different trials vary markedly because the reduction of absolute risk (i.e. the number of events avoided/number of patients treated) is very low. (Modified from ref. 22.)

Table 13.2 Interventional trials in ischemic heart disease

Factor(s) investigated	Trial	No.of patients	IHD death		Total death		Death reduction (%)		Lives saved per 1000 treated*
			Int.	Placebo	Int.	Placebo	IHD	Total	
Multiple	WHO	60 881	428	450	1325	1341	−5	−1	−0.5 (6)
	Goteborg	30 000	462	461	1293	1318	0	−1.9	−1.7 (12)
	MRFIT	12 866	115	124	265	260	−7	+2	+0.8 (7)
	Helsinki	1 222	4	4	10	5	0	+50	+8 (5)
	Oslo	1 232	6	13	16	23	−54	−30	−11 (5)
Cholesterol	WHO (clofibrate)	15 745	54	48	162	127	+13	+28	+4 (5)
	LRC-CPPT	3 806	32	44	68	71	−27	−4	−1.6 (7)
	Gemfibrozil	4 081	6	8	45	42	−25	+7	+1.5 (5)
Smoking	Whitehall	1 445	49	62	123	128	−21	−4	−7 (10)
Hypertension	(8 trials)	17 314	—	—	784	887	—	−12	−12 (—)
	MRC	17 354	106	97	248	253	+9	−2	−0.6 (5)

In the treated group (Int.) the reduction of IHD mortality ranged from 0 to 54% but mortality was higher in two trials (+13% and + 9%). Total mortality was reduced in one trial to 30% but was increased in four trials from +2 to +50%. The most striking finding was the small difference in the number of deaths per 1000 patients over the whole duration of the observation period, ranging from a reduction of 11 deaths over 5 years in the Oslo study to an increase of 8 deaths over 5 years in the Helsinki study for treated patients

*Total years of follow-up in parentheses. (From ref. 36.)

ly in most studies and actually increased in some because of higher death rates due to cancer or to an altered behavior pattern in the intervention group.[23] It decreased significantly only in trials that included individuals who had multiple risk factors and serum cholesterol levels between 290 and 400 mg% and who hence were at a high risk of premature death from IHD (for example the Oslo trial).[24] Even in this trial, which included 1232 individuals and attained a 54% reduction of IHD-related mortality and a 30% reduction of total mortality, the absolute reduction of IHD and total mortality was seven (six in the treated group versus 13 in the control group) and seven (16 versus 23) deaths respectively over the whole 5-year duration of the trial.

A greater reduction of ischemic events might be achieved in individuals at high risk by interventions started earlier, continued for longer and resulting in a greater reduction of serum cholesterol levels.[25] There may be no risk in reducing serum cholesterol levels by diet,[26] but whether more aggressive interventions would increase life expectancy in individuals with moderately elevated cholesterol levels is uncertain for three main reasons:

1. As discussed in Chapter 12, in the MRFIT study,[27] although death rates from IHD over a 7-year follow-up period in men aged between 37 and 57 years increased in a curvilinear fashion over a sixfold range with serum cholesterol levels from 120 to 300 mg%, the increase was steep only for values above 250 mg% and total mortality was increased by about 50% only for cholesterol levels in the top decile (see Fig. 12.1). A cumulative meta-analysis study indicates that total mortality can be reduced only in individuals at very high risk (see Fig. 13.12).[28]

2. There is no evidence that decreasing cholesterol levels to 160 or 140 mg% in men aged between 37 and 59 years would reduce IHD mortality according to the observational data in Fig. 13.3, just as there is no evidence that lowering systolic blood pressure levels to 120 or 100 mmHg would cause a reduction of IHD mortality according to the same observational data. No data are available on the effects of reducing cholesterol levels and total mortality in elderly men and in women.

3. A rather small increase in life expectancy from a lifelong reduction of moderately elevated cholesterol levels is also predicted by theoretical calculations (see Fig. 13.13).[29] A major unproven assumption of these theoretical calculations is that all individuals are equally susceptible to elevated values of serum cholesterol. As indicated in Fig. 12.1, a 50% population attributable risk can result from a 100% prevalence of individuals in whom cholesterol carries a risk ratio (RR) of 2, but also of a 20% or 5% prevalence of individuals with an RR of 5 and 20, respectively. Only the ability to distinguish susceptible from insusceptible individuals could allow the former to be specifically targeted for treatments that provide a much greater absolute reduction of risk, thus sparing the latter the burden and anxiety of controlling a risk factor to which they are not susceptible.

The urge to take at least some immediate practical action against IHD has led to preferential citation of trials reporting beneficial results of cholesterol lowering,[30] and to the suggestion of an indiscriminate reduction of cholesterol levels below 200 or 180 mg% for the general population in spite of the lack of data in men above the age of 65 and in women, of the log-linear relationship between cholesterol and total mortality (see Figs 12.6 and 13.13) and of the increased mortality in individuals with decreasing cholesterol levels during follow-up observed in the Framingham study.[31] Such a view has, therefore, been questioned by scientists as there may be a "risk of correcting risk."[32] It has also been seized upon by the nonmedical press: in his review article in *Atlantic Monthly*,[33] Moore wrote: "Lowering your cholesterol is next to

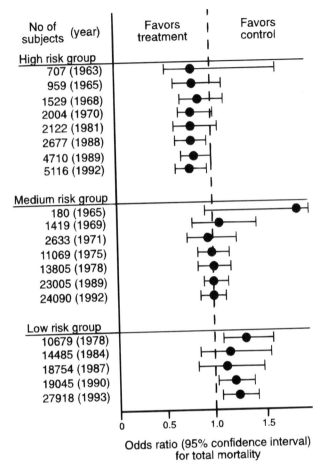

Fig. 13.12 Reduction of total mortality by lowering serum cholesterol levels is detectable only in high-risk groups. Cumulative meta-analysis of the effects of cholesterol-lowering treatment on total mortality stratified by risk (number of deaths from IHD per 1000 person-years in control subjects: high risk greater than 50, medium risk 10–50, low risk less than 10). Only in the high-risk group does the odds-ratio favor treatment with about a 20% reduction in the incidence of total mortality. (Modified from ref. 28.)

impossible with diet and often dangerous with drugs and it won't make you live longer." The results of available trials indicate that control of asymptomatic hypertriglyceridemia cannot yet be recommended conclusively for the general population.[34]

Control of hypertension. Reduction of severe hypertension is associated with a significant reduction of cerebrovascular and cardiac ischemic events. A meta-analysis of the major blood-pressure-lowering trials, which included over 45 000 patients,[35] indicates that reduction of mild hypertension, although associated with a decrease in the number of cerebrovascular events, causes only a small, often insignificant, reduction of cardiac ischemic events. This observation is in sharp contrast to the linear increase of IHD mortality with systolic blood pressure levels above 100 mmHg (see Fig. 13.3).

Multiple interventions. The results of multiple intervention trials have also been rather disappointing (see Table 13.2).[36] The reduction of IHD mortality was slight and, in some trials, not statistically significant. Total mortality was not significantly affected. Cardiac and total mortali-

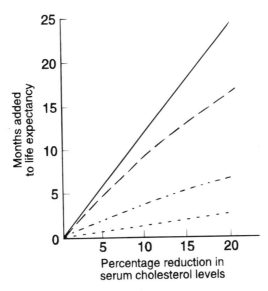

Fig. 13.13 Theoretical effect of the reduction of serum cholesterol levels on life expectancy. The calculated change in life expectancy from a lifelong reduction of serum cholesterol levels at the 90th percentile of the age- and gender-stratified population distribution (——, high-risk women; – – –, high-risk men; — — —, low-risk women; · · · · · ·, low-risk men). The months added to life expectancy are few for low-risk men and women, even for a 20% reduction. (Modified from ref. 29.)

ty actually increased in the intervention group of the Finnish study on 1222 business executives over a 10-year follow-up period.[37]

It is possible that a greater reduction of ischemic events could be obtained if risk factors were better controlled, and especially if the baseline risk was higher, but compliance with more drastic changes to the habits of a lifetime is even more difficult to achieve and maintain. The evidence of several large and well-designed trials seems, therefore, to give little support to the hope that specific interventions aimed at correcting moderate levels of multiple, known risk factors may increase life expectancy significantly except in individuals at very high risk.

Aspirin. In the United States Physicians' Health Study of 22 071 male physicians aged between 40 and 84 years and prescribed either aspirin (325 mg every other day) or placebo for a period of 5 years, there was a highly significant (44%) reduction in the incidence of MI.[38] However, in those treated with aspirin there was a slight increase in hemorrhagic stroke, and the numbers of cardiovascular deaths in the two groups were similar. In the British Doctors' Trial of 5139 male physicians aged between 50 and 78 years, two-thirds were assigned to take aspirin (500 mg daily) and the others were instructed to avoid aspirin-containing products. After 6 years there were no statistically significant differences in the combined endpoints of important cardiovascular events, MI, stroke (with a slight increase in disabling strokes in aspirin-treated subjects), or total cardiovascular mortality.[39] Given the very low absolute risk in the healthy men in these studies (about 0.7% per year), the absolute benefit of aspirin therapy was low and could not appreciably reduce total mortality.

The evidence supports the choice of between 75 and 100 mg aspirin daily for the prevention of arterial thromboembolism in all high-risk situations and is based on the following considerations:

1. This dose of aspirin is somewhat in excess of the lowest amount necessary and is sufficient to suppress thromboxane-dependent platelet activation fully.
2. Three separate, placebo-controlled trials of 75 mg daily have been completed

with the participation of over 4000 patients with cardiovascular or cerebrovascular disease, with consistently positive results.

3. Unbiased, indirect comparisons of different aspirin regimens do not demonstrate
   a larger effect of higher doses and suggest that the opposite may be true.[40]

Community medicine approach

Efforts to reduce IHD-related mortality and disability in the community should target individuals with moderate and even low levels of known risk factors because they represent the
majority of those among whom IHD will develop. General screening of the population cannot be recommended until new and more specific risk factors are identified, because of the
limited results obtained in randomized trials of high-risk individuals (such as the 3% in the
top decile of risk selected for randomization following the screening of 361 662 men in the
MRFIT study)[27] as well as the limited prognostic value of a positive ECG exercise stress test
when proven risk factors are corrected.[8]

Health authorities should, therefore, proceed with a general program of community education, starting from infancy and adolescence, in order to reduce cultural and individual
dysadaptation (which is a major cause of risk factor clustering) and to promote a philosophy of life that reduces stressful situations and improves social support and an individual's
ability to cope. Reduction of dysadaptation could, by itself, lead to:

a. the cessation of smoking
b. the adoption of healthier dietary habits
c. regular daily physical exercise
d. a decrease in hypertension
e. the control of excess body weight.

Only a global approach such as this could last throughout life and would not only reduce
the risk of IHD (and, possibly, prolong life expectancy by reducing a major cause of risk factor clustering) but would also improve the quality of life.

A partial approach against individual risk factors for IHD, such as cessation of smoking
(which is a much stronger risk factor for lung cancer and obstructive lung disease) and the
control of hypertension (which is a major risk factor for stroke), is more easily achieved than
the control of diet and the loss of weight, which, although undoubtedly useful, require an
even stronger sense of motivation. Control of diet by reduced intake of cholesterol and
unsaturated fats is a widely accepted recommendation, but fat composition, antioxidants,
fiber, as well as total caloric intake (in relation to consumption) may all be equally important. Campaigns aimed at the modification of diet should not neglect the problem of excess
body weight, which is quite prominent in affluent societies (over 30% of adolescents in the
USA are overweight) and appears to have important prognostic consequences independent
of serum cholesterol levels.[41]

Clinical approach

Individuals with markedly elevated levels of a single risk factor known to be associated with
premature death from IHD and with clustering of multiple high levels of risk factors, particularly when associated with other causes of mortality (such as cerebrovascular disease and
cancer) and/or with ECG or echocardiographic signs of left ventricular hypertrophy, should
be treated by physicians. An aggressive approach aimed at reducing known, proven risk factors should be adopted on the assumption that the individual may be susceptible to at least

one of them. Cessation of smoking and control of hypertension should be accompanied by reduction of serum cholesterol levels to about 240 mg% in a conservative approach, and to below 200 mg% in an aggressive approach, according to the recommendations of various task forces.[42,43] As the greatest benefit is to be expected in high risk patients, interventions should be proportional to the baseline risk.[43] The improvement in total and event-free life expectancy associated with a reduction in serum cholesterol levels from 240 to 200 mg% in individuals at high risk of IHD because of the clustering of other risk factors, can be assessed properly only in randomized trials.

In individuals considered at high risk, a global change of lifestyle should also be strongly advised when required. Some patients may be heavy smokers; others may be overweight, lead sedentary lives, or have very abnormal lipid profiles; still others may be in a particularly stressful period of their lives. The advice should be tailored to the patient's personality, taking great care not to create new or additional anxieties, because the correction of risk will require a lifelong effort.

Focusing uniquely on the cessation of smoking and the correction of hypertension and abnormal serum lipid patterns may not be the optimal advice for a patient if it distracts focus from the correction of all other individual risk factors and from the improvement of lifestyle. For individuals unable to cope with the stresses of their lives, the suggestion that they take periodic breaks, find some pleasant regular recreational physical activity, and reduce the pace of their activities could be as important as advising dietary restrictions for overweight individuals with unhealthy diets.

Patients considered at high risk of IHD should also be advised to take 50 mg aspirin on a full stomach, unless contraindicated. As low-dose aspirin is a fairly simple preventive measure with a low risk of side effects, the additional beneficial effects of other, less simple, forms of preventive strategies in patients at very high risk should be assessed in prospective randomized trials. The benefits of other antiplatelet agents in high-risk individuals has not been evaluated.

■ *Patients should be convinced by objective data, but they should never be panicked into becoming more compliant, as the fear and anxiety thus generated will immediately and continuously impair the quality of daily life, merely for the achievement of a future possible gain in an event-free or total life expectancy.*■

13.2.2 Secondary prevention

Prevention becomes the major goal of therapy for patients not requiring treatment for the relief of documented ischemia-related symptoms or signs. Such patients have already declared themselves at risk, but it is not known precisely which particular risk factors concurred to cause their illness. The only available strategy, therefore, is to advise them to make the changes to their lifestyle that are generally advocated in individuals at high risk. In addition, when specific known individual risk factors are identified they should be treated, as they could be causally related to the disease.

These general, long-term secondary prevention strategies should be planned carefully, as they must be continued throughout life and integrated with prophylactic drug therapy and revascularization procedures on the basis of the evidence of improved total and event-free life expectancy provided by randomized trials.

In patients with severe symptoms and prognosis, the beneficial effects of some medical and interventional treatments are so obvious that no trials are required and, hence, they generate the hope of similar beneficial effects also in patients with less severe symptoms and prognoses. In patients without severe symptoms and obvious reduction of life expectancy, the beneficial effects of treatment may not be separated easily from a spontaneous benign course of the disease and from a placebo effect; they can therefore, be assessed objectively only by prospective, controlled randomized trials. Controlled trials are also necessary in order to assess objectively any side effects and complications resulting from treatments as they contribute to the quality of life, which becomes the major endpoint of treatment when its effect on the prolongation of life is not immediately apparent. It should, however, be stressed that in low-risk patients the prognostic predictive accuracy of tests is very low and those who benefit from treatment are a very small fraction of those treated.

Review of main randomized trials

The effects of treatment on survival and secondary prevention of nonfatal IHD have been assessed in patients with specific chronic clinical syndromes, such as healed MI and resolved unstable and chronic stable angina, as well as in patients separated according to coronary and ventricular angiographic findings. Such studies provide very valuable baseline information on the benefits, as well as the side effects and risks, to be expected, in general, in a given class of patients. Unfortunately, as very broad inclusion criteria are commonly adopted, in order to enroll sufficiently large numbers of patients for statistical analysis within a short period, the groups studied often appear quite heterogeneous to practising physicians. In many trials, patients with symptoms or signs of ischemia (which in themselves require treatment) are grouped together with patients without symptoms and signs of ischemia, in whom treatment is aimed only at the improvement of prognosis.

Patients included according to only clinical criteria may have varying degrees of coronary stenosis severity, reduction of coronary flow reserve, and ventricular dysfunction and those included according to angiographic criteria may have variable severity of symptoms and signs of ischemia. Thus, significant differences in the effects of a given treatment on patients meeting the inclusion criteria may be revealed only by subgroup analysis that had not been envisaged when the trial was originally planned.

Healed MI. A recent meta-analysis study[44] identified five forms of treatment that produced statistically significant reductions in mortality by 14–22% (Table 13.3). The number of patients enrolled in the trials ranged from 5000 to 20 000 for the various forms of treatment, which included anticoagulants, rehabilitation regimens, β-blockers, and cholesterol-lowering and antiplatelet agents. It remains to be established whether the beneficial effects obtained from individual interventions apply to all patients or only to specific subgroups, and to what extent

Table 13.3 Progressive meta-analysis of secondary prevention trials in post-MI patients

Strategy	No. of trials	No. of patients	Odds-ratio	P
Anticoagulants	12	4975	0.78 (0.67–0.90)	<0.001
Rehabilitation regimen	23	5022	0.80 (0.67–0.95)	0.012
β-Blockers	17	20 138	0.81 (0.73–0.89)	<0.001
Cholesterol lowering	8	10 775	0.86 (0.79–0.94)	<0.001
Antiplatelet agents	9	13 917	0.83 (0.74–0.93)	0.002

The average reduction of mortality with different prevention strategies ranges from 14% for cholesterol-lowering agents to 22% for anticoagulants. It is not known whether all patients benefited equally from each treatment and whether the beneficial effects would be additive when applied to the same patient. The absolute risk reduction (total number of patients saved out of the total treated) with all treatments was small. (From ref. 44.)

able 13.4 Absolute benefit on mortality in long-term preventive trials post-MI

rial	Drug	No. of patients	Follow-up (months)	Annual mortality per 1000 (control group)	Annual mortality per 1000 (treated group)	Lives saved per 1000 per year	Mortality reduction (%)
HAT	β-blockers	4000	24	50	35	15	30
AVE	ACE inhibitors	2231	42	70	58	12	17
SPECT	Anticoagulants	3404	37	36	32	4	11

The absolute benefit (i.e. number of lifes saved per year per 1000 patients treated) varied in different trials. These data re examples from refs. 45–47)

the benefits obtained from one form of treatment are additive to those of others. In studies in which patients were enrolled before discharge, or soon after, the effect of treatment on time-dependent postdischarge risk, as opposed to the late constant risk, was not considered. It is also unknown whether the beneficial effects apply to patients on aspirin and/or those who received thrombolytic treatment during the acute phase.

The number of lives saved is an important element, not considered in trials that report only the percentage reduction in mortality, which varies in different trials (see Table 13.4).[45–47]

The results of subgroup analyses exemplify the possible difficulties of a straightforward application to individual patients of the average results of trials that included heterogeneous patient populations: for example, diltiazem[48] and verapamil[49] increased mortality in patients with obvious impairment of left ventricular function, but improved it in those with preserved ventricular function; the average effect, therefore, was nil. For verapamil, the results of subgroup analysis were confirmed by a trial in which only patients with preserved ventricular function were included,[50] and for diltiazem by a trial in patients with non-Q-wave infarction.[51] β-Blockers produced greater beneficial effects in patients with moderate impairment of left ventricular function than in those with good ventricular function, but this result was not tested in specific prospective trials.

For all effective treatments, the greatest absolute reduction of fatal and nonfatal ischemic events occurs early after MI, during convalescence, when the risk of reinfarction and death is greatest. Whether treatment prolonged after 6 months causes a further statistically significant improvement of survival is still not known, largely because the risk of events after the initial 3–6 months is low. Thus, a very large number of patients should be randomized and followed for many years in order to detect a possible further significant beneficial effect, but the number of patients saved per 1000 treated can only be small (see Ch. 22).

Unstable angina. In patients who had gone through a phase of unstable angina, randomized long-term follow-up studies included a mixture of cases, i.e. with or without prior infarction, with persisting symptoms and signs of ischemia, or in a quiescent phase of IHD. In these heterogeneous groups, aspirin was found to reduce the incidence of acute ischemic events by about 50% over a 12–36-month follow-up period. The effect was similar not only for doses of aspirin ranging from 325 to 1250 mg/day but also for doses of only 75 mg/day (see Ch. 19). In none of these trials have the effects of treatment on the time dependency of risk been considered adequately. Bypass surgery was found to reduce 5-year mortality rates in patients with reduced left ventricular EF, but not in those with preserved left ventricular function, as was also observed in stable patients (see below).

Chronic stable angina. There have been no prospective randomized trials on the effects of anti-ischemic drug therapy (i.e. β-blockers, calcium antagonists, or nitrates) on survival and on the development of nonfatal infarction in patients with mild chronic stable angina. The use of these drugs in patients in a quiescent phase of IHD is not based on objective data and is, therefore, theoretical. Prospective randomized trials now in progress on anti-ischemic therapy in stable, totally asymptomatic patients presenting only silent myocardial ischemia, include those with and those without a previous MI. They will, therefore, be unable to distinguish between the effects of treatment on these two groups of patients that have different baseline risks. No data are available for asymptomatic patients with no evidence of silent ischemia (i.e. who are in a quiescent phase and who are likely to be at an even lower risk) (see Ch. 17).

Results of coronary artery surgery. No specific controlled studies have been undertaken on the beneficial effects of coronary artery bypass grafting (CABG) in patients in a quiescent phase of IHD. In patients whose symptoms are mild enough to make them eligible for randomization, subgroup analysis shows that the results of CABG are superior to those of medical therapy only in the presence of either left ventricular dysfunction or three-vessel disease, particularly when the proximal LAD is stenosed. Patients with a left main coronary artery stenosis greater than 50 or 60% are also generally considered to be improved by surgery, but it is not known whether this conclusion applies to asymptomatic patients with negative exercise stress tests. On average, the steeper the decline of yearly survival in the control group, the greater the benefits of surgery. No statistically significant benefits were demonstrable in patients with rather flat survival curves and over 90% average survival at 5 years on medical

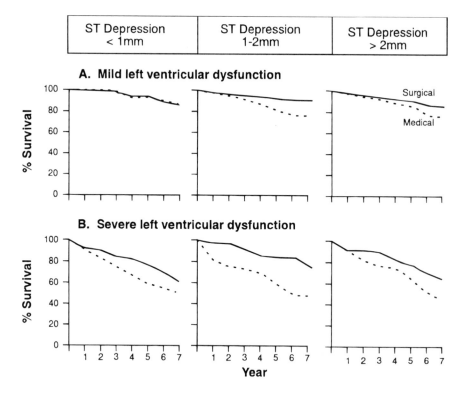

Fig. 13.14 Influence of left ventricular dysfunction and of the results of exercise stress testing on the benefits of CABG. (A) The average improvement of survival by CABG (—) is negligible in patients with a good prognosis (i.e. with mild left ventricular dysfunction and negative exercise stress test), because their 7-year survival is good also on medical therapy (– – –); hence, there is little room for improvement. **(B)** The benefit of CABG on survival is greater in patients with severe left ventricular dysfunction and positive exercise stress test who have a poor survival on medical therapy; thus, there is ample room for improvement.

therapy, in particular in those with negative exercise stress tests (see Fig. 13.14).[52] It is not known whether the improvement in survival occurred in the same patients in whom symptoms and signs of ischemia were improved (for whom surgery would have been required anyway), or whether it occurred also in those in whom surgery was performed mainly to improve prognosis. The beneficial effects of bypass surgery on survival tends to decrease after 10 years.[53]

Results of percutaneous coronary angioplasty (PTCA). The beneficial effects of PTCA in patients in a quiescent phase of IHD or with mild symptoms and signs of IHD have not been evaluated. Several prospective randomized studies comparing PTCA with medical and surgical therapy are in progress, but they include a mixture of patients with severe symptoms and signs of ischemia (which may themselves indicate the need for the procedure) and patients with mild or no symptoms and signs of ischemia submitted to the procedure only because of their coronary arteriographic findings.

Angiographic regression of coronary stenoses. The effects of cholesterol-lowering strategies and calcium antagonists on both regression of coronary stenoses and formation of new lesions were considered as possible surrogate evidence of their beneficial long-term effects on the evolution of IHD, which is more difficult to demonstrate. The effects on stenoses observed with cholesterol-lowering strategies, although statistically significant, were minimal in quantitative terms. For proximal stenoses the diameter change was from 1.910 to 1.875 mm after 2.5 years' treatment with colestipol and niacin, and from 1.910 to 1.915 mm after placebo.[54] In a recent review on the subject, Brown et al[55] concluded that these changes were insufficient to explain the reduction of ischemic events. Nifedipine failed to influence either progression or regression of stenoses, but caused a 28% reduction in the appearance of new lesions. In treated and control patients, 63% of stenoses did not change, 25% progressed and 12% regressed; 103 new lesions greater than 20% occurred in treated patients as opposed to 144 in controls.[56] Over the 3 years' duration of one of the trials, eight cardiac deaths occurred among treated patients and two occurred among patients treated with placebo. A reduction in the number of new lesions, from 27 to 15%, was observed in another study using nicardipine.[57]

The surrogate approaches that consider the effects of treatment on stenoses rather than on the development of ischemic events are limited by the uncertainties about the remodeling of stenoses with extraluminal expansion of plaques, which cannot be assessed angiographically (see Ch. 8), and by the variable relationship between stenosis progression and ischemic manifestations (see Chs 8 and 9).

Clinical approach

For patients who are in a quiescent phase of IHD or have very mild symptoms, a rational management must aim at improving both life expectancy and the quality of life, but the former can be improved only when it is obviously reduced compared with controls.

Improvement of life expectancy. A caring physician must consider all available clinical, laboratory, and investigational data that have cumulative effects on life expectancy, compared with life tables for healthy matched individuals. Only such an assessment can allow an informed choice by balancing the burden, the side effects, and the risk of each form of therapy with the magnitude of the expected improvement of life expectancy. As prognostic information has usually been collected only after considering specific determinants of prognosis, it is necessary to apply information obtained from different studies to the patient under consideration.

Many forms of medical treatment have been shown to produce a statistically significant reduction of mortality in secondary prevention trials; however, the number of patients saved per year of treatment was relatively small and the consequent average improvement of life expectancy cannot be estimated.

In an aggressive approach aimed at improving prognosis, patients without persistent ischemic manifestations also could be prescribed all forms of treatment that have proven beneficial in randomized trials; however, it is not known to what extent the beneficial effects of one form of treatment are additive to those of others, or for how long they are beneficial, nor is it known to what extent complications are increased and lifestyle affected by multiple therapy.

In individuals without a demonstrable reduction of life expectancy, therefore, lifelong preventive treatments with the least side effects and inconvenience, such as aspirin (75 mg/day), when not contraindicated should have priority. Improvement of dysadaptation, cessation of smoking, reduction of excess weight, and control of hypertension and of high levels of serum cholesterol and fibrinogen should also be considered, but the extent to which each contributes to the prolongation of an event-free and total life expectancy in any individual patient remains uncertain.

Additional preventive drug treatments, such as β-blockers, calcium antagonists, and oral anticoagulants, should be prescribed for patients with no ischemic manifestations only when such patients are considered to be at high risk; for example, during the early period after infarction or after unstable angina, ACE inhibitors should be prescribed for patients with obvious post-MI impairment of left ventricular function, but it is not clear for how long the treatment should be continued in totally asymptomatic post-MI patients.

The improvement of survival with CABG is likely to be greater with arterial conduits, which are now used widely, than with the vein grafts that were used in the trials reported above. However, the survival of medically treated patients is also likely to be better with the use of aspirin, β-blockers, and ACE inhibitors, and with the stricter control of risk factors now more widely applied. Finally, the results of surgery are not necessarily the same in all institutions and, therefore, the only results applicable to the patient under consideration are those from the center where the procedure would be carried out.

Quality of life. The quality of life is even more difficult to assess than the reduction of life expectancy, because it is influenced not only by the disability caused by disease but also by anxiety about prognosis, the inconvenience of prescribed therapy, or the resulting side effects. For low-risk patients, treatment should, therefore, be individualized also according to the patient's philosophy of life. Sound advice will be given by physicians who are capable not only of assessing the prolongation of total and event-free life expectancy produced by the various forms of treatment, as well as their possible risks and side effects, but who are also prepared to spend sufficient time trying to understand a patient's personality and attitude toward the disease, in order to offer balanced advice aimed at improving their quality of life while it remains event free.

REFERENCES

1. Myerburg RJ, Kessler KM, Castellanos A et al. Sudden cardiac death. Structure, function and time-dependence of risk. Circulation 1992;85(Suppl. 1):12.
2. US Department of Health and Human Services. Public Health Service. Agency for Health Care Policy and Research National Heart, Lung, and Blood Institute. Unstable angina: diagnosis and management. In: Clinical Practice Guideline, No. 10, 1994.
3. Neaton JD, Wentworth D for the Multiple Risk Factor Intervention Trial Research Group. Serum cholesterol, blood pressure, cigarette smoking and death from coronary heart disease. Arch Intern Med 1992;152:56.
4. Kannel WB. Some lessons in cardiovascular epidemiology from Framingham. Am J Cardiol 1976;37:269.

5. World Health Organization: MONICA Project. Geographical variation: the major risk factors of coronary heart disease in men and women aged 35–66 years. World Health Statistics Quarterly 1988;*41*:115.

6. Shaper AG, Pocock SJ, Walker M, Phillips AN, Whitehead TP, Mcfarlane PW. Risk factors for ischaemic heart disease: the prospective phase of the British Regional Heart Study. J Epidemiol Community Health 1985;*39*:197.

7. Gordon DJ, Ekelund LG, Karon JM et al. Predictive value of the exercise tolerance test for mortality in North American men: the Lipid Research Clinics Mortality Follow-up Study. Circulation 1986;*74*:252.

8. Multiple Risk Factor Intervention Trial Research Group. Exercise electrocardiogram and coronary heart disease mortality in the Multiple Risk Factor Intervention Trial. Am J Cardiol 1985;*55*:16.

9. Epstein SE, Quyyumi AA, Bonow RO. Sudden cardiac death without warning. Possible mechanisms and implications for screening asymptomatic populations. Engl J Med 1989;*321*:320.

10. Holmes DR, Davis K, Gersh BJ et al. Risk factor profiles of patients with sudden cardiac death and death from other cardiac causes: a report from the Coronary Artery Surgery Study (CASS). J Am Coll Cardiol 1989;*13*:524.

11. The Multicenter Postinfarction Research Group: Risk stratification and survival after myocardial infarction. N Engl J Med 1983:*309*:331.

12. Mock MR, Ringqvist I, Fisher LD et al. Survival of medically treated patients in the Coronary Artery Surgery Study (CASS) Registry. Circulation 1982;*66*:562.

13. Weiner DA, Ryan TJ, McCabe C et al. Risk of developing an acute myocardial infarction or sudden coronary death in patients with exercise-induced silent myocardial ischemia. A report from the Coronary Artery Surgery Study (CASS) Registry. Am J Cardiol 1988;*62*:1155.

14. Waters D, Craven TE, Lespérance J. Prognostic significance of progression of coronary atherosclerosis. Circulation 1993;*87*:1067.

15. Pekkanen J, Linn S, Heiss G et al. Ten-year mortality from cardiovascular disease in relation to cholesterol levels among men with and without preexisting cardiovascular disease. N Engl J Med 1990;*322*:1700.

16. Gruppo Italiano per lo Studio della Streptochinasi nell'Infarto Miocardico (GISSI): Long term effects of intravenous thrombolytic treatment in acute myocardial infarction: Final report of the GISSI study. Lancet 1987;*2*:871.

17. GISSI-3: Effects of lisinopril, of transdermal nitrates and of their association on six-week mortality and ventricular function among 19,394 patients with acute myocardial infarction. Lancet 1994;*343*:1115.

18. Podrid PJ, Graboys TB, Lown B. Prognosis of medically treated patients with coronary-artery disease with profound ST-segment depression during exercise testing. N Engl J Med 1981;*305*:1111.

19. Weiner DA, Ryan TJ, McCabe CH et al. Prognostic importance of a clinical profile and exercise test in medically treated patients with coronary artery disease. J Am Coll Cardiol 1984;*3*:772.

20. Rutherford JD. Coronary artery surgery, 1984. N Z Med J 1984;*97*:813.

21. Brunelli C, Cristofani R, L'Abbate A, for the ODI Study Group. Long term survival in medically treated patients with ischaemic heart disease and prognostic importance of clinical and electrocardiographic data (the Italian CNR Multicentre Prospective Study ODI). Eur Heart J 1989;*10*:292.

22. Holme I. An analysis of randomized trials evaluating the effect of cholesterol reduction on total mortality and coronary heart disease incidence. Circulation 1990;*82*:1916.

23. Muldoon MF, Manuck SB, Matthews KA. Mortality experience in cholesterol reduction trial. Lancet 1991;*324*:922.

24. Hjermann I, Velve-Byre K, Holme I, Leren P. Effect of diet and smoking on the incidence of coronary heart disease: report from the Oslo Study Group of a randomized trial in healthy men. Lancet 1981;*2*:1303.

25. Law MR, Wald NJ, Thompson SG. By how much and how quickly does reduction in serum cholesterol concentration lower risk of ischaemic heart disease? Br Med J 1994;*308:*367.
26. Law MR, Thompson SG, Wald NJ. Assessing possible hazards of reducing serum cholesterol. Br Med J 1994;*308:*373.
27. Martin MJ, Browner WS, Hulley SB, Kuller LH, Wentworth D. Serum cholesterol, blood pressure, and mortality: implication from a cohort of 361,662 men. Lancet 1986;2933.
28. Smith GD, Song F, Sheldon TA. Cholesterol lowering and mortality: the importance of considering initial level of risk. Br Med J 1993;*306:*1367.
29. Taylor WC, Pass TM, Shepard DS, Komaroff AL. Cholesterol reduction and life expectancy. A model incorporating multiple risk factors. J Am Coll Phys 1987;*106:*605.
30. James TN. Presidential Address AHA 53rd Scientific Session. Sure Cures, Quick Fixes and Easy Answers. A cautionary tale about coronary disease. Circulation 1981;*63:*1199A.
31. Anderson KM, Castelli WP, Levy D. Cholesterol and mortality. 30 years of follow-up from the Framingham Study. J Am Med Ass 1987;*257:*2176.
32. Oliver MF. Doubts about preventing coronary heart disease. Multiple interventions in middle aged men may do more harm than good. Br Med J 1992;*304:*393
33. Moore TJ. The cholesterol myth. Atlantic Monthly, September 1989.
34. Consensus Conference. Treatment of hypertriglyceridemia. J Am Med Ass 1984;*251:*1196.
35. Cruickshank JM, Fox K, Collins P. Meta-analysis of hypertension treatment trials. Lancet 1990;*235:*1992.
36. McCormick J, Skrabanek P. Coronary heart disease is not preventable by population interventions. Lancet 1988;*II:*839.
37. Strandberg TE, Solomaa VV, Naukkarunen V et al. Long term mortality after 5-year multifactorial primary prevention of cardiovascular diseases in middle-age men. J Am Med Assoc 1991;*266:*1225.
38. Steering Committee of the Physicians' Health Study Research Group. Final report on the aspiring component of the ongoing Physicians' Health Study. N Engl J Med 1989;*321:*129.
39. Peto R, Gray R, Collins R et al. Randomised trial of prophylactic daily aspirin in British male doctors. Br Med J 1988;*296:*13.
40. Patrono C. Aspirin as an antiplatelet drug. N Engl J Med 1994;*330:*1287.
41. Must A, Jacques PF, Dallal GE, Bajema CJ, Dietz WH. Long-term morbidity and mortality of overweight adolescents. A follow-up of the Harvard Growth Study of 1992 to 1935. N Engl J Med 1992;*327:*1350.
42. The Expert Panel: Summary of the Second Report of the National Cholesterol Education Program (NCEP) Expert Panel on detection, evaluation and treatment of high blood cholesterol in adults. (Adult Treatment Panel II). J Am Med Assoc 1993;*269:*3015.
43. Pyörälä K, De Backer G, Graham I, Poole-Wilson P, Wood D on behalf of the Task Force (Members of the Task Force listed in the Appendix). Prevention of coronary heart disease in clinical practice. Recommendations of the Task Force of the European Society of Cardiology, European Atherosclerosis Society and European Society of Hypertension. European Heart J 1994;*15:*1300–1331.
44. Lau J, Antman EM, Jimenez-Silva J, Kupelnick B, Mosteller F, Chalmers TC. Cumulative meta-analysis of therapeutic trials for myocardial infarction. N Engl J Med 1992;*327:*248.
45. Beta-Blocker Heart Trial Research Group. A randomized controlled trial of propranolol in patients with acute myocardial infarction. I. Mortality results. J Am Med Assoc 1982;*247:*1707.
46. Pfeffer MA, Braunwald E, Mayi LA et al. Effect of captopril on mortality and morbidity in patients with left ventricular dysfunction after myocardial infarction. Results of the Survival and Ventricular Enlargement Trial. N Engl J Med 1992;*327:*669.
47. Anticoagulants in the Secondary Prevention of Events in Coronary Thrombosis (ASPECT) Research Group. Effect of long-term anticoagulant treatment on mortality and cardiovascular morbidity after myocardial infarction. Lancet 1994;*343:*499.
48. The Multicenter Diltiazem Postinfarction Trial Research Group. The effect of diltiazem on mortality and reinfarction after myocardial infarction. N Engl J Med 1988;*319:*385.

49. The Danish Study Group on Verapamil in Myocardial Infarction. Verapamil in acute myocardial infarction. Eur Heart J 1984;5:516.
50. The Danish Study Group on Verapamil in Myocardial Infarction: Effect of verapamil on mortality and major events after acute myocardial infarction (the Danish Verapamil infarction trials II-Davit II). Am J Cardiol 1990;66:779.
51. Gibson RS, Boden WE, Theroux P et al. Diltiazem and reinfarction in patients with non Q-wave myocardial infarction. N Engl J Med 1986;315:423.
52. Weiner DA, Ryan TJ, McCabe CH et al. Value of exercise testing in determining the risk classification and the response to coronary artery bypass grafting in three-vessel coronary artery disease: a report from the Coronary Artery Surgery Study (CASS) Registry. Am J Cardiol 1987;60:262.
53. Varnauskas E and ECSSG. Twelve-year follow-up of survival in the randomized European Coronary Surgery Study. N Engl J Med 1988;319:332.
54. Brown G, Albers JJ, Fisher LD et al. Regression of coronary artery disease as a result of intensive lipid-lowering therapy in men with high levels of apolipoprotein B. N Engl J Med 1990;323:1289.
55. Brown BG, Zhao XQ, Sacco DE, Albers JJ. Lipid lowering and plaque regression: new insights into prevention of plaque disruption and clinical events in coronary disease. Circulation 1993;87:1781.
56. Lichtlen PR, Hugenholtz PG, Rafflenbeul W, Hecker H, Jost S, Deckers JW on behalf of the INTACT Group Investigators. Retardation of angiographic progression of coronary artery disease by nifedipine. Lancet 1990;335:1109.
57. Waters D, Lespérance J, Fracetich M et al. A controlled clinical trial to assess the effect of a calcium channel blocker on the progression of coronary atherosclerosis. Circulation 1990;82:1940.

Mechanisms of cardiac pain and silent ischemia

Mechanisms of ischemic cardiac pain and the significance of pain in ischemic syndromes

INTRODUCTION

Anginal pain is the symptom that usually brings patients with ischemic heart disease (IHD) to medical attention. Transient myocardial ischemia and even necrosis can, however, occur without pain, whereas severe angina-like pain can occur in the absence of detectable myocardial ischemia. Although cardiac ischemic pain is an important warning signal, it is unpleasant, alarming, and, sometimes, disabling. Hence, as for other forms of bodily responses to potentially noxious stimuli, pain can elicit a protective reaction, but it may also become a major component of the disease when its severity is disproportionate to the severity of ischemia and when it bears no relation to the prognosis of the disease.

Ischemic cardiac pain in its full-blown presentation has three components:

a. a dull, poorly localized visceral component
b. a much sharper somatic component with a well-defined dermatomeric distribution
c. a subjective component of anguish and fear of imminent death (angor animi).

Not all these features are present in all patients, nor in all ischemic episodes in the same patient. Angor animi, for instance, is present only during the most severe attacks and in a minority of patients. Ischemic cardiac pain usually begins with either the visceral or somatic component only, the latter involving a single dermatome. As the severity of the attack increases, it may gradually involve previously unaffected components and spread to other dermatomes. This evolving pattern reflects the progressive recruitment of cardiac afferent fibers converging on dorsal horn spinal neurons and/or the progressive facilitation of the transmission of ascending nervous impulses.

As described in masterly fashion by Heberden,1 in its most typical presentation ischemic cardiac pain is retrosternal with a crushing, squeezing, or burning character. It may radiate to the throat, neck, or ulnar side of the left arm, extend down to the little finger and, occasionally, to the interscapular region or epigastrium. Less frequently it radiates to both arms, or to the right arm, or to the jaw and teeth. The variations are numerous,2 however, and even radiation to the left leg has been reported.3 In some patients the pain may be confined exclusively to only one of these areas. Angina pectoris may also be associated with a strangling sensation in the upper chest and neck. The intensity of the discomfort can vary greatly, from a mild feeling of retrosternal fullness or tingling in only one dermatome to pain that is excruciating and unbearable. The total lack of pain (and also of any other symptom) represents one extreme of the spectrum of the possible clinical presentations of myocardial ischemia. Although, in general, the more severe and long-lasting the pain, the more severe the ischemia, the relationship between the severity of myocardial ischemia and pain is extremely variable: indeed, myocardial infarction (MI), as well as transient ischemic episodes, may be painless in a substantial number of cases. Conversely, even in the absence of detectable ECG changes ischemia may, very occasionally, be associated with severe pain. Neither the features of ischemic cardiac pain nor its absence are related to the actual causes of ischemia.

Recent studies have led to a better understanding of the stimuli responsible for ischemic cardiac pain and of the factors that determine its occurrence and modulate its severity. This chapter summarizes the anatomic and physiologic bases of the perception of cardiac pain and discusses its significance in the various syndromes.

14.1 ANATOMIC AND PHYSIOLOGIC BASES OF PAIN PERCEPTION

Anginal pain, as somatic pain, can be defined according to Sherrington as a conscious, unpleasant perception of a noxious event that threatens the integrity of a tissue and elicits a complaint and a protective reaction.[4] The anatomic and physiologic bases of visceral pain perception can be summarized as follows (see Fig. 14.1).

1. Noxious stimuli excite bipolar neurons, which have a peripherally directed axon terminating in the heart and a centrally directed axon innervating the spinal dorsal horn. The potentially painful messages converge together with many other afferent fibers from visceral and somatic areas of the same dermatome on the same dorsal horn spinal neurons.
2. Transmission of these potentially painful messages from the dorsal horn to the thalamus is modulated by afferent and descending impulses from supraspinal centers; transmission of the impulses from the thalamus to the cortical centers may also be modulated by afferent and descending impulses.
3. Perception of these afferent impulses is related to their decoding as a conscious unpleasant experience and, as described, elicits both a complaint and a protective reaction.

■ *Because of the variable convergence of several afferent neurons coming from different visceral organs and from somatic dermatomes on the same ascending neurons, cardiac pain can be perceived in several dermatomes and can radiate to others. In addition, noncardiac stimuli can cause pain with similar features to those of cardiac ischemic pain.* ■

14.1.1 Noxious stimuli

The nature of the stimuli that excite sensory receptors has been debated for decades. About 80 years ago it was suggested that ischemic cardiac pain might be due to stretching of the ventricular wall (the "mechanical" hypothesis);[5] then, about 60 years ago, it was proposed that it might be caused by the local intramyocardial release of various substances (the "chemical" hypothesis).[6] The cardiac receptor responsible for the transmission of these afferent stimuli may be specific only for painful stimuli (the "specificity" hypothesis), or may carry a variety of afferent impulses and cause pain only when stimulated excessively (the "intensity" hypothesis) (see below).

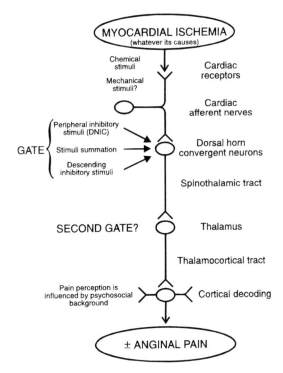

Fig. 14.1 Afferent neural pathways involved in the transmission of cardiac ischemic pain. Cardiac sensory receptors may be stimulated by chemical or mechanical stimuli. Afferent impulses project to dorsal horn convergent neurons where their progression towards supraspinal centers is modulated by peripheral or descending stimuli (the "gate" theory). Further modulation of cardiac afferent stimuli might occur in the thalamus. Pain perception takes place when cardiac afferent stimuli are decoded in the cortex and is strongly influenced by the psychosocial background. Afferent fibers from different cardiac areas and from other visceral and somatic areas converge on the same ascending neurons. The existence of specific neurons involved in only the transmission of pain (the "specificity" hypothesis) is, so far, unproven. The intense excitation of polymodal fibers, also involved in autonomic nervous control, was proposed as an alternative hypothesis (the "intensity" hypothesis). (Modified from ref. 17.)

The most likely site of ischemic cardiac pain is within the myocardium. This is certainly the case when the only cause of ischemia is an increase in myocardial oxygen consumption. It is generally accepted that free nerve endings in the myocardium, which are more abundant around small coronary vessels, are the sensory receptors, although pain receptors are also present in large coronary vessels (see below). However, patients do not usually experience pain when the subendocardium is pulled vigorously when malfunctioning pacing wires are detached, or during endomyocardial biopsies. Endocarditis, myocarditis, and myocardial abscesses are also typically painless. Our present knowledge is derived from the assessment of pseudoaffective reactions and from the results of electrophysiologic studies in animals and of clinical studies in patients with angina. Available information suggests that adenosine is a chemical mediator of pain, but pain can also be caused by intense stimulation of epicardial coronary arteries and, in some individuals under certain conditions, by mechanical stimuli.

Assessment of pseudoaffective reactions in animals

Intracoronary injection of bradykinin, a potent algogenic substance, and of veratridine, an alkaloid capable of activating both vagal and sympathetic cardiac afferent fibers, failed to induce pseudoaffective reactions in conscious dogs;[7,8] conversely, small doses of intracoronary bradykinin produced pseudoaffective reactions when injected into dogs still recovering from surgery, which indicates that summation of painful stimuli may elicit pain.[9] Similarly, sudden coronary occlusion often failed to elicit a pseudoaffective reaction, even when it resulted in infarction, in quiet relaxed dogs,[10] whereas it tended to produce pain much more frequently in nervous, excited dogs.[11] Finally, brisk stretching of coronary arteries in conscious dogs often causes pseudoaffective reactions.[12,13] These experimental observations led Malliani to hypothesize that cardiac pain results from the extreme excitation of a spatially restricted population of afferent sympathetic fibers by either chemical or mechanical stimuli.[14] This could explain why in dogs, pain is elicited by localized mechanical deformation of periarterial nerves and not by intracoronary administration of potent algogenic substances. This hypothesis is not, however, supported by the recent demonstration that the intracoronary administration of adenosine can reproduce ischemic cardiac pain in patients.[15]

Electrophysiologic studies

Recordings of electric activity from cardiac afferent nerves were used to investigate the nature of the receptors involved in the production of cardiac pain. According to the "intensity" hypothesis, pain occurs as the result of excessive stimulation of nonspecific sensory receptors that also function as chemoreceptors, mechanoreceptors, or polymodal receptors.[16] Conversely, the "specificity" hypothesis states that pain occurs as the result of the excitation of a specific type of receptor that is stimulated only by noxious stimuli (hence nociceptor). It is well known, for instance, that on the somatic side there are receptors that appear to be true nociceptors as they exhibit no background discharge, discharging only when stimulated by strong mechanical or thermal stimuli.[17] Conversely, several experimental studies, based on recordings of the electric activity from single-myelinated and nonmyelinated cardiac sympathetic fibers under normal hemodynamic conditions, have consistently shown the presence of a background discharge. The background activity of single fibers increases during hemodynamic stress and also often after chemical stimulation, indicating a polymodal function of the same fiber.[14]

The consistent failure to identify fibers with no background discharge is considered to be an argument against the presence of specific nociceptor fibers. In fact, as nociceptors would serve only to alert the body to a threat to tissue integrity, they should have no background activity and should discharge only during potentially damaging situations. However, specific pain receptors may be so sparse that they have not been identified in the experimental models utilized so far.

Evidence of chemical stimulation in man

Intracoronary infusion of adenosine consistently causes pain identical to that experienced during transient myocardial ischemia during daily life. As adenosine-induced pain has also occurred during its infusion into nonstenotic coronary branches and because it was never accompanied by ECG alterations, it is very unlikely that the pain was attributable to myocardial ischemia. The infusion of similar doses of adenosine into the right atrium failed to elicit any pain, thus showing that the pain elicited by the intracoronary infusion of adenosine originated from the heart (see Fig. 14.2).[15] Finally, theophylline, a potent antagonist of adenosine A_1 and A_2 receptors, reduced the severity of exercise-induced anginal pain for the same degree of ST-segment depression.[15] These findings are consistent with the "chemical" hypothesis because they prove that adenosine is an adequate stimulus for cardiac sensory receptors and that

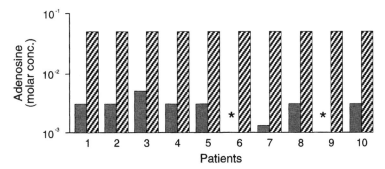

Fig. 14.2 Algogenic effects of adenosine. The minimum molar concentrations of adenosine that provoked chest pain during intracoronary infusion (■) and infusion into the right atrium (▨) are shown for each patient. All patients had chest pain during intra-atrial infusion at the doses indicated. Eight patients also had chest pain during intracoronary infusion of adenosine. The dose at which pain occurred during intracoronary infusion caused no symptoms during intra-atrial administration, showing that the algogenic effects of adenosine during intracoronary infusion originate from the heart. Furthermore, the chest pain caused by intracoronary infusion was always similar to that experienced during daily life, but it occurred in the absence of ECG changes. (Modified from ref. 15.)

endogenous adenosine is a mediator (the first hitherto identified) of ischemic cardiac pain, as proposed by Sylven et al.[18] It is worth noting that the intracoronary infusion of substance P, a potent algogenic substance, does not elicit pain at doses that produced obvious hemodynamic effects.[19]

The algogenic and vascular effects of adenosine are independent, as they are mediated by A_1 and A_2 adenosine receptors, respectively. Selective blockade of A_1 receptors by bamiphylline reduced adenosine-induced pain without affecting its vasodilator effects,[20] thus suggesting that the algogenic effects of adenosine are mediated predominantly by A_1 receptors.

Stimulation by adenosine of the afferent nerve fibers responsible for pain would explain the development of pain during ischemia, as concentrations of adenosine are known to increase markedly when oxygen supply becomes inadequate to meet demand. It could also explain the occurrence of anginal pain, even without ischemia, in patients with syndrome X, if severe prearteriolar constriction causes adenosine release as a mechanism of compensatory arteriolar dilation (see Ch. 18).

Evidence of mechanical stimulation in humans

Continuous monitoring of left ventricular volume during spontaneous or ergonovine-induced transient ischemic episodes showed that neither the rate nor the magnitude of left ventricular dilation influenced the presence or absence of anginal pain (see Fig. 14.3A,B).[21] These findings suggest that the presence or absence of anginal pain cannot be explained only by the "mechanical" hypothesis, although they do not rule out the possibility that mechanical stimuli can cause pain. This latter hypothesis is suggested by the report that, in a large proportion of patients with syndrome X, anginal pain may also be elicited by manipulation of a catheter within the cardiac chambers, by intracoronary contrast or saline injection, or by pacing at the right ventricular apex a few beats faster than the basal heart rate in the absence of ischemic ECG changes.[22–24] The very uncommon perception of pain in response to such stimuli in most anginal patients suggests a markedly enhanced perception of pain in patients with syndrome X (see Ch. 18).

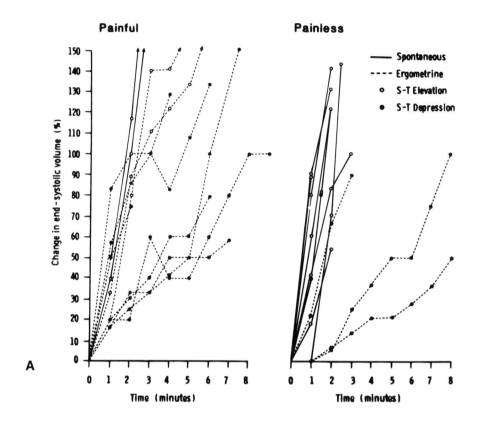

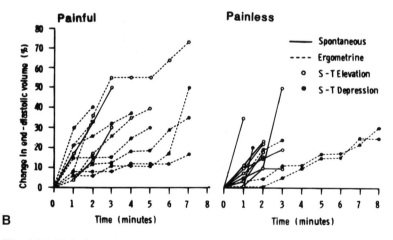

Fig. 14.3 Relation of pain to the rate or magnitude of left ventricular dilation. The rate of change and the magnitude of volume change in end-systolic volume (**A**) and end-diastolic volume (**B**) during spontaneous or ergonovine-induced transient ischemic episodes were similar in painful and painless episodes. (Modified from ref. 21.)

Nonmechanical stimuli, such as laser hot balloon angioplasty, also cause pain of such intensity that the procedure requires general anesthesia:[25] the pain must have a local vascular origin because it appears as soon as the balloon is warmed up, rather than later (as is the case during ischemia caused by balloon inflation).

Finally, mechanical alterations of the wall of large epicardial vessels can modulate the severity of pain, as the latter is more severe during percutaneous transluminal coronary angioplasty (PTCA) at higher balloon inflation pressures.[26]

14.1.2 Transmission and modulation of cardiac afferent stimuli in the dorsal horn of the spinal cord

Whatever the stimulus or receptor involved, cardiac afferent impulses travel through unmyelinated or small myelinated fibers in the cardiac sympathetic nerves to the upper five thoracic sympathetic ganglia where these neurons originate, and from there the impulses travel to the dorsal horn neurons through the white rami communicantes, the gray rami (although to a minor extent), and the upper thoracic dorsal roots.[27–29] Afferent impulses traveling through vagal fibers could explain the referred pain in the jaw, head, and neck, which was found to become more common when sympathectomy was used to cure intractable angina.[30]

The convergence of afferent nervous impulses from both visceral and somatic sensory nerves to the same dorsal horn neurons provides a plausible explanation for the somatic component of visceral pain. The poor localization of deep visceral pain is due not only to the paucity of nerve endings in visceral structures but also to the lack of a somatotopic projection of visceral pain in the cortical structure.

Convergence of cardiac afferent stimuli on dorsal horn spinal neurons

In about 70% of anginal patients, the selective infusion of adenosine into the right coronary artery elicited a pain identical to that experienced when it was infused into the left coronary artery (and, in all, the adenosine-induced pain was similar to that experienced during anginal attacks occurring in daily life).[31] This indicates that, in humans, afferent stimuli from different myocardial regions often converge on the same dorsal neurons. In the remaining 30%, the distribution of pain during adenosine infusion into the right coronary artery differed from that experienced during infusion into the left coronary artery (see Fig. 14.4). Differences in the location and radiation of anginal pain in the same patient may, therefore, be clues to the occurrence of ischemia in different areas of the heart. The reasons for this variable degree of convergence of afferent stimuli from different myocardial regions on the same dorsal horn neurons are unknown.

Modulation of afferent painful stimuli in the spinal cord

The transmission of nociceptive messages is modulated, to a very considerable extent, as early as the first relays in the dorsal horn spinal neurons. The "gate control" theory proposed by Melzack and Wall was an attempt to summarize this notion in schematic form. According to this theory, the condition, either open or closed, of the "gate" at the level of the dorsal horn neurons depends on both afferent and descending nervous impulses and determines whether a specific nociceptive message reaches supraspinal centers.[32]

Summation of subliminal nociceptive messages, from the same or different dermatomes, has been shown to result in the stimulation of neurons converging on the dorsal horn.[33] Thus, episodes of cardiac ischemic pain may occasionally appear to be associated with chronic cardiac pain originating from other visceral or somatic structures.

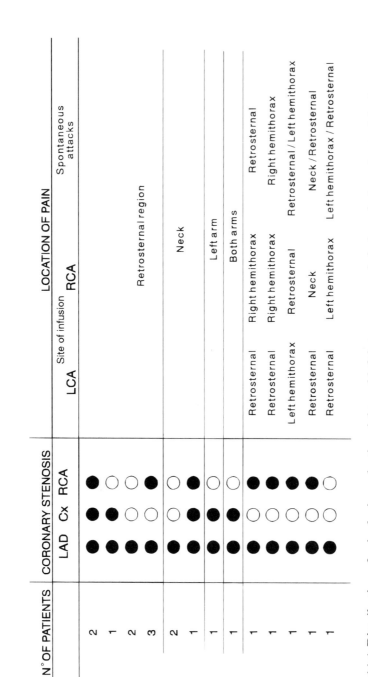

Fig. 14.4 Distribution of pain during selective right and left intracoronary infusion of adenosine and during sponta-neous anginal attacks. In 13 patients the pain induced with infusion of adenosine in the right (RCA) or left (LCA) coronary arteries occurred in the same location and was also similar to that of spontaneous attacks. In five patients the pain was perceived in different locations, indicating that afferent receptors in the territory perfused by the two arteries were coupled with different neurons in the dorsal roots. During anginal attacks not induced by adenosine, the pain was similar to that perceived during adeno-sine infusion into the RCA and/or the LCA. LAD, left anterior descending artery; Cx, circumflex artery. (Modified from ref. 31.)

Inhibition of nociceptive messages at the site of convergent neurons may involve segmental, propriospinal, supraspinal and diffuse neural systems. The latter two appear to be the most relevant and are discussed in more detail below.

It is well established that electric stimulation of brain stem structures, such as the periaqueductal gray substance and the nucleus raphe magnus, causes analgesia due to the activation of descending neural pathways that inhibit neurons converging on the dorsal horn.[34] On the basis of both anatomic and electrophysiologic evidence it is currently believed that the inhibitory effects induced by stimulation of the periaqueductal gray substance result from activation of the nucleus raphe magnus,[35] but it is not known which stimuli activate this nucleus under physiologic conditions. Such activation, however, might be important in mediating the analgesic effects caused by vagal or baroreceptor stimulation.[36,37]

The analgesic effects induced by stimulation of the nucleus raphe magnus are reduced in animals pretreated with blockers of serotonin synthesis.[38] Furthermore, the local iontophoretic application of serotonin induces depression of the dorsal-horn-convergent neuron response to noxious inputs.[39] These observations have led to postulation that the stimulation of the nucleus raphe magnus exerts its inhibitory effects by releasing serotonin.[40] Endogenous opioids could also be involved in the modulation of noxious inputs, as the systemic administration of the opiate antagonist naloxone has been shown to have a partial blocking effect on the inhibitory effects triggered by stimulation of the nucleus raphe magnus. Postulation of a spinal site of naloxone action is supported by the high density of encephalinergic terminals and opiate receptors in the upper regions of the dorsal horn, one of the principal terminal sites of projection from the nucleus raphe magnus.[41]

Nociceptive inputs from distant somatic areas can also inhibit the activity of the neurons converging on the dorsal horn. As this inhibitory system does not appear to be somatotopically organized but concerns the entire body, it has been called the "diffuse noxious inhibitory control" (DNIC).[42] Because DNIC disappears after cervical section of the spinal cord, it has been suggested that it also involves supraspinal structures;[41] morphological and electrophysiologic studies have led to the hypothesis that one of these supraspinal structures might be the nucleus raphe magnus.[42] It would appear, therefore, that both central and peripheral inhibition of nociceptive messages at the level of dorsal-horn-convergent neurons are integrated in the same supraspinal nucleus.

Modulation of cardiac afferent stimuli in anginal patients

In patients with angina, the modulation of cardiac afferent impulses at the site of neurons converging on the dorsal horn is indicated by observations not only that esophageal stimulation lowers the anginal threshold during exercise, thus suggesting the occurrence of summation of subliminal stimuli,[43] but also that transcutaneous electric nerve stimulation,[44] dorsal column stimulation,[45] or carotid sinus massage or stimulation[46] can raise the anginal threshold. Pain most often develops, after a short delay, following the onset of detectable ischemia on the ECG (see 14.1.4), but no information is available on the mechanisms and modulations of this delay.

Painful stimuli caused by myocardial ischemia and reaching the dorsal horn and thalamus may not progress to the cortex; conversely, noncardiac stimuli progressing to the cortex may be perceived as cardiac ischemic pain when they project to the same dorsal horn neurons.

14.1.3 Perception of pain and complaint

The nociceptive messages reaching the spinal dorsal horn and modulated at that site by the gate system, project to the thalamus along the spinothalamic tract and from the thalamus to the cortex. The ascending pathways of nociceptive messages beyond the thalamus are not precisely known but a recent study suggests that, during anginal pain, thalamic and cortical activation are detectable by regional cerebral blood flow measurements.[47]

The conscious perception of pain is related to the cortical decoding of afferent stimuli as unpleasant. The intensity of pain is influenced not only by the intensity of the afferent impulses reaching the cortex but also by the individual's personality, emotional status, and previous experience of pain. Nociceptive messages can apparently be modulated in supraspinal centers by inhibition or facilitation of their transmission, by opioids, and by cortical subjective attitudes such as stoicism and denial. Both the complaint and the protective reaction elicited by pain are likely to be profoundly affected by an individual's personal, social, and cultural background.[37,48]

Modulation of potentially painful stimuli in supraspinal centers

In patients who never experience anginal pain (even during severe prolonged ischemia or infarction) and in those who have predominantly painless ischemia, the failure to develop pain could be due to the absence or inhibition of transmission of cardiac afferent stimuli or to inappropriate cortical decoding. A generalized defective perception of painful stimuli was found in these subsets of patients in various studies. In general, patients with totally or predominantly painless ischemia have significantly higher thresholds of, and tolerance for, pain than patients with predominantly painful ischemia, when challenged with stimuli such as forearm ischemia, cold pressor testing, electric skin stimulation, or dental pulp stimulation (see Fig. 14.5A,B).[49–51] They also have higher thresholds for pain following intravenous injection of adenosine (see Fig. 14.6).[15] However, despite significant mean differences between groups of patients with either predominantly painless or predominantly painful ischemia, a considerable overlap in the values of pain threshold and tolerance for the various painful stimuli has been reported in all published studies. For those patients with predominantly painless ischemia who present a "normal" threshold and tolerance for pain, mechanisms other than a generalized defective perception of pain must be postulated.[52]

A generalized defective perception of painful stimuli has been attributed both to alterations of the opioid system and to psychological factors. Cardiac painful stimuli might themselves progressively modify their own central modulation, thus causing variations in each individual's susceptibility to anginal pain.[53] This hypothesis is based on the clinical observation that about 50% of patients with *silent* infarctions go on to develop a second *painful* infarction or angina, and is supported by the experimental observation that repetitive nociceptive stimuli can modify gene expression of endogenous opioids in the central nervous system.[54–56]

Role of opioids in the central modulation of cardiac afferent stimuli

Endogenous opioids have received considerable attention in relation to the central modulation of the severity of anginal pain, but available evidence is still inconclusive.

There are three main groups of endogenous opioids, derived from three different precursor molecules:

a. endorphins, predominantly secreted by the pituitary gland
b. encephalins, mainly secreted by the adrenocortical gland
c. dynorphines, the origin of which is incompletely understood.

Opioids provoke a selective suppression of dorsal horn convergent neurons through the stimulation of specific receptors. Four different types of receptors have been described so far. Endogenous opioids display varying degrees of affinity for all four classes of receptors, whereas exogenous opioids operate through the stimulation of μ receptors only.[57]

The role of endogenous opioids in the modulation of anginal pain in patients has been investigated by administration of the potent opioid antagonist naloxone; the plasma concentrations

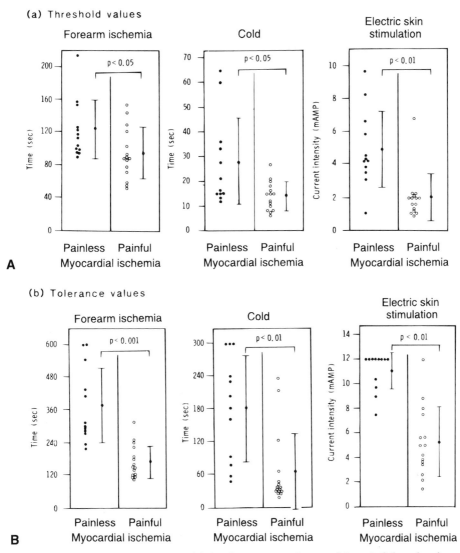

Fig. 14.5 Overlap in pain sensitivity between patients with painful and pain-less ischemia. Pain threshold (**A**) and tolerance (**B**) values for a variety of painful stimuli in patients with predominantly painless (●) or predominantly painful (○) myocardial ischemia. Although the pain threshold was, in general, significantly greater in the patients with painless ischemia, the overlap between the two groups is considerable, suggesting that factors other than a generalized defective perception of pain are also responsible for painless myocardial ischemia. (Modified from ref. 50.)

of these opioids have also been measured, but are unlikely to give an accurate picture of concentrations in the brain.

In some studies, exercise testing after naloxone administration caused earlier appearance of chest pain for a lesser degree of ST-segment depression, but this was at variance with other reports.[58–60] As naloxone has a high affinity for μ receptors only, it is unlikely to antagonize endogenous opioids efficiently, as they stimulate other receptors as well.[61] The results of studies in which plasma levels of endogenous endorphins were measured are also controversial. Similar plasma levels of endogenous opioids were found by some investigators in patients with

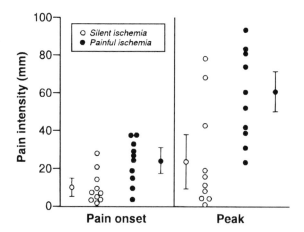

Fig. 14.6 Overlap in pain threshold during adenosine infusion between patients with painful and painless ischemia. Following intravenous administration of adenosine in patients with predominantly painless (O) or predominantly painful (●) myocardial ischemia, the severity of adenosine-induced pain (expressed as millimeters of a visual analog scale) was significantly less in the former group, but the overlap was considerable. This observation adds further evidence to suggest that factors other than a generalized defective perception of pain are responsible for painless myocardial ischemia. (Modified from ref. 15.)

either predominantly painless or predominantly painful ischemia, although the latter group had a significantly lower threshold and tolerance for experimentally induced pain;[50,60,62] higher levels were found by others in patients with predominantly painless episodes.[63–66] These discrepancies could be explained by the fact that the analgesic effects of endogenous opioids are likely to be attributable to central, rather than to peripheral, mechanisms;[67,68] plasma levels of endorphins at any one time do not, therefore, necessarily reflect their analgesic effect.

Role of complaint

Characteristic subjective and psychological personality-related features were noted in patients with predominantly silent myocardial ischemia. On a personality inventory test, patients with painless ischemia recorded significantly lower scores for nervousness and "excitability" and higher scores for "masculinity" and also had a lower tendency to complain;[53] such personality traits may explain the generalized reduction of the perception of potentially painful stimuli. Finally, denial was also proposed as a possible component of the absence of reported pain during some ischemic episodes.[48]

14.1.4 Duration of myocardial ischemia and ischemic cardiac pain

In patients with a sudden onset of transmural myocardial ischemia caused by occlusive epicardial coronary artery spasm, ischemic cardiac pain usually occurs at a late stage in the development of myocardial ischemia. The time lag between the onset of ischemia and the onset of pain is easily noted, first, in patients with variant angina, because the onset of ischemia is manifested by the very striking sudden elevation of the ST segment, and, second, during coronary angioplasty, when the presenting pain appears 30–120 s after inflation of the balloon (but in episodes without pain it is impossible to know whether it would have occurred later had the inflation been maintained.) Typically, in patients with variant angina, pain follows by some minutes the onset of metabolic, contractile, and ECG alterations (see Figs 14.7 and 14.8).[69,70] It may be absent during episodes of ischemia causing massive left ventricular dysfunction (see Fig. 14.9A–D) yet, very occasionally, may occur during very short periods of ischemia (see Fig. 14.10A–C).

In patients with variant angina or angina at rest, continuous ECG and hemodynamic monitoring has led to the following conclusions:

1. Short, transient ischemic episodes (lasting less than 3 min) causing only a minor impairment of left ventricular function (an increase of left ventricular pressure of less than 7 mmHg) are nearly always painless
2. Longer and/or more severe episodes can be either painful or painless, even in the same patient.
3. Mild, transient ischemic episodes are more likely to be painless than severe episodes, although those severe enough to cause a massive deficit of regional myocardial perfusion, and even MI, can remain completely painless.

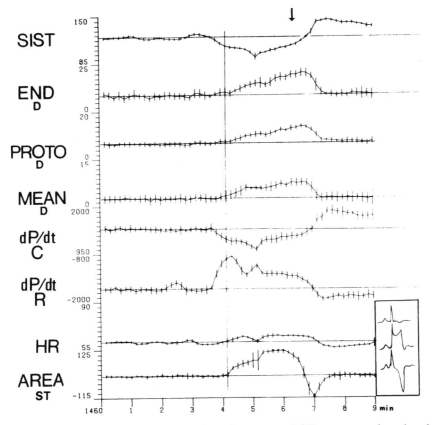

Fig. 14.7 Delayed onset of pain after the onset of ST-segment elevation in variant angina. During hemodynamic monitoring in the coronary care unit a spontaneous episode of variant angina is associated with major changes in ventricular pressure and contractile function, with massive ST-segment elevation occurring minutes before the onset of pain (arrow). The vertical line indicates the onset of ST-segment elevation. (Modified from ref. 69.)

In the human model of myocardial ischemia, represented by patients with variant angina in whom the onset of ischemia is easily identified by the dramatic elevation of the ST segment on the ECG, a critical duration (more than 3 min) and severity of ischemia (more than 7 mmHg increase in left ventricular pressure) are usually needed for the development of anginal pain; thus, ischemia is, in general, less severe in silent episodes because they are usually shorter (see Fig. 14.11).[71] These observations led to the notion that the ischemic cascade is typically characterized by left ventricular dysfunction followed by ischemic ECG

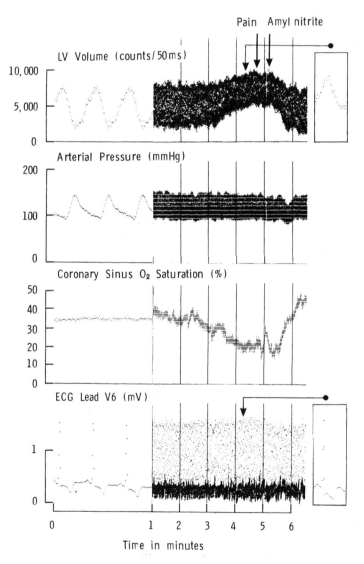

Fig. 14.8 Delayed onset of pain after the onset of ventricular dilation. During continuous monitoring of left ventricular (LV) volume by a precordial probe, a spontaneous ischemic episode is associated with an increase in LV volume and a decrease in coronary sinus oxygen saturation. Pain appears about 3 min later. (From data presented in ref. 21.)

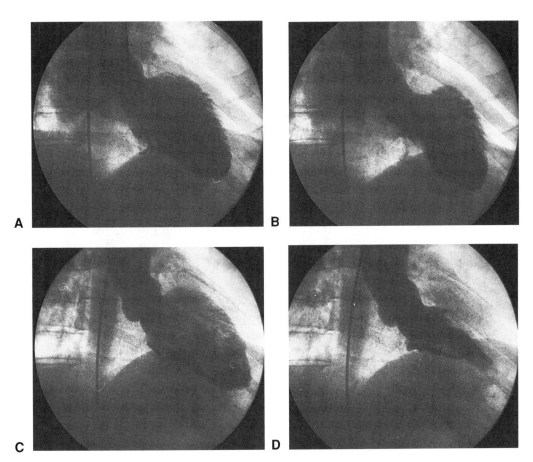

Fig. 14.9 Absence of pain during massive myocardial ischemia. Ventricular angiography performed in a patient with variant angina, proximal LAD spasm and 20 mm ST-segment elevation in the precordial leads in the absence of pain. An increase in left ventricular end-diastolic (**A**) and particularly in end-systolic (**B**) volumes compared to controls (**C, D**) can be observed.

changes and only later by pain (see Fig. 14.12). This sequence of events is typical of ischemia caused by a sudden reduction of coronary flow (see Ch. 7) but is not always the case in effort-induced ischemia.

In patients with chronic stable angina, painless ischemic episodes recorded during ambulatory ECG monitoring are, in general, shorter and associated with a lesser degree of ST-segment depression than painful episodes, but the overlap with the duration of painful episodes is quite considerable (see Fig. 14.13A,B).[72] During exercise stress testing the relationship between the onset of anginal pain and ST-segment depression is remarkably different from that usually observed in patients with variant angina, because pain often precedes (or occurs simultaneously), rather than follows the onset of, the ischemic ST-segment changes (see Fig. 14.14).[73]

The causes of the different relationships between the onset of ischemia and the onset of pain during vasospastic and effort-induced ischemia are unknown. They cannot simply be attributed to the fact that, during exercise testing, ischemia is provoked by the test, for the following reasons: first, because in patients with variant angina the onset of pain fol-

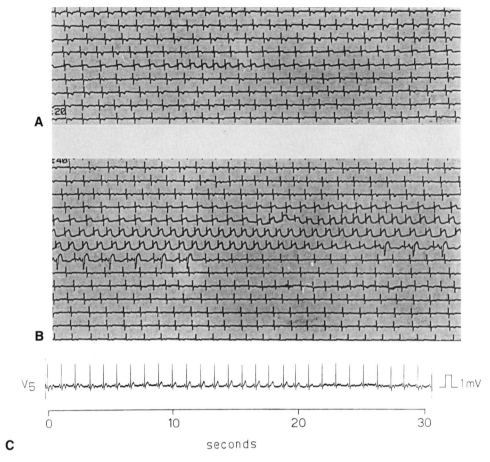

Fig. 14.10 Occurrence of pain during very short ischemic episodes. A patient with variant angina had occasional very short episodes of pain at the left sternal border in the fourth intercostal space (which he indicated with his right finger). Holter recording showed a consistent association with either very short episodes of ST-segment elevation (**A, B**) or T-wave peaking (**C**). The patient also had longer ischemic episodes with prolonged pain, but did not exhibit any delay in the perception of pain.

lows the onset of ECG changes during the ergonovine test also; second, because in patients with effort-induced angina, during PTCA the onset of anginal pain, when present, follows inflation of the balloon by several seconds (longer delays cannot be detected as the inflation is not sustained).[74]

The delayed onset or absence of pain during episodes of severe ischemia caused by epicardial coronary artery spasm or by PTCA, with obvious impairment of left ventricular function and the lack of pain in some cases of infarction, are in sharp contrast to the presence of severe anginal pain with or without transient ischemic ECG changes, but with no detectable abnormalities of contractile function in patients with syndrome X (see Ch. 18). They also contrast with the variable relationship between the onset of ST-segment depres-

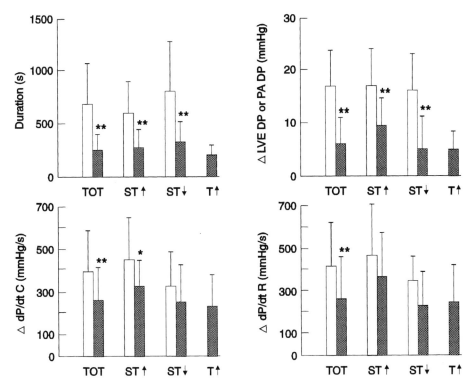

Fig. 14.11 Episodes of painless ischemia are, on average, shorter and less severe than painful episodes. The mean duration of episodes, the increases in left ventricular end-diastolic (LVEDP) or pulmonary artery diastolic (PADP) pressures and reduction of left ventricular peak contraction (dP/dt C) and relaxation (dP/dt R) were significantly greater for symptomatic (□) than for asymptomatic (■) episodes. Asterisks indicate significant differences between symptomatic and asymptomatic episodes (*$P < 0.01$; **$P < 0.001$). Asymptomatic episodes were shorter and accompanied by lesser degrees of left ventricular impairment. ST↑ or ↓, transient ST-segment elevation or depression; T↑, transient pseudonormalization or peaking of inverted or flat T waves; TOT, total. (Modified from ref. 71.)

sion and chest pain in patients with chronic stable angina during exercise testing. These findings suggest that different mechanisms of painful ischemic stimuli and/or an enhanced perception of pain are the rule in patients with syndrome X, in contrast to patients with variant angina, but they are also common in some of those with chronic stable angina. The lack of pain during some transient ischemic episodes, but not during other episodes of similar severity and duration in the same patient, can only be due to either a transient failure of the transmission of cardiac afferent impulses (closed gate) or to a transient failure of the cortex to decode them.

■ *Thus, the relationship between ischemia and anginal pain may be seen as a bell-shaped distribution in which patients with totally painless ischemia are at one extreme and patients with microvascular angina are at the other. For each individual patient the relationship varies in time because of the dynamic modulation of the perception of pain, possibly related to the gating system of afferent impulses and their central decoding (see Fig. 14.15).* ■

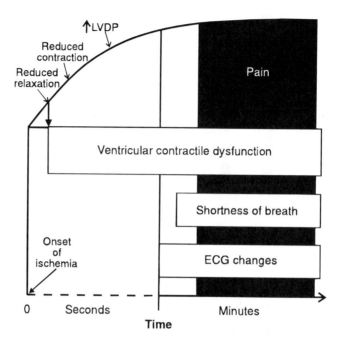

Fig. 14.12 Scheme of the ischemic cascade following sudden interruption of coronary blood flow. Relaxation and contraction velocity, increase of ventricular end-diastolic pressure and ECG changes appear within seconds of the onset of ischemia. Pain, when present, usually occurs within minutes. Shortness of breath, indicative of left ventricular failure, may precede the onset of pain.

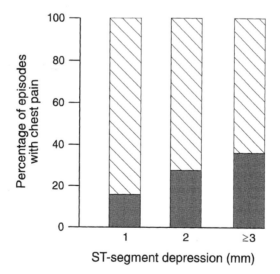

Fig. 14.13 Severity of myocardial ischemia in painless and painful episodes during ambulatory Holter monitoring in chronic stable angina. The severity of ST-segment depression was only weakly correlated with the presence of pain (■ area). The duration of painful episodes was also only slightly longer (see the data from the same study presented in Fig. 17.5). The comparison with the findings in patients with variant angina (reported in Fig. 14.11) suggest a possible difference in the perception of painful stimuli in these two ischemic syndromes. (Modified from ref. 72.)

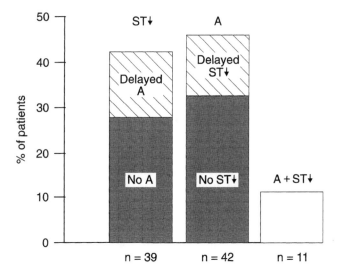

Fig. 14.14 Relationship between the onset of ischemic ECG changes and pain during exercise stress tests. In 12% of patients, chest pain (A) occurred simultaneously with the onset of ischemic changes on the ECG (ST↓); in 15% the ST↓ was delayed after the onset of pain (delayed ST↓) and in 30% there were no ST-segment changes but only chest pain (No ST↓). In only 15% did pain follow the onset of ischemic changes (delayed A). (n = number of new patients.) In 25%, ischemic ECG changes were not associated with chest pain (No A). These findings are strikingly different from those reported in Fig. 14.12. (Modified from ref. 72.)

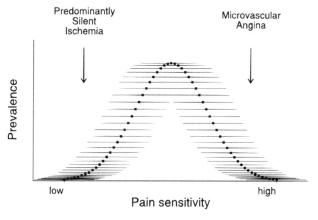

Fig. 14.15 Bell-shaped distribution of the individual perception of ischemic cardiac pain. At one extreme are patients with only silent myocardial ischemia and at the other are those with microvascular angina and no detectable ischemic dysfunction. The oscillations indicate the variability of an individual's perception of pain in time.

14.2 SIGNIFICANCE OF ISCHEMIC CARDIAC PAIN IN DIFFERENT CORONARY SYNDROMES

For an intuitive understanding of the clinical significance of ischemic cardiac pain it is useful to develop an analogy with the ringing of a doorbell, which can have various pitches and be of variable intensity. Ischemic cardiac pain is like a rather inefficient doorbell: pain indistinguishable from ischemic cardiac pain may also be elicited by nonischemic cardiac causes or by noncardiac causes, i.e. the bell rings when it should not. Ischemic cardiac pain is often not elicited by ischemia at all, i.e. the bell does not always ring when it should. The features of ischemic cardiac pain are unrelated to the cause of myocardial ischemia, and often not even to its severity, i.e. the pitch of the ring does not reveal who is ringing. However, the pattern of recurrence, together with the duration and intensity of the ringing, can provide information about who is ringing and the urgency of the call.

14.2.1 Nonischemic and noncardiac causes of anginal pain

Convergence of impulses from different receptors, organs, and tissues of the same dermatomes on the same neurons in the dorsal horn can explain the occurrence of noncardiac causes of anginal pain. Afferent fibers from the pericardium enter the spinal cord in the C_8-T_2 region; those from the stomach and the duodenum enter through T_6-T_{10}; those from the esophagus through C_7-T_{12}. The overlap with the entry of cardiac afferent nerves and the high convergence of impulses on some ascending neurons in the dorsal horn explains the possible difficulties in diagnosing ischemic cardiac pain.

Several noncardiac diseases may simulate ischemic cardiac pain (see Ch. 16). Chest pain with features similar to that described by Heberden can be associated with

a. psychiatric disorders (anxiety, depression, cardiac psychosis, self-gain)
b. gastrointestinal diseases (reflux esophagitis, esophageal spasm or rupture, peptic ulcer, cholecystitis, acute pancreatitis, distention of the splenic flexure of the colon)
c. pulmonary diseases (mediastinal emphysema, spontaneous pneumothorax) or
d. chest wall diseases (thoracic outlet syndrome, chest wall syndrome, Tietze's syndrome, herpes zoster).

Furthermore, cardiac nonischemic diseases may simulate ischemic cardiac pain. For example, the pain caused by acute pericarditis or a dissecting aneurysm of the aorta may mimic ischemic cardiac pain, and angina-like pain may be observed in valvular heart disease, cardiomyopathy, and pulmonary hypertension.[2]

■ *Transient abnormalities on an ECG recorded* during *pain are the most common means of diagnosing an ischemic, or at least a cardiac, origin (see Ch. 16).* ■

14.2.2 Relationship between the course of myocardial ischemia and ischemic cardiac pain

Myocardial ischemia involves the same sequence of biochemical, hemodynamic, and electrophysiologic events, irrespective of its causes. Thus, it should not be surprising that anginal pain or discomfort with any of the characteristic qualities described by Heberden, or ischemia without pain, can be observed in effort-related, unstable, and variant angina and in syndrome X, and can be caused by increased oxygen demand, thrombosis, coronary artery spasm, and small coronary vessel constriction. In patients with chest pain and normal coronary angiograms, and in those with angiographically detected coronary artery obstructions, no consistent differences could be found in the type of angina, the location and quality of pain, or its accompanying symptoms.[2] Painless ischemia has been described in all coronary syndromes including stable, unstable, and vasospastic angina, syndrome X, and MI and is, therefore, unrelated to the causes of myocardial ischemia (see Ch. 15). It is also common experience that patients with chronic effort-related angina (typically caused by an excessive increase of myocardial oxygen consumption in the presence of obstructive coronary atherosclerosis) experience the same type of pain during spontaneous episodes caused by coronary vasoconstriction as that experienced when they develop unstable angina or infarction caused by coronary thrombosis (at least when ischemia occurs in the same myocardial territory). Similarly, some patients with spasm superimposed on a fixed coronary stenosis experience the same type of anginal pain during episodes of coronary spasm with ST-segment elevation as that experienced during episodes of effort-induced myocardial ischemia with ST-segment depression in the same leads. Thus, myocardial ischemia, regardless of its cause, can be painful, with one of the many variations on the Heberden theme; painless, but symptomatic because of dyspnoea (due to transient left ventricular failure), palpitation, or syncope (due to transient arrhythmias); or silent, with no clinical manifestation, usually identified by transient ischemic changes on the ECG.

Painful myocardial ischemia is much more easily recognized clinically when the pain is strong, has all the typical features described by Heberden, and recurs consistently on effort (being promptly relieved by rest), than when it is mild, has only some of those features (i.e. located only in the epigastrium or jaw, or a wrist or elbow), occurs very seldom, and is not consistently referred to specific events.

Painless but symptomatic myocardial ischemia (angina equivalents, see Ch. 16) has to be confirmed by the documentation of objective signs of ischemia on the ECG, as its clinical signs (indicative of severe heart failure or severe rhythm disturbances) can also be due to nonischemic causes.

Silent myocardial ischemia (suggested by the appearance of transient ischemic changes on the ECG during exercise testing or Holter recording) by definition can only be diagnosed by techniques capable of detecting ischemia. Its diagnosis, therefore, depends entirely on the sensitivity and specificity of the techniques employed for the detection of ischemia.

The pattern of pain as a clue to the causes of myocardial ischemia

As discussed above, neither the location or radiation of ischemic cardiac pain nor the absence of pain in the same patient provide information about the causes of myocardial ischemia. Information on the causes of ischemic episodes can, however, be obtained from the pattern of recurrence, the duration, the response to sublingual nitrates, and the circumstances in which episodes of pain occur. A stable pattern of occurrence of ischemic episodes, with or without pain, over months or years, suggests a stable cause of ischemia; conversely, a recent onset and/or a rapid deterioration in the severity and duration of ischemic episodes suggests an unstable cause. A more detailed analysis of the pattern of the ischemic episodes within stable and unstable subsets of patients may often provide further useful clues about their causes.

Chronic stable, predominantly effort-related angina

Although, by definition, this form of angina is characterized by a stable pattern of symptoms over months or years, a detailed history of the circumstances in which anginal attacks develop can provide valuable information on the actual cause of the ischemia. Anginal attacks that occur predictably only when (and each time) a certain level of physical activity is exceeded, suggest a fixed impairment of coronary flow reserve; attacks that occur unpredictably during levels of effort that are usually well tolerated, suggest a variable impairment of coronary flow reserve caused by "dynamic" coronary stenoses or distal coronary vessel constriction (see Chs 16 and 17). However, the constancy of the number, duration, and severity of both painful and painless transient ischemic episodes over months or years suggests a stable cause of myocardial ischemia, no matter what that cause may be.

Chronic stable angina characterized by a long duration of attacks (30 min or longer), not relieved promptly by rest, and poorly responsive to sublingual nitrates is suggestive of a coronary microvascular cause or of a noncardiac cause (see Chs 16 and 18).

Unstable angina

The sudden onset or the sudden exacerbation of angina, with more severe and protracted attacks typically occurring spontaneously at rest, are signals of an unstable cause of ischemia and, therefore, demand prompt medical attention and aggressive management (see Ch. 19). The diagnosis of instability is easy when symptoms occur or intensify suddenly, but cannot be made merely on the basis of angina occurring at rest or unpredictably during a degree of effort that is well tolerated on other occasions. This is because a marked variability in the anginal threshold, and even occasional episodes of angina at rest, can occur over periods of months or years in patients with chronic, stable, predominantly effort-related angina.

Episodes of angina at rest with preserved effort tolerance are typical of variant angina, particularly when they occur during the early morning hours or at night, or at the same hour of the day, or occur in clusters within 30–60 min, leaving the patient free from angina during the rest of the day while conducting normal daily activities, and when they are associated with palpitations due to arrhythmias (see Ch. 20).

Acute MI

The distribution and radiation of ischemic cardiac pain associated with acute MI are as variable as those of transient ischemic episodes and, in the same patient, are usually similar to those of the stable and/or unstable angina that preceded the infarction. In acute MI, pain is usually (but not always) more severe and more frequently accompanied by angor animi. It is also frequently associated with dyspnea, sweating, nausea, and vomiting, all of which may occur during painless acute MI. The severity of symptoms is itself a reason for alarm, but even when symptoms are not severe, the unusual persistence of any of the previously described types of pain, the association with feelings and signs of distress, together with the lack of response to nitrates, demand prompt attention.

An intriguing observation of the Framingham study was that 24% of men and 33% of women who had experienced a painless infarction subsequently reported episodes of angina pectoris.[75] As the algogenic stimuli operating during MI are likely to be much more powerful than those operating during episodes of transient myocardial ischemia, these findings emphasize further how the central modulation of algogenic messages has a pivotal role in determining the perception of ischemic cardiac pain.

14.2.4 Conclusions

The relationship between myocardial ischemia and ischemic cardiac pain is elusive, for several reasons: first, because anginal pain can also result from noncardiac or cardiac nonischemic origins; second, because the severity of pain is not necessarily proportional to the

severity of ischemia; third, because ischemia occurring in different regions of the heart causes the same type of anginal discomfort in three-quarters of patients; and, finally, because
only the pattern of occurrence and the duration of pain, but none of the characteristic features or variations described by Heberden or the total absence of pain, can be related to the
actual causes of ischemia.

In some patients or in certain circumstances, the gating system at the level of the ascending dorsal root neurons, and also possibly at higher levels, can prevent the progression
towards the cortex of even the strongest afferent cardiac stimuli that develop during infarction, yet in others or under different circumstances it can allow the perception of stimuli not
associated with detectable ischemia.

In some patients, the absence of anginal pain during massive myocardial ischemia may be
caused by generalized defective perception of painful stimuli, neuropathy, or particular personality traits. In other patients, severe anginal episodes not associated with any detectable
impairment of left ventricular function must be caused by persistent chemical stimuli (such
as excessive local release of adenosine), by inhibition of the gating system, and/or by an
enhanced perception of pain. Within the same patient, the marked day-to-day variability in
the occurrence of anginal pain for ischemic episodes of similar duration and severity is most
likely related to dynamic changes of the gating system.

REFERENCES

1. Heberden W. Some account of a disorder of the breast. Med Trans 1772;*2:*59.
2. Horwitz LD. The diagnostic significance of anginal symptoms. J Am Med Assoc 1974;*229:*1196.
3. Kolettis MT, Charalambos KK, Tzannetis GC. Radiation of anginal pain to the legs. Br Heart J
   1986;*55:*211.
4. Sherrington CS. The Integrative Action of the Nervous System. Yale University Press, New
   Haven, 1906.
5. Colbeck EH. Angina pectoris: a criticism and a hypothesis. Lancet 1903;*1:*793.
6. Lewis T. Pain in muscular ischemia—its relation to anginal pain. Arch Intern Med 1932;*49:*713.
7. Pagani M, Pizzinelli P, Furlan R et al. Analysis of the pressor sympathetic reflex produced by
   intracoronary injections of bradykinin in conscious dogs. Circ Res 1985;*56:*175.
8. Barron KW, Bishop VS. Reflex cardiovascular changes with veratridine in the conscious dog. Am
   J Physiol 1982;*242:*H810.
9. Guzman F, Braun C, Lim RKS. Visceral pain and the pseudo-effective response to intra-arterial
   injection of bradykinin and other algesic agents. Arch Int Pharmacodyn 1962;*136:*353.
10. Theroux P, Ross J, Franklin D et al. Regional myocardial function in the conscious dog during
    acute coronary occlusion and responses to morphine, propranolol, nitroglycerin and lidocaine.
    Circulation 1976;*53:*302.
11. Malliani A, Pagani M, Lombardi F. Visceral versus somatic mechanisms. In: Wall PD, Melzack R
    (eds) Textbook of Pain, 2nd Edition. Edinburgh, Churchill Livingstone, 1989, p. 128.
12. Sutton DC, Leuth HC. Experimental production of pain on excitation of the heart and great ves-
    sels. Arch Intern Med 1930;*45:*827.
13. Malliani A, Lombardi F, Pagani M. Sensory innervation of the heart. In: Cervero F, Morrison JFB
    (eds) Visceral Sensations. Progress in Brain Research, Vol 67. Amsterdam, Elsevier, 1986, p. 39.
14. Malliani A. Cardiovascular sympathetic afferent fibers. Rev Physiol Biochem Pharmacol
    1982;*94:*11.
15. Crea F, Pupita G, Galassi AR et al. Role of adenosine in pathogenesis of anginal pain. Circulation
    1990;*81:*164.
16. Goody W. On the nature of pain. Brain 1957;*80:*118.
17. Burgess PR, Perl ER. Cutaneous mechanoreceptors and nociceptors. In: Iggo A (ed) Handbook
    of Sensory Physiology, Somatosensory System, Vol 2. Berlin, Springer-Verlag, 1973, p. 29.

18. Sylven C, Beerman B, Jonzon B et al. Angina pectoris-like pain provoked by intravenous adenosine in healthy volunteers. Br Med J 1986;*293:*227.

19. Crossman DC, Larkin SW, Fuller RW et al. Substance P dilates epicardial coronary arteries and increases coronary blood flow in humans. Circulation 1989;*80:*475.

20. Gaspardone A, Crea F, Iamele M et al. Bamiphylline improves exercise-induced ischemia through a novel mechanism of action. Circulation 1988;*508:*1993.

21. Davies GJ, Bencivelli W, Fragasso G et al. Sequence and magnitude of ventricular volume changes in painful and painless myocardial ischemia. Circulation 1988;*78:*310.

22. Cannon RO, Quyyumi AA, Mincemoyer R et al. Symptom benefit of imipramine in patients with chest pain despite normal coronary angiograms. N Engl J Med 1994;*330:*1411.

23. Shapiro LM, Crake T, Poole-Wilson PA. Is altered cardiac sensation responsible for chest pain in patients with normal coronary arteries? Clinical observation during cardiac catheterization. Br Med J 1988;*296:*170.

24. Cannon RO, Quyyumi A, Schenke WH et al. Abnormal cardiac sensitivity in patients with chest pain and normal coronary arteries. J Am Coll Cardiol 1990;*16:*1359.

25. Spears JR, Reyes VP, Wynne J et al. Percutaneous coronary laser balloon angioplasty: initial results of a multicenter experience. J Am Coll Cardiol 1990;*16:*293.

26. Tomai F, Crea F, Gaspardone A et al. Mechanisms of cardiac pain during angioplasty. J Am Coll Cardiol 1993;*22:*1892.

27. Brown AM. Excitation of afferent cardiac sympathetic nerve fibers during myocardial ischemia. J Physiol 1967;*190:*35.

28. Blair RW, Weber RN, Foreman RD. Characteristics of primate spinothalamic tract neurons receiving viscerosomatic convergent inputs in T3–T5 segments. J Neurophysiol 1981;*46:*797.

29. Foreman RD, Blair RW, Weber RN. Viscerosomatic convergence onto T2–T4 spinoreticular, spinoreticular–spinothalamic, and spinothalamic tract neurons in the cat. Exp Neurol 1984;*85:*597.

30. Lindgren I, Olivecrona H. Surgical treatment of angina pectoris. J Neurosurg 1947;*4:*19.

31. Crea F, Gaspardone A, Kaski JC, Davies G, Maseri A. Relationship between stimulation site of cardiac afferent nerves by adenosine and location of cardiac pain: results of a study in patients with stable angina. J Am Coll Cardiol 1992;*20:*1498.

32. Wall PD. The gate control theory of pain: a re-examination and a re-statement. Brain 1978;*101:*1.

33. Blair RW, Weber RN, Foreman RD. Responses of thoracic spinothalamic neurons to intracardiac injection of bradykinin in the monkey. Circ Res 1982;*51:*83.

34. Fields HL, Basbaum RI. Brain stem control of spinal pain transmission neurons. Annu Rev Physiol 1978;*40:*193.

35. Oliveras JL, Redjemi F, Guilbaud G et al. Analgesia induced by electrical stimulation of the inferior centralis nucleus of the raphe in the cat. Pain 1975;*1:*139.

36. Foreman RD. Organization of the spinothalamic tract as a relay for cardiopulmonary sympathetic afferent fiber activity. Prog Sensory Physiol 1989;*9:*2.

37. Fields HL. Sources of variability in the sensation of pain. Pain 1988;*33:*195.

38. Rivot JP, Chaouch A, Besson JM. Nucleus raphe magnus modulation of response of rat dorsal horn neurons to unmyelinated fiber inputs: partial involvement of serotoninergic pathways. J Neurophysiol 1980;*44:*1039.

39. Griersmith BT, Duggan AW. Prolonged depression of spinal transmission of nociceptive information by 5-HT administered in the substantia gelatinosa: antagonism by methysergide. Brain Res 1980;*187:*231.

40. Rivot JP, Chiang CY, Besson JM. Increase of serotonin metabolism within the dorsal horn of the spinal cord during nucleus raphe magnus stimulation, as revealed by in vivo electrochemical detection. Brain Res 1982;*238:*117.

41. Zorman G, Hentall ID, Adams JE et al. Naloxone-reversible analgesia produced by microstimulation in the rat medulla. Brain Res 1981;*219:*137.

42. Dickenson AH, Le Bars D, Besson JM. Diffuse noxious inhibitory controls. Effects on trigeminal nucleus caudalis neurons in the rat. Brain Res 1980;*200:*293.

43. Davies HA, Page Z, Rush EM et al. Esophageal stimulation lowers exertional angina threshold. Lancet 1985;*1:*1011.

44. Mannheimer C, Carlsson CA, Vedin A et al. Transcutaneous electrical nerve stimulation in angina pectoris. Pain 1986;*26:*291.

45. Murphy DF, Giles KE. Dorsal column stimulation for pain relief from intractable angina pectoris. Pain 1987;*28:*365.

46. Epstein SE, Beiser GD, Goldstein RE et al. Treatment of angina pectoris by electrical stimulation of the carotid-sinus nerves. N Engl J Med 1969;*290:*971.

47. Rosen SD, Paulesu E, Frith CD et al. Central nervous pathways mediating angina pectoris. Lancet 1994;*344:*147.

48. Janne P, Reynaert C, Cassiers L et al. Psychological determinants of silent myocardial ischaemia. Eur Heart J 1987;*8 (Suppl G):*125.

49. Droste C, Roskamm H. Experimental pain measurements in patients with asymptomatic myocardial ischemia. J Am Coll Cardiol 1983;*1:*940.

50. Glazier JJ, Chierchia S, Brown M et al. Importance of generalized defective perception of painful stimuli as a cause of silent myocardial ischemia in chronic stable angina pectoris. Am J Cardiol 1986;*58:*667.

51. Falcone C, Sconocchia R, Guasti L et al. Dental pain threshold and angina pectoris in patients with coronary artery disease. J Am Coll Cardiol 1988;*12:*348.

52. Maseri A, Chierchia S, Davies G et al. Mechanisms of ischemic cardiac pain and silent myocardial ischemia. Am J Med 1985;*79:*7.

53. Droste C, Roskamm H. Pain perception and endogenous pain modulation in angina pectoris. In: Kellermann JJ, Braunwald E (eds) Silent Myocardial Ischemia: A Critical Appraisal. Basel, Karger, Adv Cardiol, 1990;*37:*142.

54. Holt V, Haarmann I, Millan MJ et al. Prodynorphin gene expression is enhanced in the spinal cord of chronic arthritic rats. Neurosci Lett 1987;*73:*90.

55. Millan MJ, Czlonkowski A, Picher CWT et al. A model of chronic pain in the rat: functional correlates of alteration in the activity of opioids systems. J Neurosci 1987;*7:*77.

56. Iadarola MJ, Ruda MA, Cohen LV et al. Enhanced dynorphin gene expression in spinal cord dorsal horn neurons during peripheral inflammation: behavioral, neuropeptide, immuno-cytochemical and mRNA studies. In: Dubner R, Gebhart GF, Bond MR (eds) Proceedings of the Vth World Congress on Pain. Amsterdam, Elsevier, 1988, p. 61.

57. Basbaum A, Fields H. Endogenous pain control systems; brainstem spinal pathways and endorphin circuitry. Annu Rev Neurosci 1984;*7:*309.

58. Ellestad MH, Kuan P. Naloxone and asymptomatic ischemia: failure to induce angina during exercise testing. Am J Cardiol 1984;*54:*982.

59. Droste C, Roskamm H. A defective angina pectoris pain warning system: experimental findings of ischemic and electrical pain test. Pain 1986;*26:*199.

60. Weidenger F, Hammerle A, Sochor H et al. Role of beta-endorphins in silent myocardial ischemia. Am J Cardiol 1986;*58:*428.

61. Cohen MR, Cohen RM, Pickar D et al. Physiological effects of high dose naloxone administration to normal adults. Life Sci 1982;*30:*2025.

62. Heller GV, Ewing GC, Garber CE et al. Plasma beta-endorphin levels in silent myocardial ischemia induced by exercise. Am J Cardiol 1987;*59:*735.

63. Droste C, Meyer-Blankenburg H, Greenlee MW. Effect of physical exercise on pain thresholds and plasma beta-endorphins in patients with silent and symptomatic myocardial ischemia. Eur Heart J 1988;*9(suppl.N):*25.

64. Falcone C, Specchia G, Rondanelli R et al. Correlation between beta-endorphin plasma levels and anginal symptoms in patients with coronary artery disease. J Am Coll Cardiol 1988;*11:*719.

65. Perna G, Stanislao M, Salvatori MP. Basal plasma beta-endorphin and beta-lipotropin in patients with symptomatic and asymptomatic myocardial ischemia. Cardiologia 1988;*33:*765.

66. Opasich C, Cobelli F, Farilla C et al. Silent ischemia in post-myocardial infarction patients submitted to physical training. Eur Heart J 1988;*9(Suppl.N):*22.

67. Meisenberg G, Simmons WH. Peptides and the bloodbrain barrier. Life Sci 1983;*32:*2611.

68. Willerson JC, Sheng-Shu L, Bertagna X. Pituitary beta-endorphin not involved in pain control in some pathophysiological conditions. Lancet 1984;*2:*295.

69. Maseri A, Mimmo R, Chierchia S et al. Coronary artery spasm as a cause of acute myocardial ischemia in man. Chest 1975;*68*:625.
70. Maseri A, Parodi O, Severi S, Pesola A. Transient transmural reduction of myocardial blood flow, demonstrated by thallium-201 scintigraphy, as a cause of variant angina. Circulation 1976;*54*:280.
71. Chierchia S, Lazzari M, Freedman B et al. Impairment of myocardial perfusion and function during painless myocardial ischemia. J Am Coll Cardiol 1983;*1*:924.
72. Deanfield JE, Maseri A, Selwyn AP et al. Myocardial ischaemia during daily life in patients with stable angina: its relation to symptoms and heart rate changes. Lancet 1983;*2*:753.
73. Amsterdam EA, Martschinske R, Laslett LJ, Rutledge JC, Vera Z. Symptomatic and silent myocardial ischemia during exercise testing in coronary arterial disease. Am J Cardiol 1986;*58*:43B.
74. Wohlgelernter D, Jaffe CC, Cabin HS, Yeatman Jr LA, Cleman M. Silent ischemia during coronary occlusion produced by balloon inflation: relation to regional myocardial dysfunction. J Am Coll Cardiol 1987;*10*:491.
75. Kannel WB. Incidence, percursors and prognosis of unrecognized myocardial infarction. In: Kellerman JJ, Braunwald G (eds) Silent Myocardial Ischemia: A Critical Appraisal. Basel, Karger, Adv Cardiol, 1990;*37*:202.

Prevalence and significance of silent myocardial ischemia

INTRODUCTION

Interest in the general problem of silent myocardial ischemia originated largely from two interconnected concepts: these are, first, the possibility that episodes of silent myocardial ischemia could herald myocardial infarction (MI) and sudden ischemic cardiac death (SICD) or cause subtle damage to the heart, and second, the possibility that the abolition of silent episodes by appropriate therapy could improve prognosis. As argued in the previous chapter, myocardial ischemia not associated with symptoms may have different causes, in the same way as painful myocardial ischemia; as the location and radiation of anginal pain are independent of the actual triggers of ischemia, the absence of pain is also unrelated to the actual causes of ischemia. Thus, painless ischemia is not a separate entity and may occur in chronic stable, microvascular, unstable, and variant angina, and in MI. Painless ischemic episodes carry an obviously severe prognosis when ischemia is very severe and associated with left ventricular failure, potentially fatal arrhythmias, or myocardial necrosis (i.e. when it is painless, but not silent) (see 14.2.2).

The concept of a defective warning system obviously applies to episodes of ischemia that are painless, but symptomatic (i.e. they are associated with acute cardiac failure and arrhythmias) and those that are totally silent but caused by unstable coronary lesions, as the presence of anginal pain would normally alert the patient to rest and to seek medical attention. This concept, however, does not apply to silent ischemic episodes, not inherently life-threatening nor carrying a poor short-term prognosis, such as those occurring in syndrome X or mild chronic stable angina.

This chapter brings together aspects that are discussed in Chapters 14 and 16–19, in order to define the reality and variable importance of silent myocardial ischemia and its clinical management.

15.1 THE REALITY AND VARIABLE IMPORTANCE OF SILENT MYOCARDIAL ISCHEMIA

Evidence that severe long-lasting myocardial ischemia can be totally silent and that the absence of pain is independent of the actual causes of ischemia is presented in the previous

chapter. Silent episodes are common in all ischemic syndromes and their prognostic significance depends largely on the ischemic syndrome in which they occur.

15.1.1 Reasons for the absence of pain during ischemia

The reasons for the possible absence of pain are discussed in Chapter 14 but are summarized here. The idea of a defective warning system for the ischemic heart was popularized
by Cohn in 1981[1] and started the interest in this area; a generalized defective perception of
painful stimuli was proposed subsequently by Droste and Roskamm in 1983.[2,3] The concept
of an alarm system implies the perception and decoding of impulses as potentially noxious
and cannot, therefore, be dissociated from an individual's state of alertness, cultural background, and previous experience.[4] Although Cohn proposed that those totally asymptomatic
patients with no evidence of ischemic heart disease (IHD) who present with transient
ischemic episodes should be separated from those with a history of infarction or angina in
addition to silent episodes of myocardial ischemia, in many studies the former have been
grouped with the latter. The important limit of this generalization lies in its inability to separate anatomic neural defects, which may be present in patients who never experience cardiac ischemic pain, from functional transient alterations, which are more likely to operate in
patients who experience pain during some episodes of ischemia but not during others of
apparently equal severity and duration.

Personality traits and generalized alterations of the opioid system may modulate the
threshold for pain perception, but do not easily explain the occurrence of painless MI or
severe ischemia causing sudden left ventricular failure. They also cannot explain the occurrence, within minutes, of both painful and painless ischemic episodes of similar severity and
duration.

The following hypotheses, put forward to explain the absence of pain during ischemia, are
not mutually exclusive. The mechanisms proposed may all contribute, to different extents,
to the lack of pain in different patients and even in the same individual on different occasions.

Intensity of the stimulus

Ischemia may not last long enough to stimulate afferent fibers, as pain often develops after
a variable delay following the onset of ischemia. In patients with unstable or variant angina,
ischemic episodes of short duration are painless more often than are longer episodes (see
Ch. 14). Although this explanation is tenable in general, it can explain neither the absence
of pain in episodes of severe long-lasting ischemia and infarction, nor the presence of pain
in patients with microvascular angina and no signs of ischemia. Thus, a certain severity and
duration of ischemia are necessary—but not sufficient—conditions to explain the presence
of pain.[5]

Defective afferent neural fibers

Absence or damage of afferent cardiac fibers that carry potentially painful stimuli may
explain the absence of pain only in patients in whom it never develops, not even during MI;
however, defective afferent nervous fibers cannot be the cause of silent ischemia in those
patients who may develop pain during a second MI or who subsequently develop postinfarction angina.[6,7]

In 43% of diabetic patients who died of acute MI, at least one healed infarction was not revealed by scrutiny of the patient's clinical history.[8] Exercise stress testing caused anginal pain in only 28% of diabetic patients, but in 68% of nondiabetic patients for a similar degree of ST-segment depression. Similarly, the prevalence of only painless episodes of ST-segment depression during Holter monitoring was found to be higher among diabetic than nondiabetic patients.[9,10]

Autonomic neuropathy involving cardiac afferent nerves may explain the higher incidence of consistently painless ischemia in diabetic patients. In five such patients who died as a result of painless MI, intramyocardial sympathetic and parasympathetic nerves exhibited morphologic alterations characteristic of diabetic neuropathy, such as beaded thickening within the nerves, spindle-shaped nerve fibers, fragmentation of nerve fibers, and a decrease in the actual number of neurons.[11] ECG evidence of painless MI was found in 20% of 73 diabetic patients with peripheral neuropathy and evidence of autonomic nervous system dysfunction, but in only 4% of patients with no such evidence.[12] Although plausible, these explanations do not rule out the possible contribution of other influences that modulate the gating system for afferent, potentially painful, stimuli or the central decoding of stimuli.

The gate-control system of pain

As discussed in the previous chapter, a prominent role for afferent converging impulses, and especially for impulses descending from the brain stem and from higher structures, is a component of a general theory of visceral pain perception. A mild degree of inhibition can be sufficient to block or delay the perception of afferent impulses during short and mild ischemic episodes, whereas a greater degree of inhibition would be required to block afferent impulses generated during extensive ischemia. Strong afferent stimuli may be blocked on their way to the cortex or suppressed at the conscious level. The gating system is controlled by both afferent stimuli from the body and descending impulses from the cortex and higher centers, which depend on the patient's state of alertness and personality traits, and on the opioid system.

15.1.2 Prevalence of silent myocardial ischemia

Episodes of silent myocardial ischemia represent the largest proportion of all ischemic episodes, but the assessment of their prevalence in the various ischemic syndromes and in totally asymptomatic individuals depends on the diagnostic criteria used.

Painless episodes in patients with documented IHD

A review of the subject indicates that, on average, the frequency of painless episodes of transient ischemic ST-segment shift is about 80% of the total, both during ambulatory ECG monitoring in patients with stable angina and during in-hospital ECG monitoring in patients with variant or unstable angina; however, the prevalence of silent ischemia during exercise stress testing is only 40% (see Fig. 15.1).[13] In patients with syndrome X, many episodes of ST-segment shift are also asymptomatic.[14,15]

In the Framingham Study the incidence of painless MI was about 25% of a total of 708 infarctions discovered after periodic ECG examination, when infarctions with very atypical symptoms were also included. The percentage of painless MI was higher in women and elderly men (see Fig. 15.2). About 50% of painless infarctions were totally silent.[16]

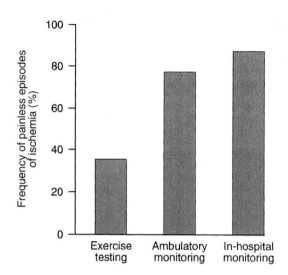

Fig. 15.1 Frequency of transient episodes of painless ischemia in patients with angina. Only about 20% of spontaneous episodes recorded during continuous ECG monitoring are associated with pain, compared to about 60% of episodes induced by exercise stress testing. This difference may be explained partly by the general awareness of the possibility that ischemia may occur during exercise testing. (Modified from ref. 13.)

In patients with chronic stable angina the proportion of silent ischemic episodes detected during ECG monitoring is quite variable in different patients and also in different recordings in the same patient.[17] A large variability in the ratio of painful to painless ischemic episodes is also frequently observed in unstable and variant angina.

The fact that ischemic episodes are often painless in each ischemic syndrome is consistent with the argument presented in Chapter 14, i.e. that the presence or absence of pain bears no relation to the actual causes of ischemia.

Silent episodes in patients without documented IHD

The prevalence of painless myocardial ischemia in totally asymptomatic individuals is unknown, but it is likely that only a few of the 40% of those individuals above the age of 50 with extensive raised fibrous atherosclerotic plaques (see Ch. 8) who are totally asymptomatic have episodes of silent ischemia. Of these few individuals, some will have only episodes of ischemia related to chronic stable coronary alterations such as those responsible for the clinical syndrome of stable angina; others may have an occasional phase of instability, such as that responsible for the clinical syndrome of unstable angina; and still others may have episodes related to the same causes responsible for microvascular angina. Totally asymptomatic patients with the equivalent syndrome of chronic stable angina can be identified at any time by exercise stress testing, because they have a reduced coronary flow reserve. In contrast, patients with the equivalent syndrome of unstable angina can be identified only occasionally if Holter monitoring is carried out during the phase of instability, which (as in its symptomatic form) should tend either to evolve rapidly towards MI, or to

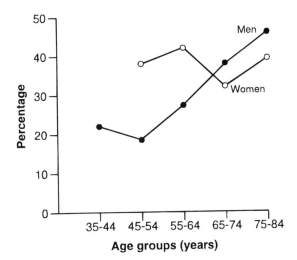

Fig. 15.2 Incidence of unrecognized MI. In the Framingham study the incidence of unrecognized (painless) MI increases with age in men, from 20% at 40–50 years of age to 45% at the age of 80, but it remains constant at about 40% in women. (Modified from ref. 16.)

subside and resolve. In asymptomatic individuals, the prevalence of silent ischemia varies with the level of risk factors for IHD. Using standard criteria, in middle-aged men the prevalence of individuals with a positive ECG exercise stress test and no angina is about 2.5%,[18,19] but in individuals in the top decile of coronary risk in the Multiple Risk Factor Intervention (MRFIT) Study the figure was 12.5% (see 15.1.3).[20] For comparison, in a low-risk group of patients with known IHD, exercise testing was positive in 38% of cases (ischemia was silent in 58%).[21]

15.1.3 Variable prognostic significance of painless myocardial ischemia

As the absence of pain bears no relation to the actual causes of ischemia, the prognostic significance of painless ischemia is as varied as that of painful ischemia, which bears no relation to the variable location and radiation of pain. The prognosis of painless ischemia is obviously severe, independent of its causes, when it is associated with symptoms of acute left ventricular failure or with arrhythmias, or when it may herald an impending MI, but when the only sign of its presence is represented by transient ischemic changes on the ECG, its prognostic significance depends on the course of myocardial ischemia.

In patients with unstable angina, the detection of totally silent ischemic episodes is an indication of persisting instability, which has an important prognostic significance and demands aggressive management. Indeed, the total duration of ischemic ST-segment depression for longer than 1 h during a 24 h recording period carries a particularly poor prognosis (see Ch. 19).[22,23]

In patients after acute MI, a positive predischarge exercise stress test has a prognostic significance independent of the presence or absence of pain. It seems reasonable to assume that the prognostic value is related to the reduction of coronary flow reserve, to the area of myocardium at risk, and to the development of potentially fatal arrhythmias (see Ch. 22).

In addition, a positive Holter recording was found to have an important prognostic significance, but it is not clear to what extent it is an independent prognostic variable.[24,25]

In patients with chronic stable angina, a positive exercise stress test in the absence of pain carries a prognosis similar to one with pain (see Fig. 13.8). Patients with a considerable reduction of coronary flow reserve and a positive exercise test at a low work load are likely to have a large number of ischemic episodes during Holter monitoring (particularly if they often exert themselves), most of which will be silent. Some studies suggest that the presence of silent ischemic episodes during ambulatory monitoring carries an independent prognostic significance above that of exercise stress testing,[26-28] but these findings require confirmation.

The cases of two patients with chronic stable angina, who were subjected to repeated Holter monitoring, illustrate the difficulties encountered when interpreting silent ischemic episodes in this syndrome. The ischemic threshold remained constant through several months in each patient, indicating that the residual coronary flow reserve, tested under standardized conditions, remained constant. Nevertheless, the number of painful and painless episodes varied considerably on different days and, in one case, an increase in the number of episodes detected by Holter monitoring was followed by MI. It was impossible to tell whether the large variations in the number of ischemic episodes that occurred from day to day were due to more frequent severe exertion or to more frequent episodes of coronary vasoconstriction (see Fig. 15.3A,B). It was also impossible to tell whether the increased number of episodes that preceded the MI in that patient were due to the usual stable mechanisms or to new unstable causes.

In totally asymptomatic individuals without known IHD, the prognosis of silent myocardial ischemia is also likely to depend on the severity of the reduction of coronary flow reserve, on the area of myocardium at risk, and on its cause. As already discussed in Chapter 13, in the MRFIT Study in individuals between 37 and 57 years of age who were in the top decile of coronary risk, a positive exercise stress test conferred about a threefold greater risk of cardiac death than a negative result, i.e. 5.0 versus 1.6% mortality rate over a 7-year period (0.7% versus 0.2% per year). This corresponds to a smaller total number of deaths in the 1601 individuals with positive exercise stress tests than in the 10 417 individuals with negative tests over the same 7-year follow-up period. A review of the predictive value of exercise stress testing[28] in about 26 000 normal individuals included in 14 studies, found an average 4.2-fold excess risk of cardiac death occurring among those with positive results, but twice as many events occurred in those with negative results, who represented the highest number of those tested. Consequently, the calculated sensitivity of the test was 37% and its specificity was 69%. Thus, a positive test result had a predictive value of only 7.5% in the

Fig. 15.3 Daily variability of silent ischemic episodes in chronic stable angina. (**A**) Multiple Holter recordings over a period of about 2 years in a stable patient show wide variability in the number of silent ischemic episodes, in the absence of any changes in exercise stress testing results. In all recordings there were only a few anginal attacks. (**B**) A series of Holter tapes recorded during a drug trial in a stable patient show a large number of predominantly silent ischemic episodes (with no changes in the value of heart rate at the onset of ischemia), which were followed by an acute MI. It is not possible to tell whether this large number of episodes reflects simply the presence of more frequent chronic stimuli, or the occurrence of new unstable stimuli (detected by chance) which lead to the development of MI. (Modified from ref. 17.)

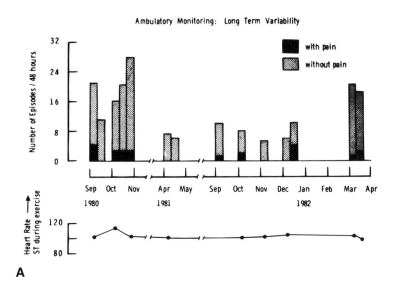

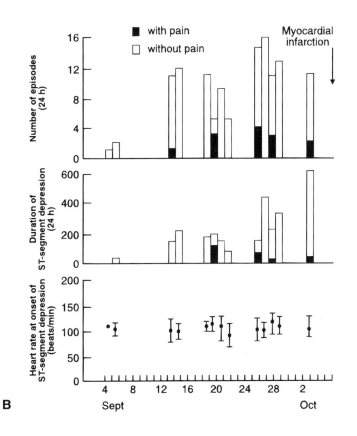

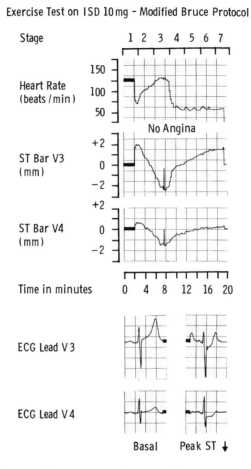

Fig. 15.4 Positive exercise stress test in a totally asymptomatic patient. Rapid, progressive development of ischemic ST-segment depression in the precordial leads at 8 min on the modified Bruce protocol after administration of sublingual isosorbide dinitrate (ISD). Multiple ischemic episodes were also detected during Holter monitoring (see also Fig. 15.5).

population studied, which mostly included individuals with high levels of risk factors for IHD.

The prognostic significance of the exercise stress test might have been greater if, instead of categorizing the results as positive or negative, the levels of effort tolerated and the area of myocardium at risk had also been considered. The number of patients identified by stricter inclusion criteria would have been even smaller.

Thus, the yield from comprehensive screening procedures such as that used in the MRFIT study appears to be extremely limited but, when encountered in clinical practise, a markedly positive exercise stress test at a low work load and with a large area of myocardium at risk may carry an important prognostic value.

A case report illustrates the possible prognostic significance of silent myocardial ischemia in a totally asymptomatic individual, detected by a routine exercise stress test that was markedly positive at a low work load.

Case report

A male patient from the Indian subcontinent, an executive aged 49 years, had no history suggestive of any cardiac disorder. He had never experienced any type of discomfort in the chest, throat, teeth, or arms that was suggestive of pain. He had a normal resting ECG but, before assignment abroad, was required to undergo exercise stress testing, which was reported as showing ischemic changes with no subjective symptoms. Other findings were as follows:

- Past medical history: vagotomy for duodenal ulcer 1982; jaundice as a child
- Social history: nonsmoker
- Physical examination: normal; BP 130/90
- Investigations: full blood count, urea and electrolytes, liver function tests, cholesterol (5.8 mM) within normal limits; hepatitis B surface antigen negative; ECG within normal limits; chest radiograph normal.

Exercise stress test on a Marquette CASE system was strongly positive and was positive also after the administration of sublingual nitrates, on both occasions in the absence of any subjective symptom (see Fig. 15.4). Holter monitoring showed several episodes of ST-seg-

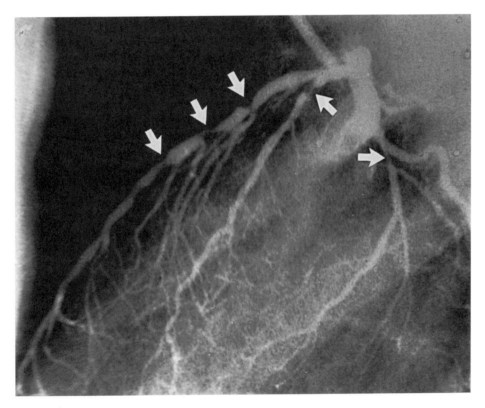

Fig. 15.5 Left coronary angiogram of a patient with totally silent myocardial ischemia. In the same patient depicted in Fig. 15.4, multiple severe stenoses are visible in the left coronary branches (arrows). A 50% diameter stenosis was also present in the right coronary artery. The patient died suddenly a few days after angiography whilst awaiting CABG, without ever in his life having experienced anginal pain or discomfort.

ment depression, all totally asymptomatic. Cross-sectional echocardiographic assessment at the end of the exercise test showed a large area of anterolateral dyskinesia. Angiography showed a normal ventricle with severe multiple stenosis of all major vessels (see Fig. 15.5).

After angiography the patient was immediately put on aspirin (325 mg/day on a full stomach) and atenolol (100 mg in the morning) and was advised to undergo urgent coronary artery bypass grafting (CABG), but he died suddenly at 07.45 h 4 days after angiography, with no symptoms and in the presence of witnesses.

15.2 CLINICAL MANAGEMENT OF SILENT MYOCARDIAL ISCHEMIA

As silent myocardial ischemia is a clinical reality and may carry a prognostic significance, it is useful to define the indications for its diagnosis and treatment.

15.2.1 Diagnostic relevance of silent myocardial ischemia

In patients with known IHD we have learned to use the pattern of anginal pain as an indicator of the stability or instability of the disease and of the response to therapy. We have also learned that, in the various ischemic syndromes, most patients respond to appropriate anti-ischemic therapy with a similar reduction in both painful and painless episodes of transient ischemic ST-segment shift. Double crossover studies in patients with variant angina showed that verapamil,[29] isosorbide dinitrate,[30] and nifedipine[31] reduced both painful and painless episodes by approximately the same percentage (see Fig. 15.6A,B). In patients with chronic stable angina, β-blockers[32,33] reduced the number of painful and painless ischemic episodes to a similar extent. Finally, successful CABG[34] and angioplasty[35] were associated with the disappearance of both painful and painless episodes of ST-segment depression during ambulatory ECG monitoring. In all these patients with different causes of ischemic episodes, therefore, silent episodes of transient ST-segment changes responded to the appropriate treatment, like painful episodes. Thus, the occurrence of a larger number of ischemic episodes, not detectable clinically, in patients taking part in clinical trials, allows a better statistical assessment of the efficacy of anti-ischemic treatment.[29]

In clinical practise, the importance of detecting silent ischemic episodes is vital for patients with unstable angina, as persistent silent ischemic episodes indicate ongoing instability and the need to intensify the treatment, even when the patient is totally asymptomatic. It is also of considerable importance for those patients with variant angina who have life-threatening arrhythmias during ischemic episodes: in such patients it is essential to eliminate not only painful episodes but also silent episodes, as they can all equally trigger fatal arrhythmias. Conversely, the additional prognostic value in patients with chronic stable angina remains to be established, as ischemic episodes (painful or painless) are caused by chronic stable coronary alterations and may not be prognostically significant unless they are inherently severe.

For individuals without known IHD, the most common diagnostic problem is the occurrence of silent ST-segment depression during routine exercise stress testing. Two questions should be asked: first, are the ECG changes really caused by ischemia; second, is the cause of ischemia stable or unstable? An ischemic cause is likely when the ECG changes occur in an individual with known risk factors and a high pretest probability of IHD, when the "ischemic" ST-segment depression is large (more than 2 mm), occurs at a low heart rate (less than 120 bpm) and is markedly improved in a test performed after sublingual nitrates.

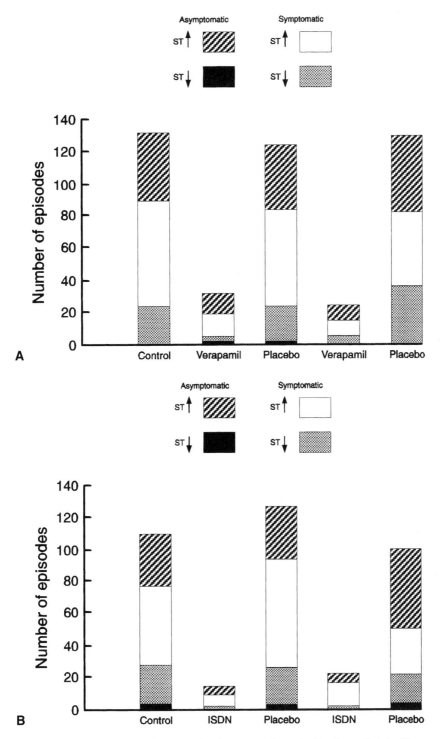

Fig. 15.6 In variant angina, medical therapy has similar beneficial effects on painful and painless ischemic episodes. In two double cross-over trials, verapamil (**A**) and isosorbide dinitrate (ISDN) (**B**) produced a similar reduction in the number of painful and painless episodes, which were characterized by either ST-segment elevation or depression. (Modified from refs 29 and 30.)

The ischemic nature is confirmed by the demonstration of associated transient regional impairment of ventricular function or myocardial perfusion. In general, a stable cause of ischemia is the most likely as unstable phases of ischemia are short lived, but the occurrence of many severe prolonged episodes of ischemic ST-segment depression during Holter monitoring not associated with tachycardia may be suggestive of an unstable phase that may need urgent treatment.

15.2.2 Practical management of silent myocardial ischemia

Painless but symptomatic myocardial ischemia causing acute ventricular failure on arrhythmias, or so persistent that it causes MI, should be managed as aggressively as painful ischemia because its immediate prognostic significance is severe, even in the absence of warning pain. Silent myocardial ischemic episodes that are not life threatening should be managed within the framework of the ischemic syndrome in which they occur (unstable, stable, or variant angina) and according to the severity of ischemia. They should be treated with antithrombotic and thrombolytic drugs when caused by thrombosis, with high doses of vasodilators when caused by occlusive coronary artery spasm, and by interruption of effort and by reduction of myocardial demand when occurring during exercise stress testing.

Efforts to detect silent ischemic episodes not inherently severe (i.e. totally silent) are appropriate in unstable angina and in variant angina when complicated by ischemia-induced arrhythmias. In such patients, continuous monitoring of the ECG leads showing ischemic changes may provide evidence of persistent anginal instability or of incomplete prevention of potentially arrhythmogenic ischemic episodes, indicating the need, therefore, for intensification of therapy and/or further investigation (see Chs 19 and 20).

In patients with mild chronic stable angina and good effort tolerance, it is not yet clear whether the detection of silent ischemic episodes during Holter monitoring has clinical implications above and beyond those provided by clinical symptoms and exercise stress testing, and whether treatment with anti-ischemic drugs aimed at preventing them improves prognosis. In stable patients, the concept of the "total ischemic burden" may not be such an independent indicator of risk as it is in unstable patients. Totally asymptomatic individuals with a positive exercise stress test at a high work load (more than 9 min on the Bruce protocol, see Ch. 17) and patients with no evidence of a large area of myocardium at risk (identified by a large myocardial perfusion defect, wall motion abnormality, or a marked reduction of left ventricular ejection fraction) have a good prognosis, but should be advised to control their risk factors (which in the MRFIT study, abolished the risk conferred by a positive exercise stress test),[20] and to take aspirin (75 mg/day on a full stomach). The additional prognostic benefit of anti-ischemic drug therapy and of revascularization procedures in low-risk patients is difficult to prove unless very large numbers of patients are randomized and followed for several years.

The number of fatal and nonfatal ischemic events avoided by any treatment per 1000 patients treated per year of follow-up can only be small because of their low baseline risk.

REFERENCES

1. Cohn PF. Asymptomatic coronary artery disease. Mod Concepts Cardiovasc Dis 1981;*50*:55.
2. Droste C, Roskamm H. Experimental pain measurement in patients with asymptomatic myocardial ischemia. J Am Coll Cardiol 1983;*1*:940.
3. Droste C, Greenlee MW, Roskamm H. A defective angina pectoris pain warning system: experimental findings of ischemic and electrical pain test. Pain 1986;*26*:199.

4. Malliani A, Lombardi F. Consideration of the fundamental mechanisms eliciting cardiac pain. Am Heart J 1982;*103*:575.

5. Maseri A, Chierchia S, Davies G, Glazier J. Mechanisms of ischemic cardiac pain and silent myocardial ischaemia. Am J Med 1985;*79(Suppl. 3A)*:7.

6. Droste C, Roskamm H. Pain perception and endogenous pain modulation in angina pectoris. In: Kellermann JJ, Braunwald E (eds) Silent Myocardial Ischemia: A Critical Appraisal. Basel, Karger, Adv Cardiol, 1990;*37*:p.142.

7. Kannel WB, Abbott RD. Incidence and prognosis of unrecognized myocardial infarction. An update on the Framingham Study. N Engl J Med 1984;*311*:1144.

8. Bradley RF, Partamian JO. Coronary heart disease in the diabetic patient. Med Clin North Am 1963;*78*:1093.

9. Nesto RW, Phillips RT, Kett KG et al. Angina and exertional myocardial ischemia in diabetic and nondiabetic patients: assessment by exercise thallium scintigraphy. Ann Intern Med 1988;*108*:170.

10. Chiariello M, Indolfi C, Cotecchia MR et al. Asymptomatic transient ST changes during ambulatory ECG monitoring in diabetic patients. Am Heart J 1985;*110*:529.

11. Fearman I, Faccio E, Melei J et al. Autonomic neuropathy and painless myocardial infarction in diabetic patients: histologic evidence of their relationships. Diabetes 1977;*26*:1147.

12. Niakan E, Harati Y, Rolak LA et al. Silent myocardial infarction and diabetic cardiovascular autonomic neuropathy. Arch Intern Med 1986;*146*:2220.

13. Rozanski A, Berman DS. Silent myocardial ischemia. I. Pathophysiology, frequency of occurrence, and approaches toward detection. Am Heart J 1987;*114*:615.

14. Kaski JC, Crea F, Nihoyannopoulos P, Hackett D, Maseri A. Transient myocardial ischemia during daily life in patients with syndrome X. Am J Cardiol 1986;*58*:1242.

15. Bugiardini R, Borghi A, Biagetti L, Puddu P. Comparison of verapamil versus propanol therapy in syndrome X. Am J Cardiol 1989;*63*:286.

16. Kannel WB, Cupples LA. Silent myocardial infarction. Incidence, prevalence and prognostic significance. In: Singh BN (ed) Silent Myocardial Ischemia and Angina. Prevalence, Prognostic and Therapeutic Significance. New York, Pergamon Press, 1988, p. 174.

17. Deanfield JE, Maseri A, Selwyn AP et al. Myocardial ischemia during daily life in patients with stable angina: its relation to symptoms and heart rate changes. Lancet 1983;*2*:753.

18. Froelicher Jr VF, Thomas MM, Pillow C, Lancaster HC. Epidemiologic study of asymptomatic men screened by maximal treadmill testing for latent coronary artery disease. Am J Cardiol 1974;*34*:770.

19. Erikssen J, Cohn PF, Thaulow E, Mowinckel P. Silent myocardial ischemia in middle aged men: long term clinical course. In: von Arnim T, Maseri A (eds) Silent Ischemia: Current Concepts and Management. New York, Springer-Verlag, 1987, p. 45.

20. Rautaharji PM, Prineas RJ, Eifler WJ et al. Prognostic value of exercise electrocardiogram in men at high risk of future coronary heart disease: Multiple Risk Factor Intervention Trial experience. J Am Coll Cardiol 1986;*8*:1.

21. Ignone G, Vona M, Scardi S on behalf of the participants. Multicenter Study on Silent Ischemia during exercise testing (SMISS). Clinical and ergometric parameters in 4389 patients with proven ischemic heart disease. G Ital Cardiol 1984;*24*:349.

22. Gottlieb SO, Weisfeldt ML, Ouyang P, Mellits ED, Gerstenblith G. Silent ischemia as a marker of early unfavourable outcomes in patients with unstable angina. N Engl J Med 1986;*314*:1214.

23. Bugiardini R, Borghi A, Pozzati A, Ruggeri A, Puddu P, Maseri A. Relation of severity of symptoms to transient myocardial ischemia and prognosis in unstable angina. J Am Coll Cardiol 1995 (in press).

24. Langer A, Minkowitz J, Dorian P et al. Pathophysiology and prognostic significance of Holter-detected ST segment depression after myocardial infarction. J Am Coll Cardiol 1992;*20*:1313.

25. Ruberman W, Crow R, Rosenberg CR, Rautaharju PM, Shore RE, Pasternack BS. Intermittent ST depression and mortality after myocardial infarction. Circulation 1992;*85*:1440.

26. Deedwania PC, Carbajal EV. Silent ischemia during daily life is an independent predictor of mortality in stable angina. Circulation 1990;*81*:748.

27. Yeung AC, Barry J, Orav J, Raby KE, Selwyn AP. Time dependent effects of asymptomatic ischemia on prognosis in chronic stable coronary disease. Circulation 1991;*83:*1598.

28. Yusuf S. Design of studies to critically evaluate if detection of asymptomatic ST-segment deviation (silent ischemia) is of medical or public health importance. In: Singh BN (ed) Silent Myocardial Ischemia and Angina. Prevalence, Prognostic and Therapeutic Significance. New York, Pergamon Press, 1988, p.206.

29. Parodi O, Maseri A, Simonetti I. Management of unstable angina at rest by verapamil. A double-blind cross-over study in CCU. Br Heart J 1979;*41:*167.

30. Distante A, Maseri A, Severi S, Biagini A, Chierchia S. Management of vasospastic angina at rest with continuous infusion of isosorbide dinitrate. Am J Cardiol 1979;*44:*533.

31. Previtali M, Salerno JA, Tavazzi L et al. Treatment of angina at rest with nifedipine: a short-term controlled study. Am J Cardiol 1980;*45:*875.

32. Chierchia S, Glazier JJ, Gerosa S. A single-blind, placebo-controlled study of effects of atenolol on transient ischemia in "mixed" angina. Am J Cardiol 1987;*60:*36A.

33. Imperi GA, Lambert CR, Coy K et al. Effects of titrated beta blockade (metoprolol) on silent myocardial ischemia in ambulatory patients with coronary artery disease. Am J Cardiol 1987;*60:*519.

34. Crea F, Kaski JC, Fragasso G et al. Usefulness of Holter monitoring to improve the sensitivity of exercise testing in determining the degree of myocardial revascularization after coronary artery bypass grafting for stable angina pectoris. Am J Cardiol 1987;*60:*40.

35. Josephson MA, Nademanee K, Intarachot V, Lewis H, Singh B. Abolition of Holter monitor-detected silent myocardial ischemia after percutaneous transluminal coronary angioplasty. J Am Coll Cardiol 1987;*10:*499.

Transient, reversible myocardial ischemia

Transient myocardial ischemia and angina pectoris: classification and diagnostic assessment

INTRODUCTION

Transient acute myocardial ischemia, whatever its cause, can manifest clinically in the following ways:

a. with chest pain (angina pectoris) or discomfort (having only some of the characteristic features of angina pectoris)
b. with sudden transient acute ventricular failure or arrhythmias (but no pain), or
c. it may remain silent altogether (a phenomenon which, on average, occurs in about 70% of episodes) (see Ch. 15).

Angina equivalents are painless, but not asymptomatic, episodes of transient ischemia associated with acute left ventricular failure or arrhythmias. *Silent ischemic episodes* are attacks of acute transient myocardial ischemia that are totally asymptomatic. *Atypical chest pain,* involving the precordial region but without the characteristic features of angina (i.e. it is elicited and/or relieved by pressure, movement, and/or respiration and can last for only a few seconds or for several hours, recurring chronically), is extremely unlikely to be caused by myocardial ischemia.

Three facts are firmly established:

1. A pain or discomfort indistinguishable from that accompanying myocardial ischemia can have other cardiac or noncardiac causes.
2. Different causes of myocardial ischemia (such as increased demand, coronary artery spasm, coronary vasoconstriction, or thrombosis) can give rise to the same type of anginal pain; thus, in an individual patient, the location and radiation of pain usually do not change when stable angina becomes unstable, and vice versa. Although the severity of angina is usually proportional to the severity and extension of myocardial ischemia, in some patients anginal pain can be mild and often absent, even in the presence of massive ischemia; in others, conversely, it can be very severe in the presence of barely detectable signs of ischemia.
3. As myocardial ischemia can result from a variety of different causes, the symptom of angina pectoris can have an extremely variable prognostic significance.

Moreover, about 50% of patients presenting with angina have other cardiovascular alternations, such as hypertension, previous MI, etc. Prognosis is largely related to the stability or instability of angina, but is also influenced by:

    a. the extension of myocardium jeopardized by ischemia

    b. the extent of preexisting myocardial damage, which makes the heart more vulnerable to new ischemic insults, and

    c. the susceptibility to ventricular arrhythmias.

■ *Angina pectoris is, therefore, a symptom like pallor. When it persists, pallor is a clue to the presence of anemia, but it is only the evidence of reduced blood hemoglobin content that confirms the diagnosis and such a reduction can occur without pallor. It is only the diagnosis of the underlying cause of anemia that provides the rational basis for its treatment and prognostic assessment. Similarly, for angina pectoris, it is necessary to use all the clues that are available from the medical history and from the results of appropriate tests to diagnose the presence of episodes of myocardial ischemia (which may also occur without pain) and, having done so, to search for their causes.*■

This chapter deals with the clinical classification of angina pectoris and the diagnostic assessment of transient myocardial ischemia.

16.1 CLINICAL CLASSIFICATION

Once the ischemic origin of the anginal pain has been established from both the pattern of attacks and the results of objective tests, the occurrence of angina should be classified into *stable* or *unstable* patterns, as the prognosis and the pathogenetic mechanisms of these two patterns of angina differ, although the location and radiation of the pain are identical.

Patients with chronic stable angina generally tend to remain stable, whereas from 5 to 20% of those with unstable angina either develop myocardial infarction (MI) or succumb to sudden ischemic cardiac death (SICD) within 6 months and, therefore, require prompt and aggressive management. Among patients presenting with stable, predominantly effort-related angina, a subgroup with angiographically normal coronary arteries can be identified and is defined as "syndrome X." Among patients presenting with unstable, predominantly spontaneous episodes of angina, a subgroup with preserved effort tolerance and recurring occlusive epicardial coronary artery spasm can be identified and is termed "variant angina." For clinical purposes, therefore, patients with angina pectoris can be classified into two major groups, each of which includes a subgroup:

    1. Chronic stable angina
        a. syndrome X
    2. Unstable angina
        a. variant angina.

A minority of patients presenting with occasional anginal attacks at rest or on effort, separated by periods of several months and even years, cannot be classified because of the lack of a detectable pattern of recurrence.

In both stable and unstable syndromes, the pathogenetic mechanisms of myocardial ischemia are composite and varied (see Fig. 16.1A–D). Moreover, many ischemic episodes occur without pain; indeed, an unknown number of individuals have only painless or silent episodes of ischemia that represent asymptomatic equivalents of these syndromes.

■ *As neither the type of pain nor its absence are influenced by the causes of ischemia, it is difficult to assess precisely when a patient passes from a stable to an unstable phase, or vice versa, in the absence of an obvious change in the pattern of attacks.* ■

16.1.1 Chronic stable angina, predominantly effort related

In patients with a chronic stable pattern of angina, the anginal attacks are predominantly, but not necessarily, effort related, are of short duration, are relieved promptly by rest and sublingual nitrates, have an unchanged pattern of occurrence over at least the last 2 months, and have no *detectable* tendency to evolve towards MI and SICD in the short term (i.e. over weeks or months) (see Ch. 17). Chronic stable angina may be the first manifestation of ischemic heart disease (IHD) or it may appear after MI or unstable angina. It may subside for years, but then become unstable or be complicated by an acute MI or by SICD.

In such patients, transient myocardial ischemia can be caused by chronic stable coronary atherosclerotic obstructions, with either a fixed or a variable residual coronary flow reserve, modulated by coronary vasoconstriction occurring at the site of coronary stenoses or in distal vessels.

Patients who for months have had a stable pattern of angina can be divided into two groups, according to the predictability or unpredictability of their anginal attacks:[1]

1. The first group comprises patients with recurrent anginal attacks that are predictably caused by a certain intensity of physical effort (such as walking a given distance at a particular pace). The constancy of the anginal threshold suggests that myocardial ischemia is caused exclusively by an excessive increase in demand in the presence of a fixed limitation of coronary blood supply. Patients who present this pattern of isolated, predictable, effort-related, angina learn to recognize the anginal threshold and to avoid efforts that may trigger angina, but such patients are rare.

Angina occurs exclusively during efforts of similar intensity (the attacks that occur after rather than during the effort cannot be caused only by increased cardiac work and myocardial oxygen consumption) and is consistently relieved by rest within 1—5 min. The duration of angina is related to the duration of the effort. The anginal threshold is fairly constant and the patient cannot tolerate more intense effort without developing angina (which does not occur for efforts of lesser intensity, except in emotional situations, in the cold, or after meals). This makes angina predictable and attentive patients can remain relatively free from angina by limiting their daily activities or by taking sublingual nitrates prophylactically before effort. These patients typically have fixed chronic flow-limiting coronary stenoses.

---

2. The second group comprises those patients who, besides recognizing an upper threshold for angina "during their good days," also present with occasional, unpredictable anginal attacks for efforts that are clearly milder than those tolerated at other times without angina or even occurring at rest. These patients may also remain stable for years: they have a *mixed form* of chronic stable angina and are the most common (see Ch. 17). The variability of the anginal threshold suggests that the cause of ischemia is a combination of a coincidentally subliminal increase in demand and a subliminal transient impairment of residual coronary flow or a sudden reduction of coronary blood supply below resting levels.

In a subgroup of patients, typically with a mixed pattern of angina, transient myocardial ischemia may be caused exclusively by inappropriate distal coronary vessel constriction in the absence of epicardial coronary artery stenoses. The size of this heterogeneous subgroup, in which angina is predominantly effort related, ranges from 5 to 50% (according to the indications used for arteriography),[2,3] and is currently defined as *syndrome X*. Patients with

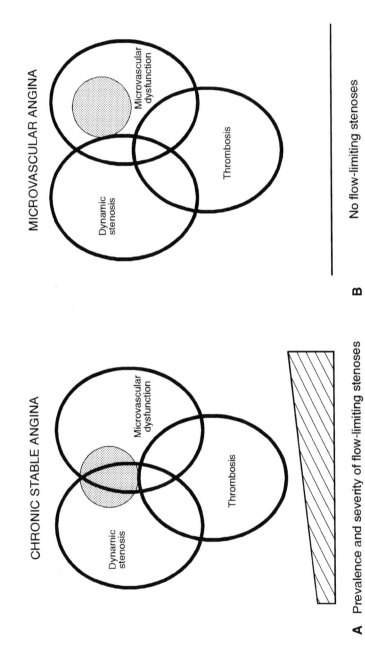

CHRONIC STABLE ANGINA

Dynamic
stenosis

Microvascular
dysfunction

Thrombosis

MICROVASCULAR ANGINA

Dynamic
stenosis

Microvascular
dysfunction

Thrombosis

A Prevalence and severity of flow-limiting stenoses   **B** No flow-limiting stenoses

Fig. 16.1 Pathogenetic components of stable and unstable anginal syndromes.
Chronic stable angina (**A**) is caused by flow-limiting coronary artery stenoses of variable severity and number, but residual coronary flow reserve can be modulated by dynamic changes in peristenotic smooth muscle tone (dynamic stenoses) or by microvascular dysfunction. Microvascular angina (**B**) is caused by coronary microvascular dysfunction. (*Figure continues.*)

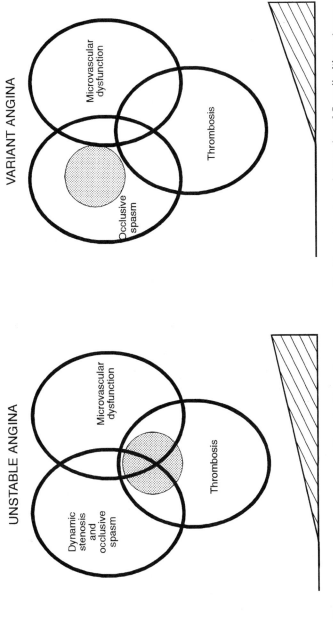

UNSTABLE ANGINA

Microvascular
dysfunction

Dynamic
stenosis
and
occlusive
spasm

Thrombosis

C Prevalence and severity of flow-limiting stenoses

VARIANT ANGINA

Microvascular
dysfunction

Occlusive
spasm

Thrombosis

D Prevalence and severity of flow-limiting stenoses

Fig. 16.1 (*Continued*) Unstable angina (**C**) is caused by a variable combination of thrombosis, dynamic stenoses, occlusive spasm and microvascular dysfunction occurring not only in the presence of flow-limiting coronary artery stenoses, but also in their absence. Variant angina (**D**) is caused by occlusive epicardial coronary artery spasm, which may occur not only at the site of flow-limiting stenoses of variable severity, but also in angiographically normal segments.

455

syndrome X may have an extracardiac, a cardiac but nonischemic, or a coronary microvascular cause of pain, i.e. microvascular angina (see Ch. 18).

The prognosis of most patients with syndrome X is virtually normal; that of patients with stable angina who have atherosclerotic obstructions of the coronary arteries is good in the short term, particularly when their ventricular function is normal. They can, however, quite unpredictably develop unstable angina or unheralded MI, or succumb to SICD. This unfavorable evolution occurs more frequently in patients with previous infarction and impaired left ventricular function, and also in those with a low effort tolerance and severe multiple coronary obstructions that jeopardize segments of myocardium.

16.1.2 Unstable angina, predominantly spontaneous

Angina is defined as unstable when it is of recent onset and/or has suddenly become much worse during the last 2 months (see Ch. 19). Anginal attacks typically have no precipitating cause, or occur on efforts that were previously quite well tolerated in the absence of extra-coronary causes affecting the myocardial demand/supply balance. Some attacks are severe and can last for over 20 min. In such patients, transient myocardial ischemia is the result of recent alterations in the coronary arteries that lead to thrombus formation and/or vasoconstriction, with sudden transient reduction of coronary blood flow (CBF), and that may evolve in the short term (i.e. days or weeks) toward MI and SICD.

Within the syndrome of unstable angina is a small subgroup of patients who present with predominantly spontaneous nocturnal, early morning, and rest angina but who have normal or good effort tolerance. This syndrome is defined as *variant angina* and includes patients with and without coronary artery stenoses, who develop transient episodes of occlusive epicardial coronary artery spasm. Variant angina also had quite a poor prognosis before the introduction of calcium antagonists and high doses of nitrates, particularly when it was associated with a history of fainting, palpitations, and prolonged chest pain (see Ch. 20).

In patients with unstable angina, a sudden reduction of CBF can be caused by mural epicardial coronary artery thrombosis, with or without a proximal or distal coronary vasoconstrictor component, or by epicardial coronary artery spasm, with or without angiographically detectable coronary stenoses (which is typical of patients with variant angina).

Some patients may progress to MI or succumb to SICD soon after the onset or exacerbation of symptoms, or may develop chronic stable angina; the majority, however, become totally asymptomatic (and remain so for months or years). Catastrophic events occur more frequently in patients whose symptoms persist and intensify in spite of medical therapy.

In patients presenting with an unstable pattern of angina, instability of the underlying coronary lesion is suggested by one or more of the following features:

a. recent (within the last few days or weeks but within 2 months at the outside) onset or recent increase in the number of spontaneous attacks, which indicate a tendency to develop a sudden reduction of coronary flow
b. sudden onset of spontaneous attacks of long duration (lasting more than 15–20 min), which indicates a tendency to persistent reduction of CBF
c. sudden reduction of the anginal threshold, which indicates a sudden development or progression of coronary stenoses, attributable to a recently formed coronary thrombosis that has become organized rather than lyzed.

Instability may occur in the following:

a. in patients who previously had a stable pattern of angina or were previously in a quiescent phase of IHD (*destabilizing unstable angina*)

b. in patients who had a recent MI (*postacute myocardial infarction unstable angina*), or

c. in individuals who were previously apparently healthy (*de novo unstable angina*).

The instability may intensify (*crescendo unstable angina*), and may do so in spite of maximal therapy (*refractory unstable angina*), and then subside (*resolving crescendo or resolving refractory unstable angina and probably resolved unstable angina*). It may evolve into MI during crescendo and refractory phases, into chronic stable angina (when incompletely lyzed thrombi cause flow-limiting stenoses), or into a quiescent phase of IHD (see Ch. 19). Destabilizing unstable angina in patients with flow-limiting coronary stenoses should be differentiated from extracardiac causes of instability, which impair the balance between demand and supply, such as anemia, hypoxemia, hyperthyroidism and uncontrolled hypertension.

In patients with angina occurring predominantly at rest, variant angina can be suspected when it occurs at night, in the early morning, or at a fixed time of day, usually but not necessarily with preserved effort tolerance. In this syndrome, angina may occur in clusters of two or more episodes within 30–60 min in the early morning hours, followed by an absence of angina for the rest of the day. The duration of the attacks is variable, seldom lasting more than 10 min; longer episodes tend to be associated with a deteriorating, less stable form of the disease. Palpitations and syncope (related to ischemia-induced arrhythmias) may occur during, or at the very end of attacks. This pattern may occasionally persist for weeks or months, with fluctuations in the number of attacks from one week to another ("good" and "bad" weeks), but sudden exacerbations of symptoms may occur with a clinical pattern indistinguishable from that of unstable angina (see Ch. 20).

16.2 DIAGNOSTIC ASSESSMENT OF TRANSIENT MYOCARDIAL ISCHEMIA

This section presents the general rationale for a stepwise diagnostic process in which there are two closely interrelated stages:

1. Identification of the ischemic or nonischemic origin of the pain on the basis of the following:
    a. the past history of IHD and the clinical presentation
    b. the differential diagnosis
    c. objective documentation.

    In those cases in which angina or angina equivalents are absent and in which the suspicion of ischemic episodes is derived only from transient changes on the ECG, the diagnostic problem becomes the identification of the ischemic or nonischemic nature of these changes.

2. Assessment of the stability or instability of the causes of ischemia on the basis of the following
    a. the clinical presentation, the duration of attacks, and the evolution of symptoms
    b. their prevailing triggering mechanisms, which can be inferred clinically from the comparison of the maximal level of exercise that can be tolerated without ischemia developing (either on good days or after the administration of sublingual nitrates) with the level of activity during which attacks occur.

The importance of obtaining an urgent definite diagnosis depends on the stability or instability of symptoms. It is more important to establish promptly the ischemic or nonischemic nature of a chest pain or type of discomfort that suggests an unstable pattern of ischemic attacks, than it is for one that has remained stable for months. Investigative techniques and tests are usually required in order to confirm the diagnosis and/or to assess the cause of ischemia and the area of myocardium jeopardized by ischemia.

16.2.1 Manifestations of transient myocardial ischemia

A brief summary of the manifestations of myocardial ischemia (see Ch. 7) may assist in the understanding of the rationale behind the available diagnostic criteria.

Ischemia is manifested in the following ways:

a. *directly* by the results of coronary sinus blood sampling, which reveal local tissue acidosis with release of H⁺, mostly in the form of lactate, other ischemic metabolites, and potassium ions, into the coronary venous effluent blood draining the ischemic myocardium
b. *indirectly* by ECG, echocardiography, radionuclide ventriculography, myocardial scintigraphy, or magnetic resonance imaging techniques, which show:
   • the sudden appearance of repolarization changes on the ECG
   • impairment of regional myocardial contractile function
   • a deficit of regional myocardial blood flow
c. *clinically* by:
   • angina pectoris
   • the sudden appearance of signs of acute, transient left ventricular failure or arrhythmias when ischemia is severe (with or without anginal discomfort).

   Myocardial ischemia can remain clinically silent and be detectable only by the techniques reported in (a) and (b) above.

The consequences of myocardial ischemia are determined by its severity, extent, and duration and are largely independent of its actual causes. ECG changes and signs of ventricular failure will be conspicuous either when a major artery is completely occluded by thrombosis or spasm, or when a massive increase in demand occurs in the presence of a proximal coronary artery obstruction that critically limits blood supply to a large part of the ventricular wall. The consequences will be minimal, or even absent, when ischemia caused by stenosis, spasm, or thrombosis of a small branch, or by patchy constriction of distal coronary vessels, involves only a small part of the myocardial wall.

Anginal pain may be very severe during episodes of mild ischemia and, conversely, may be totally absent during severe episodes; however, in the same patient, the severity and duration of pain are usually proportional to the severity and duration of ischemia (see Ch. 14).

16.2.2 Diagnosis of Ischemia

Anginal pain and the other indirect transient manifestations of ischemia may not be entirely specific for ischemia and the sensitivity of tests may be insufficient to detect mild and localized ischemia. As outlined previously, diagnosis of the ischemic or nonischemic nature of the pain (or painless transient ST-segment changes on the ECG suggestive of ischemia) is made on the basis of history, clinical presentation, differential diagnosis (all of which

Table 16.1 General criteria for diagnosing episodes of myocardial ischemia*

1. Typical anginal pain + diagnostic, transient ischemic ECG changes†
2. Typical anginal pain + transient defects of regional myocardial perfusion or contractile function (also in the absence of ECG changes)
3. Typical ischemic ST changes on the ECG + transient defects of regional myocardial perfusion, or contractile function (also in the absence of angina)
4. Very obvious transient abnormalities of regional myocardial perfusion or contractile function (also in the absence of angina and ECG changes).

*Having established the ischemic nature of painful or painless ischemic ECG changes, it is also reasonable to assume an ischemic cause for other episodes occurring in the same patient

†In patients with syndrome X, typical pain and ischemic ECG changes may not be accompanied by a detectable impairment of regional contractile function. It is not clear, however, whether this is due to a patchy distribution of ischemia or to a nonischemic cause of the syndrome (see Ch. 18)

determine the pretest probability of an ischemic cause), and objective documentation (which depends on the posttest probability of an ischemic cause). The simultaneous occurrence of very severe and/or multiple ischemic manifestations, particularly in individuals with a high pretest probability of having IHD, increases the likelihood of an ischemic cause (Table 16.1).

History and clinical presentation

In patients *with an established diagnosis of IHD,* pain or discomfort similar to that experienced in the past during an episode in which myocardial ischemia was objectively documented should be considered ischemic unless proved otherwise, particularly when its pattern is suggestive of unstable angina. The diagnosis is practically certain when it is associated with transient ischemic ECG changes. Additionally, obvious painless transient "ischemic-like" ECG changes during a stress test or ambulatory ECG monitoring should be considered ischemic until proved otherwise.

In patients *without an established diagnosis of IHD,* interpretation of the origin of anginal pain or discomfort (ischemic or nonischemic) is not straightforward. A diagnosis is easier to make when the pain has most of the characteristic features of angina and is recurrent (so that patterns of occurrence and triggering mechanisms can be recognized) and also when it occurs in individuals with risk factors for IHD.

At one extreme, the clinical diagnosis of ischemia and its underlying causes can be nearly certain. Recurrent episodes (with the characteristic qualities described by Heberden)[4] predictably produced by effort and consistently relieved by rest within 1—5 min, are highly suggestive of effort-related myocardial ischemia, particularly in individuals with known risk factors for IHD.

The diagnosis may be more difficult when episodes of pain or discomfort occur in young individuals with no known risk factors, or when such episodes lack some or most of those characteristic qualities described by Heberden. In this case, their relief by rest, when effort induced, and the response to sublingual nitroglycerin within 1—3 min, when spontaneous, become important additional clinical diagnostic elements.

A diagnosis is most difficult when only one attack has occurred, or if attacks occur so rarely that there is no recognizable pattern. In these cases, the quality of the discomfort, the circumstances in which it occurs, and its duration are the only available clues and these should be considered in association with the presence of known risk factors. The likelihood of there being an ischemic origin is greater for pain that has typical features, is severe, lasts from 1 to 10 min (or even for 20 min), and occurs in an individual at high risk of developing IHD; it is quite low for either a sharp pain lasting only a few seconds or a dull pain lasting some hours and unrelieved by nitroglycerin in an individual at low risk of developing IHD; however, although exceptions are very rare, they do occur (see Ch. 14).

In general, the duration of pain is of critical importance: recurrent episodes of pain with a typical location and radiation and lasting for 1–20 min are likely to be ischemic, whereas those lasting longer, but recurring frequently over a period of months and unassociated with reversible or evolving ECG changes, are unlikely to be ischemic. Chronically recurring, long episodes of pain, without evolving ECG changes and often poorly responsive to sublingual nitrates, are frequently observed in patients with syndrome X (see Ch. 18). Gradually worsening attacks of progressively longer duration exceeding 20 min are suggestive of unstable angina.

Differential diagnosis

Other conditions (cardiovascular and noncardiovascular) can be associated with transient anginal discomfort that has all, or only some, of the features described by Heberden.[4] Noncardiac and cardiac/nonischemic causes of anginal discomfort can occur not only in patients with normal coronary arteriograms, but also in those with coronary stenoses. The consistent association of pain with transient ST-segment/T-wave (ST–T) changes indicates a cardiac and most likely an ischemic cause (see below).

Other cardiovascular causes of anginal pain. Chronically recurring angina pectoris is a frequent presenting symptom in severe aortic stenosis. Physical signs will differentiate it from ischemia related to coronary stenoses and a correct diagnosis is essential, as patients are at risk of dying and require prompt valve surgery. Chronic angina is also common in patients with hypertrophic cardiomyopathy and, here again, the physical signs will differentiate it. Angina can occasionally occur in patients with congestive cardiomyopathy and with other types of valvular disease, systemic or pulmonary hypertension, and mitral valve prolapse. Among all these conditions, an ischemic origin of anginal pain is very likely in severe aortic stenosis when pain is caused by effort and relieved by rest, it is possible in hypertrophic cardiomyopathy, and it is uncertain in the other conditions, as it may or may not be attributable to mechanisms similar to those causing anginal pain in syndrome X. Although these causes of anginal pain are typically chronic and stable, they should be differentiated from unstable angina when pain presents for the first time. The diagnosis is often made by observing the evolution of symptoms.

Pericardial pain, which is typically sharp in nature, changes with respiration and posture, and is often associated with a friction rub and fever, should be differentiated from unstable recent-onset spontaneous angina. Echocardiography can identify pericardial fluid (as opposed to a localized area of dyskinesia attributable to regional ischemia). Aortic dissection is also an important differential diagnosis, with sudden-onset unstable angina. The possibility of aortic dissection should be considered when the pain is maximal at its very onset, rather than building up gradually, and is associated with features of Marfan syndrome, a history of hypertension, asymmetry of brachial pulses, the appearance of a diastolic murmur, and the normality of the ECG during pain (however, ECG changes typical of infarction may coexist when the origin of the coronary arteries is also involved in the dissection). A diagnosis of aortic dissection can be confirmed by chest radiography, transesophageal echocardiography and single photon emission computed tomography (SPECT).

When the pain is severe and associated with obvious signs of general distress it should never be disregarded, even if the ECG is nondiagnostic, and the patient should be kept under close surveillance. Sharp, stabbing, or pleuritic qualities do not exclude completely an ischemic etiology. In the Multicenter Chest Pain study, acute ischemia was diagnosed in 22% of patients presenting to the emergency department with sharp or stabbing pain and in 13% of patients with some pleuritic qualities accompanying the pain. Furthermore, 7% of patients whose pain was fully reproduced by palpation were ultimately recognized to have acute IHD (see Ch. 14).[5]

Noncardiovascular causes of chest pain. *Anxiety states.* These are thought to be the most common cause of atypical, nonischemic chest pain but they may contribute to an enhanced perception of pain, for example in patients with syndrome X (see Ch. 18). The pain may be stabbing or like a piercing needle, lasting a few seconds (in some very rare cases, this symptom is caused by a single extrasystole, usually ventricular, which can be demonstrated by continuous ECG recording), or aching, lasting for hours. The very short duration of pain in the first case, the usually long duration in the second, together with its association with other signs of anxiety (such as palpitations, hyperventilation, claustrophobia, and obsession with the idea of having a serious heart disease) make an ischemic origin unlikely.

Esophageal spasm. Patients with esophageal spasm can experience attacks of pain that are retrosternal, that radiate to the back, arms, and jaw, and that are similar in nature to those caused by myocardial ischemia. The pain may also be dull, or sharp and squeezing. Esophageal spasm is common in middle age; it can be caused by diverticuli and is relieved by nitroglycerin. It may occur with the ingestion of cold drinks, at night, or during anxiety and emotion and it may be precipitated by effort; it may be relieved by a few sips of water. As ischemia and esophageal spasm can coexist, a diagnosis is possible if ECG recordings show no transient ischemic changes and if radiologic and manometric studies of the esophagus are obtained during a painful attack (see Ch. 18).

Hiatus hernia and reflux esophagitis. Reflux esophagitis is caused by failure of the lower esophageal sphincter to prevent regurgitation of gastric secretion. It causes a retrosternal burning sensation, is usually long-lasting, is related to meals and posture, is associated with acid regurgitation, and is relieved by antacids. It can be associated with anxiety states and the diagnosis is confirmed by a barium swallow.

Musculoskeletal pain. This is usually chronic, superficial, long-lasting, dull, and provoked or accentuated by movements or by local pressure.

Thoracic outlet syndrome. Neural or vascular compression at the outlet of the chest, usually by a cervical rib, can cause pain in the neck, shoulder, arm, scapula, axilla, and even in the anterior chest wall, sometimes with paresthesia. The pain is chronic, long-lasting and related to posture. Clinical examination and chest radiography provide the diagnosis.

Self gain. Some patients try to mislead their physician for insurance purposes or financial benefit, or when attention seeking. In this case the definite exclusion of ischemia by ECG recordings and other investigative techniques is necessary.

The demonstration of any of these possible causes in a patient under consideration does not exclude the coexistence of an ischemic or cardiac origin of the pain, which must be disproved, rather than excluded, because of the possibility of a noncardiac culprit. Reassurance may be useful for patients with chronic symptoms and good effort tolerance, but should not be adopted for patients with recent onset of symptoms who may have unstable angina.

Objective diagnosis of ischemic episodes

An objective diagnosis of ischemia can be obtained by transient changes of the ST segment on the ECG, global or regional ventricular function, and by reversible myocardial scintigraphy perfusion defects during pain. The detection of coronary atherosclerotic obstructions makes an ischemic origin of pain more likely, but transient myocardial ischemia and even MI can occur independently of coronary artery obstructions; conversely, coronary artery obstructions may not necessarily cause ischemia (see Ch. 9).

In the Coronary Artery Surgery Study, of over 16 000 patients who were subjected to coronary arteriography for angina, 28.3% had normal or minimally diseased coronary arteries.[6] Among women the percentage was as high as 50%.[2,3] In those patients with no detectable coronary artery stenoses, angina could have been caused either by nonischemic mechanisms or by myocardial ischemia resulting from epicardial coronary artery spasm or small vessel coronary alterations, such as those responsible for microvascular angina.

The objective demonstration of the presence of acute myocardial ischemia during an attack of chest pain or discomfort (spontaneous or induced) is the first essential step in the diagnostic assessment. When myocardial ischemia is severe and extensive, it can be detected clinically by the appearance of a third or fourth heart sound, or by mitral regurgitation caused by papillary muscle ischemia, and also by most diagnostic techniques. When ischemia is mild and limited, the sensitivity of the diagnostic tests available may not be sufficient to provide a conclusive diagnosis.

As indicated above, myocardial ischemia can be detected indirectly from its electrical effects on the ST–T segment of the ECG, from its mechanical effects on regional and global contractile function, and from differences in regional myocardial deposition or washout of radioactive flow tracers.

In the catheterization laboratory, myocardial ischemia can be detected directly from markers of ischemia such as the release of lactate, hydrogen, and potassium ions and adenosine or adenosine degradation products into the vein draining the ischemic myocardium (but the sensitivity of the technique may be very low when the reduced blood flow draining the ischemic territory is diluted by the normal or increased blood flow draining the normal myocardium).

As the diagnostic sensitivity and specificity of any currently available technique for detecting ischemia are not 100%, interpretation of the results depends on the magnitude of the alteration, the presence of other clinical signs of ischemia, and the pretest probability that the patient suffers from myocardial ischemia (as indicated by past history, symptoms, and risk factors for IHD).

The Bayesian Theory states that the diagnostic or predictive value of a test (or symptoms) decreases as the prevalence of the disease (or events) diminishes in the group of individuals submitted to the test: in any group of individuals tested, the lower the probability of IHD the lower the diagnostic specificity or prognostic accuracy of any test (see Fig. 16.2 and Table 16.2).[7] The specificity of tests increases when the diagnostic criteria adopted are very stringent, but the more stringent the criteria, the lower the sensitivity of the tests.

The diagnosis of transient myocardial ischemia can be considered certain (100% specificity) when the transient changes are very obvious and are associated with the patient's usual anginal discomfort or with simultaneous changes detected by other independent techniques. However, this conclusion may not be applicable for those patients with microvascular angina who, during exercise or dipyridamole testing, present their typical pain and typical transient ischemic ST-segment depression on the ECG, in the absence of detectable changes of regional myocardial contractile function (see Ch. 18).

The diagnosis is probable when the changes are not very obvious but occur in patients with previously documented IHD or in those having a high degree of pretest probability of IHD.

A negative result may still be compatible with ischemia, albeit of an extent insufficient to cause detectable alterations, as none of the available diagnostic techniques has a sensitivity of 100%.

The application of all diagnostic techniques requires an episode of pain or transient ischemic-like ST-segment changes on the ECG, either spontaneous or induced; when the diagnosis of IHD is uncertain, anti-ischemic therapy should be withdrawn before the test.

When the history reveals that anginal pain is induced by effort and relieved by rest, an exercise stress test is the first logical step. It is more likely to be positive if performed under the conditions that are most often associated with the pain, for example after meals or with an abrupt onset of effort. The diagnosis of myocardial ischemia can be established when the exercise test reproduces the usual discomfort or painless ischemic-like ST-segment changes on the ECG, together with changes in global or regional ventricular contractile function or a reduced regional uptake or washout of a radioactive flow tracer. The absence of diagnostic changes does not rule out the presence of coronary artery stenoses that either are not severe enough to limit the increase of myocardial blood flow or are sufficiently well compensated for by collaterals. Furthermore, the absence of diagnostic changes does not exclude the presence of myocardial ischemia that is not sufficiently severe and/or extensive to be detected by the techniques used. However, in the latter case a negative maximal exercise test indicates that the patient's coronary flow reserve is sufficient to permit the attainment of the cardiac work load achieved at peak exercise, without producing detectable ischemia (see below).

When anginal attacks occur only at rest and the patient reports a preserved effort tolerance, an exercise stress test is still indicated in order to investigate the possible presence of a reduced coronary flow reserve or of effort-induced coronary artery spasm; however, when the test is negative, attempts should be made to obtain an ECG during an anginal attack. Continuous recording of the ECG is appropriate when attacks occur every day or several

---

Table 16.2 Definitions of the terminology commonly applied to diagnostic tests

Predictive value of a positive test	=	$\dfrac{\text{Number of patients with disease}}{\text{Total number of patients with a positive test}}$
Predictive value of a negative test	=	$\dfrac{\text{Number of subjects without disease}}{\text{Total number of subjects with a negative test}}$
Sensitivity	=	$\dfrac{\text{Number of patients with disease with a positive test}}{\text{Total number of patients with disease tested}}$
Specificity	=	$\dfrac{\text{Number of disease-free subjects with a negative test}}{\text{Total number of disease-free subjects tested}}$
Pretest likelihood	=	$\dfrac{\text{Number of patients with disease in the test population}}{\text{Total number of patients in the test population}}$
Posttest likelihood	=	$\dfrac{\text{Number of patients with disease showing a given test result}}{\text{Total number of subjects showing the test result}}$

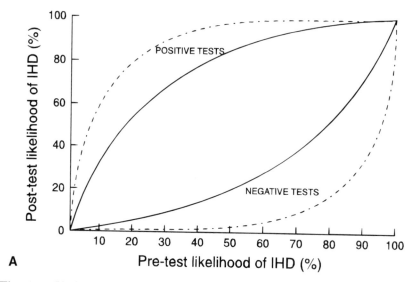

Fig. 16.2 Variable value of noninvasive tests for predicting flow-limiting stenoses according to the Bayesian theory. The predictive value of tests increases progressively with the likelihood that a patient has the disease (pretest probability). For a given pretest probability, the predictive value of a test depends on its sensitivity (percentage of positive results among patients with the disease) and its specificity (percentage of negative results among patients without the disease). The sensitivity and specificity values should be derived from a sample of patients representative of the general population.

(**A**) The posttest likelihood of a patient having the disease, using a test with 95% sensitivity and 95% specificity, is defined by the dotted lines: a positive test will correctly predict the presence of a coronary artery stenosis (a true positive test) in practically all patients with an 80% pretest probability of having the disease, but will also incorrectly predict the presence of a stenosis (a false positive test) in about 20% of patients with a 20% pretest probability of the disease. A negative test will correctly predict the absence of stenoses in nearly all patients with a 20% pretest probability of having stenoses (a true negative test), but will also incorrectly predict the absence of the disease (a false negative test) in about 30% of patients with a 90% pretest probability of the disease.

For comparison, the posttest likelihood of a patient having the disease, using a positive or negative test with 75% sensitivity and 85% specificity, is indicated by the continuous lines: such a test is nearly as good as one having 95% sensitivity and 95% specificity for predicting correctly both the presence of the disease in patients with a very high pretest probability and its absence in patients with a very low pretest probability. However, it produces many more false positive and false negative results in patients with an intermediate pretest probability of having the disease. *(Figure continues.)*

times a week; when attacks occur very rarely, and when a maximal effort test is clearly negative, provocative tests for variant angina should be performed if considered useful for the patient's management (see Ch. 20).

■ *The establishment of a definite diagnosis becomes imperative when there is the possibility that the ischemic syndrome may be unstable, or when the pain and anxiety impair the patient's lifestyle. In some difficult cases, however, a definite ischemic or nonischemic cause of chest pain cannot be identified by even the most extensive series of currently available diagnostic tests and only its evolution during the follow-up period may clarify the cause of pain.* ■

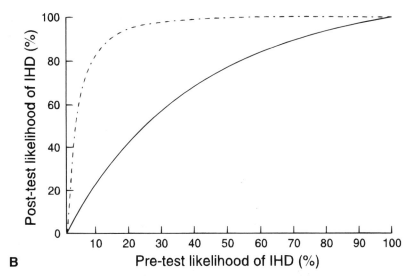

B

Fig. 16.2 *(Continued)* (**B**) Increasing the specificity of the test (e.g., by adopting stricter diagnostic criteria such as 3 mm ST-segment depression during exercise testing as opposed to 1 mm) will reduce the number of false positive results. This will increase the predictive value of a positive test for the presence of the disease, in particular in patients with a low pretest probability of the disease, as indicated by the dotted line compared to the continuous line. The increase in specificity, however, will be associated with an increase in the number of false negative results, thus decreasing both the sensitivity and the predictive value of a negative test for the absence of the disease. (Modified from ref. 7.)

The principles derived from the Bayesian theory apply also to any diagnostic approach or test designed to assess prognosis. In both cases, its positive predictive value in patients with a good prognosis is low.

16.2.3 Assessing the causes and severity of transient ischemic attacks

Besides establishing that the patient suffers from attacks of transient myocardial ischemia, it is necessary to ascertain whether the patient has a chronic stable pattern of angina or an unstable pattern, to assess the triggering mechanisms of the attacks, and to assess the area of myocardium jeopardized by ischemia.

Diagnosis of stable/unstable patterns of angina

A fairly wide range of frequency of attacks, severity of angina, and signs of transient myocardial ischemia can be observed in patients with stable and unstable angina. Once an ischemic nature is established, the diagnosis of stability or instability is clinical, but is made difficult by the fact that the location and radiation of anginal pain are the same, irrespective of the cause of ischemia.

The diagnosis of a stable pattern of angina can be made easily for patients in whom effort tolerance, the number of attacks per week, and their severity and duration have remained unchanged for months or years. The diagnosis of unstable angina can also be made easily for patients in whom anginal attacks have appeared during the last few days or weeks and have become more frequent, severe, and long-lasting (in the absence of extracoronary causes, affecting the myocardial demand/supply balance).

The diagnosis is not straightforward in a patient with known IHD who was in a quiescent, asymptomatic phase until a recent isolated attack, and it is even more difficult in a patient with no history of IHD and who has had a single, but typical, anginal attack during the last few days or weeks; in both cases, until reliable objective markers of instability become available, only the short-term evolution will allow the diagnosis to be confirmed (see below).

Triggering mechanisms of transient myocardial ischemia

In patients with either stable or unstable angina, the imbalance between myocardial oxygen consumption (demand) and CBF (supply) can be triggered by three distinct mechanisms (see Fig. 16.3):

1. The first mechanism is a fixed reduction of coronary flow reserve (due to an epicardial coronary artery obstruction that developed either very gradually over a period of months or years, or suddenly as a result of an incompletely lysed coronary thrombosis) and an excessive increase of myocardial demand.
2. Another mechanism involves the transient sudden reduction of CBF below resting levels, caused by coronary vasoconstriction (at the site of a stenosis or in distal vessels), by fresh intraluminal thrombosis, or by a combination of the two.
3. The third mechanism is the combination of a coincidental subliminal increase in demand and a transient subliminal reduction of coronary flow reserve (by one of the mechanisms outlined above), each insufficient in itself to cause ischemia.

The reduction of coronary flow reserve may jeopardize areas of myocardium of very variable size and, hence, has a variable prognostic significance (the reduction of coronary flow reserve can be assessed from the limitation of effort tolerance and from exercise stress testing—see below).

The mechanisms that modulate coronary flow reserve or cause a reduced blood supply below resting levels are stable in chronic stable angina (dynamic vasoconstriction of stable stenoses, lack of adequate dilation or constriction of distal coronary vessels) and unstable in unstable angina (mural thrombosis with or without coronary constriction or occlusive coronary artery spasm). When the reduction of baseline coronary flow reserve (in the absence of any dynamic modulation) is not severe, mechanisms (2) and (3) above can be recognized from the history and the clinical diagnosis can then be substantiated by investigative techniques (see below).

Area of myocardium jeopardized by ischemia

As indicated above, for any given reduction of coronary flow reserve the area of myocardium jeopardized by ischemia may vary, with consequent important prognostic implications. In patients with a previous MI and reduced contractile reserve, even a small area of myocardium at risk may be critical. A critical extension of the area at risk is indicated by the following:

a. the appearance of a third or fourth heart sound, mitral regurgitation, or dyspnea during ischemia
b. the failure of systolic pressure to increase, or the development of hypotension during the test

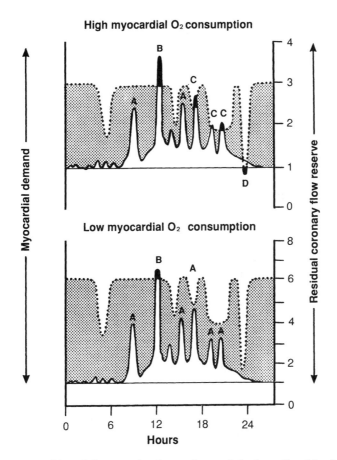

Fig. 16.3 Effect of basal flow on the dynamic modulation of residual coronary flow reserve and ischemic threshold. In the scheme depicted in the upper panel, basal flow during 24 h is double that depicted in the lower panel because of a higher basal MVO_2. The maximal residual coronary flow allowed by the most critical stenosis is the same in both the upper and lower panels but, in the upper panel, flow can increase only 3 times above baseline, as against 6 times in the lower panel. For a similar increase in myocardial demand (white area, points A) and a similar reduction of coronary flow reserve (stipled area), ischemia is less likely to occur (points C and D) when basal flow is low. The increase in MVO_2 may be insufficient to cause ischemia (A) because it does not exceed maximal residual coronary flow reserve. Myocardial demand may exceed maximal residual coronary flow reserve (B) but ischemia is more severe when basal MVO_2 is high. Basal flow can be reduced by decreasing MVO_2 and by correcting anemia and hypoxemia when present. The dynamic modulation of residual coronary flow reserve can be eliminated by preventing dynamic stenoses and inappropriate microvascular constriction. Maximal residual coronary flow can be increased by collateral development or by revascularization procedures.

c. the severity of ST-segment shifts and the number of leads in which ischemic changes develop

d. the extension of the deficit in myocardial perfusion (and the uptake of thallium by the lungs) revealed by scintigraphy

e. the severity of impairment of ventricular contractile function detected by angiography, echocardiography, and radionuclide ventriculography.

The area of myocardium at risk is largely determined by the proximal or distal location of a coronary stenosis in a major coronary artery; however, in view of the variable relation between coronary occlusion, myocardial necrosis and malignant arrhythmias (see Ch. 10), it is impossible not only to establish whether the whole area of myocardium distal to the stenosis will become ischemic but also to assess the probability of an irreversible ischemic event taking place.

16.2.4 Role of investigative techniques and provocative tests

Traditionally, in patients without anginal pain, the most relevant diagnostic problem has been considered to be the detection of flow-limiting coronary stenoses, in view of their possible therapeutic and prognostic implications. Thus, the presence or absence of flow-limiting coronary stenoses became the yardstick by which the specificity and sensitivity of non-invasive tests, developed to detect myocardial ischemia, were judged.

This traditional view should now be reconsidered because although, in general, prognosis is influenced by the number of stenosed coronary arteries, the correlation is fairly weak as prognosis is also influenced strongly by ventricular function and by the stability and instability of angina. On the one hand, stable patients with triple-vessel disease but a normal resting ECG, normal ventricular function, and normal effort tolerance have a 98% 5-year survival (see Chs 13 and 17). On the other hand, the infarct-related artery cannot be identified from the retrospective analysis of preinfarction coronary arteriograms as the occlusion often develops at the site of minor or mild stenoses, whereas other severe stenoses may remain unchanged (see Chs 8 and 9).

The selection of investigative techniques and provocative tests should, therefore, be dictated by the need to answer specific questions relevant to the management of the patient under consideration, rather than just by the wish to detect flow-limiting coronary stenoses. As discussed above, these questions concern the diagnosis of myocardial ischemia, the stable or unstable cause of ischemic episodes, the residual coronary flow reserve, and the extent of myocardium jeopardized by ischemia.

Investigative techniques can be applied during ischemic episodes occurring either spontaneously or induced by provocative tests. Arteriography can demonstrate the site and severity of organic and functional coronary abnormalities.

Spontaneously occurring ischemic episodes

The main questions about anginal episodes occurring spontaneously concern their ischemic origin, when the diagnosis is uncertain, and the severity, extent, and cause of ischemia, when their ischemic origin is already established. As discussed above, a 12-lead ECG is the most commonly available means of establishing the presence of transient ischemic changes for anginal episodes occurring in either the physician's office or in hospital. Cross-sectional echocardiography, when promptly available in the physician's office, in the emergency room, or in the coronary care unit (CCU), can be a very useful additional technique in uncertain cases. The availability of nuclear medicine techniques during spontaneous episodes is exceptional in clinical practise. Continuous ECG monitoring is required for episodes occurring out of hospital during ordinary daily life.

12-lead ECG. Transient changes of the ST segment or T waves recorded during an episode of anginal discomfort, which disappear together with the discomfort, are diagnostic of ischemia (with the possible exception of patients with syndrome X; see Ch. 18). The 12-lead ECG may be negative when ischemia is confined either to the dorsal part of the left ventricle (in which case changes may be seen only in leads V_8 and V_9 placed on the back of the chest) or to the right ventricle (in which case transient right ventricular dysfunction may be the only detectable abnormality[8]). The severity, extent and location of ischemia can be judged, with rather limited accuracy, from the degree of the ST-segment shift and the leads involved (see below).

Cross-sectional echocardiography. The prompt availability of an echocardiographic machine and an expert operator can usually provide the diagnosis, when the ECG is negative during typical pain or during painless ischemic ECG changes or when the question becomes the definition of the extent and location of ischemia.

Continuous ECG recording. Continuous recording of the ECG can be applied to patients admitted to a CCU or to ambulant patients (i.e. Holter monitoring). Continuous ECG recordings have the following advantages:

a. they can provide diagnostic information on the ischemic or nonischemic origin of chest pain when the leads monitored explore the ventricular wall that becomes ischemic
b. they can detect ischemic episodes without pain
c. they can establish whether ischemic episodes are caused predominantly by increased myocardial demand or by a reduced CBF.

Monitoring two leads, one inferior, the other anterior, at the apex detects over 95% of ischemic changes recorded by 12 leads during exercise stress testing.[9]

Excessive myocardial oxygen consumption can be assumed to be the prevailing cause of ischemia when all episodes occur at levels of heart rate (within 10–20 beats) similar to that observed during episodes of spontaneous tachycardia or at the onset of ischemia during exercise stress testing.

Significant dynamic modulation of residual coronary flow reserve should be suspected when ischemic episodes begin at a value of heart rate 20 or more beats lower than that observed at the onset of ischemia during the exercise test, or lower than episodes of tachycardia lasting more than 10 min and not associated with any signs of ischemia; however, a dynamic modulation may have a contributory role also when the differences in heart rate are less.

In some patients the cause of the transient impairment of coronary blood supply can be inferred from the direction of the ST-segment shift (depression or elevation). Transient elevation of the ST segment, associated with a clinical pattern of attacks consistent with variant angina and promptly relieved by nitroglycerin, is practically diagnostic of coronary artery spasm. However, transient ST-segment elevation can also be caused by dynamic thrombosis, with or without associated local coronary constriction. Episodes of transient ST-segment depression can be caused by increased demand, by increases in coronary vasomotor tone, or by dynamic incomplete thrombosis; they can also occur in variant angina. Only the pattern of the attacks and their evolution can provide clues to causal mechanisms.

Continuous ECG monitoring can provide useful information in patients with the following conditions:

a. unstable angina, in which continuous monitoring can assess the waxing and waning of instability, which has important implications on prognosis and management (see Ch. 19)
b. predominantly rest angina and a negative exercise stress test, in whom it may allow an objective diagnosis of ischemia to be made
c. chronic stable angina, in whom it may allow the objective assessment of the frequency of ischemia during ordinary daily life and its prevalent cause (increased demand or reduced supply) (see Chs 17, 19, and 20).

Provocative tests

In patients without spontaneous episodes or with infrequent episodes, provocative tests can be useful for the diagnosis of ischemia and for the assessment of residual coronary flow reserve, the location and extent of myocardium jeopardized by flow-limiting stenoses, and the actual mechanisms of ischemia. The information provided on these four aspects by commonly used tests and techniques varies considerably.

Diagnosis of myocardial ischemia. For patients in whom the diagnosis of ischemia remains uncertain, provocative tests should be performed while the patient is not receiving anti-ischemic therapy, in an attempt to maximize the probability that ischemia may develop during the test.

For patients presenting with effort-induced angina, the test of first choice should be the exercise test, which should be maximal and, whenever possible, performed under conditions similar to those most commonly producing the anginal discomfort during daily life (for example in the morning, after a meal, or in the cold). When the test reproduces the usual discomfort and is associated with diagnostic changes on the ECG or myocardial scintigram or during ventricular wall motion studies, a diagnosis of ischemia can be established. A negative maximal exercise stress test is compatible with a nonischemic cause, with ischemic attacks being caused by transient reduction of CBF (which did not occur during the test), or with inadequate sensitivity of the technique used to detect the ischemia. A good exercise tolerance carries an excellent prognosis, even when the results are uncertain. Exercising for longer than 6 min on the Bruce protocol carries an excellent long-term prognosis also in patients with known IHD, even when the test is positive (see Fig. 17.6). For patients in whom a maximal exercise test is negative, provocative tests of coronary spasm may be indicated when variant angina is clinically suspected (see Ch. 20).

For patients who cannot exercise, and for those with a negative but submaximal test, flow-limiting coronary stenoses can be detected by selective coronary vasodilators such as dipyridamole or adenosine, or by inotropic drugs that increase myocardial oxygen consumption, such as dobutamine. The dipyridamole test (0.5 mg/kg intravenously in 4 min, with an additional dose of 0.3 mg/kg in 4 min when negative) is diagnostic when it causes transient regional wall motion dysfunction[10] on a two-dimensional echocardiogram, or when it causes regional differences in the deposition of myocardial flow tracers.[11] Infusion of dobutamine during echocardiographic monitoring can also be used in order to induce ischemia by increasing myocardial oxygen consumption.[12]

According to the Bayesian theory, the possibility of false positive tests increases progressively when the pretest probability of the disease is low. In patients at low risk, therefore, only strongly positive tests carry relevant prognostic implications. In patients with known IHD, the major prognostic determinant is represented by the extent of left ventricular dysfunction, which becomes a multiplier of the risk conferred by the areas of myocardium jeopardized by flow-limiting stenoses and by malignant arrhythmias.

As discussed above, neither the sensitivity nor the specificity of tests for detecting myocardial ischemia can be defined precisely, for a number of reasons. First, the response to tests is considered in terms of positivity and negativity, rather than in terms of the extent of the abnormality; second, when considered in term of positivity and negativity according to arbitrary cut-off points, their predictive accuracy depends on the prevalence of IHD in the group of patients studied;[7] third, the reference standard currently used is the presence of coronary flow-limiting stenoses at angiography. This reference standard is not ideal, either when the challenging stimulus is insufficient to cause ischemia in the presence of a coronary artery stenosis (false negative for the detection of the stenosis, but correctly negative for failing to detect ischemia) or when ischemia is caused by coronary artery spasm or by small vessel coronary constriction in the absence of a coronary artery stenosis (false positive for the detection of coronary stenoses, but correctly positive for detecting myocardial ischemia). In the presence of a previous MI and ventricular dysfunction, the sensitivity and specificity of tests to detect ischemia is also not clearly known (although, by definition, the patients must have IHD) and the extent of the abnormality carries a much greater importance than just the positivity of the test. Indeed, when the alterations caused by ischemia are not obvious, the results of noninvasive tests may conflict. For example, a positive myocardial scintigram and ventricular wall motion studies may identify different segments at risk, or a positive myocardial scintigram during exercise testing may be associated with an increased left ventricular ejection fraction (EF).

During exercise stress testing, the diagnostic accuracy of the 12-lead ECG for detecting coronary artery stenoses is, on average, inferior to SPECT or myocardial scintigraphic and echocardiographic studies.[13–17] A more meaningful comparison of these techniques with the results of ECG exercise stress testing for use in clinical practise would require the group of patients in whom these differences are observed to be precisely defined; for example, patients with a normal resting ECG and a negative maximal ECG exercise stress test should be separated from those with a negative test at low or high work loads in the presence of an abnormal resting ECG; similarly, patients with a previous MI should be separated from those without.

Prospective randomized trials on the effects of more accurate diagnostic tests, on patient management, and on long-term survival and event-free survival are desirable.[17,18]

Causes of myocardial ischemia. In patients with documented ischemia, provocative tests can provide information on the prevailing mechanisms of ischemia, but not on the stability or instability of the actual causes of ischemia, which can best be assessed clinically (see above).

In patients with rest angina and preserved effort tolerance, episodes of transient ST-segment elevation on a Holter recording are diagnostic of variant angina. In patients with chronic stable angina, in order to establish whether angina during daily life is caused predominantly by increased myocardial demand, it is useful to enquire how the level of effort associated with the development of ischemia during the effort test compares with the patient's normal level of effort and with that associated with the development of angina during daily activities.

For patients who state that they never perform exercise as strenuous as that performed during the test, and in whom the test was nevertheless negative for ischemia, it is reasonable to assume that they have a coronary flow reserve sufficient for the requirements of their daily lives and that the anginal attacks are caused by a transient impairment of coronary blood supply. This conclusion may be documented by Holter monitoring (see above). Conversely, if the intensity of the effort performed during the test was similar to that usually performed during ordinary daily life, and the test was clearly positive for ischemia, the patient's residual coronary flow reserve is obviously insufficient. In daily life, ischemic attacks, occurring during effort comparable to that attained during the exercise test, are most likely to be caused only by increased myocardial oxygen consumption; attacks occurring on much lesser effort, or spontaneously, are most likely to be caused by transient impairment of myocardial blood flow. This distinction becomes difficult to make (and also rather academic) for those patients with a very reduced coronary flow reserve and a very low ischemic threshold.

Reduction of exercise tolerance following sublingual nitrates, in the absence of a marked fall in arterial blood pressure, is suggestive of microvascular angina (see Ch. 18).

Assessment of residual coronary flow reserve. In patients with documented ischemia, residual coronary flow reserve limited by organic coronary stenoses is best assessed objectively by exercise stress testing performed after the administration of sublingual nitrates (in order to minimize a dynamic component related to dynamic stenosis or to small vessel coronary constriction; see Ch. 17). This information helps not only in the establishment of the level of maximal effort that each patient can sustain during normal daily activities without ischemia, in the absence of superimposed functional components transiently interfering with coronary blood supply, but also in the selection of the first line of therapy. When assessing residual coronary flow reserve, the test should be interrupted as soon as myocardial ischemia becomes detectable from ECG changes or from the appearance of anginal pain. The prognostic value of maximal residual coronary flow reserve requires the definition of the extent of the myocardium jeopardized by flow-limiting stenoses.

Extent of myocardium jeopardized by ischemia. In patients with documented ischemia, its location and extension in the ventricular wall are best assessed by regional wall motion or myocardial perfusion studies. The degree of ischemia induced by the test must be severe in order to increase the possibility of accurate detection.

The ability of imaging techniques to identify correctly the location and extent of myocardial ischemia depends on their spatial resolution, on the severity and extent of ischemia, and on the presence of resting alterations. Precise detection is easy when the geometric resolution of the technique used is high (for example in magnetic resonance imaging), when ischemia is transmural and extensive, and when resting myocardial perfusion and ventricular wall motion are normal. It is difficult when the resolution of the technique is low (for example in planar thallium-201 scintigraphy or echocardiography with a bad thoracic window) and when ischemia is subendocardial, has a limited extent, and occurs in the presence of a previous MI. SPECT, myocardial scintigraphy and cross-sectional echocardiography appear to provide similar results in the hands of equally experienced operators.[13–16]

A critical extension of myocardial ischemia can be inferred indirectly from transient impairment of global ventricular function detected clinically, from thallium-201 accumulation in the lungs, or from a marked increase in residual end-systolic volume and a decrease in left ventricular EF detected by radionuclide ventriculography or echocardiography.

A large segment of the left ventricle jeopardized by ischemia, and the precipitation of severe global ventricular dysfunction at low work loads in patients with a previous MI, are absolute indications for coronary arteriography with a view to coronary revascularization procedures.

Coronary arteriography

The traditional indication for coronary arteriography is the detection of flow-limiting stenoses, but coronary arteriography can also have a diagnostic role in patients with functional causes of myocardial ischemia. It can demonstrate the site and extent of coronary artery spasm, the absence of stenoses that could account for the presence of effort-induced ischemia (and hence can suggest the diagnosis of microvascular angina) and the presence of fresh thrombus (and hence can indicate an unstable coronary lesion).

The indications for the test are strongly influenced by local practise. At one extreme, absolute indications for coronary arteriography are the inability of medical therapy to prevent ischemic episodes, evidence of a large segment of the left ventricle jeopardized by ischemia, or ischemia occurring at low workloads in patients with impaired ventricular function. In these patients, the site of stenoses detected by arteriography defines the area of myocardium at risk and provides the information necessary for the choice between bypass surgery or percutaneous transluminal coronary angioplasty. At the other extreme, there appear to be no indications for coronary arteriography in stable patients with good effort tolerance (more than 6 min on the Bruce protocol), as they have such a good prognosis that the possible improvement of prognosis by revascularization procedures is difficult to demonstrate. The absence of any indications, therefore, is even more obvious for patients without known IHD, with a normal resting ECG and in whom a maximal ECG exercise stress test is either nondiagnostic or negative.

Growing evidence suggests that the prognostic implications of flow-limiting coronary stenoses in patients with normal ventricular function have decreased over the years because the indications for arteriography have widened, leading to the study of a larger number of patients with less severe forms of IHD (see Fig. 16.4).[19,20] As is implied by the Bayesian theory, the inclusion of a large number of low-risk patients has led to a decrease in the prognostic specificity of coronary angiographic findings. In addition, studies in which coronary arteriography was performed systematically in patients receiving thrombolytic therapy for acute MI (e.g. the GUSTO trial)[21] or in patients with unstable angina (e.g. the TIMI IIIB trial)[22] show a low prevalence of patients with triple-vessel disease (14 and 15%, respectively). Conversely, patients who have had uncomplicated chronic stable angina for several years may have nearly twice as many flow-limiting stenoses and occlusions as patients presenting with an unheralded MI.[23]

In 1990 it was proposed that "to be considered appropriate, the procedure (coronary arteriography) had to have been performed for an indication that a panel of experts concluded was acceptable,"[24] but an obvious clue that the indications for the procedure are too broad is provided by the number of studies performed that provide no indications for revascularization procedures or that have normal results.

These uncertainties leave ample space for individual judgment based on the arguments presented in the previous paragraphs and on the physician's perception of the patient's attitude towards the disease.

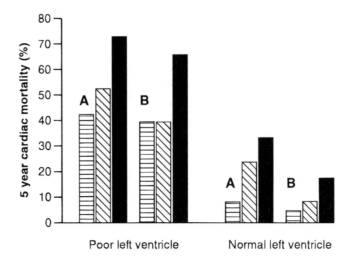

Fig. 16.4 Variable prognostic value of coronary arteriography. In patients with poor left ventricular function (poor left ventricle) the 5-year mortality rate was similar in both the Cleveland Clinic series, published in 1969 (groups A), and the CASS study, published in 1982 (groups B). In contrast, in patients with preserved left ventricular function (normal left ventricle) and only mild symptoms, mortality was about 50% lower in the CASS study. (▤ one-vessel disease; ▨, two-vessel disease; ■, three-vessel disease.) Thus, in patients with poor ventricular function, prognosis did not change over the years as it was determined mainly by left ventricular dysfunction, but in those with preserved ventricular function, the prognostic value of arteriography decreased substantially, most likely because of the inclusion of less severely symptomatic patients. (From data presented in refs 19 and 20.)

REFERENCES

1. Maseri A, Chierchia S, Kaski JC. Mixed angina pectoris. Am J Cardiol 1985;56:30E.
2. Welch CC, Proudfit WC, Sheldon WC. Coronary arteriographic findings in 1000 women under age 50. Am J Cardiol 1975;35:211.
3. King SB, Douglas JS. Coronary arteriography and left ventriculography. In: Hurst JW, Logan RB, Jeffert RC, Wengen NR (eds) The Heart. 4th edition. New York: McGraw-Hill, 1978, p. 397.
4. Heberden W. Some account of a disorder of the breast. Med Trans 1772;2:59.
5. Lee TH, Juarez G, Cook EF et al. Ruling out acute myocardial infarction. A prospective multicenter validation of a 12-hour strategy for patients at low risk. N Engl J Med 1991;324:1239.
6. Kemp H, Kronmal R, Vliestra R, Frye R et al. Seven year survival of patients with normal or near normal coronary arteriograms: a CASS registry study. J Am Coll Cardiol 1986;7:479.
7. Epstein SE. Implications of probability analysis on the strategy used for non invasive detection of coronary artery disease. Role of single or combined use of exercise electrocardiographic testing, radionuclide cineangiography and myocardial perfusion imaging. Am J Cardiol 1980;46:491.
8. Parodi O, Marzullo P, Neglia D et al. Transient predominant right ventricular ischemia caused by coronary vasospasm. Circulation 1984;70:170.
9. Lanza GA, Mascellanti M, Placentino M, Lucente M, Crea F, Maseri A. Usefulness of a third Holter lead for detection of myocardial ischemia. Am J Cardiol 1994;74:1216.
10. Picano E, Lattanzi F, Masini M, Distante A, L'Abbate A. High dose dipyridamole echocardiography test in effort angina pectoris. J Am Coll Cardiol 1986;8:848.

11. Nishimura S, Mahmarian JJ, Boyce TM, Verani MS. Equivalence between adenosine and exercise thallium-201 myocardial tomography: a multicenter, prospective, crossover trial. J Am Coll Cardiol 1992;*20:*265.
12. Cohen JL, Greene TO, Ottenweller J et al. Dobutamine digital echocardiography for detecting coronary artery disease. Am J Cardiol 1991;*67:*1311.
13. Quinones MA, Verani MS, Haichin RM, Mahmarian JJ, Suarez J, Zoghbi WA. Exercise echocardiography versus thallium-201 single photon emission computed tomography in the evaluation of coronary artery disease: analysis of 292 patients. Circulation 1992;*85:*1026.
14. Pozzoli MMA, Fioretti PM, Salustri A, Reijis AEM, Roelandt JRTC. Exercise echocardiography and technetium-99m MIBI single-photon emission computed tomography in the detection of coronary artery disease. Am J Cardiol 1991;*67:*350.
15. Nguyen T, Heo J, Ogilby JD, Iskandrian AD. Single photon emission computed tomography with thallium-201 during adenosine-induced coronary hyperemia: correlation with coronary arteriography, exercise thallium imaging and two-dimensional echocardiography. J Am Coll Cardiol 1990;*16:*1375.
16. Jain A, Suarez J, Mahmarian JJ, Zoghbi WA, Quinones M, Verani MS. Functional significance of myocardial perfusion defects induced by dipyridamole using thallium-201 single-photon emission computed tomography and two-dimensional echocardiography. Am J Cardiol 1990;*66:*802.
17. Mahamarian JJ. Clinical applications of myocardial perfusion scintigraphy. Am Coll Cardiol Learning Center Highlights 1994;*9:*4.
18. Marwick TH. Stress echocardiography: comparison with other functional tests for the diagnosis of coronary heart disease. Am Coll Cardiol Learning Center Highlights 1994;*10:*11.
19. Bruschke AVG, Proudfit WL, Sones FM. Progress study of 590 consecutive nonsurgical cases of coronary disease followed 5–9 years. II. Ventriculographic and other correlations. Circulation 1973;*57:*1154.
20. Mock MB, Ringquist I, Fisher L et al. Survival of medically treated patients in the Coronary Artery Surgery Study (CASS) Registry. Circulation 1982;*66:*562.
21. The GUSTO Angiographic Investigators. The effects of tissue plasminogen activator, streptokinase, or both on coronary-artery patency, ventricular function, and survival after acute myocardial infarction. N Engl J Med 1993;*329:*1615.
22. The TIMI IIIB Investigators. Effects of tissue plasminogen activator and a comparison of early invasive and conservative strategies in unstable angina and non-Q-wave myocardial infarction. Results of the TIMI IIIB Trial. Circulation 1994;*89:*1545.
23. Bogaty P, Brecker SJ, White SE, et al. Comparison of coronary angiography findings in acute and chronic first presentation of ischemic heart disease. Circulation 1993;*87:*1938.
24. Brook RH, Park RE, Chassin MR, Solomon DH, Keesey J, Kosecoff J. Predicting the appropriate use of carotid endarterectomy, upper gastrointestinal endoscopy, and coronary angiography. N Engl J Med 1990;*323:*1173.

Chronic stable angina

INTRODUCTION

Clinically, the syndrome of chronic stable angina is typically manifested by attacks of angina pectoris caused predominantly by effort and occurring with a stable pattern over at least the last 2 months; its essential feature is the lack of a detectable short-term evolutive tendency towards myocardial infarction (MI) or sudden ischemic cardiac death (SICD). (The use of the term "syndrome" rather than "disease" is to emphasize the very heterogeneous origins of both the obstructive lesions and the chronic dynamic components that modulate residual coronary flow reserve.)

The anginal attacks are caused by ischemic episodes related to the presence of at least one chronic stable coronary artery stenosis, which limits the increase of blood flow to the distal myocardium, i.e. it reduces the coronary flow reserve.

The residual coronary flow reserve can be fixed, but in most cases it is modulated to a variable extent by transient changes in vasomotor tone at the site of a stable coronary stenosis or in small distal vessels. Thus, coronary vasoconstriction can sometimes reduce the ischemic threshold during effort, and occasionally can cause myocardial ischemia, even at rest. The clinical terms used for some forms of angina (i.e. emotion angina, cold angina, postprandial angina, walk-through angina, decubitus angina) are purely descriptive: when recurring chronically in patients with a reasonably good effort tolerance, these ischemic episodes are most likely to be caused by transient coronary vasoconstriction; when they occur in patients with a very low effort tolerance and markedly reduced coronary flow reserve, it becomes difficult (and also rather academic) to establish whether these ischemic episodes are caused by coronary vasoconstriction, by increased demand, or by a combination of the two (as long as the pattern of the attacks is stable in time).

Ischemic attacks caused by stable coronary obstructions can occur as the first manifestation of IHD, or in patients who have a history of previous MI, or who previously had a well-defined phase of unstable angina. Although the syndrome is characterized by a stable pattern of ischemic manifestations over a period of months or years, it may exhibit quiescent phases (with total remission of symptoms lasting for years) as well as unpredictable, unstable phases, or it may evolve into totally unheralded MI or SICD.

The syndrome is characterized by all the following features:

a. stability of symptoms and signs of ischemia over at least the last 2 months
b. effort-induced transient myocardial ischemia, which is relieved within 1—5 min by rest
c. the presence of at least one flow-limiting coronary artery stenosis.

An objective angiographic confirmation of the diagnosis may not be required for the practical management of the patient, either when evidence of previous MI makes the likelihood of coronary artery stenoses very high, or when symptoms and signs of ischemia are mild and the response to treatment is so good that percutaneous transluminal coronary angioplasty (PTCA) or coronary artery bypass grafting (CABG) are not considered.

Some patients with demonstrable coronary artery stenoses may experience several anginal episodes during the day, which may be due to frequent excessive efforts or to frequent episodes of coronary constriction; others have a good effort tolerance and only a few episodes each month. The level of exercise that can be tolerated without development of angina is predictable in some patients and variable in others.

■ *Thus, the pathogenetic mechanisms of this syndrome have multiple components, all of which are stable by definition and all of which must be considered during the diagnostic assessment in order to plan the most rational therapeutic approach.* ■

17.1 PATHOGENETIC MECHANISMS

The stable coronary artery obstructions responsible for this syndrome have developed either gradually over a period of years (as a result of smooth muscle proliferation, matrix formation, and lipid deposition) or suddenly as a result of the organization of a thrombus. As outlined in Chs 9 and 16, in the presence of these obstructions ischemia can be triggered by the following:

a. an extracoronary stimulus caused by an excessive increase in myocardial oxygen consumption that cannot be met by coronary blood supply because of epicardial coronary artery obstructions and an inadequate development of collaterals
b. increased coronary vasomotor tone at the site of the stenosis or in distal coronary vessels, which transiently reduces residual coronary flow reserve, or
c. a coincidental occurrence of coronary constriction insufficient to cause ischemia at rest, and a simultaneous increase in myocardial oxygen consumption that would otherwise have been well tolerated.

The latter two causes can be detected easily only in patients with a high residual coronary flow reserve. A mixed cause of ischemic episodes is more clearly noticeable in patients with a high maximal residual coronary flow reserve (so that on "good" days, or following the administration of acute coronary dilator drugs, they develop ischemia only for maximal or submaximal efforts). Such patients can exhibit wide differences in the levels of activity they can perform, in heart rate, and in the heart rate/blood pressure product at the onset of ischemia. In contrast, in patients who have a low maximal residual coronary flow reserve and who can expend only minor effort even on good days (or after the administration of coronary dilators) without developing ischemia, the range available for modulation of coronary flow reserve is fairly narrow.

Coronary vasoconstriction is generally thought to modulate residual coronary flow reserve through changes of the residual stenotic lumen. This mechanism of dynamic stenosis is certainly plausible for pliable plaques with a preserved smooth muscle media, but it can not explain changes in residual coronary flow reserve in patients with only fixed stenosis or total occlusions, in whom residual coronary flow reserve can be modulated only by distal coronary vasoconstriction.

■ *Abnormal endothelial function, smooth muscle response, and constrictor stimuli from resident cells or autonomic nerves may be involved in dynamic changes in the lumen of pliable coronary stenoses and in constriction of distal coronary vessels, which remain stable and recur chronically over months or years. Nervous stimuli must be involved in the coronary vasoconstriction developing promptly during handgrip, cold pressor testing, and psychological stress, but the site (stenotic lumen or distal vessels) and the pathways through which this coronary constriction develops are not known.* ■

17.1.1 Development and evolution of chronic coronary obstructions

As discussed in Chapters 8 and 9, flow-limiting coronary stenoses have very variable features. They can reduce the lumen eccentrically (eccentric stenoses), concentrically (concentric stenoses) or with irregular borders (complex stenoses). The vessel wall at the site of the obstruction can exhibit a variable area of preserved media: about 50% of critical stenoses have histologic features compatible with a vasomotor potential that is greatest in mild eccentric stenoses and smallest in severe concentric lesions (see Ch. 9).

Flow-limiting stenoses may develop either very gradually, or rapidly as a result of the organization of mural coronary thrombi. The thrombotic origin of flow-limiting coronary stenoses can be suspected when patients present with a history of a prolonged episode of angina, usually at rest, following which angina recurs consistently upon mild or moderate efforts that were previously perfectly well tolerated. Such a history may have some prognostic relevance, as it suggests that the patient may have a tendency to develop coronary thrombosis.

A thrombotic origin is also likely for stenoses that exhibit very rapid progression during the interval between two angiographic studies. The angiographic progression of stenoses over a follow-up period of several years typically involves only some stenoses. It is commoner for irregular lesions than for concentric and smooth lesions, but is independent of the severity of the stenosis at first evaluation and over 50% of even complex stenoses may not change in either severity or morphology during follow-up.[1] Finally, the progression of stenoses may be independent of the clinical evolution, as progression up to complete occlusion may be observed without infarction occurring and without changes in symptoms;[2] conversely, unstable angina and MI may develop without angiographically detectable changes occurring in coronary stenoses (see Ch. 8).[3]

17.1.2 Variable coronary flow reserve and ischemic threshold

In patients with chronic stable angina pectoris and angiographically confirmed coronary artery disease, a wide variability in residual coronary flow reserve and, hence, in ischemic threshold, has been documented objectively by a large number of studies based on exercise stress testing, other provocative tests, and continuous ambulatory monitoring (see Ch. 9). However, although it may seem incredible now, until the late 1970s it was believed that it was impossible for atherosclerotic coronary arteries to constrict and that increased heart work was the only possible cause of angina.[4]

Exercise stress testing

In general, in any group of patients with chronic stable angina, the product of heart rate and blood pressure at 1 mm ST-segment depression (as determined by repeated tests performed under identical, standardized conditions) is reproducible, but this average reproducibility usually results from large variations in opposite directions in different patients. In many patients, the ischemic threshold observed in the first and a subsequent exercise test may vary by more than 25%. The reproducibility of the ischemic threshold cannot be interpreted as evidence against the presence of an important modulatory role of coronary vasomotor tone under other conditions, as the laboratory conditions under which exercise stress tests are performed are intentionally standardized.

Administration of sublingual nitrates substantially improves residual coronary flow reserve in about one-third of patients (as assessed from heart rate/blood pressure product and time to 1 mm ST-segment depression).[5] This indicates also that, under the standard conditions in which the test is performed, about 30% of patients may have an important component of coronary vasoconstriction that further reduces their residual coronary flow reserve and that can be removed by coronary dilation.

Other provocative tests

For patients who are unable to exercise, other provocative tests can also produce ischemia by increasing myocardial oxygen demand (e.g. pacing-induced tachycardia, dobutamine) or transmural blood flow steal (e.g. dipyridamole, adenosine). Tests increasing myocardial demand are positive only when coronary flow reserve is markedly reduced. Tests causing transmural coronary blood flow (CBF) steal (see Ch. 10) provide no information about the ischemic threshold, but may be useful to detect the presence of flow-limiting stenoses and the area of myocardium at risk.

Cold pressor, handgrip, hyperventilation, and ergonovine tests can also produce coronary constriction and ischemia (through different mechanisms from those of variant angina) in a variable percentage of patients with chronic stable angina and documented coronary stenoses.[6] Psychological stress was found to cause ischemia-induced left ventricular dysfunction in a large percentage of patients with stable angina.[7,8] If artificial stimuli can cause myocardial ischemia by coronary constriction in some patients in a laboratory environment, it should not be surprising that, when exposed to the varied conditions of everyday life, the residual coronary flow reserve of many patients with chronic stable angina can be substantially modulated by coronary vasoconstriction.

Ambulatory monitoring

Ambulatory monitoring of the ECG has substantiated the frequent clinical observation of a variable anginal threshold by showing that the majority of episodes of myocardial ischemia (painful or painless) occurring during ordinary daily life develop at values of heart rate much lower than those that produce myocardial ischemia during exercise stress testing (see Figs 17.1 and 17.2).[9-11] This has been confirmed by simultaneous ambulatory intra-arterial blood pressure monitoring.[12,13] Conversely, both ECG and invasive arterial blood pressure ambulatory recordings show that patients often develop sustained high levels of heart rate and of heart rate/systolic blood pressure product with no signs of ischemia. A transient impairment of CBF should certainly be considered the predominant cause of the ischemic episodes that occur at values of heart rate about 20 beats lower than those tolerated with-

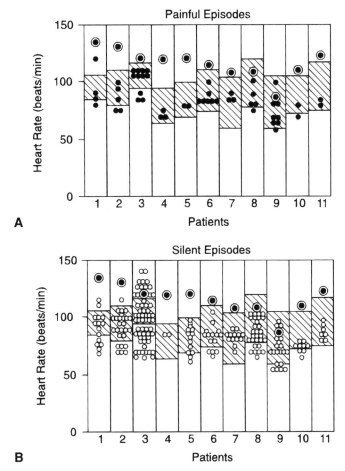

Fig. 17.1 Variable ischemic threshold in patients with chronic stable angina.
Ambulatory Holter monitoring in 11 patients showed that both painful (**A**) and pain-less (**B**) ischemic episodes began at very variable heart rates: most occurred at a lower heart rate than that achieved during exercise testing (⦿), some even occurred below the modal value of heart rate during the 24 h and many were within the range of heart rate observed during the 24 h in the absence of ischemic changes (▨). (Modified from ref. 11.)

out ischemia developing at other times of the day and for similar lengths of time, or during exercise stress testing.

A mild or moderate increase in heart rate and in arterial blood pressure can be detected before many ischemic episodes (see Figs. 17.3 and 17.4).[10–13] This increase is usually small and, therefore, insufficient per se to increase myocardial oxygen consumption beyond the ischemic threshold set by fixed stenoses as suggested by some authors,[13,14] as the doubling of heart rate/blood pressure product is required to double CBF (see Ch. 4); it suggests, rather, the occurrence of systemic activation of the sympathetic system, which could, at the same time, cause coronary vasoconstriction and increased demand.

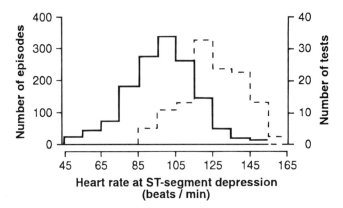

Fig. 17.2 Distribution of heart rate values at 1 mm ST-segment depression during exercise stress testing and ordinary daily life. The average value of heart rate at the onset of ischemia during exercise stress testing (------) was substantially higher than that at the onset of the episodes detected during Holter monitoring (——). In 75% of episodes occurring during ordinary daily life, heart rate was ≥ 20 beats lower than that observed at the onset of ischemia during exercise testing. (Modified from ref. 10.)

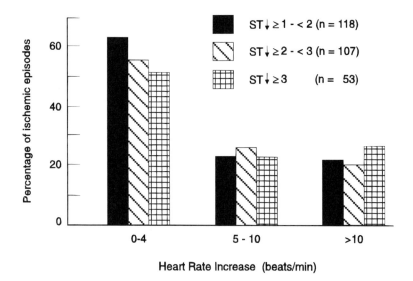

Fig. 17.3 Increase of heart rate before spontaneous ischemic episodes. During ambulatory Holter monitoring, ischemic episodes may be preceded by a variable increase in heart rate, which is not related to the severity of ST-segment depression (ST $\downarrow$). Small increases in heart rate preceding episodes occurring at a low heart rate cannot be interpreted as causal because they are insufficient to raise myocardial demand beyond residual coronary flow reserve. (Modified from ref 10.).

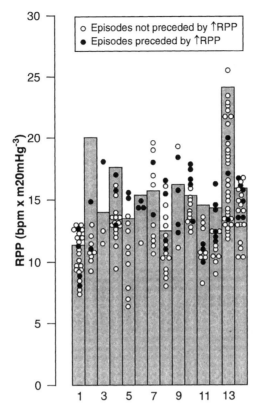

Fig. 17.4 Variable heart rate blood pressure product (RPP) at the onset of ischemic episodes during daily life. During ambulatory monitoring of brachial artery pressure and heart rate in 15 patients with chronic stable angina, most episodes occurred at lower values of RPP than that achieved during exercise stress testing (bars). Only a minority of episodes were preceded by an increase in RPP (●), and for those that occurred at low values of RPP, the increase could not have been the only cause of ischemia. (Modified from ref. 11.)

17.1.3 Prevalence, mechanisms and implications of mixed chronic stable angina

Patients who present only with fixed-threshold chronic stable angina are a minority and it is important, therefore, to define the prevalence, mechanisms, and practical implications of a mixed form of chronic stable angina in which residual coronary flow reserve is modulated by changes of coronary vasomotor tone.

Prevalence

All studies that have assessed the variability of the anginal threshold during daily life consistently report that at least 75% of patients have "mixed angina," (i.e. angina occurring during minor efforts, usually well tolerated and occasionally, also occurring spontaneously at rest).[15] During clinically stable periods the number of ischemic episodes detected by Holter monitoring usually varies considerably. This variability may reflect differences in levels of physical activity or a different incidence of ischemic episodes caused predominantly by transient impairment of CBF. This assessment has important therapeutic implications, as episodes caused by transient impairment of CBF could be prevented by vasodilator therapy and those caused by an excessive increase of demand could be reduced by limiting physical activity or by allowing the heart to work more economically.

Mechanisms of modulation of residual coronary flow reserve

As discussed in Chapter 9, in patients with coronary stenoses, residual coronary flow reserve can be dynamically modulated by changes in peristenotic vasomotor tone and by inappropriate constriction or inadequate dilation of resistive coronary vessels. Mild stenoses are more likely than severe stenoses to have a preserved smooth muscle coat and preserved pliability; however, in order to impair resting flow, increased vasomotor tone must reduce the diameter of the stenosis below about 90%. The possible role of resistive coronary vessels was demonstrated in patients with a single totally occluded coronary artery,[16] and a reduced dilator response was observed after successful PTCA in nonstenosed coronary branches also (see Ch. 9.) However, in the presence of coronary stenoses it is difficult to distinguish the role of small vessel constriction from that of increased peristenotic smooth muscle tone. In some patients with chronic stable angina, a coronary microvascular dysfunction is suggested by two similarities with patients with angiographically normal coronary arteries and microvascular angina. The first similarity is that, as in many patients with microvascular angina and also in some of those with angiographically demonstrated coronary stenoses,

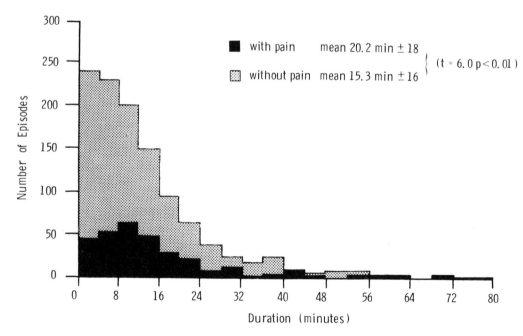

Fig. 17.5 Duration of episodes of symptomatic and asymptomatic ST-segment depression in patients with chronic stable angina. Painful episodes are slightly longer than painless episodes; some last over 30 min, and a few over 1 h. The long duration of some painful episodes is similar to that commonly observed in patients with microvascular angina. (Modified from ref. 10.)

during exercise stress testing, pain precedes the onset of ischemic ST-segment changes, which is in sharp contrast to the late appearance of pain in variant angina (see Fig. 14.14). The second similarity is that some episodes of ST-segment depression, recorded during ambulatory Holter monitoring in patients with chronic stable angina, are very prolonged, as are episodes of pain in patients with microvascular angina (see Fig. 17.5).

Practical implications

Improvement in the results of exercise stress testing is an ideal way to evaluate the anti-ischemic effect of drugs on patients in whom excessive cardiac work represents the only cause of ischemia, but ambulatory Holter recordings and angina diaries are required for patients in whom ischemic episodes are caused predominantly by a dynamic modulation of residual coronary flow reserve due to transient vasoconstriction of stenoses or resistive vessels.

Total abolition of the modulatory role of transient coronary vasoconstriction as a cause of ischemic episodes, would allow patients to experience ischemia only when their heart work increased beyond the level usually tolerated without angina on their good days.

■ *Mixed chronic stable angina can result from modulation of residual coronary flow reserve by either a dynamic stenosis or a small distal vessel coronary vasoconstriction. The prevalence and pathogenetic mechanisms of these two components of the dynamic modulation of coronary flow reserve are not precisely known but could have important therapeutic implications.* ■

17.2 DIAGNOSTIC ASSESSMENT

When considering a diagnosis of chronic stable angina, it is important to remember that the stability of symptoms implies a good short-term prognosis, and this allows time to consider and apply (with a gradual progression) diagnostic tests while assessing the patient's response to therapy.

The first diagnostic step, and the most important, is a careful clinical history. The second step is the objective documentation of effort-induced transient myocardial ischemia by exercise stress testing or, when this is impossible, by other tests. For patients with good effort tolerance, the third step is to assess the importance of a modulatory role of vasoconstriction on residual coronary flow reserve, by history, exercise testing, and (when available) ambulatory ECG monitoring, which will indicate whether most ischemic episodes experienced during ordinary daily life are caused predominantly by excessive cardiac work or by transient coronary vasoconstriction, thus helping to define the therapeutic strategy. The final step is the documentation of coronary stenosis by angiography, which is mandatory for patients with a positive exercise test at a low work load and with large segments of myocardium at risk.

17.2.1 Diagnostic clues from medical history and physical examination

Essential information can be derived from four aspects of the medical history:

a. the stable pattern of angina (indicated by the lack of change of symptoms over the last few months)
b. the severity of impairment of coronary flow reserve (indicated by the level of effort that can be tolerated without the development of angina on good days)

c. the severity and extension of myocardial ischemia (indicated by evidence of acute left ventricular failure)

d. the range of the modulation of residual coronary flow reserve by coronary vaso-constriction in patients with a good effort tolerance (indicated by the variability of the anginal threshold).

The complaint of angina pectoris, typically related to physical effort occurring during the effort itself and relieved by rest within 1–5 min, recurring repeatedly over the past months or years with a *stable pattern*, suggests stability of the underlying coronary lesions. However, even when meeting these fairly stringent criteria, the diagnostic value of the history is substantially different in patients with and without previously documented IHD.

For patients without known IHD, the probability of myocardial ischemia caused by coronary artery stenosis varies considerably with age, gender, and the presence of risk factors according to the Bayesian theory (see Ch. 16).

The probability that the symptom is caused by myocardial ischemia and coronary artery stenosis is greatest when the features of angina pectoris are typical, when the discomfort occurs daily or weekly, and when severe efforts are never tolerated and are promptly relieved by rest; the probability is least when the discomfort has less typical features, occurs rarely and unpredictably, lasts 10 or more minutes after the effort, or occurs after—rather than during—exercise. The association of undue shortness of breath together with angina alerts the physician to the possible occurrence of ischemia involving a large segment of myocardium. The next diagnostic step should be to confirm objectively that effort does reproduce the symptoms and that the symptom is, indeed, associated with diagnostic signs of myocardial ischemia. The physical examination should exclude the presence of associated aortic valvular disease or hypertrophic cardiomyopathy. A clinical differential diagnosis can be made from noncardiac causes of chest pain, as these are neither consistently related to effort nor promptly relieved by rest (see Ch. 16).

A clinical diagnosis of small vessel coronary disease can be suspected in patients with a variable anginal threshold, with prolonged duration of pain after termination of effort, and with episodes often caused by emotion (see Ch. 18). This diagnosis is supported by the finding of normal coronary arteries at angiography.

For patients with previously documented IHD, the complaint of angina pectoris with features similar to those associated with documented ischemic episodes in the past, is usually a reliable indication of myocardial ischemia related to coronary artery stenoses, unless proved otherwise.

Once it has been established that angina is caused by myocardial ischemia related to a coronary artery stenosis, and that it is stable, the patient's history can also be used to assess the *severity of the reduction of coronary flow reserve.* When a patient is a reliable historian, this information can be obtained by inquiring about the intensity of exercise tolerated without the occurrence of angina on good days or after sublingual nitrates, as this indicates the maximal residual coronary flow reserve. This is obviously impossible when patients do not exert themselves sufficiently.

A history of obvious shortness of breath during anginal attacks is suggestive of *acute left ventricular failure* due to a critical area of myocardium jeopardized by ischemia. This possibility is supported by the appearance of a fourth or third heart sound, of a pansystolic murmur, and of wheezing or crepitations on the lung field.

In patients with mixed angina, comparison of the level of exercise tolerated on good days or after sublingual nitrates, with that usually associated with the development of angina during daily life can provide a clue to the importance of the *modulation of residual coronary flow reserve caused by coronary vasoconstriction.*

Such patients most typically present with the following pattern of attacks. There is a ceiling of effort over which they can never go without experiencing angina. However, occasionally and unpredictably (particularly during bad days), they can experience angina "out of the blue" for efforts that are usually quite well tolerated, and even when resting. Attacks may also occur during the night and are more likely to do so when the maximum effort tolerance is greatly reduced. The duration of the attack is related to the duration of effort and usually lasts no longer than 1–2 min after interruption of the effort. Attacks brought on by emotion and spontaneous attacks respond promptly to sublingual nitrates. Such patients may also complain of chronically recurring postprandial angina (angina occurring after meals), of "walk-through" angina (angina occurring only at the beginning of the very first effort of the day) or "decubitus" angina (angina occurring soon after going to bed).

The key questions that will establish the range of the ischemic threshold are as follows:

1. Is your chest discomfort predictably caused by the same amount of effort? Or do you have good days (during which you can do a great deal without having angina) and bad days (during which you are very limited by angina)?
2. What is the maximum amount of exercise that you can perform without having angina on your good days or after prophylactic sublingual nitroglycerin?

In these otherwise stable patients, the maximum effort that is tolerated without the development of angina on either their good days or during exercise stress testing after sublingual nitrates indicates the fixed component of the reduction of coronary flow reserve (maximum residual coronary flow reserve). The comparison of the maximum level of effort tolerated without the development of ischemia with that associated with anginal attacks during daily life provides information on the extent to which coronary constriction can modulate coronary flow reserve. When the pattern remains unchanged for months or years and the effort tolerance is good (at least on some days), a long duration of pain and a poor response to nitrates are suggestive of microvascular angina (see Ch. 18).

17.2.2 Diagnostic value of exercise stress testing

In patients with chronic stable angina, exercise stress testing is useful for three main purposes:

a. to confirm objectively the presence of effort-induced myocardial ischemia (performed off anti-ischemic therapy)
b. to establish the residual coronary flow reserve and relate it to the efforts that usually cause angina during ordinary daily life (performed after the administration of sublingual nitrates)
c. to assess the extent of the myocardium jeopardized by ischemia (performed off anti-ischemic therapy.

Clues provided by the history can be used by performing the test under the conditions that are most often associated with the development of symptoms (for example, early in the morning, after meals, in the cold, or with abrupt onset of exercise). If the test reproduces the usual symptoms and shows that they are accompanied by ischemic ST-segment shifts, a diagnosis of effort-induced myocardial ischemia can be made with reasonable confidence.

The *diagnostic specificity* of a positive ECG exercise stress test depends on normality or abnormality of the basal tracing, on the estimated pretest probability that the patient has the disease (see Ch. 16), and on the severity of the ischemic changes, the occurrence of angina and/or signs of extensive myocardial ischemia (a fall in systolic blood pressure or the appearance of mitral regurgitation or of a gallop rhythm).

The resting ECG may sometimes reveal signs of a previous MI and, therefore, by itself provides a diagnosis of IHD. The confirmation of such a diagnosis in the absence of a clear history can be made by searching for a matching regional ventricular wall akinesia with reduced diastolic wall thickness or fixed myocardial perfusion defects. The tracing may also show ST-segment abnormalities that have persisted unchanged for months and that are not, in themselves, indicators of IHD.

When the results of ECG exercise testing do not allow a definite diagnosis to be made, myocardial scintigraphy and studies of ventricular function and wall motion can be used. For patients able to exercise maximally at high work loads, the practical importance of establishing a precise diagnosis diminishes considerably as they are at very low risk. For patients who cannot exercise, other provocative tests of myocardial ischemia may be used (see Ch. 16).

Once a diagnosis of effort-induced myocardial ischemia has been made, repeating an exercise stress test after sublingual nitrates provides an objective indication of the *maximal residual coronary flow reserve,* having minimized possible vasoconstrictor modulations (as well as reducing myocardial demand).

A comprehensive evaluation should consider both time to 1 mm ST-segment depression and the value of the heart rate/blood pressure product as an index of myocardial oxygen consumption at 1 mm ST-segment depression (see Ch. 6).

Time to angina is an unreliable index of the onset of ischemia as it is difficult to assess the time of onset of pain when it begins gradually and as it may occur only some minutes after the onset of ischemia. Time to 1mm ST-segment depression can be determined more objectively. Both measurements can be modified considerably by repeated testing, because patients who become familiar with the treadmill or the bicycle ergometer learn to exercise more economically, thus requiring lower cardiac work for the same exercise work load. Indices of myocardial oxygen consumption (such as the heart rate/systolic blood pressure product) are, therefore, more reliable as indicators of the ischemic threshold than is time alone, but such indices are influenced by changes in the heart rate response to exercise, for example, following β-blockade (bradycardia) and nitrates (tachycardia).

The patient's response to the question of how the level of exercise tolerated without angina after sublingual nitrate compares with the level of effort associated with angina during daily life, may provide an useful indication of the variability of the ischemic threshold and, hence, of the possible role of coronary vasoconstriction in modulating maximal residual coronary flow reserve.

Ischemic ST-segment changes on the ECG during exercise testing are unreliable indicators of the *severity and extent of myocardial ischemia* in the absence of the clinical signs of severe ischemia mentioned above, and are even less reliable for establishing its location. Imaging techniques are, therefore, required that are capable of detecting ischemia-related regional myocardial perfusion deficits, regional ventricular wall motion abnormalities, and global left ventricular dysfunction (see Ch. 16).

17.2.3 Diagnostic value of ambulatory ECG recording

In patients with chronic stable angina, ambulatory ECG recordings provide an indication of the number, severity, and prevailing mechanisms of ischemic episodes (both painful and painless) that occur during daily life. It also allows an objective assessment of whether episodes occur because myocardial demand increases above the limits of residual coronary flow reserve or because residual coronary flow reserve is transiently reduced by episodic coronary vasoconstriction.

The test is particularly useful for documenting ischemic episodes in patients who cannot undergo standardized exercise testing and also in those who previously had a good maximal exercise test but who complain of frequent angina with a very variable threshold. Ambulatory ECG recording is most likely to be negative in those patients with chronic stable angina who have a negative maximal exercise test.

Episodes associated with more than 1 mm ST-segment depression lasting longer than 1 min are commonly considered diagnostic of ischemia. However, similar painful and painless episodes of ST-segment depression are also common in patients with microvascular angina. Great variability in heart rate at the onset of ischemic ST-segment changes (for example from 80 to 120 bpm) indicates a reasonable maximal residual coronary flow reserve but with an important superimposed modulatory role of coronary vasoconstriction.

17.2.4 Diagnostic value of coronary angiography

Coronary angiography provides evidence of the presence of coronary stenoses and of their severity, number, and morphology, and also allows the direct assessment of changes in the stenotic lumen by vasoconstrictor or dilator stimuli.

During angiography, the operator should make use of the information provided by history and exercise testing both by adopting additional nonstandard projections when no stenoses are found in patients with a very low anginal threshold and/or a positive exercise stress test at low or moderate work loads and by introducing constrictor stimuli (such as the handgrip or cold pressor tests) and intracoronary infusion of nitroglycerin, to assess the magnitude of vasomotor changes at the site of coronary stenoses in patients with a very variable anginal threshold.

Angiography must be justified by the anticipated benefits to each patient (according to prevailing established local practise) and by the patient's wishes.

Coronary angiography is mandatory when PTCA or CABG are thought to be required in order to relieve symptoms and signs of ischemia persisting in spite of full medical therapy. A severe reduction of maximal residual coronary flow reserve (suggested by the history and documented by exercise testing after sublingual nitrates) and an estimated large area of jeopardized myocardium (suggested by signs of left ventricular failure, a decrease in systemic blood pressure during exercise, extensive and severe ST-segment depression, large areas of reduced perfusion at scintigraphy, or ventricular dysfunction during ischemia) despite full medical therapy, are mandatory indications for angiography.

Angiograpy may not be required for patients with a normal resting ECG and no evidence of previous MI, who have a positive exercise test only at a very high work load, or for those in whom anti-ischemic therapy abolishes symptoms completely and renders the exercise test negative. The prognosis for such patients is quite good and there is, therefore, no evidence that survival would be improved by either PTCA or CABG. They should, however, be reassessed very promptly whenever their anginal symptoms become worse.

In intermediate cases, the diagnostic use of angiography depends on both local practise and the wishes of the patient, as there are possible advantages, as well as disadvantages. The advantages are as follows:

a. the detection of very critical proximal stenoses, because it is possible that, in such cases, successful PTCA or CABG will improve the prognosis: very occasionally, critical proximal coronary stenoses and occlusion are found in patients with a good ventricular function and normal maximal exercise ECG stress test, but their prognostic significance in such patients has not been established
b. the demonstration that there are no flow-limiting stenoses, because this is reassuring for the patient.

The disadvantages are as follows:

a. the inconvenience, risk, and cost of the procedure
b. the urge to deal with stenoses that, in fact, may not affect symptoms or prognosis.

17.2.5 Classification of chronic stable angina

The Canadian Cardiovascular Society (CCS) clinical classification now used widely, is based on the clinical history and the maximal effort that can be tolerated without angina.[17] The New York Heart Association (NYHA) classification should not be used for angina because it is not based on the maximal physical activity that the patient can sustain, but on the circumstances in which angina may be experienced. Thus, patients with angina at rest would be classified as class IV, even if they had a good effort tolerance.

The disadvantages of the CCS classification are that it does not consider either the objective evidence of myocardial ischemia provided by the exercise test, or the possibility that patients may have a widely variable ischemic threshold (as some patients in classes I and II may occasionally experience angina at rest), or that prognosis may be influenced considerably by the impairment of left ventricular function by previous MI.

The CCS classification of patients with chronic stable angina should, therefore, be integrated with information on the following three components:

a. the degree of reduction of coronary flow reserve during exercise stress testing (as this substantiates the history)
b. the variability of the ischemic threshold (as it may affect therapy)
c. the presence and extent of previous MI (as it affects prognosis).

Table 17.1 Clinically relevant metabolic equivalent for maximum exercise

1	MET	=	resting
2	METs	=	level walking at 2 mph (~ 3.2 km/h)
4	METs	=	level walking at 4 mph (~ 6.4 km/h)
<5	METs	=	poor prognosis; usual limit immediately after myocardial infarction; peak cost of basic activities of daily living
10	METs	=	prognosis with medical therapy as good as coronary artery bypass surgery
13	METs	=	excellent prognosis regardless of other exercise responses
18	METs	=	elite endurance athletes

MET, metabolic equivalent or a unit of sitting, resting oxygen uptake; 1 MET = 3.5 ml/kg/min oxygen uptake
The actual determinants of maximal exercise capacity are multiple. Some are potentially modifiable, such as signs of ischemia, others are not, and the two may be combined in the same patient to influence prognosis

According to the *level of reduction of coronary flow reserve*, patients are categorized into four classes on the basis of the CCS clinical classification integrated with the results of exercise stress testing.

The work load during exercise testing is assessed in metabolic equivalents of resting oxygen consumption (METS), which correspond to standardized work stages on the treadmill and bicycle. According to an American Heart Association special report on exercise standards,[18] normal values of maximal oxygen uptake (expressed in METS) vary with physical fitness, age, and gender (see Tables 17.1 and 17.2).

Although a sedentary life may reduce maximal exercise tolerance considerably, an average value of 10 METS can be considered as normal between the ages of 50–59 years and 20–39 years in men and women, respectively.

■ *The results of exercise stress testing are particularly helpful for the classification of anginal patients, either when they show a good effort tolerance (because it indicates a good coronary flow reserve and puts them in a low-risk group) or when they show obvious signs of ischemia at a low work load (because it indicates a reduced coronary flow reserve, a poor prognosis and puts them in a high-risk group). It is in the intermediate group of patients that the clinical value of more complex techniques should be assessed (see Ch. 16).* ■

Table 17.2 Normal value of maximum oxygen uptake at different ages expressed as METs

	Maximum O$_2$ uptake (METs)*	
Age (years)	Men	Women
20–29	12	10
30–39	12	10
40–49	11	9
50–59	10	8
60–69	9	8
70–79	8	8

* See Table 17.1
The significance of these average values should be considered with caution, as their standard deviation from the mean is large

Thus the following classification is proposed, based on symptoms and the results of exercise testing:

1. Class I (mild reduction of coronary flow reserve): patients develop angina on their good days, only on very strenuous effort. The exercise test after sublingual nitroglycerin is negative, or they can exercise more than 10 METS.
2. Class II (moderate reduction of coronary flow reserve): patients cannot sustain the severe efforts of daily life without developing angina (climbing stairs rapidly or walking fast uphill, but they can usually walk more than 200 yards on the flat at a normal pace without developing angina). Exercise testing after sublingual nitroglycerin is positive (with or without angina) at a high work load (7–10 METS).
3. Class III (severe reduction of coronary flow reserve): patients cannot sustain ordinary daily activities (such as climbing two flights of stairs or walking 100–200 yards on the flat at a normal pace) without developing angina. The exercise test after sublingual nitroglycerin is positive (with or without angina) at a moderate work load (4–7 METS) and/or at a low heart rate.
4. Class IV (very severe reduction of coronary flow reserve): patients cannot walk on the flat for more than 50–100 yards without experiencing angina. The exercise test is positive (with or without angina) after sublingual nitroglycerin at very low workload (less than 4 METS).

When classifying patients into classes I–IV it should be specified whether or not they are on maximal tolerated medical therapy, and the results of exercise stress testing should be judged on the level of effort attained compared with that usually achieved during daily life. For the prognostic assessment and the consideration of revascularization procedures, patients should be classified while on maximal medical therapy.

The concept of residual coronary flow reserve has an inherent limitation because it is determined by the vessel with the most critical obstruction and, thus, does not discriminate between small and large areas of myocardium jeopardized by ischemia. Whenever possible, the development of ischemia should be further characterized by assessing the size of the area of myocardium at risk.

According to the *variability of ischemic threshold,* a mixed type of chronic stable angina can be diagnosed when patients report an obvious variability in effort tolerance. For example, they report with surprise that angina occasionally develops for efforts that are usually well tolerated, or that angina even occurs at rest for no apparent reason, or they report that during daily life angina occurs for efforts much lower than those that cause angina during the exercise stress test (they are surprised that they were able to perform so well during the test). A mixed type of chronic stable angina can be defined for patients in classes I and II who benefit more from prevention of inappropriate coronary vasoconstriction than from reduction of myocardial oxygen consumption. The practical relevance of this distinction becomes more difficult, and has a lesser therapeutic relevance, for patients in classes III and IV, in whom maximal medical therapy or coronary revascularization procedures are required in any case.

According to the *absence or presence of previous MI* and impairment of cardiac function, patients are classified into three groups:

Table 17.3 Classification of chronic stable angina

Class*	METs	Limitation of effort tolerance	Evidence of previous MI and left ventricular dysfunction	Ischemic threshold	Prognosis
I	>10	>Stage 3 Bruce protocol or	A, no MI	Fixed/Variable	++++
		>175 watt bicycle	B, old MI, EF ⩾40%	Fixed/Variable	+++
II	7–10	Up to Stage 3 Bruce protocol or	A, no MI	Fixed/Variable	++
		up to 175 watt bicycle	B, old MI, EF ⩾40%	Fixed/Variable	+
			C, old MI, EF <40%	Fixed/Variable	−
III	4–7	Up to Stage 3 Bruce protocol or	A, no MI		+−
		up to 100 watt bicycle	B, old MI, EF ⩾ 40%		−
			C, old MI, EF < 40%		− − −
IV	<4	<Stage 1 Bruce protocol or	A, no MI		−
		<50 watt bicycle (equivalent to	B, old MI, EF ⩾ 40%		− −
		walking at < 4 mph or 6.4 km/h)	C, old MI, EF, < 40%		− − − −

* Patients with class I angina may previously have had a small (but not a large) MI that would prevent them from exercising beyond 10 METS. In patients with classes III or IV angina it may be difficult to recognize with certainty a mixed pattern of attacks. When assessing prognosis and the indications for revascularization procedures, classification should be made when patients are on optimal medical therapy. The average prognosis is best in class I patients with no previous MI and worse in class IV patients with old MI and an EF <40%. Prospective data collection is necessary in order to quantify the gradient of risk between these two extremes. Additional noninvasive and invasive studies should allow the establishment of gradients of risk within each of these clinically defined prognostic groups

1. Group A comprises patients with no evidence of previous MI.
2. Group B comprises patients with previous MI but no evidence of impaired left ventricular function (no history of cardiac failure and no evidence of cardiomegaly) and an estimated left ventricular ejection fraction (EF) greater than 40%.
3. Group C comprises those with a documented MI with a history of left ventricular failure after the acute phase, cardiomegaly or an estimated EF less than 40%. A 40% cutoff in EF is taken as the mortality rate after MI rises steeply below this level (see Ch. 13).

The classification of patients according to their reduction of effort tolerance, baseline risk, and dynamic modulation of coronary flow reserve is summarized in Table 17.3.

The implications of this classification on treatment relate not only to the choice of first-line medical therapy for patients in the various classes (vasodilator and/or β-adrenergic blocking drugs) but also to the mandatory indications for interventional therapy for those patients who, on maximal medical therapy, are in classes IV and III, and for some in class II with a positive test, particularly when in groups C or B. Its implications for prognosis relate to a gradually worsening prognosis from classes I to IV, and from groups A to C. The prognostic implications of a mixed type of angina in classes I to II is not clear.

17.3 PROGNOSTIC ASSESSMENT

The prognosis of patients with chronic stable angina is determined by four components that, together, indicate the probability of MI and/or the vulnerability of the heart to new ischemic insults:

a. evidence of a previous (even if only a small) MI (because it may indicate that patients are susceptible to new infarctions)
b. impairment of ventricular function (because it makes the patient more vulnerable to new ischemic or necrotic episodes and to further losses of myocardium)
c. severity of reduction of coronary flow reserve (because it determines the limitation of exercise capacity and, in general, indicates the severity of coronary stenoses and the inadequate degree of compensation provided by collaterals)
d. the area of myocardium jeopardized by ischemia (because it influences the impairment of ventricular function caused by ischemia and, possibly, the area at risk of infarction).

In clinical studies, the information available on prognosis is rather fragmentary. It is usually based on only the history of angina (independent of its type, or severity, or of the presence of a previous MI) or only the results of an individual test (such as exercise ECG, myocardial scintigraphy, or coronary arteriography). As indicated in Chapter 13, this situation derives largely from the fact that diagnostic techniques are divided among different cardiologic services (i.e. the clinical service and the ECG, nuclear cardiology, echocardiographic, and catheterization laboratories), each of which may attempt to define prognosis independent of the relevant information easily available from other services. This has led to the identification of prognostic determinants based on the results of single techniques, but the relationship between any prognostic determinant and prognosis is not linear as it is also influenced by the variable prevalence and importance of other determinants of prognosis that are likely to vary in different studies according to the inclusion criteria adopted and to referral practises.

For example, the results of statistical linear regression analysis may not apply to variables that have an exponential relation with prognosis, such as age and EF. Age and impairment of left ventricular function would emerge as strong predictors of prognosis in a group that included a substantial proportion of patients above the age of 65 with a previous MI, but would not in a group below the age of 65 with no previous MI. The reciprocal influence of age, impairment of left ventricular function, reduced coronary flow reserve (and effort tolerance), and a large area of myocardium at risk (and severe coronary artery obstructions) is very considerable. The prognostic value of each of these determinants in both single and multiple statistical regression analysis obtained in different groups of patients is, therefore, strongly influenced by their prevalence, and by the presence and importance of each of the others. The additional prognostic information provided by more complex, expensive, and invasive tests must be established in groups of patients, first, with a similar history (including evidence and size of previous MI), second, with a similar response to exercise stress testing, and finally, being of similar age and gender. Imaging techniques, Holter monitoring, and coronary arteriography may add valuable prognostic information in some of these subgroups, but not in others.

17.3.1 Prognostic value of history

A careful medical history can provide valuable information, not only for the diagnosis of myocardial ischemia and its causes but also for each of the main prognostic components:

1. A history of MI is an unfavorable prognostic indicator because the patient has demonstrated a susceptibility.
2. An additional, unfavorable prognostic indicator is the history of cardiac failure or angina during the acute phase of MI, and particularly during the follow-up period.

3. A clue to a large extent of myocardium jeopardized by ischemia (or of preexisting impairment of left ventricular function) is provided by the development of undue breathlessness during ischemic episodes, which is indicative of acute left ventricular failure. When angina is only mild or is absent, effort-induced ischemia may become severer because patients continue to exercise in spite of ischemia.)
4. An indication of severe reduction of coronary flow reserve is given by the report of a poor effort tolerance because of angina even on good days or after sublingual nitroglycerin.

The severity of chest pain, in itself, is not a prognostic indicator because the intensity of pain is not necessarily related to the extension of ischemia or to its severity. The subjective nature of points 3 and 4 restricts their prognostic significance to patients who are reliable historians.

17.3.2 Prognostic value of the exercise stress test

A positive exercise stress test can provide objective evidence to support the information derived from the medical history. It can also provide information not available from the medical history when ischemia is painless, when patients do not exercise in their daily lives, or when patients are not reliable historians.

In patients with triple-vessel coronary artery disease, with and without a previous MI, the ability to exercise for only a short time carries a worse prognosis than the ability to exercise for longer, independent of a positive or negative result (see Fig. 17.6).[19]

In patients with a markedly positive exercise test, survival was found to be lowest in those with the shortest exercise duration, but the duration of exercise did not correlate with the number of acute ischemic events (i.e. unstable angina or acute MI). Those patients with the

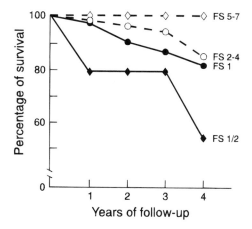

Fig. 17.6 Variable prognostic importance of triple-vessel disease. Cumulative survival rates according to the final exercise stage (FS) achieved by 572 patients with triple-vessel disease and left ventricular scores 5–9. Patients who can exercise up to and beyond stage 5 of the Bruce protocol have an excellent prognosis, even if they have triple-vessel disease, and regardless of whether they had previously suffered a small MI and/or had a positive test. Prognosis should be even better for patients with no previous history of MI and a normal ECG exercise test. (Modified from ref 19.)

shortest exercise duration, therefore, were more vulnerable because of an underlying impairment of left ventricular function as a consequence of previous MI or because of very reduced coronary flow reserve, or both (see Fig. 17.7A/B).[20]

Prognostic studies would be more informative if patients were grouped separately according to the following:

a. the amount of cardiac work needed to produce ischemia
b. the severity and extension of ischemia
c. the presence or absence of previous MI
d. an EF greater or less than 40%.

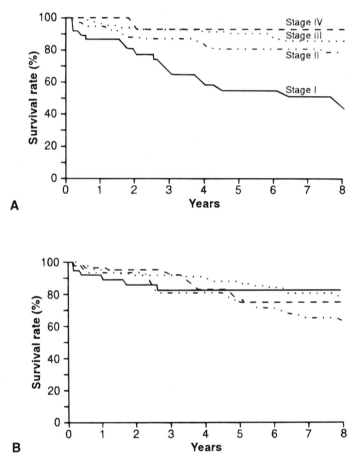

Fig. 17.7 Total and event-free survival in patients with a strongly positive ECG exercise stress test. The stage reached during exercise testing with 2 mm or more ST-segment depression influences total survival (**A**), but not event-free survival (**B**). Thus a reduced effort tolerance may also be a marker of the heart's poor response to ischemic insults, rather than of its susceptibility to such insults. The report does not specify whether a markedly reduced effort tolerance is caused by pre-existing post-MI severe left ventricular dysfunction. (------, Stage IV; ·······, Stage III; –·–·–, Stage II; ———, Stage I of the Bruce protocol) (Modified from ref. 20.)

17.3.3 Prognostic significance of ambulatory ECG recordings

Some studies suggest that the total number and duration of ischemic episodes during ambulatory recording is a prognostic indicator,[21-23] but the extent to which this prognostic information is independent of the classification of angina, the presence of previous MI(s), and the results of exercise stress testing, is not clear. The number of ischemic episodes recorded during ambulatory Holter monitoring may be correlated with the response of the exercise stress test, i.e. the lower the ischemic threshold, the larger the number and total duration of ischemic episodes during ambulatory recordings. Alternatively, the prognostic significance may relate to the number of episodes caused predominantly by coronary vasoconstriction. It would, therefore, be possible (theoretically) for a sudden large increase in the number of spontaneous episodes of silent ischemic ST-segment shift seen on repetitive ambulatory recordings to indicate the transition from stability to instability of the underlying coronary lesion (which would be undetectable clinically).

17.3.4 Prognostic significance of coronary angiography

As discussed in Chapter 13, all angiographic studies indicate that prognosis is strongly influenced by two factors:

a. the severity of impairment of left ventricular function caused by previous MIs, as estimated from the left ventricular EF (but in many cases this information will already be available from the history, 12-lead ECG, chest radiography or echocardiography)
b. the presence of a critical stenosis that reduces the original coronary diameter by at least 70% (i.e. the lumen by 90%) in one, two, or three main branches or in the left main stem (the presence of critical proximal stenoses may already have been suggested by a low effort tolerance, by the appearance of signs of left ventricular dysfunction, and by failure of blood pressure to increase during exercise.)

The risk is enhanced by the combination of impaired left ventricular function and critical stenoses. Although a gradient of risk proportional to the number of diseased vessels (i.e. single-, double-, or triple-vessel disease) was observed in all studies, the absolute risk has decreased considerably in recent studies, which included a broader range of less symptomatic patients than in the initial angiographic reports (see Fig. 16.4). The risk is very low for stable patients with normal ventricular function and good effort tolerance, even in the presence of triple-vessel disease (see Fig. 17.6).

17.3.5 Conclusions

Patients with severe symptoms and signs of ischemia (classes III and IV) require treatment that will improve their lifestyles. In mildly symptomatic patients (classes I and II), however, in whom therapy and interventions are predominantly concerned with prognosis rather than the improvement of lifestyle, it would be useful to know the extent to which the results of myocardial scintigraphy, ambulatory ECG recordings, and angiography increase the prognostic accuracy within each subgroup of patients defined according to the classification presented in Table 17.1.

The assessment of long-term prognosis should be periodically updated during regular follow-up visits, depending on the evolution of symptoms and on the results of exercise stress testing repeated every 6 or 12 months. Prolonged stability of symptoms and an unchanged exercise test result are reassuring. The gradual deterioration of symptoms and/or the results of exercise stress testing would suggest the need for therapy to be increased, for control of risk factors to be improved, and for consideration to be given to PTCA or CABG. The sudden exacerbation of symptoms should alert the physician to the possible occurrence either of extracoronary causes that increase the imbalance between myocardial oxygen demand and supply or of an unstable phase of IHD, and should be very promptly managed.

17.4 THERAPEUTIC APPROACH

The aim of therapy is twofold—the relief of symptoms without causing undue inconvenience and side effects, and the improvement of disability-free and total life expectancy. Treatment that is likely to improve prognosis by reducing risk factors, as well as treatment with aspirin, may have little or no effect on symptoms. Conversely, there is surprisingly little evidence to show that in patients with chronic stable angina prognosis is actually improved by β-blockers, calcium antagonists, and nitrates, all of which reduce the number of anginal and ischemic episodes. This may be due to the good prognosis of stable patients with good left ventricular function. In such a low-risk group, prospective randomization of very large numbers of patients and long periods of follow-up are required in order to demonstrate a possible reduction in the number of fatal and nonfatal major ischemic events.

The efficacy of treatment for relieving symptoms and signs of ischemia can be judged directly by both the patient and the attending physician; the efficacy of treatment for improving prognosis is difficult to assess when the baseline prognosis is good.

17.4.1 Assessment of the benefits of therapy

The benefits of therapy should be assessed in terms of the improvement of symptoms and signs of ischemia, the improved disability-free and total life expectancy, and the quality of life.

Improvement of symptoms and signs of myocardial ischemia

The improvement of symptoms of myocardial ischemia as a result of medical or interventional therapy can be judged easily by the patient when they are typical, frequent, and severe, but not when they are mild, atypical, and infrequent.

The difficulty in assessing the beneficial effects of anti-ischemic drugs in patients with rare episodes of ischemia is illustrated by the results of a recent multicentric trial.[24] Standardized exercise stress testing indicated that the time to ischemia was increased from 3.9 min on placebo to only 4.0 min (a 3% increase) on both propranolol and diltiazem. Angina diaries indicated that the number of anginal attacks per week was reduced from 2.3 on placebo to 1.3 by both propranolol and diltiazem (a 43% reduction). Yet ambulatory ECG recordings indicated that the number of ischemic episodes was reduced from 4.6 per 48 h during placebo to 2.0 per 48 h (a 57% reduction) during propranolol treatment and to 3.8 per 48 h during diltiazem treatment (a 17% reduction). The minimal improvement in exercise stress testing after propranolol and diltiazem is in sharp contrast to previous reports and is difficult to explain. The 17% reduction of ischemic episodes on ambulatory ECG recordings after diltiazem is clearly less than that observed with propranolol, and contrasts with the similar reduction of the two agents in weekly anginal attacks. The 57% reduction of ischemic episodes during propranolol compares well with the 63% reduction reported in a previous crossover study using atenolol. The reduction of ischemic episodes by propranolol, as seen on ambulatory ECG testing, is much greater than expected on the basis of the 3% increase of time to ischemia during exercise stress testing. This discrepancy is difficult to explain in the light of our present knowledge.

This multicentric study reports neither the heart rate at the onset of ST-segment depression during exercise, nor the maximal heart rate tolerated by each patient without the development of ischemia. The calculation of an average value of heart rate at the onset of ischemia cannot provide adequate information on the prevalence of episodes caused by an important vasoconstrictor component. The apparently different effects of propranolol and diltiazem on painful and painless episodes are also difficult to interpret. On placebo, the average number of anginal attacks per week was only 2.3; variations in a few patients having a large number of attacks might, therefore, have skewed the results, because the mean is influenced by the frequency with which, during daily life, some patients exercised beyond the ischemic threshold. (Average values are useful to identify the effects of treatment in the presence of measurement inaccuracies and biological variabilities, only when the patients included in the study and the causes of ischemic episodes are homogeneous. When this is not the case, average values may be skewed by the behavior of a few patients with a large number of episodes that can be caused either by severe effort or by episodic coronary vasoconstriction.) It is also probable that the 43% reduction in anginal attacks per week observed during both propranolol and diltiazem treatment might not differ statistically from the corresponding 57 and 17% reductions in ischemic episodes per 24 h.

These results show that the average results of anti-ischemic drugs cannot be correctly interpreted unless patients and ischemic episodes are grouped, prospectively, into homogeneous subsets and unless the prevalence of different causes of ischemia is taken into consideration.[25]

The benefits obtained with drug therapy vary in relation to the prevailing causes of ischemic episodes in the patients under consideration. For ischemic episodes caused exclusively by an excessive increase of myocardial demand, it is unreasonable to expect beneficial effects from drugs that reduce only coronary vasomotor tone, and the rational medical treatment is represented by drugs that allow the heart to work more economically. The efficacy of these drugs in preventing ischemia caused by an excessive increase of myocardial demand is best assessed by standardized exercise stress testing and by checking that the persistence of angina during daily life is not attributable to the fact that patients exercise more vigorously.

Conversely, it is inadequate to use exercise stress testing to assess the efficacy of drugs that prevent ischemia by reducing coronary vasomotor tone, for two reasons. First, evidence of a substantial limitation of residual coronary flow reserve by increased coronary vasomotor tone during standardized exercise testing can be observed in only about one-third of patients with chronic stable angina.[1] Second, during unrestricted daily life, only some episodes occur at values of heart rate and heart rate/blood pressure product similar to those at which ischemia develops during the exercise test, suggesting that the modulation of residual coronary flow reserve by coronary vasoconstriction is much more prevalent during daily life than during standardized exercise testing.

The inclusion of painless ST-segment episodes in the assessment of the anti-ischemic efficacy of drugs would improve the statistical analysis of the results when they represent ischemia, as the number of painless episodes is usually much greater than that of painful episodes. Furthermore, ECG-documented episodes can be better quantified in terms of severity and duration of ischemia than those recorded in angina diaries.

The benefits obtained by successful PTCA and CABG in patients with positive exercise stress tests and positive Holter monitoring are dramatic, as ischemic episodes either disappear completely or are greatly reduced soon after revascularization.[26,27]

Improvement in survival

The improvement in survival is easily assessed in those groups of patients with a poor prognosis, but infarction and death are relatively rare in patients with chronic stable angina. The beneficial effect of medical therapy on prognosis is, therefore, commonly inferred from its ability to prevent or reduce the number of episodes of myocardial ischemia (painful or painless) objectively documented by exercise stress testing and ambulatory monitoring, but conclusive evidence that their prevention improves prognosis is still lacking.

It is possible that the improvement in prognosis observed in those patients on chronic treatment with β-blockers and calcium antagonists who had suffered an acute MI could be related to the protective effect of the drugs at the time that such patients suddenly became unstable and/or developed severe ischemia or infarction, rather than to the antianginal effects of the drugs during the stable phase.

The effects of CABG on prognosis are obvious in patients with a markedly reduced rate of survival, typically those who can exercise for less than 6 min on a Bruce protocol or who present marked ST-segment depression (see Fig. 17.8).[28] They are difficult to assess in individuals with only a moderate reduction of life expectancy.

Quality of life

The quality of life represents a major aspect of the disease for patients with a good prognosis. Improvement in the quality of life should be assessed not only on the basis of the ability of the patient to sustain normal activities without symptoms but also on the basis of the inconvenience caused by the treatment and the emotional impact of the disease. In patients with mild symptoms and a good prognosis, a physician who knows and follows the patient in time would be the best individual to assess the balance between preventive strategies and quality of life. Fear of the disease should not be used to increase the compliance of patients with regard to controlling their risk factors, as this may cause anxiety and impair the quality of life.

17.4.2 Treatment for the relief of symptoms

The simplest treatment that relieves symptoms without causing inconvenience to the patient should be adopted. As treatment of each individual patient with chronic stable angina is, by definition, a long-term strategy, there are ample opportunities to titrate the doses of different drugs and to assess the beneficial or side effects before opting for the most efficacious and best tolerated. The first choice of treatment should be based on some rational guidelines, broadly outlined below according to the classification defined in 17.2.5. The successive empirical administration of different types of drugs (even those discarded initially on theoretical grounds) at increasing doses is acceptable in order to control symptoms and signs of myocardial ischemia.

Lowering myocardial oxygen consumption

Lowering resting myocardial oxygen consumption and, hence, resting CBF, by reducing heart rate, contractility, ventricular volume, and afterload, increases the available residual coronary flow reserve. A more economic pattern of ventricular pump function increases the amount of

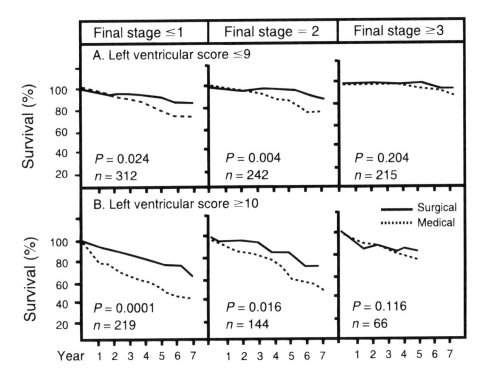

Fig. 17.8 The most significant improvement of survival with CABG occurs in patients with a poor effort tolerance. In the CASS study survival was not improved significantly by surgery (——) in patients who could exercise up to and beyond stage 3 of the Bruce protocol, regardless of the results of the test, a history of MI or angiographic findings. (**A**) shows patients with preserved left ventricular function. (**B**) shows patients with severe left ventricular dysfunction. The greatest improvement was seen in patients with severe left ventricular dysfunction who could exercise only up to stage 1 and had a poor life expectancy. Thus, an improved prognosis may be even more difficult to demonstrate in patients who can exercise longer than stage 3, have no previous history of MI and have a normal test result, because they have a good life expectancy. (·······, medically treated patients.) (Modified from ref. 28.)

physical effort that can be performed without exceeding the maximal residual coronary flow reserve. An increased residual coronary flow reserve and a more economic pattern of cardiac work also reduce the chance that occasional transient subliminal reductions of coronary flow reserve will cause ischemia, as demand is consistently lower. Lowering myocardial oxygen consumption may, therefore, be expected to reduce the number of ischemic episodes resulting not only from increased myocardial demand alone, but also from a simultaneous subliminal reduction of coronary flow reserve, a subliminal increase of myocardial oxygen demand, and a small reduction of resting flow. In contrast, lowering myocardial demand cannot be expected to prevent episodes caused by efforts well above residual coronary flow reserve or by a reduction of coronary flow well below resting levels (see Fig. 16.3).

Preventing episodes of coronary vasoconstriction

Prevention of episodic inappropriate coronary vasoconstriction would allow residual coronary flow reserve to remain constantly at its maximum, which is set by the balance between the limitation of flow caused by atherosclerotic coronary artery obstructions and the collateral circu-

lation. Rational treatment should prevent the episodic increase of vasomotor tone in the segment of coronary bed in which it takes place. However, as the causes of vasoconstriction are
multiple, involve different coronary segments, and are still unknown at present, ischemic
episodes can be prevented only by drugs, such as nitrates and calcium antagonists, that
reduce vascular smooth muscle tone nonspecifically. Prevention of local episodic coronary
vasoconstriction by a generalized sustained reduction of vascular smooth muscle tone does
not represent an optimal form of therapy. The effect of these drugs may be insufficient to inhibit completely occasional strong local stimuli or a local enhanced constrictor response, as occasionally observed in some patients with variant angina (see Ch. 20); moreover, in patients with
chronic stable angina, the causes of coronary constriction seem to differ from those responsible for occlusive spasm in variant angina (see Chs 9 and 20); the ability of calcium antagonists
to prevent coronary vasoconstriction in the former may, therefore, be less than in the latter.
The ability of calcium antagonists and nitrates to prevent small coronary vessel constriction
seems limited. In addition, coronary vasodilators cannot prevent episodes of ischemia caused
exclusively by increased demand.

In patients in classes I and II, groups A or B, deemed to be at low risk and, therefore, with
no immediate indications for PTCA or CABG to improve their prognoses, the first line of
medical treatment is determined by their pattern of angina.

For the very rare patient with only fixed, predictable effort-related angina, prophylactic
sublingual nitrates can be the first line of treatment, if this form of therapy prevents symptoms and allows the patient to lead a normal life. Typical doses are isosorbide dinitrate
(ISDN) (2.5 or 5 mg) and sublingual glyceryl trinitrite (GTN) or GTN spray taken before
exercising. In addition, β-blockers are the sustained therapy of first choice (typically atenolol
100 mg upon waking).

For patients with mixed chronic stable angina and a very variable threshold, but with a
maximal residual coronary flow reserve adequate for their daily activities, the treatment of
choice is coronary vasodilators, either calcium antagonists or nitrates. Typical starting doses
could be diltiazem retard preparation (R) (120 mg twice a day), verapamil R (120 mg twice
a day), nifedipine R (20 mg twice a day), and, if there is no history of nocturnal angina,
ISDN R (20 mg), mononitrate (10 mg), upon waking and after lunch, or percutaneous
nitroglycerin patches upon waking to be removed after dinner (in order to allow a nitrate-
free period and, thus, to avoid tolerance). The final choice is based on the improvement of
symptoms and on the side effects of the first line of therapy.

When the first line of treatment is insufficient to prevent angina, the doses should be
increased until side effects appear; calcium antagonists and nitrates should then be added
in patients with fixed threshold angina, and β-blockers in those with variable threshold angina. In the absence of side effects, full doses can be represented by atenolol (150 mg, i.e. one
and a half tablets) or diltiazem or verapamil (120 mg, four times a day). As a combination
therapy, atenolol (100 mg) can be carefully tried in association with nifedipine R (20 mg)
or with diltiazem R or verapamil R (120 mg, twice a day) plus long-acting nitrates in the
morning. A trial with these doses is indicated before considering revascularization procedures.

In patients in classes III and IV, groups A or B, with a low, fixed, or variable anginal threshold and very reduced coronary flow reserve, combination therapy of coronary dilators and
β-blockers is indicated while revascularization procedures are being considered (see above).

In patients in group C with impaired ventricular function and who are not candidates for
PTCA or CABG, anti-ischemic drugs that can further impair ventricular function should
be used judiciously, increasing the dose very gradually under careful monitoring of left ven-

tricular function. Nitrates are the therapy of first choice. These patients are also the most likely to benefit from revascularization procedures because of their inceased baseline risk.

When symptoms improve, consideration should be given to the possibilities that the patient may have entered into a quiescent phase of IHD, that they may have limited their daily activities, and/or that the ischemic episodes may have become predominantly asymptomatic. If there is any doubt, the apparent improvement should be confirmed objectively by a formal exercise test while treatment is continuing. If this is negative, a further exercise test should be performed while treatment is withdrawn, in order to assess residual coronary flow reserve. Holter monitoring may also be used to assess the possible persistence of asymptomatic ischemic episodes.

17.4.3 Treatment for the improvement of prognosis

In asymptomatic or scarcely symptomatic patients, treatment aimed only at improving prognosis should be proportional to the estimated reduction of total and event-free life expectancy, to its anticipated benefit in terms of increased life expectancy and reduced risk of infarction, and to the overall risk of complications, inconvenience, and cost relative to the treatment itself.

With the exception of those patients with previous MI and impaired left ventricular function who have ischemia at low or moderate work loads, the estimated risk of stable patients is low. Correcting known risk factors by adopting a healthier lifestyle, maintaining a stable psychological balance, improving dietary habits, taking recreational physical exercise, and reducing weight, when appropriate, should be recommended to each patient as the first, very basic, steps towards improving not only their prognosis but also the quality of their lives. Aspirin (75 mg a day after a meal) should also be prescribed for each patient, unless contraindicated (see Ch. 13).

As discussed above, prognosis is improved by surgery in patients with markedly positive exercise stress tests and/or low effort tolerance and impaired ventricular function. However, in patients who developed less than 1 mm ST-segment depression (independent of duration) or who could exercise longer than 6 min on the Bruce protocol (independent of results), the prognosis at 7 years is so good that it cannot be detectably improved by surgery. Therefore, those patients with no history of MI, with a normal resting ECG, and who can exercise longer than 6 min without signs of ischemia, should have an even better prognosis and are not candidates for CABG unless it is required to control symptoms.

A review of preliminary information from several randomized trials of PTCA compared with CABG and medical therapy in rather mixed groups of stable and unstable patients (i.e. the Randomized Intervention Treatment of Angina trial [RITA], the Veterans Administration study of Angioplasty Compared with Medicine [ACME], the Coronary Artery Bypass Revascularization Investigation [CABRI], the Emory Angioplasty Study Trial [EAST]) suggests that the differences in the results of treatments are not dramatic, except in the case of the severest forms of IHD (e.g. left main stenosis [more than 50% diameter] and proximal [more than 70% stenosis] triple-vessel disease) in which the best long-term survival results are provided by CABG. In addition, in patients who have double-vessel disease (including the left anterior descending [LAD] coronary artery), who are over the age of 65 and who have impaired left ventricular function, CABG provides improved survival compared with medical therapy. In other patients, the choice is between medicine and PTCA, with CABG reserved for those with large areas of myocardium at risk. The absolute improvement of survival (i.e. the number of lives saved out of the total of all patients treated) is greatest in those patients with an increased baseline risk (i.e. those over the age of 65 and with a reduced EF).[29]

In a conservative strategy, consideration of PTCA or CABG is mandatory for patients in whom medical therapy fails to improve symptoms and exercise stress test results adequately (so that patients remain in classes III or II), for patients in classes IV, III, or II who have signs of extensive ischemia, and for patients in group C with signs of ischemia at a low work load.

In an aggressive strategy, PTCA and CABG are more widely indicated on the assumption that they can substantially improve prognosis or the quality of life with acceptable complications.

CABG may be preferable to PTCA in patients with triple- or double-vessel disease, including a proximal LAD coronary artery stenosis. For patients with no obvious reduction of life expectancy and with mild symptoms and signs of ischemia and who have single- or double-vessel disease, the possible improvement in prognosis with arterial conduit CABG should be weighed against the increased risk of a second intervention being required should new coronary artery obstructions develop later in life.

The benefits of pharmacologic treatment should be weighed against potential side effects, cost, and the fact that therapy needs to be continued indefinitely. The benefits of interventional therapy, when not mandatory, should be considered by weighing the medical elements of the case against patients' fear of suffering an MI or succumbing to SICD unless "something is done" about their disease. Many patients are more amenable to the suggestion of a major intervention (which requires them to be a "hero" once) than to the suggestion that they change their lifestyle (thus requiring them to be a "saint" for ever).

■ *When considering interventional therapy, the anticipated success and risk of the procedure should be judged on the basis of the track record, in similar cases, of the center where the treatment will be carried out, rather than on reports in the literature.* ■

REFERENCES

1. Kaski JC, Tousoulis D, Pereira W, Crea F, Maseri A. Progression of complex coronary artery stenosis in patients with angina pectoris: its relation to clinical events. Cor Art Dis 1992;*3:*305.
2. Crake T, Tousoulis D, Kaski JK, Maseri A. Stability of symptoms in chronic angina pectoris in spite of severe coronary stenosis progression. Submitted for publication.
3. Moise A, Theroux P, Taeymans Y et al. Clinical and angiographic factors associated with progression of coronary artery disease. J Am Coll Cardiol 1984;*3:*659.
4. Friedberg CK. Diseases of the Heart, 3rd edition. Philadelphia, WB Saunders, 1966, p. 700.
5. Kaski JC, Rodriguez-Plaza L, Meran DO, Araujo L, Chierchia S, Maseri A. Improved coronary supply: prevailing mechanism of action of nitrates in chronic stable angina. Am Heart J 1985;*110:*238.
6. Crea F, Davies G, Chierchia S et al. Different susceptibility to myocardial ischemia provoked by hyperventilation and cold pressor test in exertional and variant angina pectoris. Am J Cardiol 1985;*56:*18.
7. Rosanski A, Bairey CN, Krantz DS et al. Mental stress and the induction of silent myocardial ischemia in patients with coronary artery disease. N Engl J Med 1988;*318:*1005.
8. Barry J, Selwyn AP, Nabel EG et al. Frequency of ST-segment depression produced by mental stress in stable angina pectoris from coronary artery disease. Am J Cardiol 1988;*61:*989.
9. Schang SJ, Pepine CJ. Transient asymptomatic ST-segment depression during daily activity. Am J Cardiol 1977;*39:*396.

10. Deanfield JE, Maseri A, Selwyn AP et al. Myocardial ischaemia during daily life in patients with stable angina: its relation to symptoms and heart rate changes. Lancet 1983;2:753.
11. Chierchia S, Gallino A, Smith G et al. Role of heart rate in the pathophysiology of chronic stable angina. Lancet 1984;2:1353.
12. Chierchia S, Balasubramanian V, Muiesan L et al. Transient impairment of coronary flow: a frequent cause of ischemia in chronic stable angina during daily life. J Am Coll Cardiol 1984;3:579.
13. Deedwania PC, Nelson JR. Pathophysiology of silent myocardial ischemia during daily life. Hemodynamic evaluation by simultaneous electrocardiographic and blood pressure monitoring. Circulation 1990;82:1296.
14. McLenachan JM, Weidinger FS, Barry J et al. The relationship between heart rate, ischemia and drug therapy during daily life in patients with coronary artery disease. Circulation 1991;83:1263.
15. Maseri A, Chierchia S, Kaski JC. Mixed angina pectoris. Am J Cardiol 1985;56:30E.
16. Pupita G, Kaski JC, Galassi AR, Vejar MJ, Crea F, Maseri A. Ischemic threshold varies in response to different types of exercise in patients with chronic stable angina. Am Heart J 1989;118:539.
17. Campeau L. Grading of angina pectoris (letter). Circulation 1976;54:522.
18. Fletcher GF, Froelicher VF, Hartley LH, Haskell WL, Pollock ML. Exercise standards. A statement for health professionals from the American Heart Association. Circulation 1990;82:2286.
19. Weiner DA, Ryan TJ, McCabe CH et al. Prognostic importance of a clinical profile and exercise test in medically treated patients with coronary artery disease. J Am Coll Cardiol 1984;3:772.
20. Bogaty P, Dagenais GR, Cantin B, Alain P, Rouleau JR. Prognosis in patients with a strongly positive exercise electrocardiogram. Am J Cardiol 1989;64:1284.
21. Deedwania PC, Carbajal EV. Silent ischemia during daily life is an independent predictor of mortality in stable angina. Circulation 1990;81:748.
22. Tzivoni D, Weisz G, Gavish A, Zin D, Keren A, Stern S. Comparison of mortality and myocardial infarction rates in stable angina pectoris with and without ischemic episodes during daily activities. Am J Cardiol 1989;63:273.
23. Rocco MB, Nabel EG, Campbell S et al. Prognostic importance of myocardial ischemia detected by ambulatory monitoring in patients with stable coronary artery disease. Circulation 1988;78:877.
24. Stone PH, Ware JH, DeWood MA et al. The efficacy of the addition of nifedipine in patients with mixed angina compared to patients with classic exertional angina: a multicenter, randomized, double-blind, placebo-controlled clinical trial. Am Heart J 1988;116:961.
25. Maseri A. Medical therapy of chronic stable angina pectoris. Editorial. Circulation 1990;82:2258.
26. Crea F, Kaski J, Fragasso G et al. Usefulness of Holter monitoring to improve the sensitivity of exercise testing in determining the degree of myocardial revascularization after coronary artery bypass grafting for stable angina pectoris. Am J Cardiol 1987;60:40.
27. Josephson MA, Nademanee K, Intarachot V, Lewis H, Singh B. Abolition of Holter monitor-detected silent myocardial ischemia after percutaneous transluminal coronary angioplasty. J Am Coll Cardiol 1987;10:499.
28. Weiner DA, Ryan TJ, McCabe CH et al. Value of exercise testing in determining the risk classification and the response to coronary artery bypass grafting in three-vessel coronary artery disease: a report from the Coronary Artery Surgery Study (CASS) Registry. Am J Cardiol 1987;60:262.
29. Department of Health and Human Services. Public Health Service. Agency for Health Care Policy and Research National Heart, Lung, and Blood Institute. Unstable angina: diagnosis and management. In: Clinical Practice Guideline, No. 10, 1994.

Syndrome X and microvascular angina

INTRODUCTION

This syndrome is characterized by episodes of angina (with features similar to those described by Heberden [see Ch. 14]), which recur chronically in the absence of angiographically detectable epicardial coronary artery stenoses, coronary artery spasm, or thrombosis. It manifests clinically with a pattern of chronic stable angina pectoris, often indistinguishable from that caused by organic epicardial coronary artery stenoses. The episodes usually occur during effort and on emotion, not infrequently with no apparent cause, but very seldom at night. Although the syndrome is very common, myocardial ischemia can be demonstrated convincingly in only a minority of patients. The diagnosis of myocardial ischemia is hampered because even the most typical anginal pain may not necessarily be caused by myocardial ischemia, because the specificity of ischemic ECG changes as indicators of transient myocardial ischemia in patients with a low pretest probability of having IHD is unknown, and because the sensitivity of diagnostic techniques for the detection of mild ischemia, or small areas of ischemia, is limited. Therefore, in patients in whom ischemia cannot be demonstrated, it may be difficult to establish whether the syndrome is caused by ischemia undetectable by currently available techniques, by nonischemic cardiac causes, or by noncardiac causes.

Until specific and practical diagnostic tests become available, the broad definition of syndrome X (which was introduced by Kemp in 1973),[1] should be maintained for all patients with a chronic type of angina requiring coronary angiography, in whom no fixed or dynamic flow-limiting obstructions can be detected. As indicated in Chapter 16, 10–50% of patients with angina pectoris severe enough to warrant angiography have no detectable flow-limiting coronary artery stenoses; what is not known, however, is the number of patients in whom angina pectoris is caused by coronary microvascular alterations, by other cardiac causes, or by noncardiac causes.

For patients in whom diagnostic ischemic ST-segment changes are documented during pain, a cardiac, although not necessarily an ischemic, origin of symptoms can be assumed (but the absence of ST-segment changes does not imply that a cardiac origin can be excluded).

In patients with regional myocardial perfusion abnormalities or abnormal coronary vasomotor responses, regardless of documented transient ischemic ST-segment changes, a coronary microvascular cause of symptoms can be assumed and the definition "microvascular angina" (proposed by Cannon and Epstein)[2] is appropriate; however, for patients in whom such abnormalities cannot be detected, similar causes cannot be excluded (see Fig. 18.1). Episodes of microvascular angina are usually not accompanied by detectable transient impairment of contractile function and, hence, are associated with either very limited, patchy ischemia or with no ischemia at all. Thus, the very common occurrence of episodes of anginal pain in the absence of detectable ischemia is a dominant feature of this syndrome and suggests that an increased perception of pain may be a fundamental component. The alterations responsible for microvascular angina can be multiple[3] and the percentage of patients with syndrome X in whom chronic anginal symptoms are caused by microvascular angina is not known.

This chapter defines the provisional diagnostic criteria for microvascular angina and its clinical features, discusses its pathophysiology, and provides some therapeutic guidelines.

18.1 DIAGNOSIS AND CLINICAL FEATURES

In patients with syndrome X, the diagnosis of microvascular angina requires some evidence of coronary microvascular dysfunction but not necessarily of myocardial ischemia. Also, for patients with no evidence of coronary microvascular dysfunction, a cardiac origin can be assumed when anginal pain is associated with transient ST-segment changes during induced or spontaneous anginal episodes, but it cannot be excluded when such changes are absent. The positivity of ECG exercise stress testing (which is a common inclusion criteria in many studies), is useful to narrow the possible causes of syndrome X to cardiac abnormalities, but a negative stress test can exclude neither a cardiac nor even an ischemic cause. The currently known clinical features of the syndrome are derived from various studies, some of which included incompletely characterized groups of patients. An outline of the general diagnostic principles and the main clinical features of the syndrome is also useful for a better evaluation of the variable results of pathophysiologic studies.

18.1.1 Diagnosis of microvascular angina

The sequential diagnostic steps to be followed are those outlined for the diagnosis of chronic stable angina, beginning with history and exercise stress testing (see Ch. 17). Patients with a negative maximal exercise test would not normally be submitted to coronary angiography and the differential diagnosis should be made with the other causes of noncardiac chest pain (see Ch. 16).

The demonstration of myocardial ischemic changes on the ECG may represent an indication for coronary arteriography and, when no fixed or dynamic flow-limiting obstructions in epicardial coronary arteries are evident, microvascular angina can be suspected. The diagnosis can be confirmed when myocardial scintigraphy or microvascular coronary vasomotor responses are clearly abnormal, but it cannot be excluded when the results are negative, because of the limited sensitivity of available diagnostic techniques.

When angina occurs in patients with a demonstrable coronary microvascular dysfunction, the diagnosis of microvascular angina is correct if pain is the result of the dysfunction, even when the microvascular alteration does not cause ischemia (see below).

Clinical diagnosis

In patients presenting with a mixed type of chronic stable angina, microvascular angina can be suspected clinically when pain lasts 10 min or longer after interruption of effort and

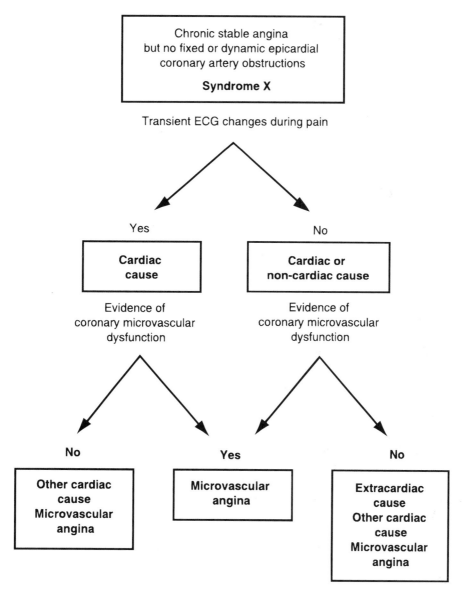

Fig. 18.1 Diagnostic classification. Patients with chronic stable angina, but no flow-limiting stenoses, with symptoms severe enough to warrant coronary arteriography are defined as *syndrome X*. (Patients with variant angina due to occlusive epicardial coronary artery spasm should be excluded.) The association of transient ECG changes with anginal pain indicates a cardiac origin of pain, but the absence of such changes cannot exclude a cardiac origin because of the low sensitivity of the ECG. Patients with evidence of a coronary microvascular dysfunction can be diagnosed as having *microvascular angina* even in the absence of detectable signs of ischemia (see text). When neither a microvascular dysfunction nor ischemia can be demonstrated they cannot be excluded because of the low sensitivity of available techniques for detecting patchily distributed ischemia and perfusion abnormalities.

when it responds inconsistently to sublingual nitrates. However, before arteriography, some patients cannot be distinguished from those having obstructive lesions of the epicardial coronary arteries. They can, however, be distinguished from patients with variant angina who typically report angina occurring spontaneously in the early hours of the morning or during the night, with a preserved effort tolerance and a prompt response to nitrates. They are also, usually, easily distinguishable from patients with unstable angina because of the chronic recurrence of their chest pain which, although often prolonged, has recurred with a stable pattern over periods of months or years. Only two-thirds of patients with positive exercise stress tests can be separated from those with flow-limiting coronary stenoses using a combination of ECG parameters,[4] but the failure of nitrates to improve the results of exercise stress testing was reported as being predictive of a normal coronary arteriogram.[5]

Demonstration of coronary microvascular alterations

Coronary microvascular alterations may be detected by positive myocardial scintigraphy, an abnormal response to coronary vasomotor stimuli, and a reduced coronary flow response.

Positive exercise myocardial scintigraphy in patients with syndrome X is a demonstration of a regional coronary microvascular dysfunction but, in this syndrome, the diagnostic sensitivity and specificity of the technique are unknown. Thus, a positive diagnosis is more reliable when regional perfusion defects are obvious and reproducible than when they are mild and not reproducible in successive tests.

An abnormal response to vasomotor stimuli includes positive dipyridamole and ergonovine tests. In patients with syndrome X, the dipyridamole test (0.5–0.8 mg/kg injection i.v. over 4–10 min) should be considered positive for microvascular angina when it reproduces the usual anginal pain, in association with transient ECG changes (indicative of the pain having a cardiac origin), even in the absence of ventricular wall motion abnormalities (see 18.2.1). In patients with syndrome X and no evidence of epicardial coronary artery spasm, the ergonovine test (up to 0.5 mg i.v.) should also be considered positive when it reproduces the usual pain, in association with even minor transient ST-segment depression or T-wave changes on the ECG (indicative of the pain having a cardiac origin).

Positive responses to these vasomotor stimuli indicate that the pain is due to a vasomotor abnormality, which can be considered to be coronary when associated with transient ECG changes. As indicated above, the absence of such changes during pain does not allow a cardiac origin to be ruled out, because of the limited sensitivity of the ECG. The vasomotor alterations may or may not cause detectable myocardial ischemia (see below).

A reduced coronary flow response to either pacing-induced tachycardia or dipyridamole is an indication of a microvascular origin when it occurs in association with the patient's usual pain and/or is associated with transient ischemic ST-segment depression, as patients with confirmed microvascular angina may have both painful and painless episodes of "ischemic" ST-segment depression.

Although an inadequate flow response has been observed in several studies (see 18.2.1), its diagnostic application is limited by the following:

a. the lack of adequate normal reference values
b. the possibility of a very unevenly distributed vascular dysfunction, or of an occasional dynamic, rather than fixed, dysfunction, or of a dysfunction predominant in a vascular bed distinct from that explored
c. the considerable inaccuracies of available methods for measuring coronary blood flow (CBF).

Detection of myocardial ischemia

The detection of myocardial ischemia is not an essential element in the diagnosis of microvascular angina, not only because the coronary microvascular dysfunction may cause anginal pain even without ischemia (see 18.2.2) but also because of the limited sensitivity of techniques available for detecting the mild or patchy distribution of myocardial ischemia resulting from a coronary microvascular abnormality.

Limited sensitivity. When ischemia is caused either by a flow-limiting stenosis or by occlusive epicardial coronary artery spasm, the 12-lead ECG may be normal even when signs of ischemia are detectable by regional myocardial scintigraphy or by ventricular wall motion abnormalities, particularly when occurring in the dorsal left ventricular wall. The ECG is not the only diagnostic tool to have a limited capacity for detecting mild or patchily distributed ischemia: myocardial scintigraphy, coronary sinus sampling, and tests for wall motion abnormalities are all also limited.

When ischemia is caused by a flow-limiting stenosis, occlusive spasm, or thrombosis of a major epicardial coronary artery, it involves evenly the whole myocardium distal to the stenosed vessel (although the subendocardial layers are involved to a greater extent). In contrast, when ischemia is caused by small vessel dysfunction not only may it have a very patchy distribution but also it may not be confined to a single vascular bed. In addition, unevenly distributed ischemia may be compensated for by increased flow and function of the interposed unaffected regions. Thus, myocardial scintigraphy can detect regional perfusion defects only when the microvascular abnormality is sufficiently uniform in its involvement of a large segment of the ventricular wall. Coronary sinus measurements can detect ischemic metabolites only when the blood drains from a homogeneously ischemic territory, because high flow from nonischemic areas dilutes the ischemic metabolites from low-flow ischemic regions. Ventricular wall motion abnormalities can also be detected only when ischemia uniformly involves a sufficiently large section of myocardial wall, as indicated in Chapter 7 (a 25% reduction of subendocardial flow caused by a flow-limiting stenosis results in only a 10% reduction of systolic thickening of the ischemic myocardium).

Limited specificity. Transient ST-segment depression during pain, although indicating a cardiac origin, may not represent myocardial ischemia as it can also be caused by ventricular repolarization alterations attributable to extracellular accumulation of adenosine and potassium ions, or by alterations of the autonomic nervous systems (see below). Furthermore, regional defects observed in exercise myocardial scintigraphy, although indicative of a perfusion abnormality, may not necessarily represent myocardial ischemia as, in patients with syndrome X, they are observed more frequently than transient regional wall motion abnormalities (see 18.2.1).

18.1.2 Clinical features

Under the broad definition of syndrome X, some studies have included a variety of patients with angina and normal coronary arteries, some of whom, however, may have had a noncardiac origin of symptoms. The inclusion of patients with a noncardiac origin of pain can be avoided by selecting patients with transient ECG changes occurring during either spontaneous or induced anginal episodes, but the presence of coronary microvascular alterations (not necessarily causing ischemia) can be demonstrated only by reversible perfusion defects detected during myocardial scintigraphy, or by an abnormal coronary vasomotor response (within the diagnostic limitations defined above). In order to reduce the possible sources of heterogeneity in the groups studied, most investigators excluded patients with any form of cardiomyopathy, a reduced ejection fraction (EF), myocardial hypertrophy, and a history of hypertension.

The exclusion of patients with ventricular hypertrophy, arterial hypertension, and other cardiac diseases narrows the field of possible causes of the syndrome but, in these patients too, angina may be caused by some form of coronary microvascular dysfunction.[6] As indicated above, the selective inclusion of patients with some evidence of a cardiac alteration occurring during pain will exclude those who may have a noncardiac origin of pain, but will not necessarily include only (or all) patients with microvascular angina. This possibility is suggested by the observation that those patients with confirmed coronary microvascular dysfunction and ECG changes occurring during pain, and most of those with no detectable ECG changes during pain, have common clinical features.

Triggering mechanisms of anginal attacks

In many patients angina is precipitated by effort, often with an extremely variable threshold,[6,7] but it can also occur spontaneously at rest. Exercise stress testing often causes asymptomatic episodes of ischemic ST-segment depression, which are also frequently observed on Holter recordings. During Holter monitoring, 61% of episodes of ischemic ST-segment depression, with or without pain, were not associated with an increased heart rate greater than 10 bpm; in contrast, many episodes of tachycardia greater than that associated with ST-segment depression during exercise stress testing were not associated with ST-segment depression.[7]

Duration of pain

Most patients with ECG changes, but also those without, report prolonged episodes of angina. In a recent review by Kaski et al,[8] 35% of patients reported episodes lasting longer than 30 min. Many patients had been admitted to hospital on several occasions for severe prolonged episodes of chest pain, at times associated with minor ECG changes, but never with elevated indices of myocardial cell necrosis. (This paradox could also be a consequence of the fact that those who develop MI are then classified in the group of patients with MI and angiographically normal coronary arteries; the possible overlap between the two groups has not yet been explored.)

Discrepancy between severity of chest pain and signs of ischemia

In patients with variant angina and transmural myocardial ischemia, about 70% of ischemic episodes are painless; when pain is present, it usually follows by some minutes the onset of ECG changes and ventricular dysfunction. These observations contrast sharply with the occurrence of severe, prolonged anginal pain with diagnostic ischemic ECG changes in the absence of detectable ventricular dysfunction during the dipyridamole and exercise stress tests in patients with angiographically normal coronary arteriograms (see below).

Inconsistent response to sublingual nitrates

An inconsistent response to sublingual nitrates is not only a common clinical observation but is also reported in most studies; although some anginal attacks do wane within 2–5 min, others persist for 10–20 min in spite of two or three doses of sublingual nitrates. Pacing-induced ST-segment depression also is not improved by nitrates;[9] similarly, the results of exercise stress testing are not improved (and can even be exacerbated) by sublingual isosorbide dinitrate (ISDN),[5] which is in sharp contrast to results in patients with flow-limiting stenoses.

Persistence of symptoms with no major ischemic events

As summarized in recent reviews,[8,10,11] patients with normal ventricular function and no left bundle branch block have a good prognosis, although their symptoms can persist for years. In patients in whom ischemia has been documented objectively, or in whom a cardiac origin of pain has been demonstrated by ischemic ECG changes, the prognosis is not detectably different from the benign course of the larger group, which is characterized by angina and normal coronary angiograms and defined broadly as syndrome X. In one study, a minority of patients without left bundle branch block had a reduced EF during follow-up, but their symptoms and coronary vasomotor responses were indistinguishable from those in patients with a normal ECG and ventricular function.[12] Such patients may present a form of microvascular dysfunction similar to that proposed for some animal models of cardiomyopathy.[13]

In contrast to the benign long-term prognosis, the persistence of anginal symptoms and the poor response to available anti-ischemic therapy cause considerable anxiety that is only temporarily relieved by reassurance or even by a further normal coronary angiogram.[14–16] Anxiety may be a major component of the syndrome, but it is not yet clear whether it is only a consequence of the chronic recurrence of angina, or whether it is one of the pathogenetic components of an enhanced perception of pain and is responsible, in part, for the initiation of a vicious circle (see 18.2.2).

18.2 PATHOPHYSIOLOGY

The results of pathophysiologic studies in patients with syndrome X are conflicting: certain patients with myocardial lactate production or transient ventricular function abnormalities during exercise stress testing had chest pain but no ischemic ECG changes; others had ischemic ECG changes but no chest pain, whereas some with both ischemic ECG changes and chest pain had no myocardial lactate production or ventricular function abnormalities. Additional confounding elements are the presence, in the same patient, of some episodes of ischemic ST-segment depression during either exercise stress testing or Holter monitoring without angina, and of angina occurring in the absence of ischemic ST-segment depression. These discrepancies may be due to differences in the patient populations studied and in the methodology used, but they may also be related to individual differences in the pathogenetic components that make up the syndrome.

18.2.1 Review of pathophysiologic studies

It is useful to consider the results of well-documented observations in order to develop a plausible pathogenetic hypothesis:

a. the dissociation of angina from ST-segment depression during the dipyridamole test
b. the evidence of a reduced coronary flow response
c. the inconsistent detection of regional myocardial perfusion defects
d. the infrequent detection of myocardial ischemia

e. the very common absence of left ventricular dysfunction
f. the possibility of noncardiac or nonmicrovascular causes of anginal pain
g. the demonstration of an enhanced perception of pain.

Most of these studies were reviewed recently by Cannon et al[17] in an article entitled "Pathophysiological dilemma of syndrome X" and the most salient features of each of these lines of research are summarized below.

Dissociation of angina from ST-segment depression during the dipyridamole test

The response to the dipyridamole test is exemplified by two studies performed in carefully characterized patients with syndrome X and no evidence of hypertension or myocardial hypertrophy or dysfunction, which took into consideration the development of both angina and ischemic ST-segment depression during the dipyridamole and exercise stress tests.

In patients with a positive exercise stress test, dipyridamole caused diagnostic ST-segment depression in 76% at a low dose (0.56 mg/kg), and in 84% at a high dose (0.84 mg/kg). It caused angina in 69 and 68%, respectively, but angina and ST-segment depression developed together in only 59 and 58%, respectively, whereas certain patients had neither ECG changes nor angina, some had only angina, and others had only ECG changes. In contrast, in patients with negative exercise stress tests, dipyridamole caused diagnostic ST-segment depression and angina in 19 and 58%, respectively. The dipyridamole test caused angina more frequently than exercise stress testing in patients with diagnostic ST-segment depression during exercise (76 versus 45%), and even more frequently in those with no diagnostic ST-segment depression during exercise (58 versus 12%).[18,19] Conversely, high doses of dipyridamole caused chest pain less frequently than ST-segment depression in a group of asymptomatic hypertensive patients (8 versus 36%).[20]

The mechanisms of action of dipyridamole are related mainly to its inhibitory effect on adenosine uptake. The resulting increase of adenosine concentrations in the myocardial interstitium causes arteriolar dilation by stimulation of A_2 receptors, and pain by stimulation of A_1 receptors, which may also cause ST-segment changes by shortening the action potential of myocardial cells and by negative chronotropic effects.[21] Thus, the accumulation of adenosine following dipyridamole administration may cause pain and ST-segment changes directly by stimulating A_1 receptors, indirectly by producing ischemia due to transmural blood flow steal[22] and an unevenly distributed prearteriolar critical closing pressure,[23] or by a combination of the two. The same mechanisms may also operate during increased endogenous adenosine production due to enhanced myocardial metabolic activity.

The results of these studies confirm the known overlap of clinical findings between patients with positive and negative exercise stress tests, which may be related not only to different causes of symptoms but also to the presence and varying severity of the microvascular dysfunction at the time that the test took place. The ability of dipyridamole testing to cause ST-segment depression and angina, whatever their significance, in patients with syndrome X, is an indication that it is, in general, as potent as exercise when causing ST-segment depression and, possibly, even more potent when causing angina.

The incomplete agreement between the results of the two tests in the same patient, in terms of the development of ST-segment depression and angina, suggests that their mechanisms of action are not identical or that the severity of the underlying cardiac alteration varied at the time that the tests were performed (for example, exercise may cause paradoxical coronary artery constriction).

■ *The discrepancy between the appearance of ST-segment changes and angina observed in many patients suggests a possible dissociation between the mechanisms that cause ST-segment depression and those that cause angina. As dipyridamole testing caused angina more often than ST-segment depression in patients with syndrome X and negative exercise stress tests, and ST-segment depression more often than angina in asymptomatic hypertensive patients, syndrome X may be associated with an enhanced perception of pain.* ■

Reduced coronary flow response

The alterations in vasomotor response can be categorized as follows:

a. a reduced response to dipyridamole and other coronary dilator agents such as papaverine and adenosine
b. an abnormal response to acetylcholine
c. a decreased CBF in response to vasoconstrictor stimuli (such as ergonovine, cold pressor and hyperventilation testing)
d. a reduced CBF in response to pacing.

A markedly reduced coronary flow response to dipyridamole in patients with syndrome X compared with controls was first reported by Opherk et al,[24] using the argon method. A smaller increase of flow during pacing-induced stress was observed by Cannon et al[25] in patients who developed chest pain during the test, and also by Camici et al,[26] using the thermodilution method. Ergonovine (0.15 mg i.v.) caused an increase in coronary vascular resistance during the pacing test in 71% of patients, accompanied by increased myocardial oxygen extraction and the development of chest pain in 91%.[25] In contrast, pain developed in only 48% of patients without a vasoconstrictor response to ergonovine. Other provocative tests, such as hyperventilation and mental stress, were found to induce angina in patients with syndrome X associated with a reduction in CBF velocity.[27]

A reduced coronary flow response to dipyridamole assessed using ^{13}N-labeled ammonia and positron emission tomography (PET) was correlated to a positive ECG exercise stress test.[18] Other studies using PET showed a reduced flow response to dipyridamole in more patients with syndrome X than in controls,[28,29] but the differences could also be related to high levels of resting flow or to the imperfect matching of controls, as was suggested recently in a study performed using ^{15}O-labeled water and PET in a large number of patients and in age- and gender-matched controls.[30]

A reduced flow response to acetylcholine was observed in about 50% of patients with syndrome X, with and without histories of hypertension, and was correlated to the reduced response to pacing and associated with a diffuse constrictor response of epicardial coronary arteries in 10% of cases.[31] A reduced coronary flow response to intracoronary infusion of acetylcholine was also observed in groups of Caucasian[32] and Japanese patients,[33] but a normal flow response to papaverine and adenosine was reported in another study.[34]

Finally, an abnormal constrictor response of epicardial coronary arteries in patients with syndrome X was detected by coronary angiography, during exercise[35] and during testing with other vasoactive stimuli in some studies[36,37] but not in others.[27,38]

Overall, these studies indicate that some form of abnormal coronary response to various vasoactive stimuli is detectable in at least some patients with syndrome X. The development of angina during pacing, and particularly after ergonovine, associated with a low CBF response and increased myocardial oxygen extraction, suggests that an abnormal coronary flow response is a common component of the syndrome. The variability of the findings in the different reports may be attributable either to the inclusion of patients with varying degrees of persisting coronary vasomotor dysfunction at the time of the study (as opposed to an occasionally triggered vasoconstriction) or to a varied prevalence of patients with different pathogenetic mechanisms in the populations studied (such as patchily increased basal tone, selective abnormal constrictor or dilator response, or variable enhancement of the perception of pain).

Inconsistent detection of regional myocardial perfusion defects

Regional myocardial perfusion defects are commonly detected in patients with syndrome X during exercise stress testing. The highest percentage was observed during stress thallium-201 myocardial perfusion scintigraphy in a study of 100 consecutive patients who had both normal coronary arteries and angina: 98 patients had detectable perfusion defects but only 30 had positive ECG evidence of ischemia during the effort.[39]

The fairly common finding of perfusion defects detected by myocardial scintigraphy is in sharp contrast to the failure to detect regional perfusion abnormalities in PET studies using ^{18}N-labeled ammonia or ^{15}O-labeled water during either the dipyridamole or pacing tests.[18,28,29] As ^{15}N-labeled ammonia kinetics are similar to those of thallium, this discrepancy could be due only to differences either in the provocative test and scintigraphic technique used, or in the patient population. An increased variability of regional myocardial perfusion was reported in only one study that analyzed very small regions of interest.[29]

The report of regional perfusion defects in exercise thallium-201 myocardial scintigraphy seems too common to be considered a methodologic artifact and suggests that some patients with syndrome X have regionally segmental coronary perfusion abnormalities. Unfortunately, no evidence exists to confirm convincingly that such perfusion abnormalities can be reproduced in successive studies. The failure of PET to detect regional myocardial perfusion defects during dipyridamole and pacing tests indicates that both ST-segment depression and angina can occur in the absence of detectable regional perfusion abnormalities, which may be unevenly distributed throughout the walls of the left ventricle or be absent altogether. Alternatively, the maximal exercise stress testing used in thallium-201 studies is a more powerful stimulus for causing detectable differences in segmental myocardial perfusion.

Detection of myocardial ischemia

Myocardial lactate production was detected during pacing stress testing in some patients in studies carried out several years ago,[24,40,41] but in none of the patients included in a recent study,[26] although in a substantial proportion of cases the flow response to pacing was reduced compared with controls. Lactate production following intracoronary infusion of papaverine in patients with syndrome X (but not in controls), reported in a recent study,[33] may not necessarily be indicative of ischemia.[42] Major limitations in the assessment of myocardial ischemia from measurements of coronary arteriovenous differences in lactate production have previously been indicated by Gertz et al.[43] These complexities are compounded with those derived from the need to sample the venous blood draining the ischemic territory, and with those derived from the possible heterogeneity of perfusion and ischemia in the myocardium from which samples are taken. However, myocardial ischemia was demonstrated convincingly in an elegant study in which coronary sinus oxygen saturation was shown to decrease progressively during incremental pacing, as typically observed in patients with flow-limiting stenoses (see Fig. 18.2).[44] Besides providing convincing evi-

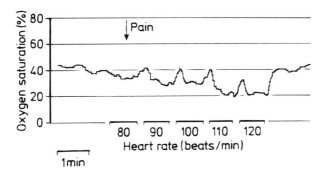

Fig. 18.2 Ischemia caused by pacing in syndrome X. A progressive drop in coronary sinus oxygen saturation developed during pacing-induced tachycardia. This response was observed in 2/10 patients who developed sufficiently extensive ischemia in the myocardial territory drained by the great cardiac vein. The ↓ indicates when pain appeared, but it was not associated with ST-segment changes, further demonstrating the low sensitivity of the ECG for detecting ischemia. (Modified from ref 44.)

dence of an inadequate coronary flow response to pacing associated with the development of pain, this study showed that, in patients with syndrome X, ECG changes may fail to occur, even when the signs of ischemia and angina were obvious.

Thus, detectable myocardial ischemia does develop in at least a minority of patients with syndrome X. Some of the differences between early and more recent studies may be due to the inclusion, in early studies, of patients with more severe degrees of coronary microvascular dysfunction as, in recent years, the indications for coronary arteriography have widened considerably, in general leading to the study of less severe forms of the disease. Alternatively, the pathogenetic mechanisms of the syndrome may vary among patients included in the different studies.

Left ventricular function studies

The results of left ventricular function studies performed during exercise, pacing, and dipyridamole testing are also conflicting. Radionuclide angiography performed during graded supine bicycle exercise was abnormal (with no change or fall in left ventricular EF) in 34, 53 and 63% of 136 patients with syndrome X and evidence of coronary microvascular dysfunction who had normal exercise stress tests, ST-segment depression, or left bundle branch block, respectively. Conversely, ventricular contractile abnormalities were noted in only 12% of 56 patients with no evidence of coronary microvascular dysfunction.[45] No alterations in left ventricular function were detected by cross-sectional echocardiography during the dipyridamole test[19] or at the end of the exercise stress test.[46] A "hyperdynamic state" was suggested both by a reduction in left ventricular diastolic pressure during the pacing test and by a high EF.[26] This finding is supported by the report of a high EF at rest (see Fig. 18.3A,B)[47] and by a decrease in end-diastolic pressure during pacing associated with reduced myocardial oxygen consumption, and is suggestive of a greater mechanical efficiency of the ventricular pump function.[26]

Thus, the opposing findings observed in different studies of the behaviour of left ventricular EF and filling pressure all suggest that there is a considerable heterogeneity among patients presenting with similar clinical features.

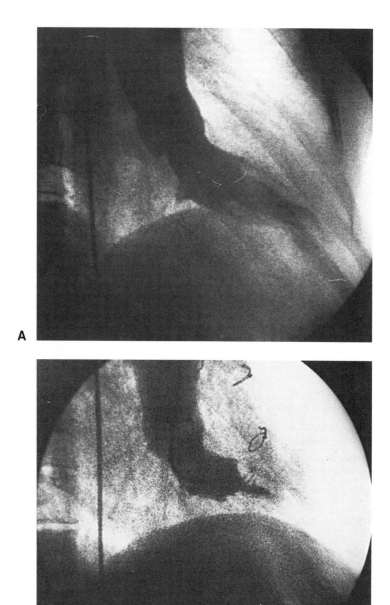

A

B

Fig. 18.3 Ventriculogram of a patient diagnosed retrospectively as having microvascular angina. The patient had disabling chronic stable angina and an exercise stress test positive at 6 min. Angiography, first performed in 1972, showed no flow-limiting stenoses and an EF of 75%. A second angiogram, performed in 1974 because of persisting symptoms, showed <50% stenosis in the mid-LAD coronary artery and an EF of 80%. The patient elected to have CABG because of the severity of his symptoms, but they did not improve. Angiography, repeated again in 1976 because of worsening effort-induced angina, showed normal patency of the graft, no new stenosis and an EF of 85%. End-diastolic (**A**) and end-systolic (**B**) frames are shown. Multiple echocardiograms failed to show any evidence of hypertrophic cardiomyopathy. The patient remained symptomatic, unresponsive to any medical therapy, for a further 10 years, when he died from a malignancy. As reported in ref. 50 a similar ventriculographic picture is common in patients with microvascular angina.

Noncardiac or nonmicrovascular causes of angina

In the search for the causes of angina in patients with syndrome X, those with no evidence of a cardiac origin of pain should be separated from those in whom pain has a demonstrable cardiac origin.

In patients with no evidence of cardiac alterations associated with the development of angina, the cause of angina severe enough to require coronary arteriography may be noncardiac. In the search for a noncardiac explanation, esophageal causes have been proposed and found in up to 60% of patients.[48–52] Any plausible explanation can be extremely helpful when it comes to reassuring patients, but the discovery of a possible extracardiac cause of angina cannot be taken as scientific proof that it represents the only, or the major, cause of symptoms. For example, reduced coronary flow velocity following esophageal exposure to hydrochloric acid was observed in the absence of epicardial coronary artery constriction.[53] The observation of coronary vasoconstriction caused by esophageal stimulation is consistent with similar findings in patients with coronary artery stenoses[54] and also with long-standing animal experiments.[55] Moreover, Cannon et al[56] found that 36% of patients with syndrome X had abnormal esophageal and cardiac test results and that 85% had the same type of chest pain during cardiac and esophageal testing. Although the studies reported above included a varying mixture of both patients with and without ECG changes during angina, they indicate that cardiac and noncardiac causes of angina may coexist in the same patient and suggest the possibility of a generalized abnormal visceral perception of pain.

In patients with transient ECG changes during angina, although the cause of pain is cardiac it may not necessarily be due to ischemia or to a coronary microvascular dysfunction.

Poole-Wilson proposed the hypothesis that an altered function of the cellular potassium pump could result in an uneven accumulation of potassium in the myocardial interstitium during increased metabolic activity, with consequent ST-segment depression and possibly anginal pain.[57] This hypothesis does not explain the frequent occurrence of perfusion abnormalities or the occasional detection of ischemia; neither does it explain easily the episodes of angina occurring at rest in the absence of increased heart rate, or the prompt relief of pain by sublingual nitrates observed at least in some episodes in a majority of patients.

Rosano et al[58] suggested that a reduced affinity of adenosine for A_2 vasodilator receptors and an enhanced affinity for A_1 receptors could explain the reduced coronary vasodilator response to the pacing and dipyridamole tests, as well as the appearance of angina and ST-segment depression. The hypothesis of reduced adenosine A_2 receptor activity does not fit the observed normal flow response to intracoronary adenosine.[34,59] The hypothesis of an enhanced affinity for A_1 receptors cannot be easily proved or disproved, but it explains neither the episodes of angina and/or silent ST-segment depression occurring at rest, with no increase in heart rate, nor the absence of angina and ST-segment depression during episodes of tachycardia occurring within a short space of time before or after episodes of angina and/or ST-segment depression. Additionally, it does not explain the relief of pain by nitrates reported by many patients, at least in some episodes.

Nonischemic metabolic alterations during pacing-induced tachycardia and angina were observed by Camici et al,[26] who reported myocardial extraction of alanine and release of pyrivate during the pacing test in syndrome X patients, a metabolic pattern differing from that observed in controls (but not compatible with acute myocardial ischemia) that so far remains unexplained.[60]

Alterations in myocytes, detected by electron microscopy, have been reported in two studies[24,61] (which included no adequate controls); however, these alterations may have been secondary to microvascular dysfunction.

Enhanced perception of pain

An increased sensitivity to, and decreased tolerance of, forearm tourniquet and electric skin stimulation were observed by Turiel et al in women with typical angina and normal coronary arteries compared with patients with coronary artery obstructions.[62] Other groups reported an exaggerated sensitivity to cardiac, potentially painful stimuli,[63,64] but also an overlap between increased sensitivity to cardiac and esophageal pain.[56] Thus, a generalized increase in somatic and visceral pain sensitivity seems to be a common feature in patients with syndrome X, but it is not known whether it is caused by an abnormal activation of pain receptors, by a defective gate control or by an exaggerated cortical decoding of afferent nervous stimuli as painful.

An enhanced perception of pain would explain the discrepancy between the common absence of detectable signs of ischemia and the presence of severe pain in these patients, putting them at the other extreme of the spectrum to those patients in whom severe myocardial ischemia and even infarction remain totally painless. An abnormal psychiatric background represented by panic disorders, anxiety neuroses, and neuroticism has been reported by several groups in patients with syndrome X and is considered to be an important component of an enhanced perception and a decreased tolerance of pain.[14–16,65–67]

18.2.2 Pathogenetic hypothesis

As Kemp wrote in 1973,[1] some observations in syndrome X "like the clues in the first half of Agatha Christie novels, may not be readily understandable, but we can be certain they are important." Distinguishing relevant from confounding clues is difficult; thus, a general working hypothesis on the pathogenetic mechanisms of microvascular angina must not only account for the salient common clinical features and the most prevalent findings of pathophysiologic studies but must also be compatible with the conflicting results of different reports.

The most salient clinical features of the syndrome are represented by the following:

a. a prolonged duration of pain with no detectable cardiac ischemic manifestations
b. the very variable anginal threshold and the common persistence of pain after interruption of effort
c. the very variable response to sublingual nitrates
d. the good long-term prognosis
e. the common unjustified anxiety about prognosis.

The most salient pathophysiologic findings are as follows:

a. the induction of angina and ST-segment depression by dipyridamole
b. the frequent episodes of ST-segment depression (with or without pain) not preceded by an increased heart rate during Holter monitoring
c. the evidence of microvascular dysfunction, which may, or may not, be associated with transient ECG changes
d. the discrepancy between anginal pain, ST-segment depression and detectable signs of myocardial ischemia
e. the enhanced perception of pain.

The most conflicting findings concern the variable prevalence of signs of both an abnormal coronary vasomotor response and ischemia.

■ *A most plausible explanation for the clinical features and pathophysiologic findings in patients with microvascular angina is provided by a pathogenetic hypothesis that considers the combination of two components—a coronary microvascular dysfunction and an enhanced perception of pain (often allied to a predisposing psychological background), (see Fig. 18.4). As indicated above, these mechanisms may operate also in those patients in whom a cardiac origin of angina cannot be demonstrated because of the low sensitivity of the diagnostic techniques available.* ■

Coronary microvascular dysfunction

A subepicardial prearteriolar constriction was proposed by Epstein and Cannon[22] because it could explain dipyridamole-induced angina by a mechanism of transmural blood flow steal (see Fig. 18.5). We extended this hypothesis[23] to include a prearteriolar vascular dysfunction that could operate in all myocardial layers across the thickness of the ventricular wall as a dysfunction of the physiologic distribution of coronary flow resistance in series (see Fig. 18.6).[68] A patchy, transmural distribution of prearteriolar constriction not only could limit CBF when myocardial demand increases but also could predispose to CBF steal within the same layers and to the critical closing pressure at the end of the most constricted prearterioles (when distending pressure becomes too low as a result of arteriolar dilation).

The causes of prearteriolar dysfunction may be multiple: they can result from a variable combination of persisting structural changes, endothelial dysfunction, smooth muscle hyperreactivity, and/or from occasional neurogenic or local autacoid-induced contrictor stimuli.

Myocardial ischemia may develop distal to the most constricted prearterioles as a result of a reduced coronary flow reserve due to persistent constriction when myocardial demand increases, of CBF steal and a critical closing pressure when arterioles dilate, for example during dipyridamole infusion or during increased metabolic activity, and/or of a sudden increase in constriction sufficient to reduce resting flow.

According to this extended hypothesis, angina and ST-segment depression can also develop in the absence of ischemia as a result of an enhanced release of adenosine distal to the most constricted prearterioles, when the degree of compensatory arteriolar dilation is sufficient to maintain adequate blood flow.

A patchy or confluent distribution of prearteriolar dysfunction associated with an enhanced perception of pain can account for the most salient clinical features and pathophysiologic findings discussed above.

Clinical features. The inconsistent relief of pain by sublingual nitrates can be explained by their varying capacity to relieve prearteriolar constriction. The very frequent occurrence of ischemic ST-segment depression without detectable ischemic manifestations may be explained by a very patchy distribution of elevated adenosine levels, with shortening of myocardial action potential and reduction of conduction velocity of the impulse. The long duration of pain may be explained by intense persistent prearteriolar constriction, with the possible development of a critical closing pressure and persistently high levels of adenosine. The long persistence of such alterations may be common because the hemodynamic effects of a very patchy distribution of coronary microvascular dysfunction differ greatly from those of a critical obstruction of a large coronary artery, which cause a uniform impairment of perfusion in the distal myocardial territory with a consequent progressive deterioration of cardiac function as a result of the multiple positive feedback mechanisms described in Chapter 7.

Pathophysiologic studies. The induction of angina by dipyridamole may be explained not only by the development of patchy areas of ischemia due to interarteriolar blood flow steal and a critical closing pressure at the end of the most constricted prearterioles, but also by the

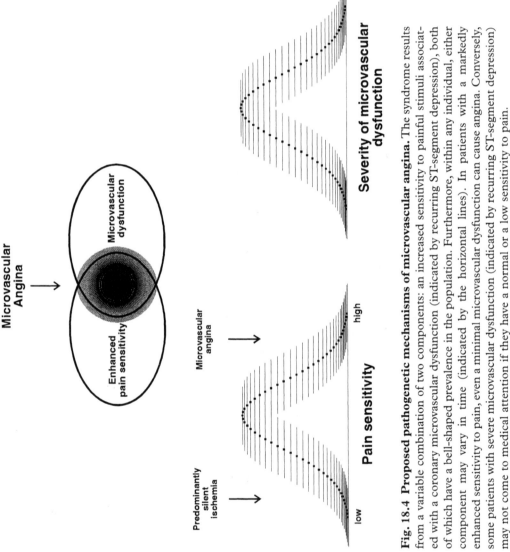

Fig. 18.4 Proposed pathogenetic mechanisms of microvascular angina. The syndrome results from a variable combination of two components: an increased sensitivity to painful stimuli associated with a coronary microvascular dysfunction (indicated by recurring ST-segment depression), both of which have a bell-shaped prevalence in the population. Furthermore, within any individual, either component may vary in time (indicated by the horizontal lines). In patients with a markedly enhanced sensitivity to pain, even a minimal microvascular dysfunction can cause angina. Conversely, some patients with severe microvascular dysfunction (indicated by recurring ST-segment depression) may not come to medical attention if they have a normal or a low sensitivity to pain.

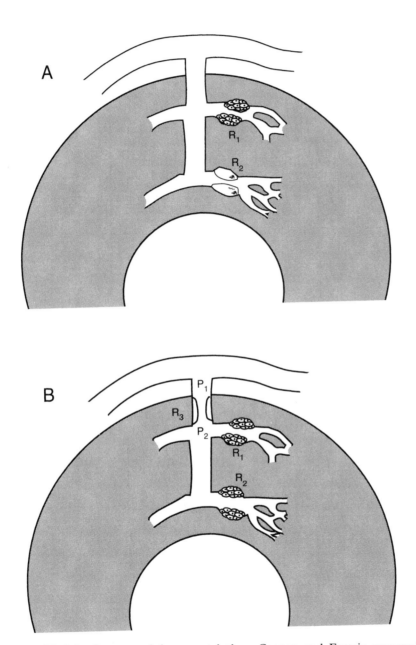

Fig. 18.5 Model of prearteriolar constriction. Cannon and Epstein proposed that, compared to normal (**A**), in patients with microvascular angina prearteriolar constriction occurs at a specific point, i.e. before subepicardial branches (**B**), causing a pressure drop ($P_2 < P_1$), which reduces coronary flow reserve in subendocardial layers and favors both transmural blood flow steal, in response to subepicardial arteriolar dilation, and a further drop of P_2. (Modified from ref. 22.)

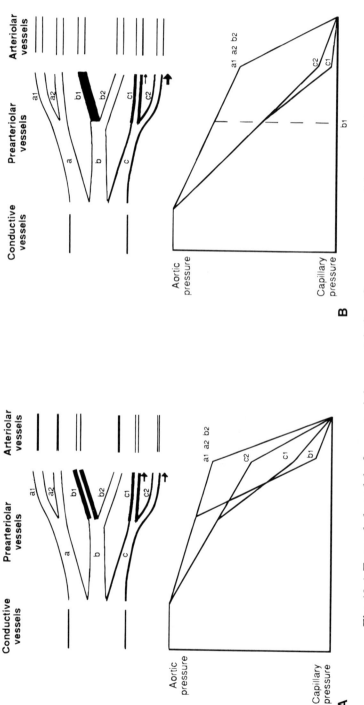

Fig. 18.6 Expanded model of prearteriolar constriction. Our group proposed that prearteriolar constriction could be patchily distributed in any myocardial layer. The regional reduction of coronary flow reserve is proportional to the severity of prearteriolar constriction and to the pressure drop at the origin of arterioles. Blood flow steal may also occur within the same myocardial layer distal to a constricted prearteriolar branching point (c). During arteriolar dilation and increase in flow, pressure at the end of prearteriolar vessels decreases further. Thus, distending pressure at the end of most constricted prearterioles may become lower than critical closing pressure (b_1). Compensatory release of adenosine distal to constricted prearterioles may be sufficient to maintain normal flow, avoiding ischemia, but, when persistent, it may cause stimulation of afferent receptors and pain when associated with an enhanced pain sensitivity. (Adapted from ref. 68.)

increased concentrations of adenosine distal to the most constricted prearterioles. The conflicting findings reported in myocardial scintigraphic and ventricular function studies, in myocardial lactate production and in the reduction of coronary flow responses to coronary dilator stimuli, can be explained by a variable confluence of the microvascular dysfunction within a segment of the myocardial wall explored. Very unevenly distributed prearteriolar abnormalities may be sufficient to cause angina and depression of the ST-segment, also in the absence of ischemia, as a result of activation of adenosine A_1 receptors and of release of adenosine and the consequent stimulation of pain receptors and local changes in action potential duration and impulse propagation. Only a confluent and regionally distributed alteration would result in a detectable reduction of coronary flow response, regional defects in myocardial scintigraphy, wall motion abnormalities, and myocardial lactate production.

A microvascular dysfunction with or without ischemic consequences can also explain the very common finding of transient silent episodes of ST-segment depression observed during Holter monitoring.

Possible causes. The microvascular dysfunction that contributes to cause the clinical syndrome is probably composed of multiple pathogenetic elements.[3] Prearteriolar dysfunction can be represented by organic structural changes and/or by persistent functional abnormalities, but the very variable anginal threshold and the common occurrence of anginal episodes at rest suggest that occasional constrictor stimuli, either neurogenic or induced by local autacoids, have a dominant role.

Structural changes of small arterial vessels in biopsy specimens were observed in some studies[3,69] but not in others.[24,61] Medial hypertrophy was observed in patients with myocardial hypertrophy and systemic hypertension.[3]

Persistent functional abnormalities include a defective endothelial production of nitric oxide (NO) and/or of other vasodilators or an enhanced smooth muscle response to physiologic constrictor stimuli.

A defective production of NO has been suggested on the basis of either a reduced dilator response or a constrictor response to acetylcholine in coronary[31–33,36] and peripheral vascular beds,[70] but these findings could also be explained by an enhanced constrictor response of the vascular smooth muscle to the direct constrictor effects of the drug. The lack of response to nitrates suggests that defective production of NO by vascular endothelium is not, in itself, a sufficient explanation because vessels with defective production of NO are hyperresponsive to exogenous nitrates (see Ch. 5). Finally, defective flow-mediated vasodilation would explain episodes occurring during increased myocardial demand, but not those occurring spontaneously at rest and not preceded by obvious changes in heart rate. Systemic alterations such as hypertension,[71] estrogen deficiency,[72] insulin resistance,[73] and a generalized enhanced constrictor response of the smooth muscle in different organs[74] could be associated with an abnormal coronary microvascular response.

With regard to *abnormal constrictor stimuli,* neurogenic stimuli could readily explain emotionally induced angina, although it could also result from an enhanced local vascular constrictor response to physiologic constrictor stimuli. Several studies have suggested the presence of an increased sympathetic tone in patients with syndrome X, as indicated by an increased heart rate during ambulatory ECG monitoring, by a rapid rise in heart rate and blood pressure at the very onset of exercise,[75] and by increased left ventricular contractility.[26,47] The sympathetic coronary vasoconstriction could be mediated either by an increased α-tone (although α-adrenergic blockers gave inconsistent results—see ahead) or by neuropeptide Y (NPY), which is predominantly distributed in coronary vessels smaller than 0.5 mm in diameter (see Chs 5 and 6).

Local autacoids, such as endothelin (which in dogs was shown to constrict selectively small coronary vessels not visible angiographically; see Ch. 6), angiotensin, and growth factors, could also produce or contribute to small coronary vessel constriction.

■ *The search for the causes of coronary microvascular dysfunction is complex because such a dysfunction may result from a variety of alterations and have a variable segmental effect on the ventricular wall, but cause the same clinical syndrome. The prevalence of different causes among groups of patients included in various studies cannot be defined precisely until markers, specific to the various alterations, are identified.* ■

Enhanced perception of pain

The reduced threshold of, and tolerance to, pain, observed in patients with syndrome X and microvascular angina, are fundamental components of the syndrome. Indeed, if such patients had a reduced perception of pain they would not come to medical attention because of the sparse evidence of cardiac dysfunction associated with the microvascular dysfunction. An abnormal psychiatric background may help to explain the enhanced sensitivity to pain and the unjustified anxiety about prognosis, but it may also contribute to the coronary microvascular dysfunction, as psychological states may influence coronary tone via brain stem pathways.[76,77] The chronic occurrence of chest pain may also represent a powerful element in a vicious circle that, on the one hand, may enhance specific mechanisms of pain perception (see Ch. 14) and, on the other, may contribute to the abnormal psychiatric background because of worries about possible prognostic implications.[78]

■ *The importance of an enhanced perception of pain and an abnormal psychiatric background as pathogenetic components of the syndrome may also be variable. In patients in whom the stimulation of potentially painful afferent stimuli is very intense because the microvascular alteration is severe and very persistent, an enhanced perception of pain and an abnormal psychiatric background may not be such necessary components of the syndrome as it is in patients in whom the microvascular alteration is mild. The enhanced perception of pain cannot be the only explanation for the syndrome at least in patients with recurrent ST-segment alterations.* ■

18.3 THERAPEUTIC GUIDELINES

In patients with syndrome X in general, and also in those with demonstrated microvascular angina, the aims of therapy are the relief of symptoms and the improvement of the quality of life, as their prognosis is known to be normal; thus, the control of symptoms should be the only endpoint of therapeutic trials. Surrogate endpoints, such as the improvement of exercise tolerance judged only from silent ST-segment changes and from the results of Holter recordings, which are often used in therapeutic trials, are not as relevant when assessing the beneficial effects of therapy because they have no prognostic significance (in sharp contrast to their established importance in patients with flow-limiting stenosis, thrombosis, or spasm).

As not only may the causes of microvascular alterations be multiple, but also the contribution made by an enhanced perception of pain may be variable, the average results obtained from therapeutic trials are influenced by the prevalence of patients with different causes and varying degrees of severity of microvascular dysfunction and an enhanced sensitivity to pain.

If patients presenting with the same syndrome have different pathogenetic components, a specific treatment may be beneficial for some and have neutral or even detrimental effects on others.

■ *Until homogeneous groups of patients can be identified with confidence, the effects of treatment on individuals with syndrome X should, therefore, be tested by multiple crossover phases in order to evaluate the consistency of the response to the treatment compared with placebo in any given patient.* ■

18.3.1 Review of therapeutic trials

The similarity between patients with chronic stable angina and those with microvascular angina with regard to symptoms and ECG changes has suggested the use of drugs used commonly in chronic stable angina to reduce myocardial work or to prevent dynamic stenoses of epicardial coronary arteries. However, the beneficial effects produced have been small and inconsistent; subsequently, more unconventional forms of treatment were tested, but again their beneficial effects were inconsistent and rather limited.

Traditional antianginal drugs

Nitrates. To date, no formal trials have been conducted on the chronic administration of nitrates in patients with microvascular angina or syndrome X. A limited beneficial effect from sublingual nitrates has been reported in about 50% of patients in most studies. Lack of a beneficial effect from sublingual nitrates, and even an adverse effect on the time to angina and to 1 mm ST-segment depression, has been observed recently during pacing[9] and exercise stress testing.[5] This contrasts sharply with the beneficial effects observed in patients with flow-limiting stenoses.

β-Blockers. β-Blockers were found to produce a mild improvement in exercise tolerance[79] and also in the results of Holter monitoring,[80] but only in patients with evidence of an enhanced sympathetic tone.

Calcium antagonists. A reduction in the number of ischemic episodes, and also in the consumption of nitroglycerin by about 40% during treatment with either verapamil or nifedipine was observed,[81] but in other studies no effect was observed with verapamil,[80] mixed results were observed with nifedipine,[82] and no effect was observed with lidoflazine.[83]

Unconventional forms of therapy

Treatments with specific aims, such as the prevention of coronary microvascular constriction and the antagonism of adenosine, as well as the reduction of the sensitivity to pain, have all been employed but have had only moderate and conflicting beneficial results.

Prevention of coronary microvascular constriction. Prazosin (an α_1-adrenergic blocker) failed to improve either symptoms or the results of Holter monitoring and exercise testing, and phenylephrine had no beneficial effects in 12 patients.[84] Conversely, doxazosin (also an α_1-adrenergic blocker) improved symptoms and exercise tolerance in 10 patients.[85] In menopausal women, estrogens had borderline effects on symptoms, but not on the results of exercise testing,[86] suggesting a prevalent effect on the perception of pain. Enalapril (an angiotensin-converting enzyme inhibitor) improved effort tolerance in 10 patients.[87]

Inhibition of stimulation of different receptors by adenosine. Aminophylline (an adenosine antagonist) improved effort tolerance in 12 patients but, because of side effects, only eight were able to complete the trial.[88] No beneficial effects were observed in another study.[89]

Reduction of sensitivity to pain. Imipramine (an analgesic drug) reduced anginal episodes and nitroglycerin consumption by about 50% in 60 patients.[90] Spinal cord stimulation improved the results of exercise testing in 12 patients.[91]

Conclusions

The partial, and often conflicting, results of therapeutic trials in patients with syndrome X are not surprising as they reflect our poor understanding of the multiple mechanisms which, in variable combinations, together produce the syndrome.

18.3.2 Clinical approach

Until substantial progress is made in our understanding of the pathogenetic mechanisms of the syndrome and in the identification of subsets of patients with the same causes responsible for their symptoms, the clinical approach to patients with syndrome X can only be empirical and highly individualized.

Reduction in the frequency and severity of pain is the main goal of therapy and should, therefore, be the yardstick against which beneficial effects are judged in individual patients.

For the interruption of anginal attacks, sublingual nitrates are the first choice and different preparations should be tried, as some patients report different benefits from sublingual nitroglycerin, ISDN, and nitroglycerin spray. It is also important to advise an immediate consumption of nitrates at the very beginning of the attack, rather than waiting for the pain to become unbearable, and the simultaneous consumption of diazepam. It may also be useful to experiment with different forms of therapy in order to prevent and interrupt particularly painful and prolonged anginal attacks that may otherwise bring the patient to the emergency room.

With chronic therapy, subjective beneficial effects are observed initially with most treatments, possibly owing to a placebo effect, but such effects gradually wane after weeks or months and very gradual dose adjustments or changes in therapy should be tried. As a first-line approach, β-blockers can be prescribed for patients with some evidence of increased adrenergic tone and calcium antagonists can be used for the others. Other drugs among those tested with inconsistent success in the trials reported above may also be tried. For patients with left bundle branch block and for those with an impaired left ventricular function, echocardiographic studies repeated at yearly intervals are indicated.

■ *For patients with normal ventricular function and no left bundle branch block, the cornerstone of therapy should remain reassurance, which helps the patient to bear the pain, but which can only be based on a good doctor–patient relationship and requires not only great patience but also time.* ■

REFERENCES

1. Kemp HG. Left ventricular function in patients with the anginal syndrome and normal coronary angiograms. Am J Cardiol 1973;32:375.
2. Cannon RO, Epstein SE. "Microvascular angina" as a cause of chest pain with angiographically normal coronary arteries. Am J Cardiol 1988;61:1338.
3. Strauer BE. The significance of coronary reserve in clinical heart disease. J Am Coll Cardiol 1990;15:775.

4. Burton P, Kaski JC, Maseri A. A combination of electrocardiographic methods represents a further step toward the noninvasive identification of patients with syndrome X. Am Heart J 1992;*123:*53.

5. Lanza GA, Manzoli A, Bia E, Crea F, Maseri A. Acute effects of nitrates on exercise testing in patients with syndrome X. Clinical and pathophysiological implications. Circulation 1994;*90:*2695.

6. Sugishita Y, Koseki S, Ajisaka R et al. Daily variations of ECG and left ventricular parameters at exercise in patients with anginal attacks but normal coronary arteriograms. Am Heart J 1986;*112:*728.

7. Kaski JC, Crea F, Nihoyannopoulos P, Hackett D, Maseri A. Transient myocardial ischemia during daily life in patients with syndrome X. Am J Cardiol 1986;*58:*1242.

8. Kaski JC, Rosano GMC, Nihoyannopoulos P, Collins P, Maseri A, Poole-Wilson PA. Cardiac syndrome X—clinical characteristics and left ventricular function—a long term follow up study. J Am Coll Cardiol 1995;*25:*807.

9. Bugiardini R, Borghi A, Pozzati A et al. The paradox of nitrates in patients with angina pectoris and angiographically normal coronary arteries. Am J Cardiol 1993;*72:*343.

10. Chambers J, Bass C. Chest pain with normal coronary anatomy. A review of natural history and possible etiologic factors. Prog Cardiovasc Dis 1990;*33:*161.

11. Assey ME. The puzzle of normal coronary arteries in the patient with chest pain: what to do? Clin Cardiol 1993;*16:*170.

12. Cannon RO, Dilsizian V, Correa R, et al. Chronic deterioration in left ventricular function in patients with microvascular angina. J Am Coll Cardiol 1991;*17:*28A.

13. Factor SM, Sonnenblick EH. The pathogenesis of clinical and experimental congestive cardiomyopathies: recent concepts. Prog Cardiovasc Dis 1990;*81:*772.

14. Bass C, Wade C, Hand D, Jackson G. Patients with angina with normal or near normal coronary arteries: clinical and psychological state 12 months after angiography. Br Med J 1983;*287:*1505.

15. Wielgosz AT, Fletcher RH, McCants CB, McKinnis RA, Haney TL, Williams RB. Unimproved chest pain in patients with minimal or no coronary disease: a behavioral phenomenon. Am Heart J 1984;*108:*67.

16. Potts SG, Bass CM. Psychosocial outcome and use of medical resources in patients with chest pain and normal or near normal coronary arteries: a long term follow-up study. Q J Med 1993;*86:*583.

17. Cannon RO, Camici PG, Epstein SE. Pathophysiological dilemma of syndrome X. Circulation 1992;*85:*883.

18. Camici PG, Gistri R, Lorenzoni R et al. Coronary reserve and exercise ECG in patients with chest pain and normal coronary angiograms. Circulation 1992;*86:*176.

19. Picano E, Lattanzi F, Masini M, Distante A, L'Abbate A. Usefulness of a high-dose dipyridamole–echocardiography test for diagnosis of syndrome X. Am J Cardiol 1987;*60:*508.

20. Picano E, Lucarini AR, Lattanzi F et al. ST-segment depression elicited by dipyridamole infusion in asymptomatic hypertensive patients. Hypertension 1990;*16:*19.

21. Lerman BB, Belardinelli L. Cardiac electrophysiology of adenosine. Basic and clinical concepts. Circulation 1991;*83:*1499.

22. Epstein SE, Cannon RO III. Site of increased resistance to coronary flow in patients with angina pectoris and normal epicardial coronary arteries. J Am Coll Cardiol 1986;*8:*459.

23. Maseri A, Crea F, Kaski JC, Crake T. Mechanisms of angina pectoris in Syndrome X. J Am Coll Cardiol 1991;*17:*499.

24. Opherk D, Zebe H, Wehie E et al. Reduced coronary dilatory capacity and ultrastructural changes of the myocardium in patients with angina pectoris but normal coronary arteriograms. Circulation 1981;*63:*817.

25. Cannon RO, Watson RM, Rosing DR, Epstein SE. Angina caused by reduced vasodilator reserve of the small coronary arteries. J Am Coll Cardiol 1983;*1:*1359.

26. Camici PG, Marracini P, Michelassi C et al. Coronary hemodynamics and myocardial metabolism in patients with Syndrome X. J Am Coll Cardiol 1991;*17:*1461.

27. Chauhan A, Mullins PA, Taylor G, Petch MC, Schofield PM. Effect of hyperventilation and mental stress on coronary blood flow in syndrome X. Br Heart J 1993;*69:*516.

28. Geltman EM, Henes G, Senneff MJ, Sobel BE, Bergmann SR. Increased myocardial perfusion at rest and diminished perfusion reserve in patients with angina and angiographically normal coronary arteries. J Am Coll Cardiol 1990;16:586.

29. Galassi AR, Crea F, Araujo LI et al. Comparison of regional myocardial blood flow in syndrome X and one-vessel coronary artery disease. Am J Cardiol 1993;72:134.

30. Camici P, Gropler RJ, Jones T et al. The impact of myocardial blood flow quantitation with PET on the understanding of cardiac diseases. Submitted for publication.

31. Quyyumi AA, Cannon RO III, Panza JA, Diodati JG, Epstein SE. Endothelial dysfunction in patients with chest pain and normal coronary arteries. Circulation 1992;86:1864.

32. Motz W, Vogt M, Rabenau O, Scheler S, Luchoff A, Strauer BE. Evidence of endothelial dysfunction in coronary resistance vessels in patients with angina pectoris and normal coronary angiograms. Am J Cardiol 1991;68:996.

33. Egashira K, Inou T, Hirooka Y, Yamada A, Urabe Y, Takeshita A. Evidence of impaired endothelium-dependent coronary vasodilation in patients with angina pectoris and normal coronary angiograms. N Engl J Med 1993;328:1659.

34. Holdright DR, Lindsay DC, Clarke D, Fox K, Poole-Wilson PA. Coronary flow reserve in patients with chest pain and normal coronary arteries. Br Heart J 1993;70:513.

35. Bortone AS, Hess OM, Eberli FR et al. Abnormal coronary vasomotion during exercise in patients with normal coronary arteries and reduced coronary flow reserve. Circulation 1989;79:516.

36. Vrints CJM, Bult H, Hitter E, Herman AG, Snoeck JP. Impaired endothelium-dependent cholinergic coronary vasodilation in patients with angina and normal coronary arteries. J Am Coll Cardiol 1992;19:21.

37. Bugiardini R, Pozzati A, Ottani F, Morgagni GL, Puddu P. Vasotonic angina: a spectrum of ischemic syndromes involving functional abnormalities of the epicardial and microvascular coronary circulation. J Am Coll Cardiol 1993;22:417.

38. Kaski JC, Tousoulis D, Galassi AR et al. Epicardial coronary artery tone and reactivity in patients with normal coronary arteriograms and reduced coronary flow reserve. J Am Coll Cardiol 1991;18:50.

39. Tweddel AC, Martin W, Hutton I. Thallium scans in syndrome X. Br Heart J 1992;68:48.

40. Greenberg MA, Grose RM, Neuburger N, Silverman R, Strain JE, Cohen MV. Impaired coronary vasodilator responsiveness as a cause of lactate production during pacing-induced ischemia in patients with angina pectoris and normal coronary arteries. J Am Coll Cardiol 1987;9:743.

41. Boudoulas H, Cobb TC, Leighton RF, et al. Myocardial lactate production in patients with angina-like chest pain and angiographically normal coronary arteries and left ventricle. Am J Cardiol 1974;34:501.

42. Christensen CW, Rosen LB, Gal RA, Haseeb M, Lassar TA, Port SC. Coronary vasodilator reserve. Comparison of the effects of papaverine and adenosine on coronary flow, ventricular function, and myocardial metabolism. Circulation 1991;83:294.

43. Gertz EW, Wisneski JA, Neese R, Houser A, Korte R, Bristow JD. Myocardial lactate extraction: multi-determined metabolic function. Circulation 1980;61:256.

44. Crake T, Canepa-Anson R, Shapiro L, Poole-Wilson PA. Continuous recording of coronary sinus oxygen saturation during atrial pacing in patients with coronary artery disease or with syndrome X. Br Heart J 1988;59:31.

45. Cannon RO. Microvascular angina. Cardiovascular investigation regarding pathophysiology and management. In: Richter JE, Cannon RO, Beitman B (eds.) Unexplained chest pain. Medical Clinics of North America. Philadelphia, WB Saunders, 1991;75:1097.

46. Nihoyannopoulos P, Kaski JC, Crake T, Maseri A. Absence of myocardial dysfunction during stress in patients with syndrome X. J Am Coll Cardiol 1991;18:1463.

47. Tousoulis D, Crake T, Lefroy D et al. Left ventricular hypercontractility and ST segment depression in patients with syndrome X. J Am Coll Cardiol 1993;22:1607.

48. Alban Davies H, Jones DB, Rhodes J, Newcombe RG. Angina-like esophageal pain: differentiation from cardiac pain by history. J Clin Gastroenterol 1985;7:477.

49. Schofield PM, Whorwell PJ, Jones PE, Brooks NH, Bennett DH. Differentiation of "esophageal" and "cardiac" chest pain. Am J Cardiol 1988;62:315.

50. Benjamin SB. The relationship between esophageal motility disorders and microvascular angina. Med Clin N Am 1991;*75*:1135.

51. DeCaestecker JS, Blackwell JN, Brown J, Heading RC. The oesophagus as a cause of recurrent chest pain: which patients should be investigated and which tests should be used? Lancet 1985;*2*:1143.

52. Richter JE. Investigation and management of non-cardiac chest pain. Baillières Clin Gastroenterol 1991;*5*:281.

53. Chauhan A, Petch MC, Schofield PM. Effect of esophageal acid instillation on coronary blood flow. Lancet 1993;*341*:1309.

54. Mellow MH, Simpson AG, Watt L, Schoolmeester L, Haye OL. Oesophageal acid perfusion in coronary artery disease: induction of myocardial ischaemia. Gastroenterology 1983;*85*:306.

55. Gilbert NC, LeRoy GV, Fenn GK. The effect of distension of abdominal viscera on the blood flow in the circumflex branch of the left coronary artery of the dog. Am Heart J 1940;*20*:519.

56. Cannon RO, Cattau EL, Yakshe PN et al. Coronary flow reserve, esophageal motility, and chest pain in patients with angiographically normal coronary arteries. Am J Med 1990;*88*:217.

57. Poole-Wilson PA. Potassium and the heart. Clin Endocrinol Metab 1984;*13*:249.

58. Rosano GMC, Lindsay DC, Poole-Wilson PA. Syndrome X: an hypothesis for cardiac pain without ischaemia. Cardiologia 1991;*36*:885.

59. Finocchiaro ML, Cianflone D, Porter AT et al. Different responses to intracoronary adenosine and dipyridamole in syndrome X and in patients with stable angina following successful coronary angioplasty. Circulation 1993;*88(Suppl. 2)*:2780.

60. Maseri A. Syndrome X: Still an appropriate name. J Am Coll Cardiol 1991;*17*:1471.

61. Richardson PJ, Livesley B, Oram S, Olsen E, Armstrong P. Angina pectoris with normal coronary arteries. Transvenous myocardial biopsy in diagnosis. Lancet 1974;*2*:677.

62. Turiel M, Galassi AR, Glazier JJ et al. Pain threshold and tolerance in women with syndrome X and women with stable angina pectoris. Am J Cardiol 1987;*60*:503.

63. Shapiro LM, Crake T, Poole-Wilson PA. Is altered cardiac sensation responsible for chest pain in patients with normal coronary arteries? Clinical observations during cardiac catheterization. Br Med J 1988;*296*:170.

64. Cannon RO, Quyyumi AA, Schenke WH et al. Abnormal cardiac sensitivity in patients with chest pain and normal coronary arteries. J Am Coll Cardiol 1990;*16*:1359.

65. Beitman BD, Mukerji V, Lamberti JW et al. Panic disorder in patients with chest pain and angiographically normal coronary arteries. Am J Cardiol 1989;*63*:1399.

66. Katon W, Hall ML, Russo J et al. Chest pain: relationship of psychiatric illness to coronary arteriographic results. Am J Med 1988;*84*:1.

67. Bass C, Wade C. Chest pain with normal coronary arteries: a comparative study of psychiatric and social morbidity. Psychol Med 1984;*14*:51.

68. Maseri A, Crea F, Cianflone D. Myocardial ischemia caused by distal coronary vasoconstriction. Am J Cardiol 1992;*70*:1602.

69. Mosseri M, Yarom R, Gotsman MS, Hasin Y. Histologic evidence for small-vessel coronary artery disease in patients with angina pectoris and patent large coronary arteries. Circulation 1986;*74*:964.

70. Sax FL, Cannon RO, Hanson C, Epstein SE. Impaired forearm vasodilator reserve in patients with microvascular angina. N Engl J Med 1987;*317*:1366.

71. Brush JE, Cannon RO, Schenke WH et al. Angina due to coronary microvascular disease in hypertensive patients without left ventricular hypertrophy. N Engl J Med 1988;*319*:1302.

72. Collins P. Role of endothelial dysfunction and oestrogens in syndrome X. Cor Art Dis 1992;*3*:593.

73. Bøtker HE, Møller N, Ovesen P et al. Insulin resistance in microvascular angina (syndrome X). Lancet 1993;*342*:136.

74. Cannon RO, Peden DB, Berkebile C, Schenke WH, Kaliner MA, Epstein SE. Airway hyperresponsiveness in patients with microvascular angina. Evidence for a diffuse disorder of smooth muscle responsiveness. Circulation 1990;*82*:2011

75. Galassi AR, Kaski JC, Crea F et al. Heart rate response during exercise testing and ambulatory ECG monitoring in patients with syndrome X. Am Heart J 1991;*122*:458.

76. Wielgosz AT. Connecting the ceruleus and the coronaries. Am J Cardiol 1988;*62:*308.

77. Cave AR, LaMaster TS, Gutterman DD. Coronary constrictor pathway from anterior hypothalamus includes neurons in rostroventrolateral medulla. Circulation 1991;*84:*98.

78. Ockene IS, Shay MJ, Alpert JS, Weiner BH, Dalen JE. Unexplained chest pain in patients with normal coronary arteriograms: a follow-up study of functional status. N Engl J Med 1980;*303:*1249.

79. Romeo F, Gaspardone A, Ciavolella M, Gioffrè P, Reale A. Verapamil versus acebutolol for syndrome X. Am J Cardiol 1988;*62:*312.

80. Bugiardini R, Borghi A, Biagetti L, Puddu P. Comparison of verapamil versus propranolol therapy in syndrome X. Am J Cardiol 1989;*63:*286.

81. Cannon RO, Watson RM, Rosing DR, Epstein SE. Efficacy of calcium channel blocker therapy for angina pectoris resulting from small-vessel coronary artery disease and abnormal vasodilator reserve. Am J Cardiol 1985;*56:*242.

82. Montorsi P, Manfredi M, Loaldi A et al. Comparison of coronary vasomotor responses to nifedipine in syndrome X and in Prinzmetal's angina pectoris. Am J Cardiol 1989;*63:*1198.

83. Cannon RO, Brush JE, Schenke WH, Tracy CM, Epstein SE. Beneficial and detrimental effects of lidoflazine in microvascular angina. Am J Cardiol 1990;*66:*37.

84. Galassi AR, Kaski JC, Pupita G, Vejar M, Crea F, Maseri A. Lack of evidence for alpha-adrenergic receptor-mediated mechanisms in the genesis of ischemia in syndrome X. Am J Cardiol 1989;*64:*264.

85. Marracini P, Camici P, Orsini E, Massi G, Gistri R, L'Abbate A. Effectiveness of alpha-1 blockade in syndrome X. Eur Heart J 1992;*13 (Abstr.Suppl.):*217.

86. Rosano GMC, Lefroy DC, Peters NS, et al. Symptomatic response to 17β-estradiol in women with syndrome X. J Am Coll Cardiol 1994;*23(Abstr.Suppl.):*6A.

87. Kaski JC, Rosano G, Gavrielides S, Chen L. Effects of angiotensin-converting enzyme inhibition on exercise-induced angina and ST segment depression in patients with microvascular angina (Abst). J Am Coll Cardiol 1994;*23:*652.

88. Emdin M, Picano E, Lattanzi F, L' Abbate A. Improved exercise capacity with acute aminophylline administration in patients with syndrome X. J Am Coll Cardiol 1989;*14:*1450.

89. Lanza GA, Cianflone D, Buffon A, Crea F, Maseri A. Terapia dell' angina microvascolare. Cardiologia 1993;*38 (Suppl. 1):*169.

90. Cannon RO, Quyyumi AA, Mincemoyer R, et al: Imipramine in patients with chest pain despite normal coronary angiograms. N Engl J Med 1994;*330:*1411.

91. Eliasson T, Albertsson P, Hardhammar P, Emanuelsson H, Augustinsson E, Mannheimer C. Spinal cord stimulation in syndrome X. Eur Heart J 1992;*13(Abstr.Suppl.):*266.

Unstable angina

INTRODUCTION

Unstable angina, like chronic stable angina, should be thought of as a syndrome rather than as a disease, because the factors that cause the instability and its evolution towards myocardial infarction (MI) may be varied. As the name suggests, its essential feature is the instability of coronary lesions, which may, unpredictably, cause MI or heal. These lesions bring about occasional episodes of myocardial ischemia due to transient reduction of coronary blood flow (CBF) caused by coronary thrombosis and/or by coronary vasoconstriction. It is frequently associated with episodic deposition of crescentic layers of mural fibrin–platelet thrombi, which may lyze spontaneously or become organized and result in a sudden increase in the severity of a preexisting stenosis or in the development of a new critical stenosis. This sudden reduction of residual coronary flow reserve by organized mural thrombi can cause ischemia upon efforts that had previously been well tolerated. The evolutive tendency towards MI is manifested clinically by recurrent and prolonged spontaneous ischemic attacks, poorly responsive to anti-ischemic therapy, which usually develop intermittently over periods of days or weeks. The tendency of some patterns of angina to evolve towards MI gave rise to several descriptive terms such as "preinfarction angina," "crescendo angina," "acute coronary insufficiency," and "intermediate coronary syndrome" until, in the early 1970s, the term "unstable angina" was proposed. This is now universally accepted and serves to alert physicians to the potentially more life-threatening nature of the condition compared with chronic stable angina.[1] However, because of its all-embracing nature, it includes patients with a wide spectrum of symptoms, preexisting disease, and prognosis.

The syndrome may occur unexpectedly in previously healthy individuals or in patients with ischemic heart disease (IHD) (chronic stable angina, quiescent IHD, or recent acute MI). Following the phase of instability, patients may either develop chronic stable, predominantly effort-related angina (or revert to it) or become quiescent.

Unstable angina is identified clinically on the basis of a combination of the following three features:

1. Anginal attacks of recent onset (i.e. within the last 2 months) occurring without apparent cause or upon efforts that had previously been well tolerated and unrelated to conditions that increase myocardial oxygen demand or reduce oxygen supply such as fever, anemia, hypoxia, tachyarrhythmias, hypertension, or hyperthyroidism. They may occur:

a. in previously healthy individuals (*de novo unstable angina*)
b. in patients with known, but stable or quiescent IHD, with or without an old MI (*destabilizing unstable angina*), or
c. within the 2 months following an acute Q-wave or non-Q-wave MI (*postinfarction unstable angina*).

2. Transient ischemic ECG ST-segment changes (depression, elevation, pseudo-normalization of T waves) occurring during an attack of angina and/or T-wave inversion or ST-segment depression recorded only minutes or hours after an episode, not previously present and which gradually return to normal within a few hours or days. This objective documentation of myocardial ischemia is essential in patients with no history of IHD, as several nonischemic causes can result in chest pain. It may not be required in patients with known IHD who recognize the features of the pain as being identical to those previously associated with documented myocardial ischemia.

3. Persistence of spontaneous ischemic episodes (painful or painless), indicating that the underlying coronary lesions continue to be active (*persisting instability*), or waxing of the instability (*crescendo angina*) and failure to respond to maximal therapy (*refractory angina*), or waning of the instability (*resolving crescendo* or *resolving refractory unstable angina* or *possibly resolved unstable angina*), until it either becomes quiescent or results in chronic stable angina.

The outcome of the syndrome depends both on its tendency to evolve towards MI (which is clinically suggested by the persistence and exacerbation of spontaneous ischemic episodes and lack of response to therapy) and on the vulnerability of the patient's heart to ischemia and infarction (which is generally determined by the degree of impairment of left ventricular function caused by previous infarctions, and also by the number and severity of preexisting coronary stenoses determining the myocardial area at risk).

Because of the very broad nature of the term, the perceived picture of the syndrome varies considerably in different institutions and also in clinical practise. Unstable angina as perceived by cardiologists in referral centers differs from that perceived by those in general hospitals and differs again from that perceived by practising family physicians. Patients admitted to referral centers because of persistent or deteriorating symptoms, possibly refractory to treatment, have more severe forms of the disease and a worse prognosis. Patients admitted to general hospitals represent the broad spectrum of the disease and reflect local referral practises. Hence, the average prognosis observed in different reports varies greatly,[2,3] according to the prevailing admission criteria.

The incidence of the syndrome is high. In the USA in 1991, there were 570 000 admissions for which the principal diagnosis was unstable angina.[4] In its most acute and aggressive form (i.e. that which precedes infarction by a few hours or days), it is also common: in about 40% of patients with acute MI, the onset of the prolonged pain that leads to hospitalization is preceded by one or more episodes of angina during the previous 24–48 h. During the first 2 months after acute MI, angina develops in about 10% of cases,[5] more often in patients who previously had chronic stable angina.

The differential diagnosis of patients presenting with pain in the emergency department is discussed in detail with that of acute MI in Chapter 21.

19.1 PATHOGENETIC MECHANISMS

In unstable angina the transient reduction of CBF responsible for recurrent ischemic episodes at rest has been demonstrated by hemodynamic monitoring, regional myocardial perfusion studies, and pacing-induced tachycardia. The ultimate mechanisms responsible for the occasional reduction of myocardial perfusion involve thrombosis and vasoconstriction, but their underlying triggering mechanisms which, according to the inclusion criteria generally adopted, can last up to 2 months, are still speculative (see Ch. 9).

19.1.1 Preexisting coronary stenoses

On average, patients with unstable angina have more complex lesions and more thrombi seen on coronary angiograms than patients with stable angina,[6] but a systematic study of patients enrolled in a large randomized trial shows that severe multivessel disease is uncommon.

The results of the TIMI IIIB trial[7] in a systematic study of 1473 randomized patients with unstable angina, hospitalized for early (within 48 h) invasive procedures or early conservative strategies, revealed no significant obstructions (less than 60% diameter stenosis) in 19% of patients, single-vessel disease in 38%, double-vessel disease in 29%, triple-vessel disease in 15%, and left main disease in 4%. These results reflect the particular population of unstable patients referred to major institutions in the USA: 85% had chronic stable angina and over 40% had suffered a previous MI. These results may not apply, therefore, to patients with de novo unstable angina, who are likely to have less extensive coronary obstructions and, by definition, have no previous MI.

Although the development of instability is often associated with the progression of coronary stenoses, about one-quarter of unstable patients subjected to repeat coronary arteriography fail to show any progression. Progression is multifocal more often in unstable than in stable patients, but 25% of stable patients may also exhibit stenosis progression in the absence of signs of instability.[8,9] Thus, no coronary angiographic findings are pathognomonic of unstable angina. Stabilization of the syndrome is not associated with the development of collaterals.[10] Only about 75% of patients were found to have fissured plaques lying under mural thrombi but, in the same patient, fissured plaques are also commonly found in noninfarct-related coronary arteries.[11–13] Fissured plaques are found less frequently in patients who died during a stable phase of IHD and in individuals who died of noncardiac causes (see Ch. 9).

Progression of stenoses is likely to be the result, rather than the cause, of the syndrome. Indeed, postmortem studies indicate that the age of mural thrombi is consistent with the time of onset of unstable symptoms. Such thrombi mostly occur at the site of fissured plaques, so that the resulting stenosis often has quite irregular and ragged contours. Irregular stenoses can be recognized angiographically in many patients with unstable angina, but not in all, and can also be observed in some patients with chronic stable angina, suggesting that such stenoses may be markers of a short-term focal process that has already taken place, rather than its actual cause. Thus, although it is well established that dynamic thrombotic and vasospastic mechanisms have dominant roles in the pathogenesis of unstable angina,[14,15] their underlying causes are still elusive[16] and it is only recently that the possible importance of a (yet unknown) inflammatory component has begun to receive attention (see Ch. 9).

19.1.2 Increased myocardial demand and reduced myocardial blood flow

As discussed in Chapter 16, episodes of prolonged, spontaneous angina, which are the dominant features of instability, are caused by a transient reduction of CBF, but some may also be caused by a sudden critical reduction of coronary flow reserve due to an organized thrombus.

Continuous hemodynamic monitoring has shown that, in patients with angina at rest, spontaneous episodes of acute myocardial ischemia are only very rarely preceded by an increase of
heart rate or blood pressure sufficient per se to cause ischemia,[17,18] and occur at values of
heart rate/blood pressure product much lower than those associated with the onset of
ischemia during the pacing test.[19] Regional myocardial perfusion studies performed during
ischemic episodes at rest have demonstrated regional deficits of thallium-201 uptake[20] similar
to those observed in patients with variant angina, confirming the dominant role of a primary
reduction of regional myocardial blood flow.

As discussed in Chapter 9, a dynamic thrombotic cause of a sudden reduction of CBF is
easier to detect than that caused by coronary vasoconstriction, as thrombi are usually more
persistent and can, therefore, be demonstrated by angiographic, angioscopic, and postmortem
studies. Direct evidence related to coronary vasoconstriction is difficult to obtain because
increased vasomotor tone is more elusive than thrombosis, being detectable only at the precise moment at which it occurs. In the presence of very tight stenoses, even a minimal change
in caliber (beyond the measuring ability of the radiographic technique) can have an important
hemodynamic significance and constriction of small coronary vessels cannot be detected
angiographically.

The currently available knowledge of the severity of coronary artery stenoses and the
thrombotic and vasoconstrictor components of unstable angina has been gathered from hospitalized patients with severe forms of the disease, who either were subjected to urgent coronary arteriography or died. The findings in different studies, therefore, are strongly influenced by local referral practises. Little information is available about the two extremes
of the syndrome, i.e. patients with a less aggressive form of the disease (who settle down
promptly and spontaneously) and those who proceed to infarction within a day. The underlying unstable stimuli in these two extreme groups could have different levels of intensity or
a different nature, but it is also possible that the vasomotor or hemostatic responses could
be the decisive elements in the evolution of the syndrome (see Ch. 9).

■ *Until the actual causes of instability can be identified, diagnosis is based on the detection of its
consequences, i.e. of the unstable ischemic manifestations. As an occasional episodic impairment of
CBF appears to be the prevalent cause of ischemia, therapy is focused on the prevention of coronary
thrombosis and vasoconstriction rather than on the reduction of myocardial oxygen demand.* ■

19.2 DIAGNOSTIC ASSESSMENT

A diagnosis of unstable angina requires the diagnosis of myocardial ischemia, the diagnosis
of the instability, and the exclusion of acute MI. Patients with clinical signs of instability may
exhibit one of three clinical manifestations, immediately recognizable by attending physicians, in which prognosis is influenced not only by the severity of the instability, but also by
that of ventricular dysfunction, of flow-limiting coronary stenoses, and, possibly, by previous treatment regimens. These are:

a. *de novo unstable angina* (occurring in patients without previous IHD)
b. *destabilizing unstable angina* (occurring in patients with documented chronic stable
   angina or those in a quiescent phase of IHD, with or without old MI, large or small)
c. *Postacute myocardial infarction unstable angina* (occurring within the first 2 months
   after acute MI, large or small).

Patients presenting with postinfarction and destabilizing unstable angina are probably
being treated with aspirin and anti-ischemic drugs (which failed to prevent the manifesta-

tion of unstable angina); in general, therefore, they may be more refractory to standard medical therapy than patients, previously untreated, presenting with de novo unstable angina. They are also likely to have more extensive left ventricular dysfunction and flow-limiting coronary stenoses.

Although, traditionally, the likehood of significant coronary artery disease is considered the major diagnostic problem for unstable patients, it does not appear to be the only short-term determinant of the evolution of the instability. The clinical diagnosis based on the patient's presentation should be confirmed by documenting the ischemic origin of pain and by the identification of the unstable cause of ischemic episodes.

19.2.1 The clinical diagnosis

General physicians or physicians in emergency departments are required to make the clinical diagnosis of unstable angina and to institute prophylactic therapy with aspirin. They decide whether patients should be admitted to a coronary care unit (CCU), or assessed as outpatients. For patients admitted to a CCU, cardiologists are called upon to confirm the diagnosis and to intensify therapy as appropriate, according to the estimated level of risk.

The urgency of establishing a provisional diagnosis depends not only on the severity of the ischemic manifestations but also on that of preexisting documented IHD. In any case, unless the diagnosis can be excluded, treatment with aspirin should be instituted and continued until the diagnosis is disproved.

■ *For patients presenting with continuing pain when first examined, the differential diagnosis with acute MI and other ischemic causes is discussed in Chapter 21.* ■

De novo unstable angina

A provisional diagnosis can be made when the patient seems to be a reliable historian, has known risk factors (such as age), and reports having at least two episodes of typical anginal pain occurring at rest, on effort or on emotion, or at least one that was associated or followed by ischemic ECG changes not present on previous tracings, during the last 2 months.

A differential diagnosis should be made with not only the first presentation of noncardiac and of possibly nonischemic causes of anginal pain (aortic stenosis, hypertrophic cardiomyopathy, etc.) but also the first presentation of ischemia not caused by unstable lesions, i.e. chronic stable angina or syndrome X. The differential diagnosis between stable and unstable causes of recent-onset angina is only possible on the basis of its evolution (see Ch. 16). The differential diagnosis with variant angina is suggested by a history of predominantly nocturnal or early morning angina with preserved effort tolerance. The diagnosis of variant angina is supported by the contrasting findings of a negative exercise test after sublingual nitroglycerin and of transient ST-segment elevation during episodes of spontaneous angina observed on a continuous ECG recording (see Ch. 20).

The diagnosis of ischemia is confirmed when transient ECG changes are recorded during pain or when the ECG shows ischemic changes, not previously present, persisting for a few hours or days. In uncertain cases, a positive exercise stress test can help to establish the ischemic nature of the pain, but a negative test cannot exclude an ischemic nature when pain is caused by transient vasoconstriction or by thrombosis (see below).

Destabilizing unstable angina

A provisional diagnosis can be made in the following circumstances:

a. a patient who was in a quiescent phase of IHD (i.e. with no anginal episodes) reports at least two episodes of angina during the last 2 months, either occurring at rest or on efforts which, until then, were quite well tolerated

b. when a patient with chronic stable angina reports a sudden obvious decrease in effort tolerance during the last 2 months, associated with the appearance of episodes of angina occurring spontaneously at rest (which were not previously present), or

c. when a patient (in a quiescent phase or with chronic stable angina) has within the last 2 months had a prolonged anginal episode lasting for more than 20 min or an episode associated with persisting changes of the ST segment or T waves that were not present on a previous tracing.

In patients with possibly destabilizing unstable angina, new causes of increased myocardial demand (such as hypertension, hyperthyroidism, fever, arrhythmias) or of reduced oxygen supply (marked hypotension, anemia, hypoxemia) should be excluded.

A history of old MI and cardiac failure and a very low effort tolerance are very strong adverse prognostic elements. Furthermore, chronic therapy with antiplatelet agents, which may be fairly common in this group, can be an adverse prognostic element compared with patients with de novo unstable angina, as it indicates that the instability could not be controlled by the inhibition of platelet function.

Postinfarction unstable angina

In patients with recent MI, a diagnosis of unstable angina can be made if they experience at least one prolonged episode of spontaneous angina lasting longer than 20 min or at least two shorter episodes, after the serum indices of myocardial necrosis have returned to baseline.

The differential diagnosis with reinfarction is based on the development of diagnostic ECG changes and/or a diagnostic rise of serum indices of myocardial cell necrosis. A differential diagnosis with non-Q-wave infarction may not be easy when serum creatine phosphokinase values are only slightly raised. In such borderline cases, the differential diagnosis is not critical because some degree of myocardial cell damage can also occur after ischemic episodes lasting only 15–20 min.[21–23] Borderline alterations of creatine phosphokinase should, therefore, be considered as further objective indications of severer ischemic episodes and, hence, of a more worrying degree of instability with a tendency to evolve towards infarction. The differential diagnosis is more difficult for patients who had chronic stable angina before the acute MI, particularly if their exercise tolerance was very low (classes III or IV).

For patients with postacute MI unstable angina, the presence of cardiac failure and/or of a reduced left ventricular EF are very important adverse prognostic elements. Their prognosis may be worse than those of patients with de novo or destabilizing unstable angina (also for comparable levels of impairment of ventricular function and similar degrees of severity of coronary flow-limiting stenoses), because the instability is already known to have caused an acute MI and was not controlled by continuing therapy.

■ *Once a provisional diagnosis of de novo, destabilizing, or postinfarction unstable angina has been made, it should be confirmed by documenting the ischemic origin of the pain and the unstable cause of the ischemic episodes.* ■

19.2.2 Confirmation of the ischemic origin of pain

Confirmation of the ischemic origin of pain can be obtained by the following:

a. The observation of transient ischemic changes on the ECG during an episode of angina.[24] (It is useful to keep the patient linked to the ECG machine in the same position, after administration of sublingual nitrates, until the pain disappears and then to repeat the tracing for comparison). Transient changes are more obvious in the presence of a previously normal resting ECG, but ischemia of the posterior myocardial wall may fail to alter the conventional 12-lead ECG. The detection of diagnostic changes on the ECG is difficult in the presence of bundle branch block or of extensive preexisting QRS or ST-segment/T-wave (ST–T) alterations. Thus, a negative ECG during very typical pain (particularly in patients with previously documented IHD or with high levels of risk factors), is not sufficient to rule out myocardial ischemia (see Ch. 21).

b. The presence of ischemic ST–T changes on a tracing recorded within a few minutes or hours of a prolonged anginal attack, which were not present on a previous tracing recorded a few days earlier, and which disappear gradually within hours or days.[25] This electrocardiographic evolution should occur in the absence of a diagnostic increase in the indices of myocardial necrosis in order to rule out infarction.

c. The documentation of transient regional ventricular dyskinesia or regional myocardial perfusion deficits during an episode of chest pain, even when the ECG is nondiagnostic.

d. The documentation of spontaneous, transient silent ischemic episodes during continuous ECG recording.

e. A positive submaximal exercise stress test. In uncertain cases of possible de novo or destabilizing unstable angina, the test should be performed when the resting ECG is normal or unchanged from those recorded previously and at least 48 h after the last reported episode of pain. It should be performed under aspirin and chronic anti-ischemic therapeutic cover in patients with possible destabilizing unstable angina, and under aspirin cover alone for those with possible de novo unstable angina. The test should not be maximal because its only function is to provide evidence of critical lesions; a maximal test may increase the risk of occlusion occurring in an unstable coronary artery. A maximal test under aspirin cover alone can be performed to assess and reassure the patient after a few weeks free from anginal episodes. Other provocative tests of ischemia may be used when clinically indicated (see 19.4.5).

f. The development of the same type of pain and/or of diagnostic ischemic changes during provocative tests for coronary artery spasm in patients with a negative exercise test and suspected variant angina (see Ch. 20).

Having established the ischemic origin of the pain during one episode, it is then reasonable to assume that all attacks of a similar pain have an ischemic cause. In the presence of a strong clinical suspicion but no objective evidence (including a negative maximal exercise test and negative tests for spasm), the diagnosis of ischemia remains presumptive of either unstable or variant angina or of some form of distal small coronary vessel disease, unless an alternative cause of pain has been documented convincingly. The possibility should be considered that a coronary thrombus may have lysed spontaneously and that the mechanisms responsible for occlusive epicardial coronary artery spasm or other forms of coronary constriction may not be susceptible to the challenging test. In suspected cases, careful follow-up and prophylactic treatment with aspirin and calcium antagonists is indicated for a period of 2 months, together with the assessment and control of risk factors. Coronary arteriography is indicated only when considered useful for the patient's reassurance (see below).

19.2.3 Diagnosis of instability

As the causes of instability are still unknown, the diagnosis of unstable angina can usually be made on a clinical basis only. Once the ischemic origin of the pain has been documented, its unstable cause is indicated by the following:

a. Clinical signs:
    • spontaneous occurrence, long duration, and poor response to sublingual nitrates of ischemic episodes
    • persistence or exacerbation of attacks despite anti-ischemic therapy
    • sudden, obvious reduction of the anginal threshold upon effort and exercise stress testing while receiving anti-ischemic therapy (in the absence of extracoronary causes)
    • occurrence of spontaneous ischemic episodes after an acute MI.
b. Gradually reversible ischemic ST–T changes (over a period of hours or days) after an ischemic episode (indicative of previously severe, prolonged myocardial ischemia).
c. A gradual increase, followed by a decrease, in the indices of myocardial cell necrosis not attaining the diagnostic threshold for MI, but indicative of severe, prolonged myocardial ischemia. Troponin-T appears to have the most suitable half-life for this purpose as it exhibits an early rise and a slow fall after the ischemic insult.[23]
d. Angiographic evidence of fresh intracoronary thrombus. Irregular lesions are compatible with, but not necessarily diagnostic of, unstable lesions because they cannot be dated and may be preexisting.

Persistence of, or increase in, the instability during either admission or the follow-up period is indicated by:

a. the persistence or exacerbation of spontaneous angina
b. the appearance of transient or prolonged ischemic changes on the standard 12-lead ECG, and/or
c. the detection of transient silent episodes of ischemic ST–T changes during continuous ECG monitoring of the leads showing the most obvious transient changes, occurring in spite of full medical therapy.

Preliminary data indicate that elevated levels of C-reactive protein (CRP) or serum amyloid A protein (SAA) also have an important short-term prognostic significance.[26]

■ *The detection of painful or painless ischemic episodes determines the continuance of patients in the category of persisting unstable angina or their movement to the categories of crescendo or refractory unstable angina (see 19.3.2). Conversely, the disappearance of angina (and the absence of ischemic ST-segment shifts during ECG monitoring when available) for 48 h in patients with crescendo or refractory unstable angina is an indication that the underlying coronary lesion may be healing, and determines the movement of patients to the categories of possibly resolved refractory or crescendo or possibly resolved unstable angina (see 19.3.2).■*

19.2.4 Diagnostic coronary arteriography

The indications for diagnostic coronary arteriography in patients who have not previously been subjected to the procedure are absolute in some cases and relative in others, being governed by local practises and by the wishes of the patient.

An absolute indication for arteriography is represented by the failure of full medical therapy to abolish ischemic episodes (so that the procedure is undertaken with a view to percutaneous transluminal coronary angioplasty [PTCA] or coronary artery bypass grafting [CABG]): this is the case, for example, when a patient has refractory unstable angina or persistent instability (in spite of full medical therapy), particularly when associated with poor left ventricular function, or when a predischarge exercise test is positive at a low work load on full anti-ischemic therapy with a large area of myocardium at risk.

A relative indication for arteriography in all patients hospitalized for unstable angina is represented by the documentation of spontaneous transient ischemic ECG changes after admission, and is based on the assumption that it may be useful in order to assess both prognosis and the possible need for revascularization procedures. In the absence of recurrent ischemic episodes, however, the information obtained from arteriography must be used judiciously, as the detection of stenoses may lead to PTCA or CABG in cases where there is insufficient evidence available from randomized trials to suggest that they improve prognosis in low-risk patients.

The relative indications for angiography are influenced markedly by local practise. For example, in the USA the costs of hospitalization in a CCU are generally very high. This factor, together with the frequency of malpractise suits, leads to aggressive patient management in which arteriography is accepted as a key diagnostic element for indicating either prompt discharge or the need for revascularization procedures to be carried out.[3]

The findings of the TIMI IIIB trial[7] suggest that, even in a group of patients with a high prevalence of a previous history of chronic stable angina and old MI, early use of cardiac catheterization, when not indicated by persisting symptoms or signs of ischemia, is best determined by the preferences of each individual patient.

During angiography, arteriograms of the culprit lesion should be taken, ideally both before and after the administration of intracoronary nitrates in order to assess the importance of the vasoconstrictor component of the stenosis. When angiography confirms the presence of fresh coronary thrombus in patients with refractory unstable angina, intracoronary thrombolysis may be considered, but the benefit of this approach has not been confirmed. When angiography fails to reveal any critical stenosis, an ergonovine test, if clinically justified, should be considered in order to assess the patient's susceptibility to coronary artery spasm and, consequently, the need for treatment with appropriate doses of calcium antagonists (see Ch. 20).

About 20% of patients with documented ischemic episodes are found to have no critical coronary stenoses and about 10% have angiographically normal coronary arteries and no inducible epicardial coronary artery spasm. In such patients it is impossible to establish whether the ischemic episodes were caused by completely lysed thrombi, by epicardial coronary artery spasm that is no longer inducible, or by small vessel coronary constriction.

19.2.5 Diagnostic uncertainties

A differential diagnosis can be made more easily when patients present with pain rather than when their symptoms have resolved. When patients present with continuing pain and the ECG shows acute ischemic changes, the differential diagnosis is with acute MI; when the ECG is nondiagnostic, the differential diagnosis is with noncardiac causes (see Ch. 21).

When symptoms have resolved, a major diagnostic difficulty in establishing a presumptive diagnosis occurs in patients with no previous history of IHD. Such patients may present with the occurrence of one or two severe and prolonged anginal episodes during the last few days or weeks, and may have a normal resting ECG tracing recorded after, but not during, the episodes of pain. Uncertainty also exists over patients hospitalized because of the apparent severity of their clinical presentation, but who experience no ischemic episodes during admission. In these cases a positive diagnosis can be made only if the predischarge exercise stress test reproduces the pain with diagnostic ECG changes. If the test is negative in the absence of anti-ischemic treatment, the diagnosis can be neither confirmed nor excluded.

When the persistence of the instability is being assessed, major uncertainty surrounds not only those patients with a previous history of chronic stable angina who continue to have episodes suggestive of mixed angina but also those who had previously been in a quiescent phase but who, after the instability has waned, are left with effort-induced angina. These uncertainties are resolved gradually over the following 2 months if no exacerbation of symptoms occurs.

There is uncertainty, also, over the length of time for which a patient should be considered unstable after the last ischemic episode. For symmetry with the period of 2 months that is now generally accepted as a diagnostic criterion, a similar period free from spontaneous ischemic episodes can be proposed as being provisionally indicative of the clinical resolution of the instability. This proposition is also justified by observational data from the Duke Cardiovascular Databank on 21 761 patients treated for IHD without interventional procedures at Duke University Medical Center between 1985 and 1992: by the end of 2 months, postdischarge mortality rates for patients admitted with unstable angina were similar to those for patients admitted with chronic stable angina.[3]

19.3 PROGNOSTIC ASSESSMENT AND CLASSIFICATION

Our knowledge of the natural history of unstable angina is rather fragmented as all patients are referred to as "unstable," although the degrees of both instability and baseline preexisting disease vary widely and evidence of the ischemic and unstable nature of the pain is not always available. Information is obtained from community-based studies (which cover the spectrum of the disease as it presents to general physicians) and also from hospital-based studies (which cover the spectrum of hospitalized patients according to prevailing local referral practise). Of cases of recent-onset angina diagnosed by general physicians among men aged between 40 and 70 years, about 10% developed an acute coronary event within 1 month of diagnosis,[27,28] but it is not known whether the development of MI was associated with previous IHD or with persistence and waxing of symptoms. In patients hospitalized for unstable angina, mortality rates varied between 1 and 8% in different studies.[2,3] The risk decreases rapidly during the first month after discharge and subsequently stabilizes (see Fig. 19.1).[3] It is also not known whether death after discharge is more common in patients with preexisting IHD and/or in those with persistent or recurrent symptoms. These differences in mortality rate are probably related to local referral practise and admission policies, but retrospective analysis is impossible as the relevant studies contain no precise information on the time dependency of risk, on the severity and persistence of symptoms, and on the relationship between the outcome and the chronic and acute determinants of prognosis.

19.3.1 Determinants of prognosis

The determinants of prognosis considered so far are multiple and their individual prognostic values vary in different reports. The major determinants of short-term prognosis most consistently recognized are the recurrence and the total duration of ischemic episodes, painful[29-33] or painless,[33-38] which were also found to have a long-term prognostic signifi-

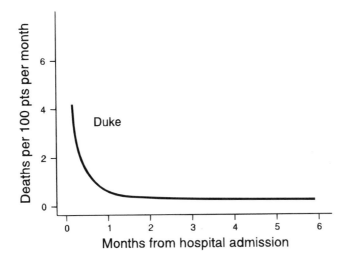

Fig. 19.1   Time-dependence of risk in patients with unstable angina. Outcome of medically treated patients with unstable angina in the Duke Cardiovascular Databank indicates that the risk of death decreased sharply during the first month. The mortality rate in other smaller groups varied between 4% and 6% during admission. (Modified from ref. 3.).

cance.[34,37] Other studies have indicated the prognostic importance of the resting ECG,[39,40] the predischarge exercise stress test in terms of both an ischemic response[39,41] and thallium-201 uptake in the lungs,[42] age,[43] previous IHD,[44] and the rapidity with which symptoms develop and progress.[45]

Serum levels of myoglobin, MB fraction of creatine phosphokinase (CKMB) and troponin-T—sensitive indicators of myocardial necrosis—were found to be elevated in unstable patients[21-23] and troponin-T values were found to be prognostic for MI and mortality.[23] Elevated serum levels of CRP and SAA protein, two acute-phase reaction proteins, were found to be highly predictive of subsequent MI and refractory unstable angina requiring urgent revascularization, in the absence of elevated levels of troponin-T (see Fig. 9.26).[26] The prognostic value of elevated levels of CKMB and troponin-T can be interpreted as reflecting severe, prolonged episodes of myocardial ischemia causing small foci of necrosis (and hence have a similar significance to prolonged episodes of painful or painless myocardial ischemia). The reasons for the very high prognostic values of CRP and SAA are still unknown.

None of the individual prognostic predictors considered are linearly related to prognosis, because of their variable intensity and their relationship with other prognostic determinants. Thus, in any given study, the importance of one determinant may emerge because it reflects its prevalence and intensity in the group of patients under consideration compared with that of other predictors. For example, if only patients within a narrow age range and with no significant impairment of ventricular function are included in the study, age, left ventricular ejection fraction (EF), and thallium uptake in the lungs may not emerge as important prognostic indicators. If only a minority of patients with very prolonged episodes of pain or persistent ST–T changes are considered, elevated levels of troponin-T may not emerge as a significant predictor of prognosis. Conversely, the statistical importance of an abnormal resting ECG and of

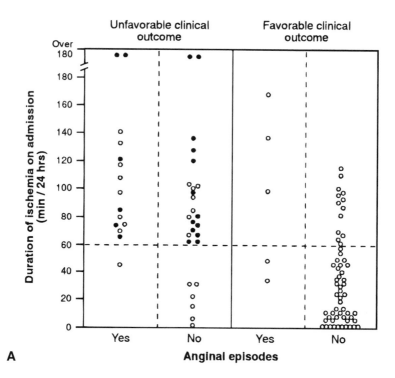

A   **Anginal episodes**

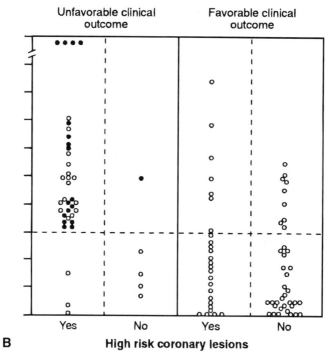

B   **High risk coronary lesions**

Table 19.1   General classification of patients presenting with unstable angina

Clinical presentation of angina	Baseline determinants of prognosis*	Acute determinants of prognosis
De novo		Persisting instability
	Chronic stable angina	Crescendo unstable angina
Destabilizing	Old MI, EF >40%	Refractory unstable angina
	Old MI, EF <40%	Resolving crescendo
Post-acute MI	EF >40%	Resolving refractory unstable angina
	EF <40%	Possibly resolved unstable angina

* Age is also a major determinant of absolute risk as mortality for MI increases exponentially. The increase is very steep after the age of 65

Patients are classified according to clinical presentation and to baseline determinants of prognosis. In each subgroup, defined by clinical presentation and by baseline determinants of prognosis, the importance of acute determinants of prognosis is indicated by the waxing and waning of the ischemic manifestations, as described in detail in Fig. 19.3

thallium uptake in the lungs may appear much greater in studies that include many patients with previous MI, than in studies including only patients with de novo unstable angina. The complex overlap between duration of ischemia, coronary artery anatomy, and symptoms can be appreciated from the data presented in Fig. 19.2A,B.

The additional prognostic value of tests, above that provided by the clinical presentation, should be assessed in homogeneous subgroups of unstable patients, classified according to a history of chronic stable angina or previous MI and the impairment of left ventricular EF (which indicate their preexisting baseline determinants of prognosis), and to the waxing and waning of anginal attacks (which indicate the acute determinants of prognosis), as indicated in Table 19.1 and described below.

Acute determinants of prognosis

The tendency to evolve towards MI is suggested not only by the exacerbation of spontaneous anginal attacks recurring in spite of adequate medical therapy and prolonged episodes lasting over 20 min (spontaneous angina is defined as angina not precipitated by any strong emotion or significant effort, but occurring unexpectedly at rest or during everyday activities) but also by the sudden, persistent, obvious reduction of the ischemic threshold during effort in the absence of extracoronary causes (see below) (indicative of the sudden development or worsening of a coronary artery stenosis as a result of recent thrombosis).

Fig. 19.2   Multiple predictors of outcome in unstable angina. A total duration of ischemia for >60 min during the first 24 h after admission detected by continuous ECG recording is a more important predictor of outcome than the total number of both anginal attacks (**A**) and high risk angiographic coronary lesions (**B**). Some asymptomatic patients had an unfavorable clinical outcome, whilst others with high risk lesions had a favorable outcome. Basal ECG and left ventricular function, two additional important determinants of prognosis, were not considered in this analysis. Thus, prolonged ischemia, without pain, has the same prognostic significance as recurring, prolonged anginal attacks. (● fatal or non-fatal MI, ○ other clinical outcomes) (Modified from ref. 38.)

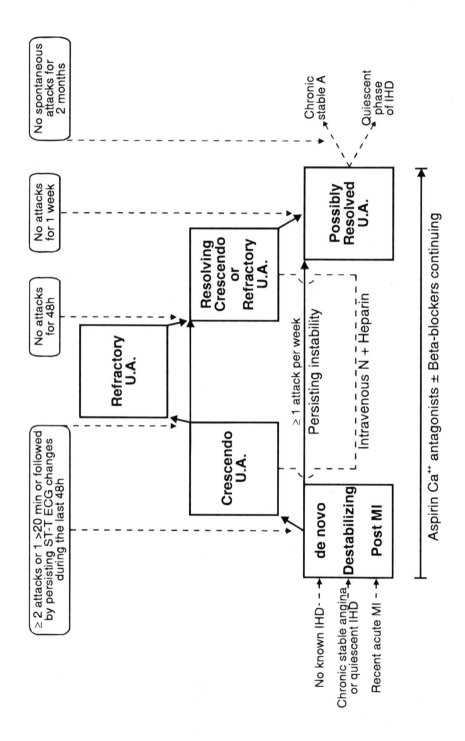

Preexisting baseline determinants of prognosis

The chronic preexisting determinants of the vulnerability of the heart to ischemic insults are represented by the severity of preexisting left ventricular damage (which makes the heart more vulnerable to further losses of myocardium and to ischemia-induced arrhythmias), by the site and severity of coronary stenoses (which determine the amount of myocardium at risk), and by the exponentially increasing mortality from acute MI with increasing age. As such, these chronic determinants of prognosis represent constant baseline prognostic factors during the changing phases of instability and the follow-up period. Impairment of left ventricular function may be present to a variable extent in patients with destabilizing and postinfarction angina, but is unlikely in patients with de novo unstable angina.

19.3.2 Classification

For patients with any of the three types of clinical presentation of instability defined above (i.e. *de novo unstable angina, destabilizing unstable angina* or *postacute MI unstable angina*) a prognostic classification should not be based only on a "still photograph" taken when the patient is examined initially, as is the case in the widely adopted classification proposed by Braunwald:[1] it should also consider the persistence or waning of the condition and the preexisting baseline determinants of prognosis, which are the baseline multipliers of the risk conferred by the severity of instability (see Table 19.1 and Fig. 19.3).

Acute determinants of prognosis (i.e. the waxing and waning of instability)

According to the *persistence and waxing of symptoms,* patients are divided into three classes, as follows:

a.   *persisting instability (class 1)* if at least one spontaneous ischemic episode (painful or painless) occurred during the last week (either on or off anti-ischemic therapy).

◄───

Fig. 19.3   Flow diagram of the dynamic classification of unstable angina. Patients with no known IHD (de novo unstable angina), with chronic stable angina or with quiescent IHD (destabilizing unstable angina) and those with recent acute MI (post MI unstable angina) who meet the definition of unstable angina and continue to have at least one ischemic episode a week, in spite of aspirin and oral anti-ischemic therapy, are defined as "persisting" unstable angina. According to the baseline risk conferred by any previous MI they are classified as groups A (no previous MI), B (left ventricular EF >40%) and C (EF <40%). When they remain free from ischemic episodes for 1 week they are redefined as "possibly resolved" unstable angina. Patients who had two or more ischemic episodes or an episode lasting >20 min or an episode followed by persistent ST-T changes during the last 48 h, are classified as "crescendo" unstable angina and require the addition of intravenous nitrates and heparin: such patients are reclassified as "refractory" unstable angina if they continue to present ischemic episodes. Following these acute phases, patients are reclassified as "resolving crescendo" or "resolving refractory" unstable angina when they remain free from ischemic episodes (painful or painless) for 48 h, as "persisting" unstable angina if they present at least one episode a week, and as "possibly resolved" unstable angina if they present no episodes for 1 week. Patients experiencing no spontaneous ischemic episodes for 2 months are reclassified as "resolved" unstable angina.

b. *crescendo unstable angina (class 2)* if, during the last 48 h, while on first-line treatment (with aspirin and anti-ischemic therapy), at least two spontaneous ischemic episodes occurred, or one episode occurred and lasted more than 20 min, or episodes occurred that were followed by persistent ischemic changes on the ECG. As soon as a diagnosis of crescendo unstable angina is made, intravenous nitrates and heparin should be added to the therapeutic regimen. Patients not on aspirin and anti-ischemic therapy should be treated promptly and classified as crescendo unstable angina as soon as they meet the above criteria.

c. *refractory unstable angina (class 3)* if, during the last 48 h, ischemic episodes occurred in spite of full therapy with aspirin, intravenous nitrates and heparin, calcium antagonists, and/or β-blockers (i.e. at least two spontaneous ischemic episodes occurred, or one episode occurred and lasted longer than 20 min, or episodes occurred that were followed by persistent ischemic changes on the ECG). Patients continue to be classified as refractory if they continue to present ischemic episodes in spite of full medical therapy.

According to the *waning of symptoms and signs of ischemia*, patients are divided into two categories, as follows:

a. *resolving crescendo* or *resolving refractory unstable angina,* if no episodes of ischemia occurred for periods from 48 h to 1 week (which suggests that healing of the unstable lesions is taking place)

b. *possibly resolved unstable angina,* if no ischemic episodes occurred for periods from 1 week to 2 months (which suggests that the unstable coronary lesions may have healed).

After 2 months with no signs of instability, patients enter or revert to either a quiescent phase or to chronic stable angina.

■ *Episodes of myocardial ischemia influencing the dynamic classification of instability may be painful or painless (i.e. detectable only by continuous ECG monitoring).* ■

Preexisting baseline determinants of prognosis

Patients with destabilizing or postinfarction unstable angina are classified into three groups (A, B, and C) according to either the absence or presence of previous MI, and to the severity of impairment of ventricular contractile function:

a. *group A:* no evidence of previous MI
b. *group B:* evidence of previous MI, old or recent, with no history of cardiac failure and a left ventricular EF greater than 40% (as mortality begins to increase steeply below this value; see Ch. 13)
c. *group C:* evidence of previous MI, old or recent, with a history of cardiac failure or with a left ventricular EF less than 40%.

Chronic baseline determinants of prognosis multiply the effects of acute determinants of prognosis in each category of instability.

■ *Thus, a patient can be classified either according to the clinical syndrome, as having de novo, destabilizing, or postinfarction unstable angina, or according to their baseline risk, as belonging to groups A, B, or C or according to the acute determinants of risk, as having persisting, crescendo, or refractory unstable angina or resolving crescendo, resolving refractory, or possibly resolved unstable angina.* ■

Estimation of the average risk defined on the basis of chronic and acute determinants of prognosis requires prospective data collection, but the gradient of risk is likely to be continuous: at lowest risk would be patients under 65 years of age with de novo, possibly resolved unstable angina; at highest risk would be patients over the age of 65 in group C with refractory unstable angina.

A clinical diagnosis of crescendo angina (class 2) for patients on aspirin and anti-ischemic therapy, or of possible crescendo angina for those with de novo unstable angina, not yet on therapy, calls for admission to a CCU. Patients with persistent instability (class 1) and those with possibly resolved unstable angina can be managed, after the appropriate tests have been performed, out of hospital, but should be advised to seek medical attention immediately should their symptoms recur or deteriorate.

■ *Future prospective studies may suggest that the inclusion criteria in each of the clinically defined prognostic groups, as well as the time intervals proposed in the above classifications, should be modified on the basis of new prognostic evidence and, possibly, of new blood markers of instability.* ■

19.4 MANAGEMENT

Until the clinical value of some blood markers of instability becomes established, the presence and intensity of the instability can be judged only from the waxing and waning of ischemic episodes (painful and painless). Until the causes of instability are elucidated, therapy is intended primarily to reduce its consequences, i.e. to oppose the local thrombotic and vasoconstrictive tendencies. This can be achieved only by interfering with the systemic hemostatic equilibrium, in order to prevent coronary thrombosis and increase fibrinolysis, and by reducing the vasomotor tone of the whole body, in order to prevent occasional episodes of coronary vasoconstriction. Such therapy may be ineffective when local thrombogenic and vasoconstrictor stimuli are very intense. In patients with a critical reduction of coronary flow reserve, therapy is intended also to reduce myocardial oxygen consumption (and possibly ischemia-induced arrhythmogenesis) by reducing β-adrenergic sympathetic tone and left ventricular afterload and preload. For patients failing to respond adequately to these forms of medical therapy, urgent PTCA or CABG are the only alternatives available.

Therapy should be proportional to both the estimated severity of the instability and the risk conferred by chronic baseline determinants of prognosis and, therefore, graded according to the clinical classification of risk presented above. The results of therapeutic trials cannot always be applied readily to clinical practise because the inclusion criteria and the duration of follow-up adopted in different studies are often too broad and too variable.

19.4.1 Results of Therapeutic Trials

The most convincing and dramatic short- and long-term improvement of prognosis in patients with a history of unstable angina was obtained with aspirin.[46–49] The reduction in the incidence of both MI and mortality was similar for doses of 75–1250 mg/day (see Fig. 19.4). A similar reduction in mortality rate and in the incidence of nonfatal events has also been observed with ticlopidine (250 mg/twice daily).[50] During the hospital phase a significant reduction of MI was observed with intravenous infusion of heparin.[49,51] CABG improved long-term survival in high-risk patients with unstable angina.[52]

In contrast, although they reduced symptoms, anti-ischemic drugs produced only a very small improvement in prognosis compared with aspirin and heparin.[53,54] A reduction in the number of ischemic episodes was observed with intravenous nitrates[55,56] and by combining

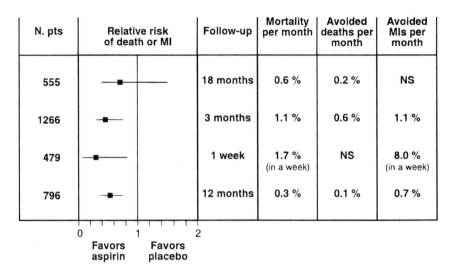

N. pts	Relative risk of death or MI	Follow-up	Mortality per month	Avoided deaths per month	Avoided MIs per month
555		18 months	0.6 %	0.2 %	NS
1266		3 months	1.1 %	0.6 %	1.1 %
479		1 week	1.7 % (in a week)	NS	8.0 % (in a week)
796		12 months	0.3 %	0.1 %	0.7 %

0   1   2
Favors   Favors
aspirin   placebo

Fig. 19.4   Time-dependent beneficial effects of aspirin. The beneficial effects of aspirin were statistically significant in all studies, but the absolute benefit (i.e. the number of events prevented per 100 patients treated per month) was lowest in those trials with long periods of follow-up, which also had the lowest average mortality rate per month due to the rapid time-dependency of decreased risk and the consequent dilution effect by the low mortality in subsequent months. (From data presented in refs 46–49.)

β-blockers and calcium antagonists, but nifedipine alone was found to have adverse effects on prognosis.[57] Verapamil produced a larger reduction of painful and painless ischemic episodes than propranolol in patients with a vasospastic component.[58] A reduction in the number of attacks was also observed with picotamide, but not with aspirin.[59]

Thrombolysis failed to improve prognosis in unstable patients,[7,60–62] although it reduced the incidence of intracoronary thrombosis; it also increases the risk of intracranial bleeding. This failure is not surprising, not only because thrombolytic drugs are not used for reestablishing CBF, as acute coronary occlusion is only a transient feature of unstable angina, but also because the drugs cannot prevent thrombotic stimuli from recurring after the lytic effects have worn off.

The variable beneficial effects of anti-ischemic therapy reflect the heterogeneous nature of the patients included in the various studies, the intensity of recurring coronary thrombotic and vasoconstrictor stimuli, and, possibly, an enhanced thrombotic and constrictor response.

Emergency PTCA and CABG are associated with increased morbidity and mortality in comparison with elective PTCA or CABG,[63–66] but the increased risk is justified for patients with refractory unstable angina or a markedly reduced coronary flow reserve and large areas of myocardium at risk.

The preliminary results of several recently completed or partially completed trials of medical therapy, CABG, and PTCA are applicable only to patients eligible for randomization, but not to patients with refractory unstable angina who would not be eligible. For those who are eligible, the results of the TIMI IIIB trial indicate that in uncertain cases the choice is determined by local practise, surgical expertise, and the wishes of the patient.[3]

19.4.2 Management of persisting (class 1) and possibly resolved unstable angina

Patients may come to medical attention with a history compatible with persisting or possibly resolved unstable angina. On the basis of the estimated risk, patients can be assessed either as outpatients or during hospitalization.

Immediately a provisional diagnosis has been made, a loading dose of aspirin (325 mg) should be administered on a full stomach (unless contraindicated because of hypersensitivity, active bleeding, or the risk of severe bleeding), followed by a maintenance dose (75 mg/day). Ticlopidine (250 mg, twice a day) can be prescribed to patients with hypersensitivity to aspirin.

In addition, a calcium antagonist that does not increase heart rate, such as long-acting diltiazem or verapamil (120 mg, 2–4 times a day) should be administered. Patients with destabilizing unstable angina who are receiving β-blockers should continue on the same dosage, but calcium antagonists of the dihydropyridine type, such as nifedipine retard (20 mg, 3 times a day), should be added as a first choice. The persistence of occasional attacks, even without a crescendo pattern, indicates that therapy should be increased. A maintenance dose of aspirin (75 mg/day on a full stomach) should be prescribed in the possibly resolved phase of unstable angina, but the maintenance dose of ticlopidine remains the same (250 mg/twice a day).

Therapy should be withdrawn as soon as the diagnosis of unstable angina can be excluded confidently. It should, however, be continued for 2 months at the same level if the diagnosis can neither be ruled out nor confirmed. If anginal attacks recur, the patient should be reassessed promptly.

■ *Ischemic episodes should be treated promptly with sublingual or intravenous nitrates, repeating the dose every 2–3 min if the episode persists (unless a significant fall in arterial blood pressure is observed). Ischemia that persists despite repeated boluses of intravenous nitrates indicates the need for immediate thrombolytic therapy (see below).* ■

Investigations

Routine blood tests of chemistry, hemoglobin, and serum indices of myocardial necrosis should be obtained in order to investigate the possible occurrence of episodes of subclinical myocardial necrosis during the preceding days. Levels of CRP should also be measured, if its high short-term prognostic value is confirmed.

A standard chest radiogram (PA and LL) and either a cross-sectional echocardiogram or radionuclide angiogram should be obtained to form part of the baseline reference information (particularly for patients with destabilizing or post-MI unstable angina). A 48 h Holter recording and submaximal ECG stress test can be useful to confirm the diagnosis and to assess the severity of the instability and the area of myocardium at risk.

■ *Patients in class 1 and those with possibly resolved unstable angina, groups A and B, with negative tests for ischemia are at low risk. They should be followed carefully as outpatients, should correct any risk factors and should have a maximal ECG exercise stress test at 2 months. Humoral markers of susceptibility to recurrent episodes of instability and of a possible unfavorable outcome of the instability are needed in order to identify those relatively few patients at risk of a short-term relapse.* ■

19.4.3 Management of crescendo unstable angina (class 2)

Patients presenting to the emergency department with a history suggestive of crescendo unstable angina should receive a loading dose of aspirin (325 mg) and full anti-ischemic therapy, as described above. Those developing a crescendo pattern of angina while receiving aspirin and anti-ischemic therapy should be managed in a CCU and prescribed intravenous nitrates and heparin (in addition to the full oral therapy indicated above). Intravenous therapy either should be continued as long as the attacks persist or should be withdrawn gradually after the patient has remained free from ischemic episodes (painful or painless) for 48 h.

The dose of intravenous heparin should increase activated partial thromboplastin time (aPTT) by between 46 and 70 s. This applies to those institutions with a mean control aPTT of about 30 s; in others, aPTT should be increased by approximately 1.5–2.5 times control. This is usually achieved with a bolus of 80 units/kg followed by an intravenous infusion of 18 units/kg/h.[67]

Serial hemoglobin and platelet levels should be measured each day in order to monitor the development of heparin-induced thrombocytopenia (which may occur in 10–20% of patients). Contraindications to heparin infusion are active bleeding, the risk of severe bleeding, recent stroke, and a history of heparin-induced thrombocytopenia.

The dose of intravenous nitrates (nitroglycerin 0.01–0.1 mg/min or isosorbide dinitrate (ISDN) 0.05–0.3 mg/min) should be titrated to bring about a fall in systolic blood pressure of 10–20 mmHg, and increased as necessary to maintain this drop in pressure in order to overcome the problem of tolerance. It should also be boosted by intravenous boluses whenever a new ischemic episode occurs.

Individual ischemic episodes should be treated aggressively, as for class 1 patients.

In patients with resolving crescendo or resolving refractory unstable angina, after an interval of 48 h from the last ischemic episode, heparin and intravenous nitrates should be tapered off gradually over a 6 h period, as sudden interruption can cause rebound effects with recurrence of ischemic episodes.[68,69]

Thrombin inhibitors, such as hirudin[70] and platelet adhesion receptor blockers,[71] are now under clinical investigation. Appropriate clinical trials in carefully classified subgroups of patients are required to assess the additional benefits of these new agents, compared with currently established treatment regimens, and to provide guidelines readily applicable to clinical practise.

Investigations

In class 2 patients, the indices of myocardial cell necrosis should be measured daily and aPTT monitored as indicated above, in addition to the tests indicated for class 1 patients. Assessment of baseline left ventricular function and its deterioration during ischemic episodes can provide useful information on the extent of jeopardized myocardium.

■ *Patients with crescendo unstable angina unresponsive to aspirin and full anti-ischemic therapy are at very high risk and may benefit from continuous ECG ST-segment monitoring, as the recurrence of ischemic episodes indicates that they are refractory to medical therapy.* ■

19.4.4 Management of refractory unstable angina (class 3)

Refractory unstable angina occurs in about 10% of hospitalized patients, as most patients may respond to maximal medical therapy prolonged over several days.[72]

Thrombolytic therapy should be considered whenever a patient presents with an ischemic episode with obvious acute ST-segment elevation or depression on the ECG that does not subside within 30 min despite repeated intravenous boluses of nitrates (i.e. impending infarction). The failure of trials of thrombolytic therapy in unstable angina to obtain statistically significant beneficial effects may be related to the inclusion criteria, as there is no obvious rationale for giving a short-acting thrombolytic drug to patients who may not, at that time, have continuing acute occlusive coronary thrombosis (even though they may have had one in the past and may have another in the future). In patients with persistent ischemia, emergency PTCA is indicated when a major coronary artery supplying a critical area of myocardium is acutely occluded (see Ch. 22).

Urgent PTCA or CABG should be considered whenever ischemic episodes recur in spite of maximal medical therapy. The indications for revascularization procedures in other patients, and, to some extent, the choice between PTCA and CABG, will continue to be influenced by local practise and levels of expertise until compelling evidence favoring either becomes available from randomized trials.

19.4.5 Predischarge assessment

Patients with possibly resolved unstable angina are considered for discharge depending on their previous symptoms, their response to therapy, the severity of preexisting IHD, and local practise.

In the choice of predischarge tests consideration should be given to the following:

a.   the severity of preexisting left ventricular dysfunction
b.   the residual coronary flow reserve as assessed by previous exercise stress testing and the findings of coronary arteriography (when performed prior to the unstable phase)
c.   the in-hospital evolution and response to therapy of symptoms and signs of myocardial ischemia (the more frequent, severe, and prolonged the ischemic episodes on full therapy, the more guarded the prognosis and, hence, the more aggressive the investigations, the more intensive the therapy, and the closer the follow-up)
d.   the patient's attitude towards the disease (the need for reassurance at one extreme and the urge to control risk factors at the other).

Choice of tests

A submaximal ECG exercise stress test should be performed on aspirin alone in patients in whom no episodes of ischemia occurred during hospitalization and with no previous evidence of IHD.

In patients with a confirmed ischemic origin of pain (i.e. diagnosed during admission), or with previous evidence of IHD, the test should be performed on full medical therapy at least 72 h after the last spontaneous ischemic episode, as its sole aim is to assess residual coronary flow reserve; a positive result on full therapy, particularly at a low work load, would be an absolute indication for assessing the area of myocardium at risk using imaging techniques or, when these are not easily available, coronary arteriography (see Ch. 16). The exercise test should be performed on a very gradual protocol (such as the modified Bruce protocol) and should be terminated as soon as diagnostic ischemic ST-segment shifts, pseudonormalization of an inverted T wave (with or without angina), or a fall in blood pressure appear.

A negative submaximal exercise test on anti-ischemic therapy is a good prognostic indicator, but the test should be repeated after 2 months, off anti-ischemic therapy (but continuing aspirin), until the maximal predicted heart rate is achieved. In the presence of a good left ventricular function (EF more than 40%), a negative maximal exercise test, off anti-ischemic therapy, is a good prognostic indicator and may dispense with the need to perform elective coronary arteriography (unless required for patient reassurance) because, in patients with a good EF and good effort tolerance, there is no evidence that the prognosis can be improved by revascularization procedures, even when they have multivessel coronary disease (see Figs 17.6 and 17.8). In patients who cannot exercise because of physical limitations, the dipyridamole test should be considered, although, during the acute phase, it is not without risk.[73] Predischarge Holter monitoring and radionuclide techniques have been shown to produce a reasonably good risk stratification.[74] However, it is not clear whether these findings would apply also to low-risk groups such as patients without post-MI unstable angina, with a good EF, and with a negative submaximal ECG exercise stress test.

Anti-ischemic treatment should be continued for at least 2 months and low-dose aspirin indefinitely. Patients should be reassessed as outpatients within 2 months of discharge, but instructed to seek immediate readmission if their symptoms recur. In totally asymptomatic patients with a negative maximal exercise stress test performed off anti-ischemic treatment, therapy may be reduced gradually and possibly discontinued unless required for control of arterial hypertension or ventricular remodelling. Such patients are eligible for the long-term management plan discussed in Chapter 13 for patients who enter a quiescent phase of IHD.

■ *The development of humoral markers of instability and of a patient's susceptibility to develop unstable angina are necessary steps in the identification of patients at risk, based not merely on the appearance or recurrence of symptoms.* ■

REFERENCES

1. Braunwald E. Unstable angina. A classification. Circulation 1989;*80:*410.
2. Julian DG. The natural history of unstable angina. In: Hugenholtz PG, Goldman BS (eds) Unstable Angina. Current Concepts and Management. Schattauer, New York, 1985.
3. U.S. Department of Health and Human Services. Public Health Service. Agency for Health Care Policy and Research National Heart, Lung, and Blood Institute. Unstable angina: diagnosis and management. In: Clinical Practice Guideline, No. *10,* 1994.
4. Graves EJ. National hospital discharge survey: annual summary, 1991. National Center for Health Statistics. Vital Health Statistics. Series 13, Number *114.* Washington: Public Health Service, 1993.
5. Volpi A, De Vita C, Franzosi MG et al. Determinants of 6-month mortality in survivors of myocardial infarction after thrombolysis. Results of the GISSI-2 data base. Circulation 1993;*88:*416.
6. Ahmed WH, Bittl JA, Braunwald E. Relation between clinical presentation and angiographic findings in unstable angina pectoris, and comparison with that in stable angina. Am J Cardiol 1993;*72:*544.
7. The TIMI IIIB Investigators. Effects of tissue plasminogen activator and a comparison of early invasive and conservative strategies in unstable angina and non-Q-wave myocardial infarction. Results of the TIMI IIIB Trial. Circulation 1994;*89:*1545.
8. Moise A, Theroux P, Taeymans Y et al. Unstable angina and progression of coronary atherosclerosis. N Engl J Med 1983;*309:*685.

9. Crake T, Tousoulis D, Kaski JC, Maseri A. Stability of symptoms in chronic angina pectoris in spite of severe coronary stenosis progression. Submitted for publication.

10. Neill WA, Ritzmann LW, Selden R. The pathophysiologic basis of acute coronary insufficiency. Observations favoring the hypothesis of intermittent reversible coronary obstruction. Am Heart J 1977;*94:*439.

11. Davies MJ, Thomas A. Thrombosis and acute coronary-artery lesions in sudden cardiac ischemic death. N Engl J Med 1984;*310:*1137.

12. Falk E. Morphologies of unstable atherothrombotic plaques underlying acute coronary syndromes. Am J Cardiol 1989;*63:*114E.

13. Arbustini E, Grasso M, Diegoli M et al. Coronary atherosclerotic plaques with and without thrombus in ischemic heart syndromes: a morphologic, immunohistochemical, and biochemical study. Am J Cardiol 1991;*68:*36B.

14. Willerson JT, Campbell WB, Winniford MD et al. Conversion from chronic to acute coronary artery disease: speculation regarding mechanisms. Am J Cardiol 1984;*54:*1249.

15. Fuster V, Badimon L, Badimon JJ et al. The pathogenesis of coronary artery disease and the acute coronary syndromes (2). N Engl J Med 1992;*326:*310.

16. Maseri A, Crea F. The elusive cause of instability in unstable angina. Am J Cardiol 1991;*68:*16B.

17. Chierchia S, Lazzari M, Simonetti I, Maseri A. Hemodynamic monitoring in angina at rest. Herz 1980;*5:*189.

18. Figueras J, Singh BN, Ganz W, Charuzi Y, Swan HJC. Mechanism of rest and nocturnal angina: observations during continuous hemodynamic and electrocardiographic monitoring. Circulation 1979;*59:*955.

19. Berndt TB, Fitzgerald J, Harrison DC, Schroeder JS. Hemodynamic changes at the onset of spontaneous versus pacing-induced angina. Am J Cardiol 1977;*39:*784.

20. Uthurralt N, Davies GJ, Parodi O, Bencivelli W, Maseri A. Comparative study of myocardial ischemia during angina at rest and on exertion using thallium-201 scintigraphy. Am J Cardiol 1981;*48:*410.

21. Biagini A, Mazzei MG, Carpeggiani C et al. Myocardial cell damage during attacks of vasospastic angina in the absence of persistent electrocardiographic changes. Clin Cardiol 1981;*4:*315.

22. Botker HE, Ravkilde J, Sogaard P et al. Gradation of unstable angina based on a sensitive immunoassay for serum creatine kinase MB. Br Heart J 1991;*65:*72.

23. Hamm CW, Ravkilde J, Gerhardt W et al. The prognostic value of serum troponin T in unstable angina. N Engl J Med 1992;*327:*146.

24. Lee TH, Cook EF, Weisberg M et al. Acute chest pain in the emergency room. Identification and examination of low-risk patients. Arch Intern Med 1985;*145:*65.

25. Lee T, Cook EF, Weisberg MC et al. Impact of the availability of a prior electrocardiogram on the triage of the patient with acute chest pain. J Gen Intern Med 1990;*5:*381.

26. Liuzzo G, Biasucci LM, Gallimore JR et al. Prognostic value of C-reactive protein and serum amyloid A protein in severe unstable angina. New Engl J Med 1994;*331:*417.

27. Fulton M, Duncan B, Lutz W et al. Natural history of unstable angina. Lancet 1972;*1:*860.

28. Duncan B, Fulton M, Morrison SL et al. Prognosis of new and worsening angina pectoris. Br Med J 1976;*1:*981.

29. Conti CR, Brawley RK, Griffith LS et al. Unstable angina pectoris: morbidity and mortality in 57 consecutive patients evaluated angiographically. Am J Cardiol 1973;*32:*745.

30. Bertolasi CA, Tronge JE, Mon GA, Turri D, Lugones MI. Clinical spectrum of "unstable angina." Clin Cardiol 1979;*2:*113.

31. Cairns JA, Fantus EG, Klassen GA. Unstable angina pectoris. Am Heart J 1976;*92:*373.

32. Mulcahy R, Daly L, Graham I et al. Unstable angina: natural history and determinants of prognosis. Am J Cardiol 1981;*48:*525.

33. Romeo F, Rosano GMC, Martuscelli E, Valente A, Reale A. Unstable angina: role of silent ischemia and total ischemic time (silent plus painful ischemia), a 6-year follow-up. J Am Coll Cardiol 1992;*19:*1173.

34. Gottlieb SO, Weisfeldt ML, Ouyang P, Mellits ED, Gerstenblith G. Silent ischemia as a marker for early unfavorable outcomes in patients with unstable angina. N Engl J Med 1986;*314:*1214.

35. Langer A, Freeman MR, Armstrong PW. ST segment shift in unstable angina: pathophysiology and association with coronary anatomy and hospital outcome. J Am Coll Cardiol 1989;*13*:1495.
36. Arnim THV, Gerbig HW, Krawietz W, Höfling B. Prognostic implications of transient—predominantly silent—ischaemia in patients with unstable angina pectoris. Eur Heart J 1988:*9*:435.
37. Nademanee K, Intarachot V, Josephson MA, Rieders D, Vaghaiwalla F, Singh BN. Prognostic significance of silent myocardial ischemia in patients with unstable angina. J Am Coll Cardiol 1987;*10*:1.
38. Bugiardini R, Borghi A, Pozzati A, Ruggeri A, Puddu P, Maseri A. Relation of severity of symptoms to transient myocardial ischemia and prognosis in unstable angina. J Am Coll Cardiol 1995 (in press).
39. Severi S, Orsini E, Marraccini P, Michelassi C, L'Abbate A. The basal electrocardiogram and the exercise stress test in assessing prognosis in patients with unstable angina. Eur Heart J 1988;*9*:441.
40. Nyman I, Areskog M, Areskog NH, Swahn E, Wallentins L and the RISC Study Group. Very early risk stratification by electrocardiogram at rest in men with suspected unstable coronary heart disease. J Intern Med 1993;*234*:293.
41. Wilcox I, Freedman SB, Allman KC et al. Prognostic significance of a predischarge exercise test in risk stratification after unstable angina pectoris. J Am Coll Cardiol 1991;*18*:677.
42. Brown KA. Prognostic value of thallium-201 myocardial perfusion imaging in patients with unstable angina who respond to medical treatment. J Am Coll Cardiol 1991;*17*:1053.
43. Cairns JA, Singer J, Gent M et al. One year mortality outcomes of all coronary and intensive care unit patients with acute myocardial infarction, unstable angina or other chest pain in Hamilton, Ontario, a city of 375 000 people. Can J Cardiol 1989;*5*:239.
44. White LD, Lee TH, Cook EF et al. Comparison of the natural history of new onset and exacerbated chronic ischemic heart disease. The Chest Pain Study Group. J Am Coll Cardiol 1990;*16*:304.
45. Betriu A, Heras M, Cohen M, Fuster V. Unstable angina: outcome according to clinical presentation. J Am Coll Cardiol 1992;*19*:1659.
46. Lewis HDJ, Davis JW, Archibald DG et al. Protective effects of aspirin against acute myocardial infarction and death in men with unstable angina. Results of a Veterans Administration Cooperative Study. N Engl J Med 1983;*309*:396.
47. Cairns JA, Gent M, Singer J et al. Aspirin, sulfinpyrazone, or both in unstable angina. Results of a Canadian multicenter trial. N Engl J Med 1985;*313*:1369.
48. Wallentin LC. Aspirin (75 mg/day) after an episode of unstable coronary artery disease: long-term effects on the risk for myocardial infarction, occurrence of severe angina and the need for revascularization. Research Group on Instability in Coronary Artery Disease in Southeast Sweden. J Am Coll Cardiol 1991;*18*:1587.
49. Theroux P, Waters D, Qiu S et al. Aspirin versus heparin to prevent myocardial infarction during the acute phase of unstable angina. Circulation 1993;*88*:2045.
50. Balsano F, Rizzon P, Violi F et al. Antiplatelet treatment with ticlopidine in unstable angina. A controlled multicenter clinical trial. The Studio della Ticlopidina nell'Angina Instabile Group. Circulation 1990;*82*:17.
51. Telford AM, Wilson C. Trial of heparin versus atenolol in prevention of myocardial infarction in intermediate coronary syndrome. Lancet 1981;*1*:1225.
52. Sharma GV, Deupree RH, Khuri SF et al. Coronary bypass surgery improves survival in high-risk unstable angina. Results of a Veterans Administration Cooperative study with an 8-year follow-up. Veterans Administration Unstable Angina Cooperative Study Group. Circulation 1991;*84*:III260.
53. Held PH, Yusuf S, Furberg CD. Calcium channel blockers in acute myocardial infarction and unstable angina: an overview. Br Med J 1989;*299*:1187.
54. Lubsen J. Medical management of unstable angina. What have we learned from the randomized trials?. Circulation 1990;*82*:II82.
55. Roubin GS, Harris PJ, Eckhardt I et al. Intravenous nitroglycerin in refractory unstable angina pectoris. Aust N Z J Med 1982;*12*:598.

56. Kaplan K, Davison R, Parker M et al. Intravenous nitroglycerin for the treatment of angina at rest unresponsive to standard nitrate therapy. Am J Cardiol 1983;51:694.

57. Lubsen J, Tijssen JG. Efficacy of nifedipine and metoprolol in the early treatment of unstable angina in the coronary care unit: findings from the Holland Interuniversity Nifedipine/Metoprolol Trial (HINT). Am J Cardiol 1987;60:18A.

58. Parodi O, Simonetti I, Michelassi C et al. Comparison of verapamil and propranolol therapy for angina pectoris at rest: a randomized, multiple-crossover, controlled trial in the coronary care unit. Am J Cardiol 1986;57:899.

59. Neri Serneri GG, Gensini GF, Poggesi L et al. The role of extraplatelet thromboxane A$_2$ in unstable angina investigated with a dual thromboxane A$_2$ inhibitor: importance of activated monocytes. Cor Art Dis 1994;5:137.

60. van den Brand M, van Zijl A, Geuskens R, de Feyter PJ, Serruys PW, Simoons ML. Tissue plasminogen activator in refractory unstable angina: a randomized double blind placebo controlled trial in patients with refractory unstable angina and subsequent angioplasty. Eur Heart J 1991;12:1208.

61. Bär FW, Verheugt FWA, Col J et al. Thrombolysis in patients with unstable angina improves the angiographic but not the clinical outcome: results of the UNASEM, a multicenter, randomized, placebo-controlled, clinical trial with anistreplase. Circulation 1992;86:131.

62. Freeman MR, Langer A, Wilson RF, Morgan CD, Armstrong PW. Thrombolysis in unstable angina. Randomized double-blind trial of t-PA and placebo. Circulation 1992;85:150.

63. Goldman BS, Katz A, Christakis G, Weisel R. Determinants of risk for coronary artery bypass grafting in stable and unstable angina pectoris. Can J Surg 1985;28:505.

64. Myler RK, Shaw RE, Stertzer SH et al. Unstable angina and coronary angioplasty. Circulation 1990;82:II88.

65. de Feyter PJ, Serruys PW, Suryapranata H, Beatt K, van den Brand M. Coronary angioplasty early after diagnosis of unstable angina. Am Heart J 1987;114:48.

66. Cowley MJ, Corros G, Kelsey SF, van Raden M, Detre KM. Acute coronary events associated with percutaneous transluminal coronary angioplasty. Am J Cardiol 1984;53:12C.

67. Raschke RA, Reilly BM, Guidry JR et al. The weight-based heparin dosing nomogram compared with a "standard care" nomogram. Ann Intern Med 1993;119:874.

68. Figueras J, Lidon R, Cortadellas J. Rebound myocardial ischemia following abrupt interruption of intravenous nitroglycerin infusion in patients with unstable angina at rest. Eur Heart J 1991;12:405.

69. Theroux P, Waters D, Lam J et al. Reactivation of unstable angina after the discontinuation of heparin. N Engl J Med 1992;327:141.

70. Topol EJ, Fuster V, Harrington RA et al. Recombinant hirudin for unstable angina pectoris. A multicenter, randomized angiographic trial. Circulation 1994;89:1557.

71 Simoons ML, Jan de Boer M, van den Brand MJBM et al. Randomized trial of a GPIIb/IIIa platelet receptor blocker in refractory unstable angina. Circulation 1994;89:596.

72. Grambow DW, Topol EJ. Effect of maximal medical therapy on refractoriness of unstable angina pectoris. Am J Cardiol 1992;70:577.

73. Zhu YY, Chung WS, Botvinick EH et al. Dipyridamole perfusion scintigraphy: the experience with its application in one hundred seventy patients with known or suspected unstable angina. Am Heart J 1991;121:33.

74. Marmur JD, Freeman MR, Langer A, Armstrong PW. Prognosis in medically stabilized unstable angina: early Holter ST-segment monitoring compared with predischarge exercise thallium tomography. Ann Intern Med 1990;113:575.

20 | Variant angina

INTRODUCTION

The syndrome of variant angina is characterized by ischemia caused by recurrent transient occlusive spasm of a segment of epicardial coronary artery, with or without flow-limiting stenoses, usually associated with transmural reduction of myocardial blood flow and ST-segment elevation and usually with no recognizable trigger.

This "variant" form of angina was described in 1959 by Prinzmetal et al[1] who reported 12 cases of angina occurring predominantly at rest, rather than during effort, without apparent cause, and characterized by elevation, rather than depression, of the ST segment. He argued that these spontaneous attacks of angina were caused by a transient increase of tonus at the site of a subcritical coronary artery stenosis, rather than by an excessive increase in myocardial oxygen consumption which, at the time, was the only accepted cause of angina. He defined this form of angina as "variant." The possibility that coronary artery spasm could be a cause of angina had been proposed by several clinicians nearly a century before, but the concept had fallen into such disrepute that in the 1950s Prinzmetal dared not use the term "spasm," describing it instead as "an increased coronary tonus." Occlusive epicardial coronary artery spasm became a proven hypothesis only in the mid-1970s, and our report, which initially encountered considerable difficulty in finding acceptance on an internationally recognized journal, subsequently became a citation classic.[2] (For a historical review see reference 3.)

Although, as Prinzmetal correctly surmised, spasm usually occurs at the site of a noncritical coronary artery stenosis, it can also occur at the site of a very severe stenosis or even in the absence of any angiographically detectable stenosis: Prinzmetal's angina in patients with angiographically normal coronary arteries was described as a "variant of the variant" form of angina in the early 1970s.[4]

Clinically, variant angina has the following essential features:

a. recurrent ischemic episodes occurring predominantly at rest (usually in the early morning), mostly without apparent cause and usually characterized by ST-segment elevation, sometimes associated with arrhythmias and/or syncope
b. preserved effort tolerance

c. spontaneous or induced spasm of a major branch of an epicardial coronary artery, usually localized, but occasionally involving multiple branches either segmentally or diffusely

d. waxing or waning of symptoms over a period of weeks or months, but occasionally, persistence of symptoms for years whenever therapy is withdrawn.

Patients with variant angina may also present with ST-segment elevation during or soon after the end of an exercise stress test, but the test becomes negative after sublingual nitrates; ergonovine and hyperventilation tests are usually positive when performed during an acute phase of the disease.

The syndrome can present very acutely with several attacks a day, making it difficult to distinguish from unstable angina, or more chronically with episodes occurring once or twice every week or once every few weeks, with intervening asymptomatic periods of several weeks.

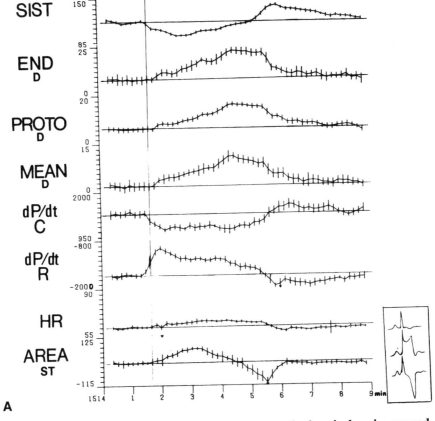

Fig. 20.1 Sequence of hemodynamic changes during ischemia caused by occlusive coronary artery spasm. A. illustrates the computerized analysis of a typical ECG and hemodynamic recording of a painless ischemic episode in a patient with variant angina. The vertical line indicates the onset of ST-segment elevation which, after about 2 min, is followed by the development of negative T-waves. A decrease in peak contraction (C) and relaxation (R) left ventricular dP/dt precedes the onset of ECG changes; a decrease in systolic (SIST) and an increase in end-, proto and mean diastolic pressures (End D, Proto D, and Mean D) follow the onset of ECG changes. *(Figure continues.)*

Occlusive coronary artery spasm may also contribute to other unstable ischemic syndromes characterized by different clinical presentations and which, therefore, may have underlying pathogenetic mechanisms differing from those responsible for the most typical, and much less frequent, variant form of angina, which is the vasospastic syndrome most clearly identifiable because of its "chronic" pattern of recurrence and distinctive clinical features (see Ch. 9).

In the 1970s, the revival of coronary artery spasm,[5] by demonstrating a rare cause of angina, helped to dispel the traditionally accepted belief that increased myocardial demand was the only "respectable" cause of angina pectoris.[6]

20.1 DEMONSTRATION OF SUDDEN REDUCTION OF CORONARY BLOOD FLOW

It has now been clearly established that variant angina is caused by a sudden reduction of myocardial blood flow caused by localized occlusive spasm of a segment of a major epicardial coronary artery.

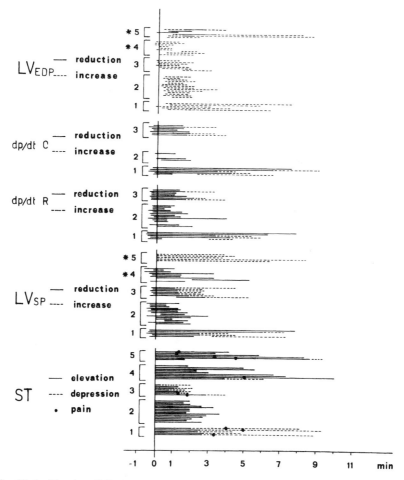

Fig. 20.1 *(Continued)* **B.** illustrates the sequence of events for all the episodes recorded in 5 patients. LV_{EDP} and LV_{SP} = left ventricular end-diastolic and end-systolic pressures, respectively. In patients 4 and 5 diastolic pulmonary artery pressure was measured instead of left ventricular pressure. The elevation of the ST segment begins at time 0. Pain, when present, occurs minutes later. (From data presented in ref. 8.)

20.1.1 Hemodynamic monitoring

Continuous hemodynamic recordings, in patients hospitalized in a coronary care unit (CCU) with variant angina and very frequent episodes of ischemia, failed to detect an increase of the hemodynamic determinants of myocardial oxygen consumption.[7] They actually showed a sequence of events identical to those observed in the experimental animal following acute coronary occlusion by ligature and following balloon occlusion of a coronary artery during percutaneous transluminal coronary angioplasty (PTCA) (see Fig. 20.1A,B).[8] Episodes characterized by ST-segment elevation may be followed by episodes of ST-segment depression (see Fig. 20.2).

The development of myocardial ischemia not preceded by any increase in myocardial oxygen consumption must be the result of a sudden reduction of regional coronary blood flow

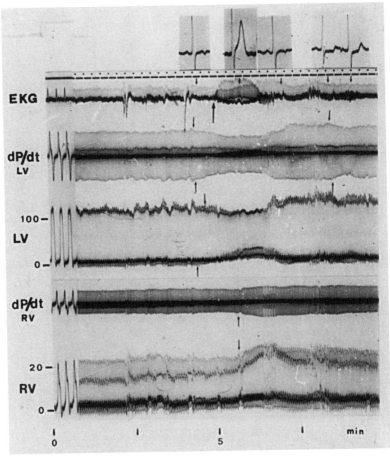

A

Fig. 20.2 Episodes of ST-segment elevation due to occlusive spasm may alternate with episodes of ST-segment depression caused by nonocclusive spasm.
Low-speed playback of a typical hemodynamic recording in a patient with variant angina (**A**) and a computerized analysis of another segment of the same recording (**B**). In (**A**), a painless episode of ST-segment elevation with peaking of T waves on the ECG (EKG) is followed by an episode of ST-segment depression, both associated with transient impairment of left ventricular (LV) function (arrows). (*Figure continues.*)

(CBF) associated with a compensatory increase in myocardial oxygen extraction, and is indicated by a sudden, very rapid drop in coronary sinus oxygen saturation (see Fig. 20.3A,B).[9] In full-blown spontaneous ischemic episodes, this is accompanied by a massive transmural reduction in regional myocardial perfusion (see Fig. 20.4).[10] Similar changes are also observed during ischemic episodes induced by provocative tests of coronary spasm in susceptible patients.

20.1.2 Angiographic findings

During coronary arteriography, spontaneous spasm typically reveals a localized total or subtotal occlusion with no (or only very slow) distal dye progression (see Fig. 20.5A/B). Localized spasm can occasionally involve two segments of the same branch, simultaneously or during different episodes, or two different arterial branches (for example, left anterior descending and right coronary arteries) with corresponding elevation of the ST segment on both inferior and anterior ECG leads. This observation indicates the possibility that, in some

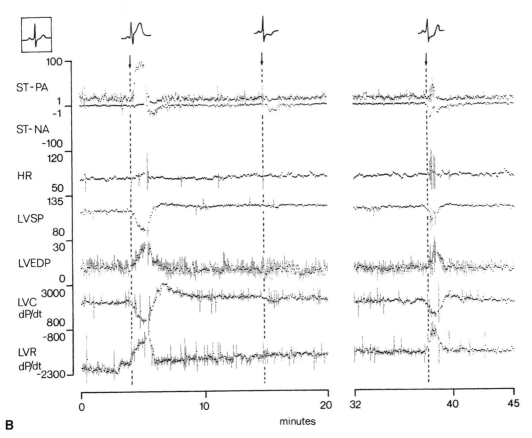

B

Fig. 20.2 *(Continued)* In (**B**), two painless episodes of ST-segment depression follow one of ST-segment elevation (ST−PA = positive area of the ST segment, ST−NA = negative area), but only the second is associated with obvious impairment of left ventricular function. (LVSP, LVEDP, LVC, LVR = left ventricular systolic pressure, end-diastolic pressure, contraction and relaxation peak dP/dt, respectively). (From data presented in ref. 8.)

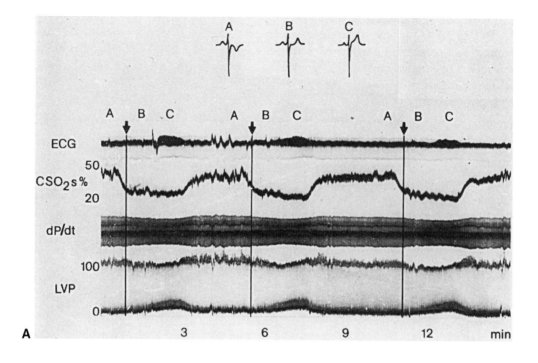

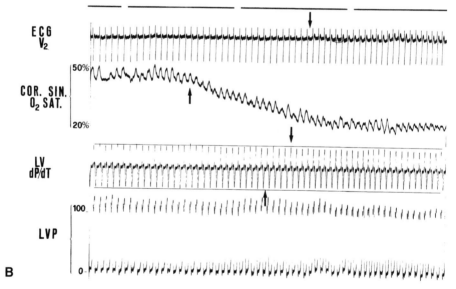

Fig. 20.3 **A decrease in coronary sinus oxygen saturation (CSO$_2$) is the first detectable change in ischemic episodes caused by occlusive spasm. A.** shows the low-speed playback of a hemodynamic recording during three successive painless ischemic episodes in a patient with variant angina. The ECG changes, consistently characterized by pseudonormalization of T waves followed by ST-segment elevation, are preceded by a large drop in CSO$_2$ and by obvious impairment of left ventricular contractile function. All three episodes resolved spontaneously. **B.** shows the high-speed playback of the beginning of an episode and the arrows indicate the onset of the changes. (LVP, left ventricular pressure). (Modified from ref. 9.)

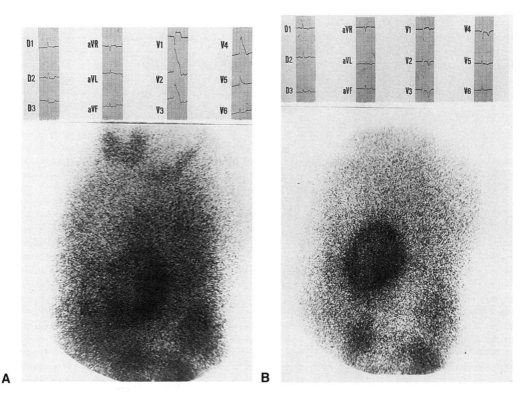

Fig. 20.4 Transmural anterior perfusion defect during occlusive spasm of the left anterior descending (LAD) coronary artery. A large anterior scintigraphic defect is detectable during an ischemic episode caused by occlusive spasm of the LAD and associated with anterior ST-segment elevation (**A**), compared to the basal [201]thallium scintigram in a patient with variant angina in whom the basal ECG showed persistent inversion of T waves in leads $V_2 - V_4$ (**B**). (Modified from ref. 10.)

patients, more than one segment of a coronary artery may be hyperreactive to the same constrictor stimulus.[11] Subocclusive and occlusive spasm can be caused by exercise stress testing, resulting in ST-segment depression and elevation, respectively (see Fig. 20.6A–C)[12] and may extend from a few millimeters to several centimeters along the coronary artery. Less frequently, diffuse intense constriction of all coronary artery branches can be observed, but this may not have the same pathogenesis as the more typical, segmental, spasm (see Chs 6 and 9). In our original series of 107 consecutive patients subjected to coronary angiography, angiographically normal arteries were found in 8%, and greater than 50% diameter stenoses in one artery were observed in 36%, in two arteries in 32%, and in three arteries in 24%. Multivessel disease was commoner in patients with a long history of angina.[11] The prevalence of flow-limiting stenoses or of angiographically normal arteries in different reports probably reflects the varying indications for provocative tests of spasm, i.e. in all patients with a suggestive clinical history or only in those with no detectable stenoses.

The occurrence of spasm at the site of angiographically normal arterial segments is more common in Japanese than in European or American patients, in whom occlusive spasm is usually observed at the site of a plaque.[13] In addition, multifocal and diffuse spasm[14] and increased basal tone[15] appear to be common in Japanese patients, but no increase in basal tone has been observed in Caucasians.[16] It remains to be established whether or not this dif-

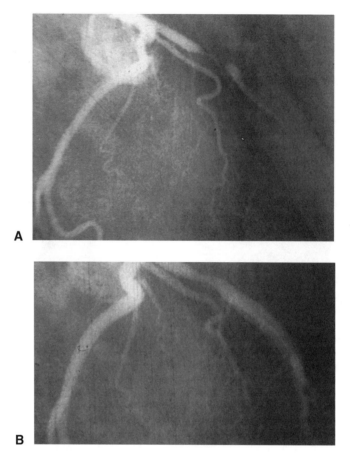

Fig. 20.5 Typical occlusive spasm of the left anterior descending (LAD) coronary artery in a patient with variant angina. Segmental occlusive spasm of the LAD, with only limited and faint distal dye progression, occurred spontaneously during angiography in a patient with variant angina (**A**). Following administration of intracoronary nitrates the spasm resolved, leaving a mild residual stenosis. The other branches were also dilated by nitrates (**B**).

ference is related to a lower prevalence of an "atherosclerotic" coronary background in Japanese patients, or whether two different diseases produce similar clinical pictures.

20.1.3 ECG Findings

The development of ischemia in patients with variant angina is typically characterized by elevation of the ST segment, which elevation can range from 1 or 2 mm to 20 or 30 mm. The beginning of such ischemic episodes is usually characterized by the peaking of T waves, or, in patients with negative T waves, by flattening and then by their pseudonormalization (see Fig. 20.3). During some short or mild episodes, peaking or pseudonormalization of T waves may be the only changes that can be observed. The voltage of R waves also frequently increases in the leads showing ST-segment elevation. Transient Q waves may occasionally develop, but disappear at the end of the episode.[17] Nonmechanical ST-segment alternance has also been reported.[18] Deep, negative T waves can occasionally be observed

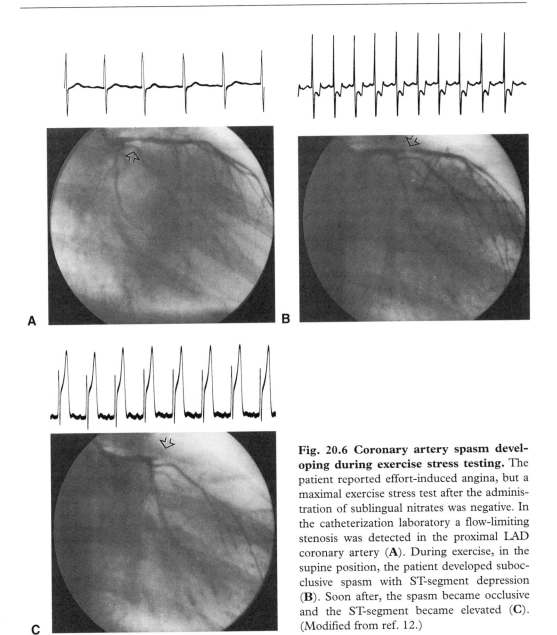

Fig. 20.6 Coronary artery spasm developing during exercise stress testing. The patient reported effort-induced angina, but a maximal exercise stress test after the administration of sublingual nitrates was negative. In the catheterization laboratory a flow-limiting stenosis was detected in the proximal LAD coronary artery (**A**). During exercise, in the supine position, the patient developed subocclusive spasm with ST-segment depression (**B**). Soon after, the spasm became occlusive and the ST-segment became elevated (**C**). (Modified from ref. 12.)

transiently at the end of an episode (see Figs 10.6 and 20.1). ST-segment depression can also alternate with ST-segment elevation (see Fig. 20.2). In patients with variant angina, like those with unstable angina, persisting negative T waves are usually the result of a previous prolonged ischemic episode with or without elevation of serum indices of myocardial necrosis. Over a period of days these negative T waves become progressively less deep, then become flat, and finally return to normal, but a sudden transient return to normal (pseudo-normalization) over a period of a few minutes is an indication of acute myocardial ischemia. Exercise-induced spasm (occurring during or immediately after the test) occurs in about 50% of patients during the "hot" phase (see below).[19]

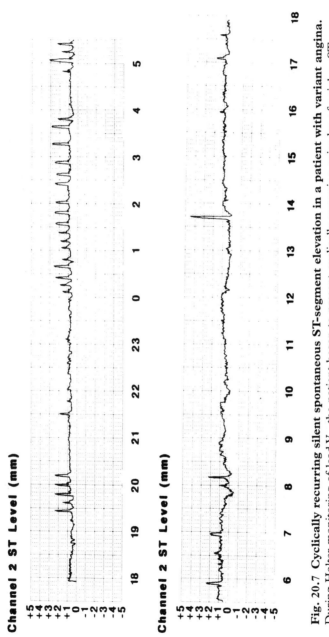

Fig. 20.7 Cyclically recurring silent spontaneous ST-segment elevation in a patient with variant angina. During Holter monitoring of lead V_5, the patient began to present cyclically recurring episodes of painless ST-segment elevation at 0000 h, continuing with a similar periodicity, although with a different amplitude, until 0400 h. Other bursts of episodes occurred at about 0200, 0500, 0700 and 0800 h. The spontaneous cyclical recurrence of episodes suggests a possible local trigger related to a marked local hyperreactivity of the vascular smooth muscle.

In some cases, occlusive spasm can be compensated for by preexisting collaterals and may not cause ischemia at rest (see Fig. 10.1).

20.1.4 Postmortem observations

In patients with variant angina who come to postmortem examination, histologic findings in the segments shown to undergo spasm during life are variable. Most commonly reported are nonspecific alterations consisting of atherosclerotic plaques with a preserved smooth muscle coat,[20-22] but normal histology has also been reported.[4,23] A persistence of local constriction post mortem was observed in some cases, as the outer diameter of the vessel wall was segmentally narrowed at the spastic site compared with both proximal and distal segments.[24,25] The prevalence of spasm persisting post mortem is unknown as it may be detected only by systematic comparison of the outer caliber at the spastic site with that in proximal and distal coronary segments. Specific alterations have been reported in some studies and include perineural infiltrates,[26] mast cell infiltration[27] and fibromuscular dysplasia.[28] Contraction bands in the media of coronary arteries have also been proposed as markers of antemortem spasm.[29] The prevalence of these alterations, however, cannot be determined until prospective studies are initiated.

20.2 PATHOGENETIC MECHANISMS OF OCCLUSIVE CORONARY ARTERY SPASM

The susceptibility to occlusive coronary artery spasm varies widely between patients and also in the same patient over a period of days or weeks. It may lead on to persistent coronary occlusion and myocardial infarction (MI), or it may wane temporarily or permanently. The cause of a patient's susceptibility to spasm is still unknown, but it has been demonstrated that a variety of stimuli acting on different receptors can precipitate spasm in hyperreactive arterial segments (see Ch. 9).

20.2.1 Local coronary hyperreactivity and constrictor stimuli

In the mid-1970s we proposed that, in patients with variant angina, occlusive coronary artery spasm was caused by the interaction of two components:[10]

a. a local alteration in a segment of epicardial coronary artery making it hyperreactive to constrictor stimuli
b. a variety of triggering stimuli causing occlusive spasm in the same segments.

For a review of the topic see references 30 and 31.

The localized nature of the alteration was suggested by the common recurrence of ST-segment elevation in the same ECG leads and spasm in the same arterial segment. It was subsequently demonstrated by the effect of intracoronary injection of ergonovine, which caused occlusive or subocclusive spasm in the hyperreactive coronary segment, but only mild constriction in all other coronary branches.[32] It was also demonstrated during spontaneously occurring occlusive spasm,[33] because it was consistently associated with mild diffuse constriction of all coronary branches, suggestive of a local hyperreactivity to a generalized constrictor stimulus producing only mild constriction elsewhere. In Japanese patients presenting with variant angina, a diffuse increase in resting coronary tone, relieved by nitrates, has been reported[15] but was not found in Caucasians.[16]

Table 20.1 Relative efficacy of provocative tests in relation to the dose of ergonovine

Test	Ergonovine i.v. dose (μg)		
	<100 ($n = 18$)	200 ($n = 6$)	300 ($n = 3$)
Hyperventilation	8	2	2
Histamine	4/9	1/2	2/3
Exercise	4	4	—
Cold pressor	3	—	—
Handgrip	2	—	—
Pitressin	1/5	1/3	—

The frequency of a positive result of most provocative tests is related to the dose of ergonovine required to cause spasm (<100 μg in 18 cases, 200 μg in 6, 300 μg in 3), in particular cold pressor and handgrip testing are likely to be positive in patients who respond to the lowest dose of ergonovine. In one patient with a positive ergonovine test at <100 μg, all the tests were positive

The triggering stimuli of spontaneous spasm are multiple[31] and have been indicated by the triggering of spasm in susceptible patients by a variety of pharmacologic agents (such as histamine, serotonin, dopamine, acetylcholine, and norepinephrine) acting on different receptors, as well as by physiologic provocative tests such as exercise, handgrip, and cold pressor (see below). The comparative potency of some stimuli in relation to ergonovine is presented in Table 20.1.

The occurrence of spasm in some patients within seconds of the onset of the handgrip or cold pressor tests indicates that it can be triggered by nervous stimuli. Conversely, the delay of minutes between the intravenous injection of ergonovine or histamine and the development of spasm, together with the demonstration that ergonovine, serotonin, and acetylcholine cause segmental occlusive spasm when injected selectively into the spastic coronary artery, indicate that some stimuli, acting on different receptors, can trigger spasm directly possibly because of postreceptoral alterations (see below).

During the hyperventilation test, which increases the arterial pH to 7.65 or 7.70, spasm usually develops minutes after the test has ended, when the arterial pH has already returned to normal values.[34-36] This delay is compatible with the gradual increase of calcium in the hyperreactive smooth muscle and a consequent reduction in the spastic threshold. Attacks of variant angina associated with alcohol ingestion, subarachnoid hemorrhage, and peripheral venospasm have been reported,[37-39] but the mechanisms by which these stimuli trigger spasm are unknown.

In spite of this evidence, which supports the view that a local alteration in a segment of coronary artery has a major role, the pathogenetic hypotheses that have been put forward so far have focused largely on parasympathetic, α-adrenergic, and serotoninergic mechanisms, as well as on an imbalance between thromboxane A_2 and prostacyclin.[40-44] None of these hypotheses has stood the test of time, as the use of specific blockers (such as atropine, phentolamine, prazosin, ketanserin, aspirin, and prostacyclin) has consistently failed to prevent coronary artery spasm (see ahead). This failure is not surprising, as blockade of a single receptor/agonist interaction would leave other receptors unopposed and capable of eliciting spasm.

20.2.2 Changing levels of vascular hyperreactivity

The frequency of occlusive spasm and the response to provocative tests may vary considerably, not only among patients, but also within the same patient over periods of a few days or a few weeks, with or without a recognizable periodicity. Waxing of angina is associated with periods of psychological distress and inability to cope.

When patients are in a *"cold" phase* of the disease, they may become unresponsive to a dose of ergonovine 20 times greater than that sufficient to elicit spasm during a "hot" phase.[45] This variable susceptibility to the same stimulus suggests that changing local coronary artery reactivity has a major pathogenetic role, not only in the genesis of coronary artery spasm, but also in its persistence and resistance to vasodilators.

During *"hot" phases,* a circadian distribution of painful and painless ischemic episodes, with a peak in the early morning hours (i.e. between 04.00 and 06.00 h) is fairly common in patients with variant angina. This appears to be associated with higher vasomotor tone in the early morning hours, which could lower the threshold for vasoconstrictor stimuli in susceptible coronary arterial segments.[46] In some patients, attacks recur at the same hour of the day, not necessarily early in the morning but sometimes late in the evening or after a meal. In particularly hot phases, spasm may recur cyclically every 10–20 min, for hours (see Fig. 20.7). Indeed, recurrence of angina in clusters of two to four episodes within 20–30 min was also noted in the original report by Prinzmetal and is not uncommon. This cyclic recurrence suggests that when the local vascular reactivity becomes extreme, spasm might also be generated by the same mechanisms responsible for the maintenance of local coronary artery smooth muscle tone.

The causes of the circadian modulation of coronary vascular reactivity are not clear because the biologic and physiologic variables that exhibit a circadian variation, with peaks or troughs in the early morning hours, are fairly numerous (see Ch. 9). The causes of the enhanced coronary vascular reactivity associated with periods of psychological distress are also unknown.

20.2.3 Possible causes of coronary vascular hyperreactivity

The causes of local coronary artery hyperreactivity to a variety of constrictor stimuli acting on different receptors are still speculative. Theoretically, they could be related to a primary alteration involving the endothelium, the smooth muscle, some resident cells in the arterial wall, or the local nerve supply. Fairly common alterations such as hypercholesterolemia, the presence of a raised plaque, a plaque fissure, or a local loss of endothelium have been proposed, but it is obvious that such a very rare syndrome as variant angina cannot be explained simply on the basis of very common alterations such as hypercholesterolemia or atherosclerotic plaques. Plaque fissure or loss of endothelium are also incompatible with the frequent chronic persistence of the disease for months or even years. Furthermore, animal models, in which some stimuli consistently cause a hyperreactive response to some agents, do not mimic closely enough the very rare and variable occurrence of hyperreactivity to a wide variety of stimuli observed in patients with variant angina (see Chs 6 and 9).

The occlusion of spastic segments in response to a variety of constrictor stimuli acting on different receptors (see review contained in reference 31) is more compatible with a smooth muscle postreceptor alteration (for example, at the level of the G-protein transduction system) than with abnormal nervous or resident cell behavior. Growth factors are potent vasoconstrictors and can be produced directly by smooth muscle cells in the proliferative phenotype, but they should be involved chronically to account for the hyperreactivity that can last for several years in some patients. Whether the local fibromuscular hyperplasia reported in some cases is the cause or the effect of spasm in variant angina remains unknown, but the severity of the angiographically observed stenosis may remain unchanged for several years, in spite of the persisting activity of the disease.[47]

The distribution of risk factors for ischemic heart disease (IHD) in patients with variant angina is similar to that observed in patients with other ischemic syndromes,[11] the notable exception being that extremely high levels of cholesterol have not been reported. In many patients no known risk factors can be recognized, as is the case in other forms of IHD. No family clustering of the disease has been found, except in isolated case reports. Cigarette smoking was reported to be common,[11,48] particularly in women,[49] but as smoking is fairly common its specificity is rather low.

■ *Rational forms of therapy and prevention will be developed only when the causes of the underlying coronary vascular hyperreactivity to a variety of constrictor stimuli are elucidated. Meanwhile, we are forced to use drugs that persistently reduce smooth muscle tone in the whole body (possibly causing reactive vasoconstriction) in order to prevent occasional episodes of spasm. It is not surprising, therefore, that nitrates and calcium antagonist drugs, which nonspecifically lower the threshold for smooth muscle contraction, are much more effective in preventing spasm than any specific receptor blocker, as triggering stimuli can be multiple during ordinary daily life and blockade of a specific stimulus would leave unopposed all the other varieties of constrictor stimuli that act on different receptors. ■*

20.3 DIAGNOSTIC AND PROGNOSTIC ASSESSMENT

The incidence of variant angina in its most easily recognizable clinical form is very low compared with that of chronic stable angina. The male:female ratio is similar to that found in other ischemic syndromes, but the incidence seems to be higher among oriental races than among Caucasians.

In Pisa during the 1970s, before calcium antagonists became widely used and as interest in the syndrome increased, over a 6-year period we documented about 200 cases (about 2% of all patients subjected to angiography for IHD). During the 1980s, at the Hammersmith Hospital in London, the syndrome was documented in about 60 cases (about 0.5% of patients subjected to angiography) and at the Policlinico Gemelli in Rome during 1992–1993, 24 cases of variant angina have been diagnosed out of 1952 patients subjected to angiography.

The frequency with which the syndrome is recognized depends on several factors:

a. the awareness of its existence
b. the care with which the medical history is taken
c. referral practise
d. the proper use of diagnostic tests (see below).

It also depends on the recurrence of angina over a sufficiently long period, so that the patient seeks medical attention, and on the disease remaining in an active phase while the patient is subjected to continuous ECG monitoring and provocative tests. It is likely that the present wide-spread use of calcium antagonists and nitrates in all anginal syndromes causes abatement of symptoms in the majority of patients, making referral and hospitalization less frequent.

The clinical diagnosis of variant angina is made on the basis of medical history and response to therapy. The diagnosis is confirmed by ECG tracings during spontaneous ischemic episodes, exercise stress testing, or provocative tests of spasm, and also by coronary arteriography during spontaneous or induced spasm.

20.3.1 Clinical diagnosis

A clinical diagnosis of variant angina should be considered when patients with good effort tolerance present with anginal pain occurring unpredictably, particularly at night and in the early morning, and lasting only a few minutes (usually less than 10). A provisional diagnosis can be made after considering a possible differential diagnosis with nonischemic and other ischemic causes.

The differential diagnosis with nonischemic causes is more difficult for variant than for chronic stable angina, in which the discomfort is typically caused by effort and relieved promptly by rest. The most difficult differential diagnosis is with esophageal spasm, which should be suggested by the pain being related to meals, swallowing, or acid stomach, and by its prompt relief after a few sips of water.

An ischemic origin is strongly suggested by the following:

a. the association with palpitations, with fainting, suggestive of ischemia-induced arrhythmias, or with transient dyspnea, suggestive of ischemia-induced left ventricular failure
b. the recurrence of the discomfort at night, in the early morning, or at the same time of day, particularly in clusters of two to three episodes
c. the prompt relief of pain following sublingual nitrates (although they can also relieve esophageal spasm).

The most difficult differential diagnosis with other causes of ischemia is that with transient coronary thrombosis, with mixed chronic stable angina (class I or II patients), and with microvascular angina.

The differential diagnosis with unstable angina can be made because patients with variant angina usually present not only with a recurrence of ischemic episodes over a period of days and weeks with preserved effort tolerance (whereas, in unstable angina, recurrent coronary thrombosis often causes the sudden exacerbation of coronary stenoses and reduction of coronary flow reserve) but also with brief ischemic episodes that respond promptly to nitrates. However, the differential diagnosis may be difficult when patients with variant angina present with a rapidly deteriorating course.

The differential diagnosis with mixed chronic stable angina should be considered for those patients with flow-limiting stenosis who represent the vast majority among Caucasians. The differential diagnosis is based on a careful history; the preserved effort tolerance, at least during good days or after sublingual nitrates, and the occurrence of spontaneous episodes during the night, in the early morning, or at rest are highly suggestive of variant angina.

The differential diagnosis with syndrome X by definition should be considered when coronary angiography is normal, but in syndrome X anginal attacks are usually effort or emotion related, are long lasting (10–30 min), are never associated with arrhythmias, occur predominantly during the daytime, and often do not respond promptly to sublingual nitrates.

In all cases the differential diagnosis should be confirmed objectively by appropriate tests, as the documentation of occlusive epicardial coronary artery spasm calls for therapy with high doses of calcium antagonists and nitrates.

20.3.2 Objective documentation of the diagnosis

In patients without known IHD, the diagnosis of an ischemic origin is confirmed by the documentation of transient ischemic ST-segment shifts during a spontaneous or induced anginal episode. Transient elevation of the ST-segment is virtually diagnostic of coronary artery spasm when documented in patients with a negative exercise stress test off therapy or after administration of sublingual nitrates. In such patients, transient ST-segment depression could be compatible with a spastic origin, but only if the clinical history supports it. Occlusive spasm of the circumflex artery may cause only minimal ST-segment elevation and increase of R-wave voltage in inferior leads, depression in lateral precordial leads, and a large deficit of perfusion in the posterior wall (see Fig. 20.8A–D).

Inverted T waves, appearing after a prolonged episode of angina and gradually returning to normal over a period of days, with a pattern similar to that observed following transient coronary thrombosis in patients with unstable angina, can also be observed in variant angina. Transient flattening or pseudonormalization of these inverted T waves is also an indication of acute transient myocardial ischemia when it is promptly reversed by sublingual nitrates, and it may suggest a spastic origin if the clinical history supports it (see Fig. 20.3).

During routine angiography, coronary artery spasm can be detected fortuitously by injecting contrast dye into the coronary arteries during episodes of angina and/or transient silent ischemic ST-segment changes. The chances of detecting spontaneously occurring spasm in patients with variant angina is greater if angiography is performed following the withdrawal of nitrates and calcium antagonists. The criteria for diagnosing spasm during angiography are the same as those for spasm induced by provocative tests (see below).

Provocative tests and the arteriographic demonstration of spasm are required in the following circumstances:

a. when the clinical presentation and ECG findings are nondiagnostic
b. when the response to calcium antagonists and nitrates is not prompt and complete
c. when the maximal exercise stress test is positive on therapy.

In addition, when symptoms and/or signs of ischemia persist for days or weeks in spite of adequate therapy, or when a precise diagnosis is clinically desirable, such tests are useful. The resulting confirmation of the diagnosis then justifies the administration of progressively increasing doses of calcium antagonists and nitrates until all ischemic episodes have been abolished, a course of action that is needed for patients with ischemia-induced arrhythmias and for those unresponsive to standard doses.

The sequence of tests differs for patients in a hot phase who have frequent attacks, and for those who have only one or two episodes per week or less.

For patients with daily attacks, continuous 24 or 48 h ECG monitoring (in hospital or ambulatory) is the first step. Patients should be instructed to press the event button and take sublingual nitrates at the first appearance of pain. It is desirable to monitor leads V_3, V_6, and aVF, or V_3 and aVF. If the history is typical, the observation of transient ST-segment elevation or pseudonormalization of inverted T waves coincident with an event marker, confirms the diagnosis of variant angina. The detection of asymptomatic, clearly diagnostic, transient ischemic ST-segment shifts also suggests an ischemic origin of pain, but ST-segment elevation provides the most positive indication of coronary artery spasm. If the recording is negative, a maximal exercise test, off therapy, should be performed.

If the exercise test is positive, with typical ST-segment elevation occurring during or a few minutes after the end of the test, and if it reproduces the patient's symptoms, an ischemic origin

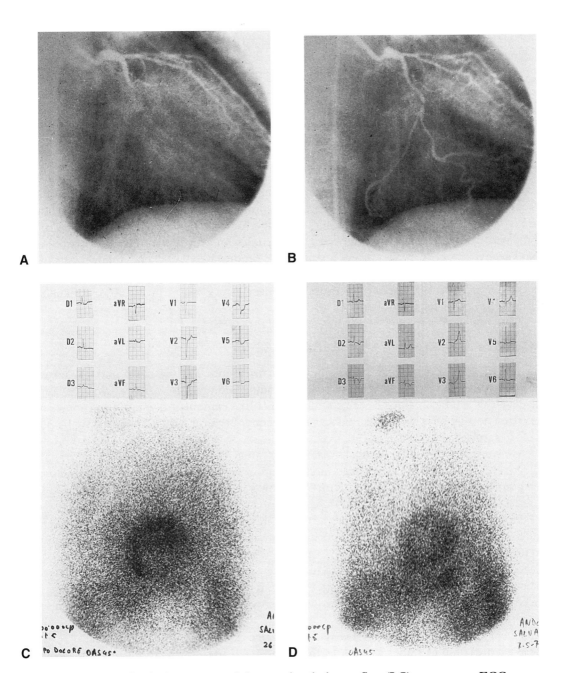

Fig. 20.8 Occlusive spasm of the proximal circumflex (LC) may cause ECG changes not diagnostic of spasm. An occlusive proximal LC spasm (**A**) in the absence of a flow-limiting stenosis (**B**) caused a transmural posterolateral [201]thallium defect in the left lateral scintigram, but only pseudonormalization of inverted T waves in inferior leads and ST-segment depression in anterior leads (**C**) compared to basal (**D**).

can be confirmed. The test should then be repeated after sublingual nitrates. If it becomes negative, a diagnosis of coronary artery spasm can be confirmed. If the test is positive with ST-segment depression and becomes negative at a much higher work load after sublingual nitrates, a diagnosis of variant angina can be suspected if it is compatible with the clinical presentation.

When anginal attacks are rare, both ECG monitoring and exercise testing are likely to be negative, in which case provocative tests of coronary spasm may be required to confirm the clinical diagnosis.

20.3.3 Provocative tests of spasm

A wide variety of provocative tests for coronary artery spasm are in use,[34–36,43,50–57] but the ergonovine and hyperventilation tests are practised most widely. They can be performed in the CCU or in noninvasive stress testing or catheterization laboratories, with minimal risk to the patient if the correct procedures are followed. Ergonovine was originally employed as a provocative test of "coronary artery insufficiency" in the late 1940s[58] and, following its use in the catheterization laboratory,[59–62] was introduced into the CCU and noninvasive laboratory.[45,63] Exercise stress testing also causes coronary artery spasm in 20–40% of patients during, or immediately after, the test.[19,45,46,64]

Indications for, and choice of, provocative tests

Provocative tests of spasm are contraindicated in patients with frequent and prolonged ischemic episodes—particularly those not responding promptly to nitrates—first, because the diagnosis can be obtained by the combination of ECG ambulatory monitoring and exercise stress testing after sublingual nitrates and second, because induced spasm may be difficult to resolve.[65]

Performing the tests in the catheterization laboratory presents two advantages: first, the ability actually to demonstrate spasm and its location and extent; second, the possibility of using intracoronary nitrates and calcium antagonists in cases where it cannot be promptly reversed by intravenous drugs.

Performing the tests in the CCU or in the noninvasive exercise stress testing laboratory under continuous 12-lead ECG monitoring is safe and practical for patients with negative exercise tests following nitrates and for those in whom arteriography has already demonstrated either normal arteries or mild to moderate coronary artery disease.

For patients who come to medical attention with a typical history but who have experienced no symptoms during the last few weeks, provocative tests can be negative, even off therapy.

In theory, the hyperventilation test is slightly safer than the ergonovine test because the spasmogenic stimulus wanes as soon as the intracellular pH returns to normal, but severe arrhythmias have been observed in hyperventilation-induced ischemic episodes; this is because the consequences of ischemia are independent of the form of provocation. Hyperventilation is fairly demanding: it requires the patient's full cooperation and is less frequently positive than ergonovine; in general, therefore, ergonovine is the test of choice.

■ *Studies in a very large series of patients indicate that the tests are safe when the indications for them are correctly followed.*[66,67] ■

Table 20.2 Interpretation of ergonovine and hyperventilation tests performed in a coronary care unit*

Result	Diagnosis
Transient ST-segment elevation + angina	Certain
Transient ST-segment elevation and no symptoms	Certain
Transient diagnostic ST-segment depression, painful or painless	Possible subocclusive spasm
Angina and no ECG changes or only minor changes	Negative for variant angina–possible microvascular angina

Cautionary notes: (1) ischemia of the dorsal left ventricular wall or right ventricle may fail to cause ST-segment or T-wave changes, which may be detected by monitoring left ventricular function by echocardiography, nuclear ventriculography, or by myocardial scintigraphy; (2) a positive test may be caused by segmental single-vessel, multivessel or diffuse epicardial coronary spasm; (3) a negative test cannot rule out variant angina because the patient may be in a cold phase of the disease

Protocol of provocative tests

Provocative tests should be performed according to well-established protocols in the institution concerned and should be accompanied by continuous ECG monitoring and frequent blood pressure measurements. Intravenous nitrates and calcium antagonists, and standard facilities for cardiopulmonary resuscitation, should be immediately available.

The hyperventilation test is performed by the patient breathing as deeply as possible about 30 times a minute for 5 min, so that the arterial pH increases to about 7.60 or 7.70. The alkalinization process can be increased by the infusion of Tris buffer (300 ml) over 15 min.[34-36]

The ergonovine test is performed with the intravenous injection of incremental doses, beginning with 25 μg, followed at 5 min intervals by 50, 100, and 300 μg.[45,63] The test should be interrupted as soon as diagnostic ischemic changes appear on the ECG or when the patient complains of pain or other side effects (such as malaise, nausea, and/or hypertension). Alternatively, a fixed dose can be used during coronary arteriography: this latter protocol has been followed without significant complications being reported.[66,67] Intracoronary injection of ergonovine,[32] acetylcholine,[43,56] and serotonin[57] has also been used. The choice should be based on the investigating team's previous experience. The criteria for interpreting the test are summarized in Tables 20.2 and 20.3.

Table 20.3 Interpretation of ergonovine and hyperventilation tests performed in a catheterization laboratory*

Results	Diagnosis
Transient ST-segment and T-wave changes with symptoms and reduction of peak dP/dt and increase in end-diastolic pressure	Positive
Complete or subtotal occlusion of one or more segments of coronary artery, with or without detectable stenotic plaque	Positive
Segmental reduction of 50% or more of the diameter of an angiographically normal coronary artery segment	Positive

*See footnote to Table 20.2

20.3.4 Prognostic assessment

The variable evolution of variant angina is related to the following:

a. the evolution of the alteration responsible for the segmental coronary artery hyper-reactivity

b. the possible coexistence of local endothelial activation or plaque fissure and a pro-thrombolytic state

c. the arrhythmic response of the heart to ischemic stimuli

d. the severity of the preexisting impairment of left ventricular function and of coronary artery obstructions, which make the heart more vulnerable to ischemic insults.

At one extreme, the disease can be mild and fairly chronic, although occasionally waxing; at the other extreme, the disease either may evolve immediately after its first onset towards MI or sudden ischemic cardiac death (SICD) or may rapidly become quiescent and wane.

The disease can obviously be recognized easily only when it persists; initially, therefore, only the severest and most classic cases were recognized and reported. As a result, a 30% mortality rate was reported in 1971, over an average follow-up period of 19 months,[68] before the use of calcium antagonists and nitrates in high doses became widely adopted. In the late 1970s, hospital mortality was about 3% and the incidence of MI about 20%.[11] Mortality during long-term follow-up was low in patients with no significant coronary artery stenoses, in spite of the possible occurrence of MI, and was highest in patients with previous MI and multiple coronary artery stenoses (see Fig. 20.9A,B).[69–71] The number of symptomatic patients decreased gradually over a 4-year follow-up period. None of those with a normal coronary angiogram had episodes of pain during the last 6-month follow-up at 4 years (see Fig. 20.9A/B).

After the patient's discharge from hospital on a drug regimen of calcium antagonists and nitrates, the average frequency of angina decreases progressively (see Fig. 20.10A,B), but a minority of patients with no angiographically detectable stenoses can continue to have occasional anginal episodes with waxing and waning over periods of several years.[72,73] Other patients may manifest a recurrence of angina after an interval of several years. MI and SICD are less common in Japanese patients: only 18 patients out of 349 followed for an average period of 3 years developed MI (fatal in two cases) and only five succumbed to SICD.[74]

The complications to be feared are MI and potentially fatal arrhythmias.

Development of MI

In patients with "chronic" forms of variant angina, MI develops almost exclusively during the waxing of symptoms, its occurrence out of the blue during apparently quiescent phases being very rare. Although patients with severe and extensive coronary artery disease have a greater chance of developing MI, it can also occur in patients with angiographically normal coronary arteries.[11,74] Persistent coronary artery occlusion can result from either persistent spasm or thrombosis initiated by occlusive spasm, or by a combination of the two (see Ch. 9). Activation of the hemostatic system during spasm in patients with variant angina was suggested by the marked elevation of plasma levels of fibrinopeptide A in venous blood that occurred during episodes of occlusive spasm and was reported by two Japanese groups,[75,76]

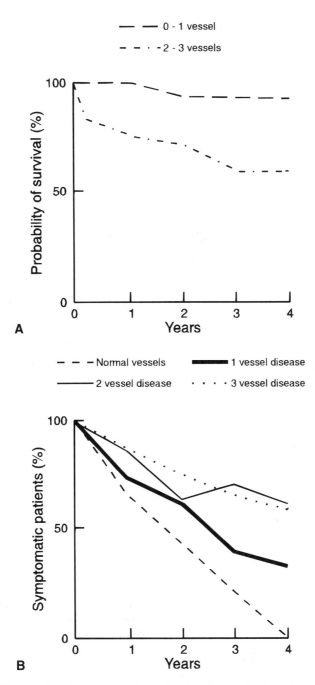

Fig. 20.9 Survival and symptoms in patients with variant angina according to the number of stenosed coronary arteries. Survival (**A**) and persistence of symptoms (**B**) is worse in patients with double- or triple-vessel disease, particularly during hospitalization and the first month postdischarge. Symptoms (**B**) decreased after discharge on medical therapy and all surviving patients with no flow-limiting stenoses were symptom free at 4 years. (Modified from ref. 69.)

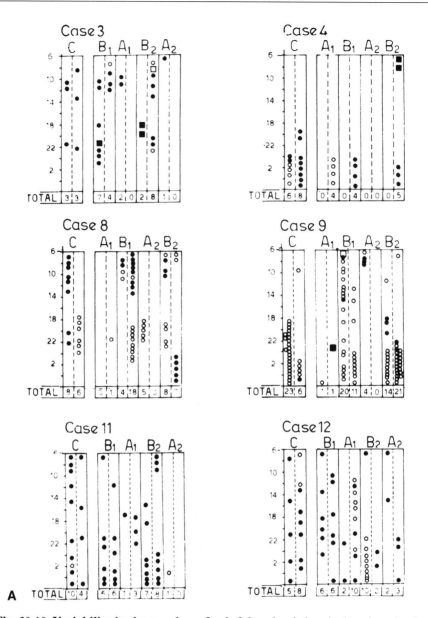

Fig. 20.10 Variability in the number of painful and painless ischemic episodes during successive continuous ECG recordings in patients with variant angina. A. shows the results of Holter recordings obtained in a double cross-over trial of verapamil and placebo for periods of 48 h. (C = control, A = active, B = placebo, circles = episodes of ST-segment elevation, with pain (●) or painless (○) and squares = episodes of ST-segment depression, with pain (■) or painless (□)). *(Figure continues.)*

but much lower peak values were detected in the coronary sinus in a subsequent study,[77] raising doubts about possible sampling artifacts. If thrombin activation occurs consistently each time that occlusive spasm develops, it cannot, by itself, have a major causative role in MI because occlusive spasm usually resolves spontaneously. As discussed in Chapter 9, the rarity of MI compared with the frequency of occlusive spasm indicates that MI must be the result of a very rare combination of events.

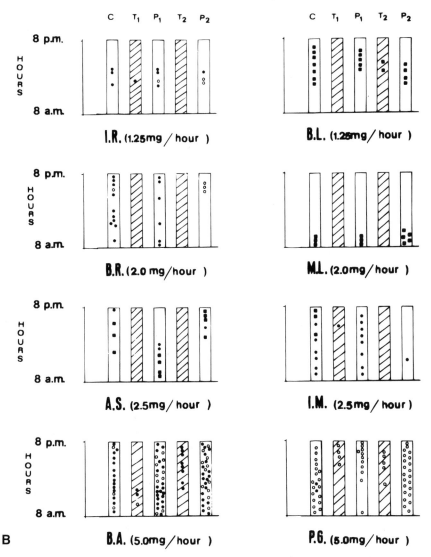

Fig. 20.10 *(Continued)* (**B**) shows the results obtained during a double cross-over trial in patients with predominantly nocturnal attacks with infusion of ISDN (T) or placebo (P) compared to control (C). Episodes of ST-segment elevation with pain are indicated by ● and those without by ○.

In all patients a large variability in the number of painless and painful episodes is common during control, placebo and treatment periods. This variability makes the assessment of drug efficacy in individual patients difficult unless they have a large number of episodes and are studied during multiple cross-over phases. (Modified from refs 89 and 88.)

Development of SICD

Potentially fatal ventricular tachyarrhythmias are much commoner in patients with variant angina than in those with chronic stable angina.[69–71,74,78,79] In the same patient, tachyarrhythmias may occur either during ST-segment elevation or at the very end of an ischemic episode during the reperfusion phase. Complete A–V block is observed less frequently, usually only during ST-segment elevation in inferior leads.

As discussed in Chapter 10, arrhythmias tend to recur in some patients and to be notably absent in others, irrespective of either the frequency, severity, and duration of ischemic episodes or the presence or absence of pain. SICD has been found to be about six times more common in patients who had exhibited episodes of ventricular fibrillation (VF), ventricular tachycardia (VT) or A–V block during ischemic episodes, than in those who did not.[79] SICD occurs more frequently in patients with severe coronary stenoses, but it can occur also in patients with angiographically normal arteries; thus, it does not seem to be related only to the severity of coronary atherosclerosis or to previous MI. However, even in patients who are prone to arrhythmias, VT and VF occur in only a small minority of anginal episodes, usually, but not necessarily, those of longer duration and greater ST-segment elevation.[79] Whether some patients have a specific susceptibility to ischemia-induced arrhythmias remains to be established (see Ch. 10) but, in patients with a history of ischemia-induced malignant arrhythmias, antivasospastic therapy must be capable of abolishing all painful and painless episodes.

20.4 THERAPEUTIC APPROACH

As long as the actual causes of coronary artery hyperreactivity to constrictor stimuli remain unknown, the main goal of therapy is to reduce, nonspecifically, the responsiveness of hyperreactive epicardial coronary artery segments to any vasconstrictor stimulus.

Prompt relief of coronary artery spasm can be achieved by sublingual nitrates and calcium antagonists. Complete or substantial prevention of ischemic episodes can also be obtained in about 80% of patients by administration of appropriate doses of these drugs, but the remainder continue to develop ischemic episodes in spite of extremely high doses.

So far, all attempts to block individual stimuli specifically have been unsatisfactory, either because the blockers used were inappropriate or insufficient or, more likely, because other constrictor stimuli were left unopposed.[31] α-Adrenergic and serotoninergic blockers failed to reduce the number of attacks.[80–82] Blockers with wider, more complex mechanisms of action, such as guanethidine and clonidine, were effective in case reports of refractory variant angina, but only when added to massive doses of calcium antagonists and nitrates (see below). Aspirin in low doses failed to reduce the number of attacks,[83] which actually increased at high dose levels of aspirin.[84] Intravenous infusion of prostacyclin also failed to reduce ischemic attacks.[85] However, in view of the observation that coronary thrombosis can be a contributory factor in persistent coronary occlusion in patients with variant angina, it is our practise to add aspirin (75 mg) to the treatment because of its antiplatelet effects. β-Blockers were generally thought to have detrimental effects in patients with variant angina, on the assumption that increased α-adrenergic tone may favor the development of coronary artery spasm. A longer duration of attacks, but not an increased frequency, was reported in one study.[86] We never observed adverse effects when blockers were added to calcium antagonists and nitrates in patients who also suffered from migraine, an association observed commonly only in an isolated report.[87] Conversely, very early multiple crossover studies with drugs that reduce coronary vasomotor tone aspecifically, such as nitrates,[88] verapamil,[89] and nifedipine,[90] showed consistently reproducible decreases in the number of painful and painless attacks (see Fig. 15.6A,B).

PTCA should be considered only for patients with segmental spasm at the site of a flow-limiting coronary stenosis and a positive exercise test on full therapy at a low work load, because the incidence of postangiography restenosis occurs in over 50% of cases.[91] Coronary artery bypass grafting (CABG) should be considered only when the patient has severe multivessel disease and a positive exercise stress test at a low work load. Reviews of the evolution of medical therapy in variant angina can be found in references 92 and 93.

20.4.1 Drugs and doses

For prompt relief of ischemic episodes the preparations most commonly used are sublingual nitroglycerin tablets, isosorbide dinitrate (ISDN) (5 mg), nifedipine (10 mg) and oral nitroglycerin spray, all repeatable within 2–3 min if symptoms persist. As differences in individual responses are common, each patient should learn to use the most rapidly effective preparation that has the fewest side effects. In resistant cases, nitroglycerin (0.1–0.4 mg), ISDN (2–10 mg), verapamil (5–20 mg) or diltiazem (5–20 mg) can be injected intravenously. The lowest dose of each drug can also be administered directly into the coronary artery when spasm occurs during angiography (see below). Patients with a history of fainting and/or of malignant arrhythmias should be advised to interrupt the attack immediately at its very onset by taking a second or third dose within 1 min when the attack does not subside promptly.

For the chronic prevention of ischemic episodes, the most commonly used calcium antagonists are diltiazem (120 mg), verapamil (120 mg), and nifedipine (20 mg), all to be taken 2 to 4 times a day. Thus, the maximum commonly used chronic daily doses are 480 mg for diltiazem and verapamil and 80 mg for nifedipine. The choice between these drugs depends on their efficacy and side effects, as assessed by each patient through trial and error. The above doses can be increased in resistant cases (see below).

The most common preparations for the chronic administration of nitrates are ISDN (20–40 mg) or isosorbide mononitrate (10–20 mg) twice a day and scheduled to cover the period when ischemic episodes tend to occur most frequently (for example, evening and early morning, or early morning and lunch time, or lunch time and evening) but leaving a drug-free interval of 10–14 h.

The efficacy of treatment is much more easily judged when ischemic episodes occur frequently, than when they occur only a few times a week. An additional confounding element in variant angina is the common spontaneous variability in the frequency of symptoms (see Fig. 20.10A,B).

Ischemic episodes may disappear in response to treatment or because of spontaneous waning of the local coronary susceptibility to vasoconstrictor stimuli. Conversely, ischemic episodes may become more frequent, not because treatment is ineffective but because the patient's susceptibility increases. Thus, in such a variable disease, convincing evidence of the efficacy of treatment is best obtained by multiple crossover clinical trials.

When ischemic episodes disappear, provocative tests may be used to assess the efficacy of treatment in preventing induced spasm.[94] However, only a positive test is a clear indication of inadequate treatment; conversely, a negative test does not offer any guarantee that treatment will be sufficient to abolish all spontaneous attacks during daily life.

Doses can be reduced gradually when patients have been free from ischemic episodes for 1 month, but should be promptly increased to the previously tolerated maximal levels if they recur.

Patients who continue to present with ischemic episodes, in spite of maximal commonly recommended doses of calcium antagonists and nitrates, are considered to be nonresponders (see below).

20.4.2 Patients unresponsive to conventional treatment

Occasionally, spasm cannot be relieved by sublingual or intravenous nitrates but only by the intracoronary administration of high doses of nitroglycerin, ISDN, or nifedipine.[65] About 10% of patients with variant angina are refractory, for a limited period, to the maximal doses of drugs indicated above. In the past, such patients have been subjected to cardiac denervation, with uncertain results,[95] and even to cardiac autotransplantation, with considerable levels of mortality.[96,97] Patients with malignant arrhythmias during episodes of coronary spasm have also been treated with implantable defibrillators.

In our experience, patients with refractory variant angina can be best managed without interventional therapy: instead, they should be under careful medical control as, in most cases, symptoms do eventually wane. Our present policy is to increase the dose of calcium antagonists gradually until all episodes have been abolished. The highest doses that we have used so far are diltiazem (960 mg/day) or verapamil (800 mg/day), each associated with nifedipine (100 mg) and ISDN (80 mg) in the evening. In three cases these doses were insufficient and complete control was obtained only by the addition of either guanethidine (10 mg) or clonidine (5 mg) three times a day (the latter two drugs were ineffective by themselves). In all three cases, therapy was gradually reduced to normal levels within 3 months.[98,99] Using the regimens discussed above, patients under our care without severe coronary stenoses have never been subjected to interventional therapy.

REFERENCES

1. Prinzmetal M, Kennamer R, Merliss R, Wade T, Bor N. Angina pectoris. I. The variant form of angina pectoris. Am J Med 1959;27:375.
2. Maseri A. Coronary artery spasm. Citation Classic. Current Contents 1991;38:10.
3. MacAlpin R. Coronary arterial spasm: a historical perspective. J Hist Med All Sci 1980;35:288.
4. Cheng TO, Bashour T, Kelser GA, Weiss L, Bacos J. Variant angina of Prinzmetal with normal coronary arteriograms. A variant of the variant. Circulation 1973;47:476.
5. Meller J, Pichard A, Dack S. Coronary arterial spasm in Prinzmetal's angina: a proved hypothesis. Am J Cardiol 1976;37:938.
6. Maseri A. The revival of coronary spasm. Am J Med 1981;70:752.
7. Guazzi M, Polese A, Fiorentini C et al. Left ventricular performance and related haemodynamic changes in Prinzmetal's variant angina pectoris. Br Heart J 1971;33:84.
8. Maseri A, Mimmo R, Chierchia S, Marchersi C, Pesola A, L'Abbate A. Coronary spasm as a cause of acute myocardial ischemia in man. Chest 1975;68:625.
9. Chierchia S, Brunelli C, Simonetti I, Lazzari M, Maseri A. Sequence of events in angina at rest: primary reduction in coronary flow. Circulation 1980;61:759.
10. Maseri A, Parodi O, Severi S, Pesola A. Transient transmural reduction of myocardial blood flow, demonstrated by thallium-201 scintigraphy, a cause of variant angina. Circulation 1976;54:280.
11. Maseri A, Severi S, De Nes DM et al. "Variant" angina: one aspect of a continuous spectrum of vasospastic myocardial ischemia. Am J Cardiol 1978;42:1019.
12. Brunelli C, Lazzari M, Simonetti I, L'Abbate A, Maseri A. Variable threshold of exertional angina: a clue to a vasospastic component. Eur Heart J 1981;2:155.
13. Maseri A, Kaski JC. Pathogenetic mechanisms of coronary artery spasm. J Am Coll Cardiol 1989;14:610.
14. Fujii H, Yasue H, Okumara K et al. Hyperventilation-induced simultaneous multivessel coronary spasm in patients with variant angina: an echocardiographic and arteriographic study. J Am Coll Cardiol 1988;12:1184.
15. Hoshio A, Kotake H, Mashiba H. Significance of coronary artery tone in patients with vasospastic angina. J Am Coll Cardiol 1989;14:604.
16. Kaski JC, Tousoulis D, Gavrielides S et al. Comparison of epicardial coronary artery tone and reactivity in Prinzmetal's variant angina and chronic stable angina pectoris. J Am Coll Cardiol 1991;17:1058.
17. Meller J, Conde CA, Donato E et al. Transient Q waves in Prinzmetal's angina. Am J Cardiol 1975;35:691.
18. Rozanski J, Meller J, Kleinfeld M et al. Non-mechanical ST segment alternance in Prinzmetal's angina. Am Int Med 1978;89:76.

19. Specchia G, De Servi S, Falcone C et al. Coronary arterial spasm as a cause of exercise-induced ST-segment elevation in patients with variant angina. Circulation 1979;*59:*948.

20. Silverman ME, Flamm MD. Variant angina pectoris. Anatomic findings and prognostic implications. Ann Intern Med 1971;*75:*339.

21. Trevi GP, Thiene G, Benussi P et al. Prinzmental's variant angina: clinical, angiographic and pathologic correlations in two typical cases. Eur J Cardiol 1976;*4:*319.

22. Rizzon P, Rossi L, Calabrese P, Franchini G, Di Biase M. Angiographic and pathologic correlations in Prinzmetal variant angina. Angiology 1978;*29:*486.

23. Auzepy F, Blondeau H, Albessard F. Aspects électrocardiographiques suggestifs d'un angor de Prinzmetal avec artères coronaires normales a l'autopsie. Arch Mal Coeur 1974;*9:*1107.

24. El-Maraghi NRH, Sealey BJ. Recurrent myocardial infarction in a young man due to coronary arterial spasm demonstrated at autopsy. Circulation 1980;*61:*199.

25. Roberts WC, Curry RC, Isner JM et al. Sudden death in Prinzmental's angina with coronary spasm documented by angiography. Analysis of three necropsy patients. Am J Cardiol 1982;*50:*203.

26. Rossi L, Thiene G. Recent advances in clinicohistopathologic correlates of sudden cardiac death. Am Heart J 1981;*102:*478.

27. Forman MB, Oates JA. Robertson D, Robertson RM, Roberts LJ, Virmani R. Increased adventitial mast cells in a patient with coronary spasm. N Engl J Med 1985;*313:*1138.

28. Petitier H, De Lajartre AY, Geslin P et al. Dysplasie fibreuse intimale coronaire et angor de Prinzmetal. Arch Mal Coeur 1978;*71:*1053.

29. Factor SM, Cho S. Smooth muscle contraction bands in the media of coronary arteries: a postmortem marker of antemortem coronary spasm? J Am Coll Cardiol 1985;*6:*1329.

30. Maseri A, Chierchia S. Coronary artery spasm: demonstration, definition, diagnosis and consequences. Prog Cardiovasc Dis 1982;*25:*169.

31. Maseri A, Davies G, Hackett D, Kaski JC. Coronary artery spasm and vasoconstriction. The case for a distinction. Circulation 1990;*81:*1983.

32. Hackett D, Larkin S, Chierchia S, Davies G, Kaski JC, Maseri A. Induction of coronary artery spasm by a direct local action of ergonovine. Circulation 1987;*75:*577.

33. Kaski JC, Maseri A, Vejar M, Crea F, Hackett D. Spontaneous coronary artery spasm in variant angina results from a local hyperreactivity to a generalized constrictor stimulus. J Am Coll Cardiol 1989;*14:*1456.

34. Yasue H, Wagas M, Omote S, Takizawa K, Tanaka S. Coronary arterial spasm and Prinzmetal's variant angina induced by hyperventilation and Tris-buffer infusion. Circulation 1978;*58:*56.

35. Girotti LA, Crosatto JR, Messuti H et al. The hyperventilation test as a method for developing successful therapy in Prinzmetal's angina. Am J Cardiol 1982;*49:*832.

36. Weber S, Pasquier G, Guiomard A et al. Application clinique du test de provocation par l'alcalose du spasme artériel coronaire. Arch Mal Coeur 1981;*74:*1389.

37. Fernandez D, Rosentel JE, Cohen LS et al. Alcohol-induced Prinzmetal variant angina. Am J Cardiol 1973;*32:*238.

38. Toyama Y, Tanaka H, Nuruki K et al. Prinzmetal's variant angina associated with subarachnoid hemorrhage: a case report. Angiology 1979;*30:*211.

39. Dagenais G, Gundel W, Conti C. Peripheral venospasm associated with signs of transient myocardial ischemia. Am Heart J 1970;*80:*544.

40. Yasue H, Touyama M, Kato H, Tanaka S, Akiyama F. Prinzmetal's variant form of angina as a manifestation of alpha-adrenergic receptor mediated coronary artery spasm: documentation by coronary arteriography. Am Heart J 1976;*91:*148.

41. Ricci DR, Orlick AE, Cipriano PR, Guthaner DF, Harrison CD. Altered adrenergic activity in coronary arterial spasm: insight into mechanisms based on study of coronary hemodynamics and the electrocardiogram. Am J Cardiol 1979;*43:*1073.

42. Tada M, Kuzuya T, Inoue M et al. Elevation of thromboxane B_2 levels in patients with classic and variant angina pectoris. Circulation 1981;*64:*1107.

43. Yasue H, Horio Y, Nakamura N et al. Induction of coronary artery spasm by acetylcholine in patients with variant angina: possible role of the parasympathetic nervous system in the pathogenesis of coronary artery spasm. Circulation 1986;*74:*955.

44. Endo M, Hirosawa K, Kaneko N, Hase K, Inoue Y, Konno S. Prinzmetal's variant angina: coronary arteriogram and left ventriculogram during angina attack induced by methacholine. N Engl J Med 1976;294:252.

45. Maseri A, Severi S, Chierchia S, Parodi O, Biagini A. Characteristics, incidence and pathogenetic mechanism of "primary" angina at rest. In: Maseri A, Klassen GA, Lesch M (eds) Primary and Secondary Angina Pectoris. New York, Grune & Stratton, 1978, p. 165.

46. Yasue H, Omote S, Takizawa A, Nagao M, Miwa K, Tanaka S. Circadian variation of exercise capacity in patients with Prinzmetal's variant angina: role of exercise-induced coronary arterial spasm. Circulation 1979;59:938.

47. Kaski JC, Tousoulis D, McFadden E, Crea F, Pereira WI, Maseri A. Variant angina pectoris. Role of coronary spasm in the development of fixed coronary obstructions. Circulation 1992;85:619.

48. Scholl JM, Benacerraf A, Ducimetière P et al. Comparison of risk factors in vasospastic angina without significant fixed coronary narrowing to significant fixed coronary narrowing and no vasospastic angina. Am J Cardiol 1986;57:199.

49. Caralis DG, Deligonul U, Kern MJ, Cohen JD. Smoking is a risk factor for coronary spasm in young women. Circulation 1992;85:905.

50. Raizner AE, Chahine RA, Ishimori T et al. Provocation of coronary artery spasm by the cold pressor test. Hemodynamic, arteriographic and quantitative angiographic observations. Circulation 1980;62:925.

51. Ginsburg R, Bristow MR, Kantrowitz N, Baim DS, Harrison DC. Histamine provocation of clinical coronary artery spasm: implications concerning the pathogenesis of variant angina pectoris. Am Heart J 1981;102:819.

52. Crea F, Chierchia S, Kaski JC et al. Provocation of coronary spasm by dopamine in patients with active variant angina. Circulation 1986;74:262.

53. Kaski JC, Crea F, Meran D et al. Local coronary supersensitivity to diverse vasoconstrictive stimuli in patients with variant angina. Circulation 1986;74:1255.

54. Shimokawa H, Okamatsu S, Taira Y, Nakamura M. Cimetidine induces coronary artery spasm in patients with vasospastic angina. Can J Cardiol 1987;3:177.

55. Okumura K, Yasue H, Matsuyama K, Morikami Y, Ogawa H. Effect of H_1 receptor stimulation on coronary artery diameter in patients with variant angina: comparison with the effect of acetylcholine. J Am Coll Cardiol 1991;17:338.

56. Miwa K, Fujita M, Fjiri M, Sasayama S. Usefulness of intracoronary injection of acetylcholine as a provocative test for coronary artery spasm in patients with vasospastic angina. Heart Vessel 1991;6:96.

57. McFadden EP, Clarke JG, Davies GJ, Kaski JC, Haider AW, Maseri A. Effect of intracoronary serotonin on coronary vessels in patients with stable angina and patients with variant angina. N Engl J Med 1991;324:648.

58. Stein I. Observations on the action of ergonovine on the coronary circulation and its use in the diagnosis of coronary artery insufficiency. Am Heart J 1949;37:36.

59. Higgins CB, Wexler L, Silverman J et al. Spontaneous and pharmacologically provoked coronary arterial spasm in Prinzmetal variant angina. Radiology 1976;119:521.

60. Heupler F, Proudfit W, Razavi M, Shirey E, Greenstreet R, Sheldon W. Ergonovine maleate provocative test for coronary arterial spasm. Am J Cardiol 1978;41:631.

61. Helfant RH. Coronary arterial spasm and provocative testing in ischemic heart disease. Am J Cardiol 1978;41:781.

62. Schroeder JS, Bolen JL, Wuint RA et al. Provocation of coronary spasm with ergonovine maleate: new test with results in 57 patients undergoing coronary arteriography. Am J Cardiol 1977;46:487.

63. Waters DD, Theroux P, Sziacheic J. Ergonovine testing in a coronary care unit. Am J Cardiol 1980;46:922.

64. Waters DD, Chaitman BR, Dupras G et al. Coronary artery spasm during exercise in patients with variant angina. Circulation 1979;59:580.

65. Buxton AE, Goldberg S, Hirshfeld JW et al. Refractory ergonovine induced coronary vasospasm: importance of intracoronary nitroglycerin. Am J Cardiol 1980;46:329.

66. Bertrand MD, LaBlanche JM, Tilmant PY et al. Frequency of provoked coronary arterial spasm in 1089 consecutive patients undergoing coronary arteriography. Circulation 1982;65:1299.

67. Harding MB, Leithe ME, Mark DB et al. Ergonovine maleate testing during cardiac catheterization: a 10-year perspective in 3,447 patients without significant coronary artery disease or Prinzmetal's variant angina. J Am Coll Cardiol 1992;20:107.

68. Silverman ME, Flamm MD Jr. Variant angina pectoris. Ann Intern Med 1971;75:339.

69. Severi S, Davies G, Maseri A, Marzullo P, L'Abbate A. Long-term prognosis of "variant" angina with medical treatment. Am J Cardiol 1980;46:226.

70. Waters DD, Miller DD, Szlachcic J et al. Factors influencing the long-term prognosis of treated patients with variant angina. Circulation 1983;68:258.

71. Bott-Silverman C, Heupler FA. Natural history of pure coronary artery spasm in patients treated medically. J Am Coll Cardiol 1983;2:200.

72. Girotti AL, Rutizky B, Schmidberg J, Crosatto J, Rosenbaum MB. Spontaneous remission in variant angina. Br Heart J 1981;45:517.

73. Waters DD, Bouchard A, Théroux P. Spontaneous remission is a frequent outcome of variant angina. J Am Coll Cardiol 1983;2:195.

74. Nakamura M, Takeshita A, Nose Y. Clinical characteristics associated with myocardial infarction, arrhythmias, and sudden death in patients with vasospastic angina. Circulation 1987;75:1110.

75. Irie T, Imaizumi T, Matuguchi T et al. Increased fibrinopeptide A during anginal attacks in patients with variant angina. J Am Coll Cardiol 1989;14:589.

76. Oshima S, Ogawa H, Yasue H et al. Increased plasma fibrinopeptide A levels during attacks induced by hyperventilation in patients with coronary vasospastic angina. J Am Coll Cardiol 1989;14:150.

77. Oshima S, Yasue H, Ogawa H, Okumura K, Matsuyama K. Fibrinopeptide A is released into the coronary circulation after coronary spasm. Circulation 1990;82:2222.

78. Kerin NZ, Rubenfire M, Naini M et al. Arrhythmias in variant angina pectoris. Relationships of arrhythmias to ST segment elevation and R wave changes. Circulation 1979;60:1343.

79. Maseri A, Severi S, Marzullo P. Role of coronary arterial spasm in sudden coronary ischemic death. Ann NY Acad Sci 1982;382:204.

80. Chierchia S, Davies G, Berkenboom G, Crea F, Crean P, Maseri A. Alpha-adrenergic receptors and coronary spasm: an elusive link. Circulation 1984;69:8.

81. Freedman SB, Chierchia S, Rodriguez-Plaza L, Bugiardini R, Smith G, Maseri A. Ergonovine-induced myocardial ischemia: no role for serotonergic receptors? Circulation 1984;70:178.

82. De Caterina R, Carpeggiani C, L'Abbate A. A double-blind, placebo-controlled study of ketanserin in patients with Prinzmetal's angina. Evidence against a role for serotonin in the genesis of coronary vasospasm. Circulation 1984;69:889.

83. Chierchia S, De Caterina R, Crea F, Patrono C, Maseri A. Failure of thromboxane A2 blockade to prevent attacks of vasospastic angina. Circulation 1982;66:702.

84. Miwa K, Kambara H, Kawai C. Exercise-induced angina provoked by aspirin administration in patients with variant angina. Am J Cardiol 1981;47:1210.

85. Chierchia S, Patrono C, Crea F et al. Effects of intravenous prostacyclin in variant angina. Circulation 1982;65:470.

86. Robertson RM, Wood AJ, Bernard Y et al. Exacerbation of ischemia in vasotonic angina pectoris by propranolol. Am J Cardiol 1981;47:463.

87. Miller D, Waters DD, Warniers W et al. Is variant angina the coronary manifestation of a generalized vasospastic disorder? N Engl J Med 1981;304:763.

88. Distante A, Maseri A, Severi S, Biagini A, Chierchia S. Management of vasospastic angina at rest with continuous infusion of isosorbide dinitrate. Am J Cardiol 1979;44:533.

89. Parodi O, Maseri A, Simonetti I. Management of unstable angina at rest by verapamil. A double-blind cross-over study in CCU. Br Heart J 1979;41:167.

90. Previtali M, Salerno JA, Tavazzi L et al. Treatment of angina at rest with nifedipine: a short-term controlled study. Am J Cardiol 1980;45:875.

91. Bertrand ME, Lablanche JM, Fourrier JL, Traisnel G. Percutaneous transluminal coronary angioplasty in patients with spasm superimposed on atherosclerotic narrowing. Br Heart J 1987; 58:469.

92. MacAlpin R. Treatment of vasospastic angina. In: Goldberg S (ed). Coronary Artery Spasm and Thrombosis. Philadelphia, F A Davis, 1983, p. 129.
93. Maseri A, Parodi O, Fox KM. Rational approach to the medical therapy of angina pectoris: the role of calcium antagonists. Prog Cardiovasc Dis 1983;*15*:269.
94. Waters D, Szlachcic J, Theroux P, Dauwe F, Mizgala H. Ergonovine testing to detect spontaneous remissions of variant angina during long term treatment with calcium antagonist drugs. Am J Cardiol 1981;*47*:179.
95. Bertrand ME, Lablanche JM, Rousseau MF, Warembourg H Jr, Stankowiak C, Soots G. Surgical treatment of variant angina: use of plexectomy with aortocoronary bypass. Circulation 1980;*61*:877.
96. Bertrand ME, Lablanche JM, Tilmant PY, Ducloux G, Warembourg H Jr, Soots G. Complete denervation of the heart (autotransplantation) for treatment of severe, refractory coronary spasm. Am J Cardiol 1981;*47*:1375.
97. Clark DA, Quint RA, Mitchel RL, Angell WW. Coronary artery spasm: medical management, surgical denervation, and autotransplantation. J Thorac Cardiovasc Surg 1977;*73*:332.
98. Frenneaux M, Kaski JC, Brown M, Maseri A. Refractory variant angina relieved by guanethidine and clonidine. Am J Cardiol 1988;*62*:832.
99. Lefroy DC, Crake T, Haider AW, Maseri A. Medical treatment of refractory coronary artery spasm. Cor Art Dis 1992;*3*:745.

Irreversible myocardial ischemia

21 Acute myocardial infarction: development and diagnosis

INTRODUCTION

Acute myocardial infarction (MI) is caused by necrosis of a portion of myocardium, developing over a period of hours as a result of severely and persistently inadequate blood flow supply relative to local metabolic requirements, whatever its causes.

The extension of necrosis can be extremely variable, ranging from a few grams of tissue to 50% of the left ventricular wall. Acute MI is more easily recognized clinically when it is large and involves the full thickness of the left ventricular wall (transmural) than when it is small and involves only the inner layers (subendocardial). Postmortem studies show that in about 10% of cases MI may involve the atrial walls and, in about 50% of cases of inferior MI, necrosis also involves segments of the right ventricular wall. Occasionally, in the presence of right ventricular hypertrophy, infarction may involve only the right ventricular wall.

The in-hospital prognosis of acute MI depends on the extent of necrosis and on the presence of preexisting ventricular damage, as well as on the age and gender of the patient. Fatal arrhythmias can, however, develop within the first few hours of the onset of symptoms, irrespective of the size of infarction, leading to a substantial number of patients with acute MI dying before they reach hospital. This may be because symptoms are often not typical, are not recognized promptly or are absent altogether; such cases are classified as sudden ischemic cardiac death (SICD). Patients with acute MI have always been treated with great determination because of their possible severe short-term prognosis, but the focus of treatment has changed dramatically over the years. It is instructive to review the different treatment strategies as they reflect our prevailing understanding of the disease and the therapeutic options currently available.

Until the early 1960s, patients with MI were confined to bed for 3 weeks, which may have been beneficial to those with very large infarcts; however, in those with very small infarcts it would certainly have been unnecessary, and even detrimental by encouraging the development of venous thrombosis and pulmonary embolism.

In the mid-1960s the concept of arrhythmic death, in hearts "too good to die," led to the widespread development of coronary care units (CCU), where continuous ECG monitoring would lead to prompt detection and treatment of potentially lethal arrhythmias. The focus of interest was on admitting patients with confirmed MI; thus, in many CCUs, enzymatic proof of myocardial necrosis was often required as a criterion for admission.

In the early 1970s, the concept of preventing pump failure by limiting infarct size became the dominant focus of attention. Thus, besides antiarrhythmic therapy, interventions intended to protect the ischemic myocardium became fashionable. These forms of treatment were clearly more successful in experimental animal models than in patients.

Then, in the early 1980s, the concept of early coronary recanalization led to the now widespread use of thrombolytic agents, with the aim of reperfusing potentially viable myocardium and preventing persistent coronary occlusion. Thus, patients with threatening MI or unstable angina also acquired preferential access to CCUs.

The fifth therapeutic era for acute MI in the 1990s awaits a better understanding of the specific predisposing and precipitating factors and of the susceptibility to various complications in each individual patient. In particular, answers need to be found for the following questions:

1. Why do coronary arteries without critical stenoses suddenly occlude?
2. Why is MI that develops distal to severe flow-limiting stenoses obviously not protected by a collateral circulation?
3. Why do about 20% of occluded arteries fail to recanalize in spite of thrombolytic treatment and 10–20% reocclude soon after recanalization, but with no evidence of reinfarction in most cases?
4. Why do some patients, but not others, develop fatal arrhythmias soon after the onset of symptoms?
5. Why does the mortality rate for acute MI increase exponentially with age, and why is it greater in women?

A close collaboration of basic and clinical research is necessary to provide answers to these questions.

The atherosclerotic background, the ischemic stimuli that may cause MI, and the cardiac response to the necrotic insult are discussed in Chapters 8–10. A brief summary of the development and consequences of infarction is useful to define some guidelines for the diagnostic assessment of individual patients. The management of MI is discussed in Chapter 22.

21.1 DEVELOPMENT AND CONSEQUENCES OF ACUTE MYOCARDIAL INFARCTION

As discussed in Chapter 7, the extent of myocardial necrosis within the area at risk depends on the determinants of infarct size, which also influence the speed with which necrosis develops, as well as the systemic and hemodynamic consequences.

21.1.1 Determinants of infarct size

The area of myocardium at risk of becoming necrotic depends on the area originally perfused by the occluded vessel: it is maximal when the occlusion is proximal. Within this area at risk, the actual infarct size is determined by the following:

a. the rapidity with which the occlusion develops
b. its duration
c. the intermittent reopening of the vessel
d. the presence and function of collaterals distal to the occlusion
e. the level of myocardial oxygen consumption.

Besides these well-established determinants, there are other modulatory factors, such as the individual myocardial and microvascular biologic response to the ischemic insult, which, so far, have received little attention (see Chs 7 and 10).

Sudden persistent occlusion of the left anterior descending coronary artery proximal to the first septal and diagonal branches can cause infarction of the anterolateral and apical left ventricular wall; part of the septum and the anterior papillary muscle and inferior apical wall can also be involved.

Occlusion of the proximal dominant circumflex coronary artery can cause infarction of the lateral and inferoposterior wall.

Occlusion of the proximal dominant right coronary artery can cause infarction of the inferoposterior left ventricular wall, of the inferoposterior part of the septum, and of the posteromedial papillary muscle, and often of the right ventricle.

Interventions that delay irreversible tissue damage can prolong the period in which restoration of blood flow can limit necrosis; thus, limitation of infarct size is a race against time. Once necrosis has extended to the entire area at risk, the reopening of the occluded artery and, hence, reperfusion, is unlikely to have substantial beneficial effects. Within the area at risk, the infarct may be limited when the occlusion is recanalized within 1–6 h, or when it is intermittent, and when myocardial oxygen consumption is low, but there may be no detectable MI when the artery occludes gradually and intermittently in the presence of both collaterals and a low myocardial oxygen consumption. When necrosis involves only a fraction of the area at risk because of either early reopening of the occluded artery or an increase in collateral blood flow, Q waves may develop in only a few leads initially showing ST-segment/T-wave (ST–T) elevation, or may not develop at all (non-Q-wave MI) (see below).

In the area at risk, when the infarction is incomplete the myocardium spared by the necrotic process may be susceptible to new episodes of ischemia and necrosis. A new episode of ischemia or infarction occurring within the area at risk within a few days of the MI is termed "infarct extension," and should not be confused with the term "infarct expansion," which implies expansion of a particular segment of the ventricular wall as a result of the wall being stretched during the repair process and associated with remodeling of the ventricular wall and cavity (see below).

Infarct extension detectable clinically by recurrent prolonged chest pain, new persisting ECG changes, and secondary peaks on the curves of serum indices of myocardial necrosis, occurs in about 15% of cases within 2–10 days of admission.[1]

21.1.2 Variable evolution of necrosis and ischemia

In patients, unlike experimental animals in which coronary occlusion occurs in a normal coronary bed and is complete and continuous from time zero, occlusion develops in the presence of variable combinations of factors that together cause sudden coronary artery occlusion. It is very often intermittent[2,3] and may follow previous shorter ischemic episodes. The different pathogenetic components are likely to influence the response of the heart to the ischemic insult and, hence, the evolution of necrosis.

In clinical practise, the evolution of myocardial necrosis can be judged from the evolution of chest pain, from the ECG changes, and from the elevation and time course of the blood markers of myocardial cell necrosis.

■ *As the development of MI after the onset of symptoms is much more variable in patients than in experimental animals, the time in which reperfusion can limit infarction also varies.* ■

Healing of myocardial necrosis

About 48 h after extensive myocardial necrosis has occurred, neutrophilic infiltration becomes prominent at the periphery and proceeds towards the center of the necrotic zone for about 10 days after the occlusion. During this time the infarcted wall becomes progressively thinner as necrotic debris is removed by mononuclear cells. Replacement of the dead muscle by granulation tissue and formation of a firm shrunken scar takes place during the following 4–10 weeks.

The repair of the necrotic zone by fibrous tissue is accompanied by several parallel processes:

a. the changing distribution of shear stress in the walls surrounding the scar tissue
b. a distorted timing and pattern of contraction
c. the lengthening and hypertrophy of remaining fibers (which is required to compensate for the loss of contractile elements, for the increased end-diastolic volume, and for the distortion of the pattern of contraction).

In *small transmural infarcts,* the infarcted segment of the wall may shrink as a result of scar formation and the end-systolic and end-diastolic ventricular volumes may remain within normal limits.

Subendocardial infarcts can also impair contraction as the residual scar can impair the normal shortening of the overlying subepicardial muscle, distorting the physiologic pattern of contraction and relaxation.

In *large infarcts,* the infarcted segment expands before the scar is firm enough to oppose the pull from the adjacent normal segment of the ventricular wall ("infarct expansion").[4] Infarct expansion can be considerable in large transmural infarcts, particularly in elderly patients with myocardial atrophy, and is reduced in hypertrophic hearts. It can lead to the formation of aneurysm in the ventricular wall, and is about four times more frequent in apical and anterior MI than in inferior MI.[5] The formation of a fibrotic aneurysm seems to carry a worse prognosis than the mere expansion of a large infarct, because it is associated with a worse prognosis for comparable values of ejection fraction (EF).[6]

Remodeling of the ventricular wall and cavity takes place during the initial few months as a consequence of infarct expansion and of lengthening and hypertrophy of myocytes in the normal myocardium. As the residual ventricular walls must perform the same amount of external work under nonphysiologic conditions, the myocardial mass of contractile elements required for external work must exceed that lost during the necrotic process (see Ch. 7). Hearts with evidence of an old MI often have a markedly increased weight post mortem, also in the absence of other causes of hypertrophy.

■ *The extent of remodeling and hypertrophy is proportional to the size of the infarct.* ■

Early myocardial reperfusion

As demonstrated in experimental animals, the fraction of ischemic myocardium that becomes necrotic following sudden coronary occlusion can be markedly restricted by early reperfusion (spontaneous or drug-induced), as the extension of necrosis increases progressively between 1–6 h if the occlusion persists. The earlier the reperfusion, the greater the mass of ischemic myocardium salvaged; however, in experimental animals, reperfusion even within 3–6 h was seen to reduce necrosis. In patients, a substantial amount of myocardium may be salvaged at an even later stage if the occlusion was intermittent, if collateral flow was present, and if oxygen requirements were low. However, reperfusion may also accelerate the death of irreversibly damaged myocardial and vascular cells and it is still not clear whether it could damage cells not yet doomed (see Ch. 7). Sudden late reperfusion may also favor the development of hemorrhage in already necrotic segments of the ventricle and lead to cardiac rupture, particularly in elderly patients. A number of interventions aimed at improving the benefits of reperfusion by reducing reperfusion damage have been proposed and are under investigation, but no convincing results have so far been obtained in patients.

Within the area at risk, the coronary vascular bed recovers its physiologic function gradually; similarly, nonnecrosed reperfused myocardium recovers contractile function over a period of hours and days, particularly when ischemia was long lasting or recurrent (myocardial stunning) (see Ch. 7).

21.1.3 Systemic consequences

Pain, fear, and anxiety, as well as hemodynamic and systemic neurohumoral consequences of myocardial ischemia and necrosis, may influence the cardiac response to the ischemic insult. To date, attention has focused mainly on stimulation of the autonomic nervous system, which is the factor most easily assessed.

In some patients, usually those with inferior MI, the response is characterized initially by increased vagal tone with bradycardia and hypotension, possibly resulting from stimulation of receptors more prevalent in the inferior wall of the heart. In patients with anterior MI, the most apparent feature usually is considerable adrenergic stimulation with tachycardia and hypertension. This response is more common after the initial 1–2 h. Hyperglycemia usually occurs as a result of adrenergic stimulation and increased glucocorticoid hormone production. Vagal stimulation, when not resulting in hypotension, can reduce myocardial oxygen consumption by lowering heart rate and afterload. However, increased vagal tone can cause bradycardia and hypotension, impair A–V conduction and encourage ventricular escape tachyarrhythmias.

When MI is extensive, adrenergic stimulation provides essential circulatory support for the maintenance of perfusion to the brain and kidneys by increasing heart rate, systemic peripheral resistance, and inotropism of the normal myocardium. Conversely, increased vagal tone is detrimental.

When impairment of ventricular function is mild to moderate, increased vagal tone has a protective role. Conversely, increased sympathetic tone has deleterious effects on the extent of necrosis by increasing heart rate, inotropic state, and systemic arterial blood pressure. Increased concentrations of catecholamines in the blood are associated with the occurrence of severe tachyarrhythmias, which are also encouraged by catecholamine-induced increases in free fatty acids. α-Adrenergic stimulation also increases platelet aggregability and, hence, can favor thrombosis.

■ *The necrotic process in the myocardium causes local production of cytokines with a systemic acute-phase response[7] with fever and leukocytosis, which affect considerably the coronary and myocardial response to ischemia. The study of this component of the systemic response in man, which may be influenced by the inflammatory process that contributed to cause MI, has, so far, received scant attention.* ■

21.1.4 Hemodynamic consequences

As discussed in Chapter 7, myocardial necrosis and ischemia impair contractile function, not only through the loss of contractile elements but also through the disruption of both physiologic coordination and the sequence of regional ventricular contraction and relaxation. The impairment includes systolic, diastolic, and global ventricular function, as well as pulmonary circulation and lung function.

Systolic function

The changes in systolic function caused by infarction, ischemia, stunning, and hibernation are potentially reversible and are manifested by the following:

a. hypokinesis (reduction in the extent of contraction)
b. akinesis (lack of contraction)
c. dyskinesis (systolic bulging)
d. dyssynchrony (uncoordinated contraction of different segments of the wall with abnormal distribution of tensile stress)
e. hyperkinesis (increased compensatory contraction of the normal segments of the wall).

■ *The ultimate consequence of systolic dysfunction is represented by reduced systolic emptying and a consequent increase of end-systolic volume (ESV).* ■

Diastolic function

The ischemic myocardium has a reduced rate of early postsystolic relaxation which, together with the larger residual ESV, causes impairment of early diastolic filling. Late filling is also impaired because the ventricle is on the steep part of the late diastolic compliance curve in order to maintain an adequate stroke volume (SV) in spite of the increased ESV, at the expense of a larger end-diastolic volume (EDV) (see Ch. 2). End-diastolic compliance may later decrease further because of fibrous scar tissue and hypertrophy.

■ *Thus, as both early and late systolic filling are impaired, diastolic pressure must increase to maintain the SV.* ■

Global ventricular dysfunction

The consequences of systolic and diastolic dysfunction are an increased ESV and EDV, associated with a reduction of EF. For a given residual ESV, EF decreases in proportion to SV: with an ESV of 100 ml, EF will be 50% when SV is 100 ml, but will be 33% when SV is 50 ml. EDV will be 200 ml in the first case and 150 ml in the second. Filling pressure is a major determinant of EDV for a given ESV (see Ch. 2).

The impairment of ventricular function increases as ischemia and infarction extend; it is maximal when the whole area at risk is ischemic or necrotic and when adrenergic stimulation is exhausted, and it decreases as peri-infarction ischemia and stunning resolve and as compensatory hypertrophy and ventricular remodeling take place over the following weeks and months.

The severity of ventricular dysfunction depends not only on the extent of the necrotic or ischemic area but also on the degree of preexisting ventricular damage. In previously normal ventricles, when infarction involves more than 25% of the myocardium, clinical signs of heart failure are usually present; when it involves more than 40%, cardiogenic shock is common.[8]

■ *When, in spite of an elevated filling pressure, SV is reduced, tachycardia remains the only way in which an adequate cardiac output can be maintained. When cardiac output falls, oxygen delivery can be maintained only by increased oxygen tissue extraction and greater venous desaturation.*[9] ■

Pulmonary hemodynamics and lung function

Increased diastolic filling pressure is associated with increased left atrial and pulmonary vascular pressures. It is also associated with interstitial fluid accumulation and alveolar edema when left atrial blood pressure is persistently above 20–25 mmHg, pulmonary lymphatic drainage is impaired, and pulmonary capillaries are leaky.

Increased pulmonary intravascular pressure and interstitial fluid accumulation lead to increased lung stiffness and reduction of the dynamic lung compliance, which increases the work of respiratory muscles. The actual volume of blood in the pulmonary circulation is only slightly increased when left atrial pressure is markedly elevated. Thus, the lung congestion seen on radiographic films is due largely to interstitial fluid accumulation and decreased lung volume, which account for the time lag in their development when left atrial pressure rises and their resolution when it falls. Lung volume and vital capacity decrease and respiration rate increases. Blood flow is diverted towards the less dependent parts of the lungs and the upper lobes and a ventilation/perfusion mismatch develops. Respiratory gas exchange can become altered sufficiently to reduce arterial oxygen saturation; usually, arterial carbon dioxide tension is reduced as a result of the hyperventilation and ventilation/perfusion mismatch. Occasionally, bronchoconstriction develops, with wheezing and paroxysmal dyspnea. Clinical pulmonary edema develops when there is sufficient intra-alveolar fluid accumulation.

The increased pulmonary artery pressure increases the work load of the right ventricle, thus impairing right ventricular systolic emptying, particularly when the infarction involves also the right ventricular myocardium.

21.1.5 Classification of the Severity of the Hemodynamic Dysfunction

As MI predominantly involves the left ventricular wall, the most common and dominant alterations involve left ventricular function, which is influenced not only by the extension of infarction, by preexisting dysfunction, and by the neurohumoral control of fluid retention, but also by the extent of sympathetic or vagal stimulation.

The commonly used classification proposed by Killip and Kimball,[10] is based only on clinical criteria, and its prognostic value could be greatly improved by considering also the results of investigations nowadays widely available in CCUs, such as the results of 12-lead ECG, chest radiographic films, and echocardiographic assessment of left ventricular function.

■ *An integrated clinical classification is useful because it provides guidelines for treatment in the early phases of acute MI.* ■

Class 1

This indicates a hemodynamic state without clinically detectable signs of failure: heart rate may be normal or increased as an expression of an hyperdynamic circulation. There is no detectable impairment of left ventricular pump function (there is an EF more than 50% and clear lungs on chest radiography).

Class 2

This class of hemodynamic dysfunction involves moderate but clearly detectable impairment of left ventricular pump function. Clinically, there may be third or fourth heart sounds and signs of lung congestion at the bases, (usually an EF more than 40% but less than 50% and signs of interstitial fluid accumulation on chest radiography). Initially, this state is also compatible with severe impairment of left ventricular pump function compensated for by intense adrenergic stimulation.

Class 3

In this, there is severe obvious impairment of left ventricular pump function, indicated by tachycardia with gallop rhythm, orthopnea, crepitations over the whole lung field, elevated jugular venous pressure, but adequate peripheral perfusion (usually an EF more than 20% but less than 40% estimated by echocardiography; chest radiography reveals signs of venous congestion and interstitial and intra-alveolar fluid accumulation).

Class 4

Hemodynamic dysfunction of this type includes hypotension and peripheral hyperperfusion with shock, associated with all the features described in class 3. This condition results from an extreme reduction of cardiac output due to severe impairment of left ventricular function. Clinically, in patients with this degree of dysfunction, gallop rhythm, orthopnea, and crepitation over the whole lung field are associated with elevated venous pressure, hypotension (less than 90 mmHg), signs of peripheral hypoperfusion, and oliguria (usually EF less than 20% estimated by echocardiography, and chest radiography showing alveolar edema).

Predominant right ventricular infarction

In addition to this classification, which is largely based on left ventricular function, some patients with inferior MI, due to proximal right coronary artery occlusion, may present with prevailing signs of acute right ventricular failure resulting from infarction of a large segment of the right ventricular wall. When the involvement of the right ventricular wall is more extensive than that of the left, the impairment of right ventricular function becomes the limiting hemodynamic factor characterized by signs of right-sided failure (see Fig. 21.1).[11–13] Clinically, such patients present with markedly elevated right atrial jugular venous pressure, no orthopnea, clear lungs, often with hypotension, and, occasionally, with shock. They have normal or mildly elevated pulmonary wedge pressure and low cardiac output and can develop a severe drop in cardiac output and hypotension when treated with nitrates and diuretics.

■ *As a guide to patient management in the acute phase, the clinical findings and the results of chest radiography may have priority over estimates of left ventricular EF, as ventricular failure may*

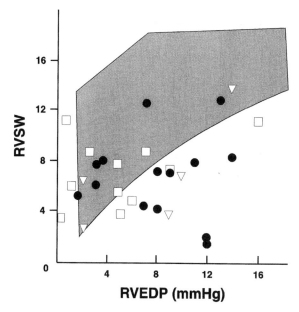

Fig. 21.1 Hemodynamic findings in right ventricular MI. When right ventricular end-diastolic pressure (RVEDP) is plotted against right ventricular stroke work (RVSW), most patients with inferior MI (●) or inferolateral MI (▽) were below the normal zone (shaded area), indicating an impaired right ventricular function. Most patients with anterior or anterolateral MI (□) are within the shaded area. (From data presented in ref. 11.)

be influenced considerably by systemic accumulation of fluid and the response of the autonomic nervous system.

During hospitalization, patients move from higher to lower classes as they are treated, but many also move from lower to higher classes as necrosis and ischemia extend and as adrenergic stimulation is reduced. At the predischarge assessment the classification should be based on the value of left ventricular EF, which is a major commonly available prognostic indicator, and on the requirement of diuretics to control signs of cardiac failure. ■

21.2 DIAGNOSIS AND INITIAL ASSESSMENT

About 75% of deaths from acute MI occur within the first day, the remaining 25% occurring between days 2 and 28. In-hospital deaths are caused mainly by ventricular failure, cardiac rupture (particularly in elderly patients), or arrhythmias in the setting of an extensive MI. Of all deaths, 50% occur within the first 2 h of the onset of symptoms, usually from ventricular fibrillation, largely outside hospital and independent of the size of the MI. The greatest therapeutic impact, therefore, can be gained from the prevention of very early arrhythmias and from reduction of infarct size. For these reasons, a very prompt diagnosis of the onset of MI is imperative and should not be delayed. When the diagnosis is uncertain, a provisional diagnosis should be made and the patient kept under close scrutiny until it can be confirmed or refuted. This early diagnosis is necessary for emergency management by the first attending physician, and should be followed by subsequent diagnostic confirmation and evaluation of infarct size and complications during admission to the CCU.

As limitation of infarct size is a race against time, it is essential that the first physician with which the patient has contact is familiar with the possible forms of presentation of acute MI, the initial clinical diagnosis, the confirmation of the diagnosis, and the differential diagnosis.

21.2.1 Clinical presentation

The presentation of acute MI may be typical, atypical, or silent but its subsequent evolution is largely independent of the form of presentation. In general, the more severe the pain, the more rapidly the patient seeks medical attention. Atypical presentation, stoicism, and denial can all delay the call for medical help. A previous history of IHD and identification of the pain as ischemic by the patient, based on past experience, considerably increase the likelihood of an ischemic cause, but the presence of cardiovascular risk factors has only a modest predictive value.[14,15] General schemes of decision support (based on computer programs) for the diagnosis of acute ischemic syndromes have been proposed,[16,17] and they may be useful in uncertain cases.

Typical presentation

Typically, patients present with persistent, very severe anginal pain, which may be accompanied by diaphoresis, nausea, and severe distress. If the patient is already an angina sufferer, the pain is usually similar in character but much more severe; it is often similar to that of previous infarction(s), if any. The pain usually builds up gradually and may persist with the same intensity, may be intermittent, or may wax and wane. About 40% of cases are preceded by short isolated episodes of similar, usually less severe, pain during the previous hours or days.

Atypical presentation

Atypical presentations of acute MI are particularly common in elderly patients but are not uncommon in middle-aged and young individuals. Discomfort can be epigastric and frequently confused with indigestion, or associated with nausea, profound weakness, diaphoresis, and a sudden onset of dyspnea or palpitations. In the Multicenter Pain Study,[18] acute IHD was ultimately diagnosed in 22% of patients presenting to the emergency department with stabbing sharp pain, in 13% with a pleuritic type of pain, and in 7% of patients whose pain was reproduced by palpation.

Silent MI

It is estimated that about 25% of infarctions occur in the absence of any pain. Symptoms can be characterized by the appearance of weakness, fatigue, or frank signs of cardiac failure, but they can also be mild and atypical and diagnosed only by a subsequent ECG assessment. In about 15% of cases, MI can be totally silent (see Ch. 14).

21.2.2 Early confirmation of the diagnosis

A clinical diagnosis of acute MI requires immediate confirmation by an emergency 12-lead ECG tracing during pain, and differential diagnoses should be considered only when the ECG is negative. In uncertain cases, the diagnosis can be confirmed only by the evolution of symptoms, serial ECGs, serum markers of myocardial necrosis, and the demonstration of a new regional ventricular dysfunction.

12-lead ECG diagnosis of ischemic origin of symptoms

A 12-lead ECG may immediately confirm the clinical diagnosis when it shows a typical lesion wave in multiple leads. It meets the standard accepted diagnostic criteria of acute MI when it shows elevation of more than 2 mm in three adjacent precordial leads or in two standard limb leads.

■ *When the ECG shows no obvious lesion wave in multiple leads, there is less urgency to consider immediate recanalization of the infarcted artery. When the ECG is not diagnostic, there is time for the application of other diagnostic techniques and for the consideration of possible differential diagnoses with unstable angina or with nonischemic causes.* ■

The following guidelines can be useful:

1. In all patients presenting with symptoms suggestive of acute myocardial ischemia, efforts should be made to record an ECG during the pain or discomfort and before the administration of sublingual nitrates which, in 5–10% of cases, may cause the disappearance of even the most obvious ST-segment elevation. When the ECG is nondiagnostic, it should be repeated after the administration of sublingual nitrates, as changes may become apparent if reversible acute ischemia is associated with pseudonormalization of T waves—a situation not unusual in patients who recently have had a further prolonged episode of pain.
2. The detection of ischemic ST-segment depression or T-wave changes not present on a previous tracing are sufficient indications for admission to a CCU for further assessment, as it is suggestive of crescendo unstable angina or of very early MI.
3. When the ECG tracing recorded during pain is normal and no changes appear after the administration of sublingual nitrates, or when it is abnormal but unchanged from tracings obtained days, weeks, or months earlier, possible differential diagnoses should be considered; however, the critical questions remaining are whether the symptoms were, indeed, caused by acute myocardial ischemia that was no longer present at the time that the ECG tracing was recorded, or was not detectable by the ECG, or whether the symptoms had other causes. An unchanged ECG in the presence of previous MI, conduction abnormalities, or aspecific ST-segment and T-wave changes does not exclude ischemia unless normal or unchanged regional ventricular wall motion or myocardial scintigraphic studies can be demonstrated during pain. Furthermore, a normal ECG recorded during typical pain does not exclude an acute MI as in two studies,[19,20] between 1 and 6% of patients presenting to the emergency department with typical cardiac ischemic pain and a completely normal ECG were subsequently found to have had acute IHD.

■ *Although a normal ECG recorded during severe pain is a very strong indication against a cardiac ischemic origin of pain, severe myocardial ischemia can be excluded only by the demonstration of normal ventricular wall motion by echocardiography.* ■

Other diagnostic techniques

In the presence of a typical ischemic pain but a nondiagnostic ECG tracing, prompt assessment of regional ventricular function by echocardiography during pain is the most widely available option. In addition, myocardial scintigraphy during pain can establish the diagnosis of acute ischemia by demonstrating new regional alterations of myocardial contractile function or perfusion, but this is possible only in well-equipped and well-organized centers.

A normal or unchanged echocardiogram recorded after the pain or discomfort has subsided does not exclude the possibility that symptoms were caused by acute transient myocardial ischemia that subsided completely, leaving no persistent changes. Determination of serum indices of myocardial necrosis provide the conclusive diagnosis that MI has occurred, but only after about 6–8 from the onset of symptoms.

Assessment of the very early evolution of MI

Time from the onset of symptoms is usually taken as the only criterion for considering thrombolysis; however, in many cases, the magnitude of ST-segment elevation, the depth of Q waves and loss of R waves can provide rough indications of the very early evolution of MI and can offer clues to the extent of the jeopardized myocardium that could still be salvaged by prompt coronary artery recanalization. Persistent elevation of the ST segment with small Q waves and preserved R waves is an indication for thrombolytic therapy, independent of the time from onset of symptoms; conversely, the presence of Q waves and the large loss of R waves indicates that the benefits of reperfusion may be limited. The presence of an old MI, conduction disturbances, and hypertrophy makes it difficult to assess the evolution of MI and the extent of jeopardized myocardium.

21.2.3 Very early differential diagnosis

When symptoms have disappeared before an ECG recording has been made, and when the 12-lead ECG tracing is normal or unchanged from a previous tracing, patients with known IHD who recognize the pain or discomfort as being ischemic but of longer duration and/or greater frequency than usual, as well as other individuals with fairly typical chest pain, should be assumed provisionally to have unstable angina (see Ch. 19). Conversely, when the ECG during pain is normal or unchanged from previous tracings, and when ventricular wall motion studies are normal or unchanged, other differential diagnoses should be considered, as follows:

1. Acute aortic dissection should be considered, particularly in patients with a marfanoid aspect or a history of hypertension. An abrupt onset of pain, most severe initially, differences in brachial arterial pulses, and enlargement or double contour of the aortic knob on standard chest radiography are suggestive of aortic dissection and call for esophageal echocardiography, computed tomography, or magnetic resonance imaging.

2. Acute pericarditis usually presents with fever, with very sharp pain which becomes worse with respiration, pressure, and changes of posture, and with pleural and pericardial friction rub. The elevation of the ST segment is widespread but modest with, initially, positive T waves. An echocardiogram may reveal pericardial fluid.

3. Acute pulmonary embolism is associated with increased jugular venous pressure and a loud pulmonary valve closure sound, but no signs of left ventricular failure, and sometimes with the appearance of incomplete right bundle branch block on the ECG. In the later phases, it can present with pleuritic chest pain. Arterial blood gases will show a typical reduction of carbon dioxide partial pressure out of proportion to the reduction in the partial pressure of oxygen, and lung scintigraphy will show segmental perfusion defects.

4. Esophageal or gastric and abdominal conditions should be considered (see Ch. 16).
5. Inflammation of costochondral–sternal articulation is usually associated with local tenderness (see Ch. 16)
6. Finally, some patients with typical pain and none of the above syndromes may have small coronary vessel disease (see Ch. 18). This possibility cannot be substantiated or disproved easily because of the lack of adequate diagnostic criteria.

21.2.4 Late confirmation of diagnosis in the CCU

In uncertain cases, the diagnosis can be confirmed within hours or days of the acute event by serial ECG changes, by the increased concentration of markers released by injured myocardial cells into the blood, and by the appearance of persistent segmental ventricular wall motion abnormalities. Imaging techniques of the necrotic tissue may also be used in uncertain cases, when available. The delayed confirmation of MI, although coming too late for thrombolysis to be considered, is useful for the subsequent patient management strategy.

Acute evolution of the ECG

The gradual development of Q waves and loss of R waves, together with the appearance of inverted T waves over a period of a few days, are diagnostic of MI, even when no tracing documenting the ST-segment elevation in the very acute phase are available. The appearance of T-wave and/or ST-segment changes in the hours following a prolonged episode of chest pain is not necessarily indicative of cell necrosis, but is indicative of an ischemic origin of symptoms and diagnostic of unstable angina (see Ch. 19). In some cases, diagnostic elevation of the serum markers of myocardial cell death can occur in the absence of Q waves on the 12-lead ECG. Non-Q-wave MI is a widely used descriptive clinical term that does not represent a precise clinical entity, as there is no clear-cut relationship between the transmural extension of myocardial necrosis, the presence or absence of Q waves, and the patency of the infarct-related artery. In addition, some Q-wave MIs may involve only a small fraction of the area at risk and, conversely, some non-Q-wave MIs may be quite extensive (see below).

Serum markers of myocardial cell death

Such markers, released by irreversibly injured myocardial cells, become detectable only some hours after the onset of symptoms. For routine use, the choice among the various indices of myocardial necrosis should be confined to serum activity of creatine kinase (CK) as an early index of necrosis and to lactic dehydrogenase (LDH) as a late index of necrosis.

In patients with recent onset of chest pain, samples for CK activity should be taken every 8 h for at least 48 h, as CK activity raised above the normal range 4–8 h after the onset of pain reaches a peak at about 24 h and declines to normal values 3–4 days after the onset. For a similar infarct size, wide variations in the CK time/activity curve can be observed, depending on the evolution of the infarction and on the clearance of the enzyme from the blood. Early recanalization of the infarct-related artery is associated with an earlier, higher peak of CK. Intermittent progression of the infarction results in multiple peaks, detected by frequent sampling of myoglobin,[3] and reinfarction within 3–4 days causes a well-defined, isolated, secondary peak of total CK. In uncertain cases in which the CK elevation could be related to noncardiac causes, such as electric defibrillation, muscle diseases, trauma, intramuscular injections, vigorous exercise, or alcohol intoxication, the MB isoenzymes of CK should be measured.

In patients with an episode of severe prolonged chest pain a few days before admission, LDH activity should be measured as it exceeds the normal range within 24–48 h, reaching a peak at 3–6 days and returning to normal levels 8–12 days after the onset of MI. In uncertain cases the LDH-1 isoenzyme could be measured. Troponin-T seems to be another sensitive marker of cell necrosis, with a long plasma half-life.

Imaging techniques

Imaging techniques of the necrotic tissue are valuable for diagnostic purposes, only when they provide additional information not available from routinely available tests, but they can be valuable for research purposes for the assessment of the location and size of the MI (see below).

21.2.5 Assessment of infarct location and size

The location of the infarction in the wall of the heart can be detected by the ECG and imaging techniques. Its size is indicated by clinical signs of impaired ventricular function, by the degree of the elevation of serum concentrations of markers of myocardial cell necrosis, by the extension of Q waves on the ECG, and by imaging techniques.

The *ECG assessment* of the location of the MI as either anterior or inferior is usually reasonably accurate for clinical purposes when previous tracings were normal. It is less accurate (and even uncertain) in cases of dorsal and lateral necrosis, as well as in the presence of previous MI or conduction disturbances.

Several studies have suggested that the ECG is incapable of indicating whether ST-segment depression in leads not showing Q waves is related to ischemia in myocardial segments not perfused by the infarct-related artery, or whether it is just the electric reflection of ischemia surrounding the infarcted area.[21–23]

Elevation of the ST segment in leads V_1 and V_3R–V_6R in association with an inferior MI is indicative of right ventricular MI caused by proximal right coronary artery occlusion. However, these changes are often minimal because of both the thinness of the right ventricular wall and the coexisting inferior and dorsal lesion waves. Right atrial MI can also be suspected in patients with inferior MI and elevated jugular venous pressure but no signs of left ventricular failure, from the appearance of depression or elevation of the PQ segment associated with atrial arrhythmias.

Cross-sectional echocardiography is now widely available in CCUs for assessing global and regional contractile dysfunction. Regional impairment of contractile function can result from myocardial necrosis, ischemia, stunning, or hibernation (see Ch. 22), but a localized dysfunction and a preserved EF are good indications of a small MI. Echocardiography is particularly valuable for interpreting uncertain changes on the ECG, as the presence of a normally contracting wall rules out the presence of necrosis or severe ischemia.

Chest radiography is useful to evaluate the presence of interstitial fluid accumulation in the lungs, which indicates the presence of previous severe and prolonged impairment of left ventricular contractile function. Improvement of the radiographic picture may not become apparent until 12–24 h after improvement of ventricular dysfunction, because of the time lag required for the signs of pulmonary congestion to clear. In addition, gradual deterioration of left ventricular function may only become evident 6–12 h later, because of the time lag required for the interstitial fluid to accumulate in the lung. In the acute phase of MI, cardiomegaly usually indicates the presence of a previous heart disease, but a normal-sized left ventricle does not necessarily imply a small MI, as it is compatible with a small SV and an increased end-systolic volume (i.e. a low EF).

With regard to *enzyme* determination, under ideal conditions the size of the infarction correlates with the area below the CK or CK-MB time/activity curves. However, in practise, this correlation is influenced by a variety of circumstances that interfere with the release of the enzyme from the necrotic tissue and with its clearance from the blood. The peak of the CK and CK-MB curves, in general, is reasonably well correlated with the size of the infarction (although it is even more affected by the factors cited above) and has a semiquantitative value when interpreted together with clinical, ECG, and echocardiographic data.

Radionuclide myocardial imaging techniques are much less widely available than echocardiography, but are valuable for research purposes as they can provide information on the extent of both myocardial necrosis and reduced perfusion. Positron emission tomography (PET) has the potential to detect more accurately the location and extent of necrosis than is currently possible by single-photon cameras, but it should remain clearly confined to the domain of research until the additional information that it provides, above that available from clinical and other generally available techniques, becomes established.

Myocardial necrosis can be imaged by positive indicators that show the infarction as a "hot spot" as they are selectively taken up by the irreversibly damaged myocardium. These tracers are represented by ^{99}Tc-labeled pyrophosphates, which bind to the calcium that has accumulated in necrotic cells, and by ^{99}Tc-labeled antimyosin antibodies, which bind to the myosin exposed by the loss of sarcolemma in necrotic cells; however, the correlation between binding sites and the extent of necrosis may not always be a linear one.

Negative indicators are represented by thallium-201 and other myocardial perfusion tracers. They visualize the necrotic hypoperfused ventricular wall as a "cold spot" attributable to low tracer uptake. As the hypoperfused area includes both necrotic and ischemic myocardium, very early images with flow tracers in acute MI indicate the total extent of ischemic and necrotic myocardium. In later images, 48 h or more after the onset of symptoms, the fraction of the wall that is hypoperfused usually corresponds more closely to the necrotic area, which accumulates positive indicators of necrosis. As the spatial resolution of single-photon and also PET is limited, positive indicators selectively accumulating in necrotic tissue are capable of detecting much smaller areas of necrosis than negative tracers, but the variable uptake of positive indicators by irreversibly damaged tissues prevents an accurate quantification of the extent of necrosis. The spatial extent of necrosis is overestimated by positive indicators and underestimated by negative indicators because of the limited geometric resolution of detecting instrumentation. Magnetic resonance imaging has a much higher geometric resolution than PET and is a promising research tool.[24,25]

Estimates of infarct size useful in clinical practise

Clinical assessment based on a combination of generally available data usually allows a semiquantitative evaluation of infarct size into small, medium, large, and massive, which, in patients with previously normal hearts, should correspond to the classification of left ventricular impairment into classes 1–4. Discrepancies are sometimes observed between classes 1–4 (defined in 21.1.5) and signs of necrosis on the ECG or values of peak CK.

In patients with previously normal hearts, a markedly reduced left ventricular EF in the presence of low values of peak CK suggests the presence of viable noncontractile myocardium. Conversely, a preserved EF in spite of high values of peak CK suggests very early coronary reperfusion and a consequent small loss of myocardium.

21.2.6 Complete versus incomplete MI in the area at risk

In theory, an incomplete MI within the area at risk distal to the culprit coronary stenosis represents the potential anatomic substrate for new episodes of myocardial ischemia and necrosis, possibly associated with malignant arrhythmias. Incomplete MIs are commonly thought to be represented by "non-Q-wave" infarctions, which are, in general, more often nontransmural and associated with a patent infarct-related artery than "Q-wave" infarctions.

The descriptive ECG term "non-Q-wave MI" has been used widely in an effort to help practising physicians to assess prognosis and as a therapeutic guide.[26-28] However, in spite of some average differences, patients with Q-wave or non-Q-wave MI represent heterogeneous groups that cannot be clearly distinguished on the basis of either the transmural or nontransmural distribution of necrosis, or according to the occlusion or patency of the infarct-related artery.[29-31]

Thus, the separation of patients with Q-wave or non-Q-wave MI is as broad as the separation of patients with anterior or inferior MI: although, in general, patients with anterior MI have a worse prognosis than those with inferior MI, a large inferior MI carries a worse prognosis than a small anterior MI.

The similar long-term prognosis of Q-wave and non-Q-wave MI reported in some studies is probably related to patient selection. Non-Q-wave MIs are certainly incomplete, small, and carry a good prognosis, when no Q-waves develop in any of the ECG leads showing ST-segment elevation during the acute phase, when peak CK values are low, and when patients have no post-MI angina and have a negative predischarge ECG exercise stress test. However, those patients also in whom Q-waves develop in only a few of the leads initially showing ST-segment elevation, with low peak CK values, have an incomplete MI within the area at risk and may have a similarly good prognosis when they have no post-MI angina and have negative tests. Conversely, when no new Q waves can be detected in patients with old MI(s) in spite of elevated markers of myocardial cell necrosis, prognosis may be as severe as that of patients with a large Q-wave MI, if associated with a reduced EF.

■ *The definition of both the size of infarction (into small, medium, large, or massive) and, when possible, its final extent compared with the area initially at risk (as complete or incomplete), with or without persisting post-MI ischemia, may be more useful for the management of individual patients than simply categorizing them as either anterior and inferior MI, or as Q-wave and non-Q-wave MI.* ■

REFERENCES

1. Muller JE, Rude RE, Braunwald E et al. Myocardial recurrence, outcome, and risk factors in the Multicenter Investigation of Infarct Size. Ann Intern Med 1988;*108*:1.
2. Hackett D, Davies G, Chierchia S, Maseri A. Intermittent coronary occlusion in acute myocardial infarction. Value of combined thrombolytic and vasodilator therapy. N Engl J Med 1987:*317*:1055.

3. Kagen L, Scheidt S, Butt A. Serum myoglobin in myocardial infarction: the "staccato phenomenon." Is acute myocardial infarction in man an intermittent event? Am J Med 1977;62:86.

4. Hutchins GM, Bulkley BH. Infarct expansion versus extension: two different complications of acute myocardial infarction. Am J Cardiol 1978;47:1127.

5. Abrams DL, Edelist A, Luria MH, Miller AJ. Ventricular aneurysm: A reappraisal based on a study of 65 consecutive autopsied cases. Circulation 1963;27:164.

6. Meizlish JL, Berger HJ, Plankey M et al. Functional left ventricular aneurysm formation after acute anterior transmural myocardial infarction: incidence, natural history, and prognostic implications. N Engl J Med 1984;311:1001.

7. De Beer FC, Hind CKR, Fox KM, Allan RM, Maseri A, Pepys MB. Measurement of serum C-reactive protein concentration in myocardial ischaemia and infarction. Br Heart J 1982;47:239.

8. Cutovitz AL, Sobel BE, Roberts R. Progressive nature of myocardial injury in selected patients with cardiogenic shock. Am J Cardiol 1978;41:469.

9. DaLuz PL, Cavanilles JM, Michaels S et al. Oxygen delivery, anoxic metabolism and hemoglobin-oxygen affinity (P50) in patients with acute myocardial infarction and shock. Am J Cardiol 1975;36:148.

10. Killip T, Kimball JI. Treatment of myocardial infarction in a coronary care unit. A two year experience with 250 patients. Am J Cardiol 1967;20:457.

11. Maseri A, Pesola A, Contini C, L'Abbate A, Donato L. Hémodynamique pulmonaire et coronarienne dans la phase aiguë de l'infarctus du myocarde. Arch Mal Coeur 1973;66:401.

12. Isner JM, Roberts WC. Right ventricular infarction complicating left ventricular infarction secondary to coronary artery disease: frequency, location, associated findings and significance from analysis of 236 necropsy patients with acute or healed myocardial infarction. Am J Cardiol 1978;42:885.

13. Lopez-Sendon J, Coma-Canella I, Gamallo C. Sensitivity and specificity of hemodynamic criteria in the diagnosis of acute right ventricular infarction. Circulation 1981;64:515.

14. Chaitman BR, Bourassa MG, Davis K et al. Angiographic prevalence of high-risk coronary artery disease in patient subgroups (CASS). Circulation 1981;64:360.

15. Pryor DB, Shaw L, McCants CB et al. Value of the history and physican in identifying patients at increased risk for coronary artery disease. Ann Intern Med 1993;118:81.

16. Goldman L, Cook EF, Brand DA et al. A computer protocol to predict myocardial infarction in emergency department patients with chest pain. N Engl J Med 1988;318:797.

17. Aase O, Jonsbu J, Liestol K et al. Decision support by computer analysis of selected case history variables in the emergency room among patients with acute chest pain. Eur Heart J 1993;14:433.

18. Lee TH, Cook EF, Weisberg MC et al. Impact of the availability of a prior electrocardiogram on the triage of the patient with acute chest pain. J Gen Intern Med 1990;5:381.

19. McCarthy BD, Wong JB, Selker HP. Detecting acute cardiac ischemia in the emergency department: a review of the literature. J Gen Intern Med 1990;5:365.

20. Rouan GW, Lee TH, Cook EF et al. Clinical characteristics and outcome of acute myocardial infarction in patients with initially normal or nonspecific electrocardiograms (a report from the multicenter chest pain study). Am J Cardiol 1989;64:1087.

21. Ferguson DW, Pandian N, Kioschos JM et al. Angiographic evidence that reciprocal ST-segment depression ducing acute myocardial infarction does not indicate remote ischemia: analysis of 23 patients. Am J Cardiol 1984;53:55.

22. Little WC, Rogers EW, Sodums MT. Mechanisms of anterior ST segment depression during acute inferior myocardial infarction. Ann Intern Med 1984;100:26.

23. Lew AS, Weiss AT, Shah PK et al. Precordial ST segment depression during acute inferior myocardial infarction: early thallium-201 scintigraphic evidence of adjacent posterolateral or inferoseptal involvement. J Am Coll Cardiol 1985;5:203.

24. Johnston DL, Mulvagh SL, Cashion RW et al. Nuclear magnetic resonance imaging of acute myocardial infarction within 24 hours of chest pain onset. Am J Cardiol 1989;64:172.

25. Ratner AV, Okada RD, Newell JB, Pohost GM. The relationship between proton nuclear magnetic resonance relaxation parameters and myocardial perfusion with acute coronary arterial occlusion and reperfusion. Circulation 1985;71:823.

26. Nicod P, Gilpin E, Dittrich H et al. Short-and long-term clinical outcome after Q wave and non-Q wave myocardial infarction in a large patient population. Circulation 1989;*79:*528.

27. O'Brien TX, Ross J. Non-Q-wave myocardial infarction: incidence, pathophysiology, and clinical course compared with Q-wave infarction. Clin Cardiol 1989;*12(Suppl. III):*3.

28. Lavie CJ, Gersh BJ. Acute myocardial infarction: initial manifestations, management and prognosis. Mayo Clin Proc 1990;*65:*531.

29. Phibbs B. "Transmural" versus "subendocardial" myocardial infarction: an electrocardiographic myth. J Am Coll Cardiol 1983;*1:*561.

30. Levine HD. Subendocardial infarction in retrospect: pathologic, cardiographic, and ancillary features. Circulation 1985;*72:*790.

31. Spodick DH. Q-wave infarction versus S-T infarction: nonspecificity of electrocardiographic criteria for differentiating transmural and nontransmural lesions. Am J Cardiol 1983;*51:*913.

CHAPTER 22

Acute myocardial infarction: management

22.1 INITIAL MANAGEMENT

When a cardiac ischemic origin of acute symptoms is diagnosed, irrespective of whether acute myocardial infarction (MI) or unstable angina are suggested, patients should be referred promptly to an emergency department where a precise diagnosis can be made. When the ECG diagnosis of acute MI is certain, appropriate treatment should be started, even before admission if possible, because the goal is to recanalize the infarct-related artery within as short a time as possible, ideally within 1 h of the onset of symptoms.

1. Aspirin should be administered as soon as the diagnosis is suspected (unless contraindicated).
2. Analgesics should be administered as required.
3. Thrombolytic treatment should be considered as soon as the diagnosis of acute MI is confirmed by an ECG tracing.
4. Additional measures capable of limiting infarct size should then be implemented.
5. Specific treatment for pump failure, arrhythmias and complications should be instituted when appropriate.

22.1.1 Prehospital care and immediate management by the first attending physician

All patients with suspected MI should receive aspirin (325 mg as a loading dose) (unless contraindicated by allergy to salicylic acid or by a very recent history of gastric or duodenal ulcer), because it has been shown to reduce the rate of mortality in both acute MI and unstable angina. In patients with contraindications, other antiplatelet agents can be administered (see Ch. 19).

All patients who are in pain, and in whom the ECG is diagnostic of acute ischemia, should receive sublingual nitroglycerin (0.25–0.75 mg), nitroglycerin spray, or intravenous nitroglycerin, or sublingual or intravenous isosorbide dinitrate (ISDN) (5–20 mg). The initial dose should be repeated within 2–3 min if no effect is achieved, until either the systolic arterial pressure has fallen by 20 mmHg or severe headache develops. The relief of pain by sublingual nitrates indicates that an improvement in ischemia has taken place and they should, therefore, be the treatment of first choice, as they also abolish the cause of pain and indicate the reversibility of ischemia. Careful attention should be given to patients with suspected right ventricular MI, as the reduction in venous return caused by nitrates could cause a marked reduction in cardiac output and systemic blood pressure.

If the pain is not relieved within 3–5 min by reducing or abolishing ischemia with nitrates, morphine sulfate (2–4 mg i.v.) should be administered in order to reduce the perception of pain and can be repeated every 5–10 min (up to a limit of 10–30 mg i.v.) until either the pain has subsided or side effects occur (depression of respiration, vomiting, hypotension). The vagomimetic effects of morphine can be reduced by atropine (0.5–1 mg i.v.).

Very early intravenous administration of β-blockers is indicated in order to reduce the risk of prehospital sudden ischemic cardiac death (SICD) and is reasonably safe in patients with no obvious signs of cardiac failure or bradycardia (see ahead). When in doubt, the decision should be deferred until after admission to the coronary case unit (CCU), where any undesirable side effects can be treated promptly. The prophylactic use of lidocaine has failed to reduce the incidence of SICD before admission and, therefore, can not be recommended.[1]

Oxygen should be administered only to patients with arterial oxygen desaturation and central cyanosis attributable to alteration of pulmonary gas exchange, either preexisting or caused by acute left ventricular failure. In patients with normal arterial saturation, inhalation of oxygen does not increase its arterial content to any significant extent because of the shape of the oxygen dissociation curve.

Thrombolysis should be initiated, even before admission to hospital, in all patients with acute MI, diagnosed by 12-lead ECG, with unequivocal evidence of a sizable area of myocardium at risk: these are usually those patients coming to medical attention within 1–2 h following the onset of symptoms, with extensive ST-segment elevation and no loss of R waves in multiple leads (particularly V_1–V_6) (see below). Such patients obtain the greatest benefit from prompt coronary thrombolysis, which can even prevent MI[2] or reduce the extent of necrosis within the area at risk, and reduce mortality (see below). In patients not coming to medical attention until several hours after the onset of symptoms, and in those without extensive ST-segment elevation, deferring thrombolysis until they have been admitted to CCU and assessed thoroughly is not as critical as for the former group.

In addition to these general forms of treatment, emergency symptomatic treatment may be required in some patients for vasovagal syndrome with hypotension and bradycardia, hypertension, or acute left ventricular failure:

1. The vasovagal syndrome should be treated with intravenous injection of atropine.
2. Hypertension should be treated with sublingual nitrates, sublingual nifedipine, or intravenous β-blockers (or infusion of nitroprusside for patients already in hospital), depending on both the circumstances and on the response.
3. Acute left ventricular failure should be treated with morphine, sublingual nitrates (as above), and furosemide (20–40 mg i.v.).

Thrombolysis, treatment of arrhythmias, pump failure, and reduction of infarct size are discussed in detail below.

2.1.2 Admission policies, organization, and general patient management in CCU

The appreciation of the importance of unstable angina as a prodromal symptom of MI, together with the preventive efficacy of aggressive therapy in both unstable angina and in the very early phases of acute MI, are responsible for the changes taking place in CCU admission policies. Up to the late 1970s and early 1980s, nearly all patients admitted to a

CCU had to have confirmed MI; nowadays, a substantial proportion of patients have unstable angina. This change in admission policies implies some functional and technical reorganization and some changes in general patient management. The prompt admission of patients with acute MI implies organizational aspects of early diagnosis and referrals.

Admission policies

Prevention and limitation of infarction to the smallest possible fraction of the area at risk and prevention of reinfarction are as important goals as the management of arrhythmic and hemodynamic complications in patients with established MI. A more accurate identification of unstable patients at high risk would be useful when establishing admission policies, because less than 20% of patients presenting to hospital with a typical history of chest pain, but with normal ECGs, will have an infarction, and of these, less than 1% will have complications.[3,4] Elevation of both troponin T and C-reactive protein could be useful markers for identifying high-risk patients (see Chs. 9 and 19).

Organizational aspects of early diagnosis and referral. A call for a doctor at an early stage, or self-referral by a patient to an emergency department, results either from unbearably severe symptoms or from the awareness that the symptoms, although not severe, are suggestive of acute myocardial ischemia and have a severe prognostic significance. The educational and organizational aspects of referral and self-referral are, therefore, of critical importance.

Community education programs are undoubtedly the first essential step, as they should, on the one hand, improve recognition of symptoms and, on the other, overcome the frequent reaction of denial in patients who, although recognizing that the symptoms could be suggestive of acute myocardial ischemia, do not immediately accept such a possibility. Community education programs should also include the training of the general population in cardiopulmonary rescuscitation methods.

The collaboration of general physicians and family doctors must be elicited, as they have key roles in prompt diagnosis, early intervention, and emergency admission. A portable 12-lead ECG recorder is an essential tool for establishing a diagnosis; however, when this is not available, aspirin and nitroglycerin (unless contraindicated) should be administered in suspected cases while admission to an accident and emergency department is being arranged. When the diagnosis has been established, the administration of thrombolytic therapy should be considered while admission to a CCU is being arranged.

Ambulance services and paramedic personnel are useful for facilitating admission to hospital emergency departments and CCUs and, not least, possibly also for prompt emergency care. Ambulances staffed with physicians or with trained paramedics and connected by telephone to a CCU (as well as having facilities available for transmission of the ECG) can reduce the time taken to admit a patient and provide prompt emergency diagnosis and therapy. However, not only is their cost considerable and, therefore, dependent on the use of volunteers but also their efficacy depends on the traffic conditions of the territory served, as well as on the development of community education programes.

Reorganization of hospital emergency departments is essential in order to expedite the objective diagnostic assessment and the prompt initiation of thrombolytic therapy, when appropriate. When a patient arrives at an emergency department with a suspected MI, an ECG should be recorded immediately and repeated after administration of sublingual nitrates. Therapy should then be started as the immediate transfer to a CCU is being organized. To this purpose, a set of general guidelines for the staff of the emergency department, issued by the cardiologist in charge of the CCU, can be useful.

Functional and technical organization of CCUs

The need for beds equipped with invasive monitoring facilities can be reduced considerably by favoring the use of subintensive care beds equipped with only ECG monitoring equipment (including that for detecting ischemic ST-segment shifts) and with lower nurse:patient ratios (and hence much lower costs).[5] The reduction in the number of intensive care beds and in the need for invasive hemodynamic monitoring equipment is the result of the following:

a. the reduced proportion of patients admitted with complications, of the total number admitted, as a consequence of changes in admission policies
b. the considerable amount of clinical correlations accumulated from extensive invasive hemodynamic monitoring in the 1970s
c. the increasing use of two-dimensional and Doppler echocardiography
d. the need to limit ever-increasing costs.

Careful clinical and ECG monitoring is sufficient in all patients with no severe hemodynamic complications. Patients admitted with early MI or unstable angina require reliable monitoring equipment for the detection of ST-segment shifts, in order to indicate the evolution of their ischemic episodes and the occurrence of silent ischemic episodes, as well as to detect any potentially life-threatening arrhythmias.

Nowadays, in the hands of expert cardiologists, only those patients assessed as in class 4, as defined in 21.1.5, require invasive hemodynamic monitoring. However, if patients requiring invasive monitoring are admitted infrequently, the familiarity of the staff with invasive procedures is unlikely to be optimal. Coordinated stratified systems are desirable, therefore, whereby complicated cases requiring hemodynamic monitoring can be transferred to institutions that have a central sophisticated CCU with facilities for intensive care and interventional procedures. A lower tier of CCUs, equipped with only ECG monitoring facilities but sufficient for the vast majority of patients, should liaise with the few centralized units. Within any CCU, patients with acute or impending MI require careful clinical follow-up of the evolution of their symptoms in terms not only of ischemic changes in the early phases, the possible recurrence of ischemia, and the extension of MI, but also of the development of life-threatening arrhythmias and of hemodynamic impairment.

Adequate monitoring of the development of symptoms and signs of myocardial ischemia is essential and is provided by the waning, waxing, and recurrence of ischemic pain and of ST-segment changes on the leads monitored and on the 12-lead ECG.

Reliable and simple alarm systems for life-threatening arrhythmias are also essential. More sophisticated arrhythmia monitoring is optional as its practical value has not been convincingly demonstrated, except for research purposes.

Careful and frequent (every 15–30 min) clinical observation can also provide a valuable assessment of the circulatory conditions of patients in a critical condition. Trends in respiratory rate, heart rate, arterial pressure, temperature of the feet, and urine output, recorded by nurses and notified to doctors, and changes in jugular venous pressure and heart and lung signs, can provide adequate noninvasive hemodynamic monitoring for most patients.

Echocardiography provides a most valuable and immediate objective assessment of the site and extension of ventricular wall motion abnormalities and of overall ventricular function. Used in conjunction with blood gas analysis and portable chest radiographic equipment, it can often be a substitute for invasive hemodynamic monitoring.

General patient management

The emotional impact of emergency hospitalization and the anxiety caused by the fear of MI calls for a calm, friendly explanation of the nature of the illness and for reassurance (diazepam, 2–5 mg orally, 2–4 times a day may be given as required). Patients should be comfortable in bed and allowed to sit in an armchair by the bed at any time that is compatible with their clinical condition. They should walk about the room for brief periods as soon as continuous ECG monitoring is not considered necessary or a telemetric system is available.

Patients with confirmed MI should be kept on a liquid diet for the initial 24 h, and on a low-calorie diet during the days following. Full blood tests, including cholesterol concentrations,[6] should be obtained on admission. A 12-lead ECG (including right precordial leads for inferior MIs) should be obtained on admission, and repeated every 8 h for the first 48 h and also during new episodes of recurring chest pain, and daily subsequently. An echocardiogram should be obtained on admission, and repeated before discharge and whenever required for interpreting symptoms or for therapeutic decisions.

Electrolyte imbalance, particularly hypokalemia, if present should be corrected. Heart rate, respiration rate, and blood pressure (cuff manometer) graphs, as well as jugular venous pressure, by inspection, should be checked frequently.

22.1.3 Coronary thrombolysis

There is overwhelming evidence that thrombolysis reduces both the rate of mortality and infarct size, particularly when carried out soon after the onset of symptoms, independent of age. Intravenous thrombolytic drugs should be given in association with aspirin because of the proven benefits of this drug combination (see below). The additional risk carried by thrombolytic treatment in patients with no contraindications (i.e. those who could be included in large trials), is fairly small. Time from onset of symptoms is commonly taken as the only guideline for thrombolysis, but the standard 12-lead ECG is an additional useful tool with which to estimate the extent of potentially salvageable myocardium. The major unresolved limitation of thrombolytic therapy is its partial success in prompt and complete reestablishment of vessel patency (Thrombolysis in MI [TIMI] Grade 3) in infarct-related arteries, which can be observed in only 50% or less of cases (see below). (TIMI Grades 1 and 2 indicate patency with very low distal filling and delayed distal filling, respectively.) This limitation may be due to the administration of an inadequate dose of thrombolytic drug, presence of inhibitors of fibrinolysis, persistent local coronary vasoconstriction, or persistent thrombogenic stimuli.

■ *Until the actual thrombotic stimuli can be identified and prevented, or until the precise mechanisms leading to occlusive thrombosis are identified, major reductions in MI mortality and morbidity are more likely to come from organizational improvements that allow earlier use of available drugs than from more efficacious new thrombolytic strategies.* ■

Results of major thrombolytic trials in acute MI

Major trials have demonstrated convincingly that intravenous thrombolytic therapy reduces the rate of mortality in patients with acute MI.[7,8] Although, in theory, sudden reperfusion might damage injured, but not doomed, myocardium, and although recanalized arteries might reocclude, in practise the reduction in hospital mortality obtained with thrombolytic therapy compared with placebo is maintained at 1 year, even without subsequent PTCA or coronary artery bypass grafting (CABG) (see Fig. 22.1).[9] Patients with evidence of reperfusion were shown, at 6 months, to maintain the benefits initially gained from thrombolysis (see Fig. 22.2).[10]

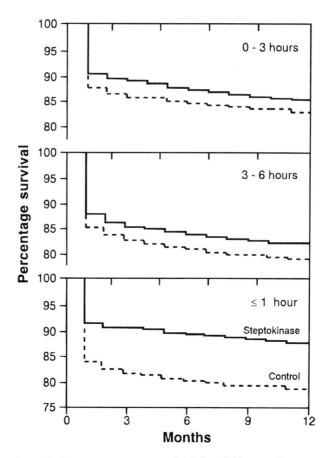

Fig. 22.1 Cumulative percentage survival for different times to start treatment from onset of symptoms to randomization. Thrombolysis achieved the greatest gain in patients treated within 1 h but for all patients the gain was maintained at 1 year. A small time-dependent excess of mortality during the early 1–6 month period compared to the late 7–12 month period was apparent in all groups except for patients thrombolyzed within 1 h. Less than 2% of thrombolyzed patients underwent CABG or PTCA. On average, therefore, in patients saved by early thrombolysis the risk of death during the first year is no greater than in nonthrombolyzed patients. (——— = streptokinase, ----- = control.) (Modified from ref. 7.)

Preliminary data suggest that treatment started before hospitalization by the first attending physician is feasible, safe, and advantageous.[11,12] The advantages are likely to be greatest in those patients presenting very early and with signs of extensive MI, but no development of Q waves.

Rationale. The extent of myocardium that can be salvaged by thrombolysis depends on two factors:

a. the fraction of the jeopardized ischemic myocardium, perfused by the obstructed vessels, that is not yet irreversibly damaged (determined by the time from the onset of symptoms, the intermittency of the occlusion, collateral flow, and low myocardial oxygen demand)

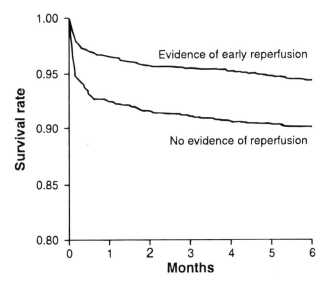

Fig. 22.2 6-month survival of thrombolyzed patients according to ECG evidence of early coronary reperfusion. The survival of thrombolyzed patients with a 50% reduction in the sum of ST-segment elevation in involved leads within 4 h of thrombolysis (evidence of reperfusion—top curve) was significantly better than in patients with no evidence of reperfusion (bottom curve). Both groups of patients showed a progressive time-dependent decrease in mortality during the first 3 months, after which the two curves become practically parallel. No excess mortality rate is apparent in patients with evidence of reperfusion, also if only a tiny percentage of patients had been subjected to revascularization procedures. (Modified from ref. 10.)

b. the active role of persistent thrombosis in impairing coronary flow and its susceptibility to lysis.

As the fraction of ischemic myocardium that becomes necrotic increases with time after the initial occlusion, it is not surprising that, on average, the earlier the reperfusion and the larger the area of myocardium at risk, the greater the benefit with regard to both infarct size and mortality.

However, the temporal relation between coronary occlusion and development of necrosis may vary. At one extreme, in some patients occlusion develops slowly in the presence of collaterals, is intermittent, and is associated with low myocardial oxygen consumption; thus large areas of myocardium may not be irreversibly damaged for several hours after the onset of ischemic pain. At the other extreme, in some patients with sudden persistent occlusion, with no collaterals, with high myocardial oxygen consumption, or with a delayed onset of ischemic pain, the area of myocardium left to be rescued 2–3 h after the onset of symptoms may be small.

Reduction in mortality. The largest reductions in mortality were observed in patients treated within 1–3 h of the onset of symptoms (see Table 22.1)[13] and in those in whom thrombolytic treatment was associated with aspirin.[8] Aspirin (160 mg) was found to produce a reduction of mortality similar to that produced by streptokinase and the benefits of the two drugs are additive (see Fig. 22.3).[8]

In unselected patients the reduction of mortality achieved with streptokinase and recombinant tissue-type plasminogen activator (t-PA) (both with and without heparin) was similar and unrelated to gender or age.[14,15]

Table 22.1 Reduction of mortality by hours from onset of symptoms by treatment with streptokinase compared to placebo

| Time after onset of symptoms (h) | Mortality rate (% [deaths/number treated]) | | Reduction in mortality rate (%) | Statistical significance (P) |
	Streptokinase group	Control group		
<3*	9.2 (278/3016)	12.0 (369/3078)	25.0	0.0005
>3–6	11.7 (217/1849)	14.1 (254/1800)	8.3	0.03
>6–9	12.6 (87/693)	14.1 (93/659)	—	NS
>9–12	15.8 (46/292)	13.6 (41/302)	—	NS
<1*	8.2 52/635	15.4 99/642	46.8	0.0001

NS = not significant

* Patients treated within <1 h are also included in the group treated within <3 h

The greatest percentage reduction of mortality was achieved in patients treated within 1 h (46.8%). In this sub-group, the randomization of 1277 patients was sufficient to achieve a highly statistically significant result (P >0.0001, about 7 patients saved per 100 treated). Larger numbers of patients were required in order to achieve a similar degree of statistical significance when the absolute benefit was smaller (two patients saved per 100 treated) among the 3649 patients randomized within 3 and 6 h (8.3% reduction)

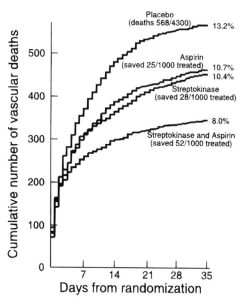

Fig. 22.3 Beneficial effects of aspirin and streptokinase on cumulative cardiovascular mortality in acute MI. The four curves describe mortality in patients allocated streptokinase and aspirin, streptokinase only, aspirin only, or placebo. The number of lives saved reached 5 per 100 treated with a combination of aspirin and streptokinse compared to placebo. (Modified from ref. 8.)

In the Global Utilization of Streptokinase and Tissue Plasminogen Activator for Occluded Coronary Arteries (GUSTO) trial, patients who received treatment within about 6 h of the onset of symptoms were found to benefit from the accelerated administration of t-PA and intravenous heparin (approximately nine lives were saved per 1000 patients treated, compared with strep-tokinase).[16] The greatest benefit was observed in patients under 75 years of age, presenting with an anterior MI within 4 h from the onset of symptoms. In a subsequent reanalysis of the results of the study by the authors, the benefit in patients presenting within 4 h (as opposed to the whole group) was no longer found to be statistically significant.[17] In the angiographic arm of the same trial,[18] accelerated administration of t-PA was associated with a greater percent-age of coronary infarct-related artery patency at 90 min (81 versus 54% for streptokinase with subcutaneous or intravenous heparin), but complete reperfusion (TIMI Grade 3) was observed in only 54 versus 29 and 32%. Reperfusion rates at 180 min were similar for all treatment groups (76 versus 73 and 74%). In addition, the average differences in left ventricular ejection fraction (EF) at 5–7 days were significant, but small (59 versus 57 and 58%).

Patients presenting with Killip classes II, III, and IV did not appear to benefit from thrombol-ysis in terms of mortality both in hospital and at 1 year,[9] possibly because they received throm-bolytic therapy too late or because its beneficial effects in some patients were offset by detri-mental effects, such as hemorrhage into the necrotic tissue caused by late reperfusion, in others. Patients with anterior MI and obvious signs of left ventricular failure, who reached hospital within 3 h from the onset of symptoms, were found to benefit more from primary PTCA than from thrombolytic therapy,[19–22] possibly because better reperfusion (TIMI Grade 3) was achieved faster and in a much larger proportion of these high risk patients.

Heterogeneity of patients. The varied results of thrombolytic trials as a function of time from the onset of symptoms can be explained by the inclusion of different types of patients. The inclusion of some patients presenting with complete MI within 2–3 h of the onset of symp-toms, or those in whom occlusion cannot be relieved by thrombolysis, may account for the incomplete benefit gained from treatment started less than 3 h after the onset of symptoms. The inclusion of patients with ST-segment elevation and only a small loss of R waves may account for the average benefits gained from thrombolytic treatment started 6–12 h after the onset of symptoms.[8,23] Such benefits may be common in patients with persisting severe ischemia, but may be obscured by the possible deleterious effects related to hemorrhage into suddenly reperfused necrotic myocardium, and may be diluted by the neutral effects in patients with completely necrosed myocardium who had no deleterious effects.

Possible reperfusion damage. Animal models (see Ch. 6) have suggested potential adverse effects from early coronary reperfusion for the following reasons:

a. sudden exposure of the ischemic tissue to oxygen and calcium has a detrimen-
    tal effect on irreversibly damaged cells, which suddenly swell, possibly obstruct-
    ing the microcirculation
b. intramyocardial hemorrhages can also develop, but these are confined to ne-
    crotic areas
c. life-threatening reperfusion arrhythymias may develop (see Ch. 7).

In patients, however, these detrimental effects are, on average, outweighed by the benefi-cial effects of early reperfusion, and reperfusion arrhythmias occur much less frequently in patients than in anesthetized animals (see Ch. 10).

A decrease of over 50% of the sum of ST-segment elevation in the leads showing signs of acute MI at 4 h was found to be predictive of coronary recanalization and, hence, of possibly salvageable myocardium potentially at risk.[10] This type of analysis could be performed in about 60% of patients enrolled in the GISSI-2 study and showed that patients with ECG changes suggestive of recanalization (66.7%) had a lower mortality at 1 and 6 months (3.5 and 5.7% versus 7.4 and 9.9%, respectively) and fewer combined events, including heart failure and an EF less than 35% (16.2 versus 22.9%). They had only a slightly higher incidence of recurrent MI (2.1 versus 1.9%) and early post-MI angina (10.4 versus 7.8%), Thus, on average, in thrombolyzed patients early coronary reperfusion leading to salvage of myocardium at risk does not, by itself, increase substantially the risk of reinfarction and SICD and the initial benefit is maintained, at least up to 6 months. During the hospital phase, ventricular fibrillation (VF) and sustained ventricular tachycardias (VT) were also less frequent in patients with evidence of early reperfusion than in those without (5.4 versus 7.5% for VF and 2.9 versus 3.8% for sustained VT).

Possible coronary reocclusion. Angiographic studies in 2431 patients enrolled in the GUSTO trial revealed a 5–6% rate of reocclusion of recanalized stenoses at 5.7 days, irrespective of either the thrombolytic strategy or the severity of residual stenoses. During hospitalization, the average incidence of detectable reinfarction following thrombolysis in all major trials is lower than that of coronary reocclusion, as it occurs in only about 3–4% of cases.

During the initial 3 months, reocclusion of recanalized arteries, patent at 48 h, may occur in over 25% of patients but, as in early reocclusion, the incidence of reinfarction is much lower: in a group of 248 patients randomized to receive placebo, aspirin, or oral anticoagulants, reocclusion rates at 3 months of arteries patent at 48 h were similar (25–32%), but reinfarction was lowest in patients treated with aspirin (3 versus 8% on oral anticoagulants and 11% on placebo).[24] The prognostic implications of late reocclusion of the infarct-related artery occurring without detectable reinfarction are unknown.

Reocclusion, reinfarction and post-MI angina may be related to incomplete lysis of the thrombus or to the same unknown coronary process that triggered the initial occlusion, and the discrepancy between coronary reocclusion and reinfarction may be accounted for by the development of collaterals.

Time from onset of symptoms and initial ECG

Patients presenting with wide, deep Q waves, with complete or near-complete loss of R waves, may have a completed MI, independent of time from onset of symptoms. Conversely, patients presenting with ST-segment elevation, small Q waves and preserved R-wave amplitude may have a sizable segment of ischemic, but not yet necrotic, myocardium, independent of time from onset of symptoms.

Thus, thrombolytic therapy should be considered in the following situations:

a.   when a patient is seen within about 6 h of the onset of symptoms with persisting ST-segment elevation and preserved R waves on the ECG, or when the ECG tracing is difficult to interpret in terms of the extent of necrosis and ischemia because of either conduction abnormalities or the presence of old MI
b.   when a patient is seen more than 6 h after the onset of symptoms, but the pain had been intermittent and the ECG still shows ST-segment elevation with preservation of R waves.

Thrombolytic therapy is unlikely to reduce infarct size significantly when the ECG shows signs of completed MI with a wide Q–S complex and loss of R-wave amplitude, even if the patient is seen early after the onset of symptoms.

In patients presenting with depression, rather than elevation, of the ST segment, thrombolysis was found to be ineffective in reducing mortality.[14,15] This average result may not apply to those patients in whom the ST-segment depression is not merely the consequence of a preceding ischemic episode, but is the expression of ongoing ischemia, refractory to nitrates and heparin (see Ch. 19).

■ *The benefit of prehospital thrombolysis is likely to be greatest when the percentage reduction of the time lag from the onset of symptoms to recanalization is considerable (for example, 1 h for patients seen within 2–3 h or 2 h for those seen within 4–5 h), and when the extent of myocardium at risk is large (for example, in patients showing ST-segment elevation in all precordial leads or in inferior and lateral leads).* ■

Contraindications to thrombolytic therapy

In large trials involving tens of thousands of patients, the major complications that occurred following intravenous therapy with streptokinase were major bleeding in 0.3% of cases and cerebrovascular accidents in about 1% of patients, which was virtually the same as in untreated patients. A slight excess of stroke was observed with t-PA.[25] Minor complications and adverse reactions were observed in about 10% of treated patients. Complications were found to be only slightly more common in elderly patients.

Absolute contraindications to thrombolytic therapy in large trials were considered to be the following:

a. a cerebrovascular accident within the last 2 months
b. surgery within the previous 10 days
c. a recent bleeding problem
d. uncontrolled hypertension
e. other life-threatening conditions.

(Previous treatment with streptokinase is a contraindication to repeated use of the same drug.)

Relative contraindications to thrombolytic therapy were considered to be a history of active gastric or duodenal ulcer and other gastrointestinal tract diseases (which could possibly cause hemorrhage) and possible pregnancy.

Weighing the potential benefits and risks is necessary for patients with relative contraindications. The main consideration that affects the decision to use thrombolytic therapy is the extent of myocardium in jeopardy, which could influence survival or the quality of life of the patient if the MI were to become complete. Patients in whom prompt coronary recanalization should definitely be attempted are those with large segments of potentially salvageable myocardium (for example, with persisting ST-segment elevation and preserved R waves in all precordial leads or in inferior, lateral and dorsal leads) and those with ventricular pump failure due to a previous MI, even if the ECG estimate of the salvageable myocardium is small.

Patients with contraindications for thrombolysis should be considered for emergency percutaneous transluminal coronary angioplasty (PTCA).

Choice of treatments

As soon as the diagnosis is suspected, all patients should receive aspirin unless contraindicated (see Ch. 19). As soon as the diagnosis is confirmed, thrombolytic therapy should be considered.

The most widely used thrombolytic drugs include the following:

a. streptokinase (1.5 megaunits i.v. administered over 1 h)
b. t-PA (administered in an accelerated manner, initially 15 mg i.v. given as a bolus, followed by infusion of 0.75 mg/kg of body weight over a period of 30 min [to a maximum of 50 mg] and then infusion of 0.5 mg/kg of body weight over a period of 60 min [to a maximum of 35 mg]. This form of administration of t-PA should be associated with heparin [5000 IU i.v. given as a bolus, followed by a continuous infusion of 1000 IU/h])
c. acetylated streptokinase (APSAC) (100 mg given as a bolus)
d. urokinase (1 $\times$ 10^6 units bolus plus 1 MU over 1 h), which is used in some European countries.

Streptokinase is the oldest and least expensive thrombolytic drug. It has a long duration of action, but it is not thrombospecific and may be neutralized by natural antibodies. t-PA has a rapid duration of action and it is thrombospecific; thus, in theory, it should produce fewer bleeding complications for the same degree of lytic power. APSAC has the advantage that it can be administered as a single bolus because it has a long duration of action. Streptokinase and APSAC cannot be used more than once in the same patient because of their antigenicity.

Streptokinase should be the first choice because its cost is one order of magnitude lower than others with similar beneficial effects on global mortality and EF and because its adverse effects are similar to those of others. Accelerated administration of t-PA, associated with intravenous heparin, should apply to patients with contraindications to streptokinase and can be considered also for those with very large infarctions who are less than 75 years old and who present within 4 h of the onset of symptoms. There is no strong evidence to suggest that either intravenous or subcutaneous infusion of heparin confers additive beneficial effects when used with streptokinase.[14,15]

Emergency PTCA should be considered for patients with acute MI and large areas of myocardium at risk, in whom thrombolysis is contraindicated. Primary PTCA can also be considered for patients in classes 2–4 with very large segments of myocardium at risk, when the procedure can be performed within 2–3 h of the onset of symptoms by an experienced team. The results of primary PTCA performed early in patients with large anterior MI and in patients in classes 3 or 4 are superior to those of thrombolysis because of the shorter delay in achieving full patency (TIMI Grade 3) in a greater percentage of cases.[19–22] As patients with indications for emergency PTCA may arrive at times when neither the catheterization laboratory nor the angioplasty team are available immediately, this approach is applicable in only a small minority of hospitals to a minority of patients.

Patients not eligible for thrombolysis because they present with completed MI should receive aspirin and be treated like thrombolyzed patients as dictated by symptoms, hospital course, and classification.

Failure of reperfusion

Failure of reperfusion is observed in a variable percentage of cases, depending on the drug doses used and on the method of administration. Full patency at 90 min was achieved in only 54% of patients receiving accelerated t-PA, and in an even smaller percentage of those receiving streptokinase, in the GUSTO trial.[18] The reasons for this failure, even when treatment is started within 2 h of the onset of symptoms, are still not clear; an inadequate dose of thrombolytic drugs, the presence of fibrinolytic inhibitors, or a persistent strong thrombogenic stimulus and coronary constrictor response could be responsible for the failure either to reperfuse or to achieve full patency (TIMI Grade 3).

Patients not responding to intravenous thrombolytic agents within 1 h may be considered for emergency PTCA, when an experienced team is readily available, when a large amount of myocardium appears to be potentially salvageable. The results of "rescue" PTCA, particularly in patients in shock, are favorable.[22] Conversely, the results of indiscriminate, systematic emergency PTCA immediately after thrombolysis in a large randomized trial have been discouraging.[26]

22.1.4 Development of arrhythmias and their management

Arrhythmias of varying severity occur in about 80% of patients during the first 1–2 h after the onset of symptoms of MI, irrespective of its size. After this time, arrhythmias become more frequent and severe in extensive MIs. Arrhythmias develop as a result of the interaction of the arrhythmogenic effects of myocardial ischemia and necrosis with preexisting myocardial scarring, with the response of the autonomic nervous system and with electrolyte imbalance.

Myocardial ischemia and necrosis can cause bradyarrhythmias, by producing blocks along the conduction system, or tachyarrhythmias, by increasing automaticity and excitability and/or by favoring the development of reentry circuits (see Ch. 7). The onset of bradyarrhythmias is facilitated by increased vagal tone; that of tachyarrhythmias is facilitated by increased adrenergic stimulation and electrolyte imbalance.

Unless they are treated promptly, VF and asystole cause immediate death. Nonfatal arrhythmias can cause hemodynamic dysfunction, thus contributing to necrosis of ischemic, but not irreversibly damaged, myocardium and may predispose to fatal arrhythmias.

Bradyarrhythmias due to A–V conduction disturbances

First- and second-degree type I A–V block occurs in about 10% of patients and third-degree block in about 5%. The block is caused more often by ischemia or edema than by necrosis and is often precipitated by both increased vagal tone and morphine administration. The block usually occurs above the bundle of His, with a narrow QRS, and is usually reversible within 48–72 h.[27] More rarely, the block occurs below the A–V node with a broad QRS, is sometimes preceded by Moebitz type II block (in less than 1%), and is usually associated with a large anterior MI and a poor prognosis. The prognosis of patients with A–V block is related to the degree of bradycardia (less than 40 beats/min, depending on symptoms) and, when this has been corrected, to the extent of myocardial necrosis. Asystole as a primary arrhythmia secondary to A–V conduction disturbances (i.e. not as a terminal complication) occurs in only about 3% of patients admitted to a CCU.

Bradyarrhythmias, including sinus bradycardia, should be monitored carefully but treated only when they cause clinically detectable hemodynamic impairment, as indicated by hypotension and peripheral hypoperfusion (because the increase of stroke volume [SV] is not sufficient to maintain cardiac output) or when they cause escape rhythms. The first line of treatment is atropine sulfate (i.v. injection of 0.5 mg) as necessary in order to increase heart rate to about 60 beats/min (bearing in mind that atropine may cause urinary retention in elderly men). Pacing may be required if atropine fails. Sequential atrioventricular pacing may be beneficial for the few patients in whom the contribution of atrial contraction is critical for the maintenance of an adequate cardiac output.[28] Prophylactic use of a temporary pacemaker is indicated in patients with acute anterior MI who develop Moebitz type II block or new bifascicular block. In patients in whom asystole or complete low-frequency A–V block develops suddenly, and in those in whom bradyarrhythmias necessitate prompt pacing, a noninvasive external pacing device is extremely useful before emergency temporary intracardiac pacing can be inserted.[29] Prophylactic insertion of a temporary right ventricular pacemaker electrode is indicated when external pacing devices are not available, in order to prevent its emergency insertion at night or during weekends. The benefits of prophylactic permanent pacemaker insertion in patients exhibiting transient second-degree type II or third-degree A–V block during the acute phase are not yet clearly established.[29,30]

Ventricular tachyarrhythmias

Increased automaticity and excitability is caused directly by partial depolarization of injured cells, with fragmentation and activation delays resulting in electric gradients occurring during diastole. These alterations make the myocardium more susceptible to the arrhythmogenic effects of circulating catecholamines released from nerve endings in the ischemic region. Adrenergic stimulation can also increase the automaticity of ischemic Purkinje fibers. The fragmentation, the regional delays in activation, and the altered duration of depolarization and of the refractory period facilitate the establishment of reentry circuits. Disruption of adrenergic nerves by infarction enhances the dispersion of the duration of the action potential and refractory period, both basally and in response to catecholamines. Reentry tachyarrhythmias may be more common than increased automaticity arrhythmias in the very early hours of MI.

Ventricular extrasystoles occur in almost all patients but their prognostic significance seems less certain now than a decade ago. As they carry a severe prognostic significance in extensive infarctions, they may also be indirect markers of the severity of the condition. Indeed, primary VF occurs in the absence of warning arrhythmias in over 50% of cases and is often precipitated by a late isolated extrasystole, rather than by an R on T type. Conversely, frequent and complex ventricular extrasystoles are common in patients who never develop VF. Accelerated idioventricular rhythm, defined as ventricular rhythm with a rate of 60–120 beats/min, occurs in about 10% of patients, usually as an escape rhythm. Its prognostic significance is still controversial but it is not severe.

Nonsustained VT, defined as three or more ventricular beats with a rate above 120 beats/min, lasting less than 30 s, occurs in about 20% of patients. Its prognostic significance is severe when it occurs in patients with a large MI. Whether this arrhythmia has an important prognostic significance also in the absence of severe impairment of left ventricular function is still uncertain. The development of ventricular tachycardia is greatly favored by hypokalemia as it is about four times more common when concentrations of serum potassium measure 2.5 mmol/l than when they measure 4.5 mmol/l. VF occurs in about 10% of patients admitted to CCUs, but it is by far the most common cause of early death occurring outside hospital. Among thrombolyzed patients enrolled in the GISSI-2 study, VF and VT occurred in 5.4 and 2.9% of patients with evidence of early coronary reperfusion, respectively, and in 7.5 and 3.8% of those without.[10] In CCUs, VF is seen in patients with either anterior or inferior transmural MI, but rarely in those with non-Q-wave MI. It usually occurs unpredictably in the absence of left ventricular failure within the first 4 h (60% of cases) or 12 h (80% of cases) of the onset of symptoms (primary VF). In about 20% of cases it occurs as a terminal event in patients with severe cardiac failure and shock (secondary VF). Late VF occurring within 1–6 weeks of infarction is also favored by hypokalemia but, in most cases, the factors that cause the arrhythmia remain unknown. The prognosis of patients who survive primary VF is much better than that of those who survive late VF, and in both cases it is worse in the presence of impairment of ventricular function.[31,32]

VF should be treated promptly by electric countershock (possibly within 1–2 min), with an initial shock of 200 watt-seconds, increasing to 400 if the first is unsuccessful. When the highest voltage is ineffective it should be repeated after intravenous or endotracheal injection of epinephrine (1 mg). Patients with accelerated idioventricular rhythm should be carefully monitored, as the indications for interruption of the arrhythmia are determined only by hemodynamic instability. Patients who, within the first few hours of infarction, display episodes of either VT or frequent ventricular arrhythmias should have their plasma potassium levels measured in order to correct hypokalemia and should be monitored assiduously. It has not been confirmed clinically that reduction of such arrhythmias necessarily prevents VF; however, when they are frequent or prolonged they may compromise cardiac pump function and should be treated with β-blockers (metoprolol 5 mg i.v. repeated every 5 min up to 15 mg) unless contraindicated. Those patients in whom β-blockers are contraindicated should receive lidocaine (100 mg loading dose followed by a maintenance dose of 1–3 mg/min). When lidocaine is ineffective or contraindicated (because of allergy), procainamide (100 mg bolus every 5 min up to 10 times, followed by a maintenance dose of 2–5 mg/min), should be given. Lidocaine is the only one of these drugs not to have a negative inotropic effect.

In patients with secondary and late ventricular arrhythmias, high doses of intravenous amiodarone should be considered, as it has no negative inotropic effects and the possible side effects result only from prolonged therapy.[33–35] Oral therapy should be continued through convalescence and stopped, possibly after 3–6 months, in order to avoid possible side effects.

Supraventricular rhythm disturbances

Severe sinus bradycardia occurs in about 30% of patients in the first hour after the onset of symptoms, particularly in patients with inferior MI. It occurs as part of a vagal reaction to pain and to stimulation of cardiac afferent fibers and may be associated with hypotension with the features of a vasovagal syncope. It should be treated with atropine (0.5 mg i.v.), repeated if required. Sinus tachycardia occurs in about 30% of patients at some stage during the days following MI. During the initial hours it is most frequently caused by pain and anxiety (hyperdynamic circulatory syndrome), but it could also be caused by acute left ventricular failure when SV is so low that tachycardia is required to maintain cardiac output; later, it can be caused by fever, cardiac failure, pericarditis, or other complications. When sinus tachycardia is not caused by acute left ventricular failure, treatment with β-blockers is indicated. Atrial extrasystoles occur in about 50% of patients and they may herald atrial fibrillation (which occurs in about 10% of cases), atrial flutter (which occurs in about 3% of cases), or paroxysmal supraventricular tachycardia (which occurs in about 3% of cases). Atrial arrhythmias may be caused by atrial distension (due to severe ventricular failure), atrial ischemia, necrosis (and are more common in extensive anterior MI), or by pericarditis in its late stages. Their prognostic significance is related largely to the severity of ventricular failure. The development of atrial fibrillation complicating an anterior MI is associated with a severer prognosis.

Paroxysmal atrial tachycardia should be treated with vagal stimulation, verapamil, or adenosine (6–12 mg bolus i.v. for a 70 kg patient),[36] and atrial fibrillation and flutter should be treated with propanolol (1–7 mg i.v.) or verapamil (5–10 mg bolus i.v., repeatable after 10 min); digoxin (0.25–0.5 mg i.v.) can be used to increase the degree of A–V block. Electric countershock (50–200 watt-seconds) should be used when the arrhythmias cause major hemodynamic impairment and need to be terminated immediately.

Hemodynamic and myocardial consequences of cardiac rhythm disturbances

Alterations of the normal sinus rhythm and heart rate become hemodynamically significant only when they are persistent and severe, and when the preexisting impairment of ventricular function is so severe that an adequate cardiac output can be maintained only within a narrow range of sinus heart rate. This could be 90–100 beats/min, which optimizes filling time, with moderate stretching and tension of ischemic myocardium and only a moderate increase in myocardial oxygen consumption. Increasing the heart rate above this range would reduce cardiac output because of reduced filling time, would raise myocardial oxygen consumption excessively, and would exacerbate ischemia in the area around the infarction. Decreasing the heart rate below this range would reduce the cardiac output (as SV cannot increase), would increase ventricular filling and pulmonary intravascular pressures, and would increase the wall tension of the injured myocardium. In the presence of impaired ventricular function, loss of atrial contribution could reduce the SV by up to 25% and increase the mean filling and intravascular pulmonary pressures.[28]

22.1.5 Management of impaired cardiac pump function

Impairment of pump function can result from myocardial necrosis, ischemia, stunning, hibernation, and inadequate left or right ventricular filling pressures. When caused predominantly by impairment of left ventricular function, the main clinical finding is orthopnea and lung congestion due to increased left atrial pressure, which is associated with hypotension and peripheral hypoperfusion when the patient is in cardiogenic shock. When ventricular pump failure is caused predominantly by inadequate left ventricular filling pressure (usually associated with relative or absolute hypovolemia, vagal stimulation, or right ventricular MI), the main clinical findings are hypotension and peripheral hypoperfusion; jugular venous pressure is normal or low in hypovolemia and elevated in right ventricular MI. Comparison of right and left ventricular filling pressures helps to interpret the predominant cause of elevated jugular venous pressure (see Ch. 21).

General therapeutic guidelines can be defined on the basis of the classification outlined in 21.1.5.

Class 1

Patients should be treated only with general measures to reduce infarct size, including β-blockers (see 21.1.7).

Class 2

Patients should be treated with diuretics, frusemide (20–40 mg p.o.) and intravenous nitrates in order to reduce infarct size (see 22.1.7). β-Blockers should be used with caution. Attention should be given to patients with inferior MI, who may develop reduced cardiac output due to right ventricular MI and relative hypovolemia, particularly in response to nitrates.

Class 3

Patients should be treated with intravenous diuretics, such as frusemide (20–40 mg). Nitroprusside should be one of the drugs of first choice during the initial hours and days, as it has the very remarkable advantage of immediate action and a very short half-life. The infusion rate can be titrated from 0.03 to 3 mg/min according to systemic arterial blood pressure, heart rate, respiratory rate, and the patient's general clinical condition (checked every 5 min), or according to the results of hemodynamic monitoring, when clinically required and easily available. If the fall in blood pressure is excessive, it can be restored promptly by lowering the rate of infusion. For subsequent longer-term vasodilation and reduction of preload, oral nitrates (to cover the daytime hours during which arterial pressure is higher and the patient is more physically active) and angiotensin-converting enzyme (ACE) inhibitors, to reduce afterload, should be titrated in order to avoid hypotension. Clinical and echocardiographic assessment of left and right ventricular function and of possible mechanical complications (such as mitral regurgitation) is necessary in these patients.

Class 4

Patients with elevated venous pressure and severe lung congestion and shock should be treated in the same way as patients in class 3 but much more aggressively, as the condition of hypoperfusion (or frank shock) must be relieved promptly before it becomes irreversible. In addition, they should receive inotropic agents: dobutamine (2–10 μ/kg/min) is the first choice. In these patients, monitoring of pulmonary artery wedge pressure and of intra-arterial systemic pressure is desirable for the titration of nitroprusside and dobutamine. However, when invasive hemodynamic monitoring is not feasible and when patients cannot be transferred to better-equipped centers, these drugs can be administered at gradually increasing doses under continuous careful clinical monitoring of heart rate, systemic blood pressure by cuff manometer, respiration rate, urine output, and peripheral skin temperature.

When the inadequacy of right or left ventricular filling pressure is relative rather then absolute (i.e. when left filling pressure, although higher than normal, is insufficient to generate an adequate SV), plasma expanders should be infused until an adequate arterial pressure and peripheral perfusion are reestablished or until pulmonary wedge pressure begins to rise rapidly or signs of left ventricular failure (increased respiration rate, moist rales) become apparent. In this case, the infusion should be stopped and inotropic drugs administered. Monitoring of pulmonary wedge pressure, when easily available, helps to titrate the infusion of plasma expanders.

When maximal therapy fails to resolve the condition of cardiogenic shock, the use of balloon intra-aortic counterpulsation should be considered in order to gain time in those cases in which the degree of left ventricular impairment seems disproportionate to the infarct size as estimated from markers of cell necrosis, and/or in which the condition might be relieved by interventions such as PTCA of a critical coronary stenosis or surgical correction of acute mitral valve regurgitation of an intraventricular septal defect. For patients in whom shock is caused exclusively by extensive or critical necrosis of the myocardium, there is no convincing evidence that counterpulsation improves prognosis, unless undertaken as a bridge to cardiac transplantation. In patients presenting in classes 3 and 4 very early after the onset of symptoms, emergency PTCA can considerably reduce mortality.

Cardiac surgery in patients with an acute MI is associated with a high perioperative mortality, particularly in patients with an EF less than 50%. The increased risk is highest during the first week and decreases progressively up the fourth or fifth weeks (see 22.2.4)

22.1.6 Limitation of infarct size

Limitation of myocardial necrosis within the area at risk should be considered separately from reinfarction, which occurs only when an early recanalized artery reoccludes. Measures to limit infarct size can have a beneficial effect in the very early hours of coronary occlusion and/or during early reperfusion, when irreversible damage to viable myocardial cells jeopardized by ischemia may still be avoided.

Ischemia can be abolished by restoring myocardial oxygen supply, or reduced by improving collateral blood supply and by reducing myocardial oxygen demand until flow is restored. Ischemia-induced myocardial and microvascular damage may be delayed, and possibly reduced, by metabolic interventions, at least in animal models (see Ch. 7). Efforts to limit infarct size should be initiated as soon as possible after diagnosis and continued for the first 12–24 h after infarction.

Results of trials

A meta-analysis of randomized trials in patients who have not received thrombolytic therapy shows that very early administration of β-blockers produced a 13% reduction in mortality during hospitalization, corresponding to seven lives saved per 1000 patients treated (among those eligible for randomization over the first 7 days).[13] This reduction was achieved during the initial 3 days and was caused by a lower incidence of SICD and cardiac rupture. A meta-analysis of randomized trials of intravenous nitroprusside and nitroglycerin showed a reduction in mortality of about one-third, corresponding to six lives saved per 100 patients treated over the first few days of hospitalization. The higher number of lives saved, compared with early β-blockade, over the short period of intravenous therapy, is due to the selective inclusion of patients with severe left ventricular dysfunction and high short-term baseline mortality (18%), compared with the inclusion criteria adopted in the β-blocker trials of patients who had much milder ventricular dysfunction and, hence, much lower baseline mortality. A meta-analysis of trials of the effects of calcium antagonists administered early after the onset of symptoms failed to show any beneficial results, because the beneficial effects in patients with good ventricular function were balanced by detrimental effects in those with signs of cardiac failure (see Ch. 13).[13]

Two recent large multicentric trials[37,38] showed that oral nitrates and magnesium treatment during the first 5 weeks post-MI failed to influence early mortality and that ACE-inhibitors resulted in, respectively, 8 and 4 lives saved per 1000 patients treated. Previous smaller trials[39] failed to achieve short-term statistical significance, most likely because of the small absolute benefit produced by the treatment. One of these trials,[40] showed a significant benefit from early ACE-inhibitor treatment after MI at 1-year follow-up (41 lives saved per 1000 patients treated), possibly related to a late reduction in MI observed in post-MI patients.[41] It is possible that the improvement in survival occurred predominantly in patients with large infarctions, as suggested by the improvement in long-term survival documented in trials that included patients with cardiac failure and/or with reduced left ventricular EF.[42,43] The absolute and percentage benefit observed in trials in patients with very recent MI are reported in Table 22.2. Clinical trials with antioxidants are in progress.[44]

The results of prospective randomized trials that adopted broad inclusion criteria are more difficult to apply to clinical practise, because it is impossible to identify those patients who are most likely to benefit from interventions (see Ch. 13). There is, therefore, ample scope for therapeutic strategies to be individualized according to the general rational guidelines outlined below.

Myocardial oxygen supply can be improved by thrombolysis, which, when performed early after coronary occlusion, is by far the most effective way of providing adequate myocardial perfusion, or by coronary vasodilators, which may dilate the residual culprit stenosis, may prevent constriction of distal coronary vessels, and may increase collateral blood supply. Nitrates (nitroglycerin, 0.01–0.1 mg/min i.v. or ISDN, 0.03–0.3 mg/min i.v.) should be

Table 22.2 Absolute benefit on mortality soon after MI

Trial	Drug	Number of patients	Follow-up	Mortality (per 1000) Control group	Treated group	Lives saved (per 1000) treated group	Mortality reduction (%)	Statistical significance (P)
ISIS 1	β-blockers	16105	1 week	46	39	7	15	0.04
ISIS 2	SK	8600	5 weeks	132	104	28	21	0.00001
ISIS 2	ASA	8595	5 weeks	132	107	25	19	0.00001
ISIS 2	SK + ASA	8592	5 weeks	132	70	52	39	0.00001
GISSI 3	ACE-inhibitors	19314	5 weeks	71	63	8	11	0.03
ISIS 4	ACE-inhibitors	58000	5 weeks	73	69	4	5	0.04

Mortality in the control group influences the number of lives saved for any given percentage reduction in mortality. When the number of lives saved per 1000 patients treated is small, large numbers of patients must be enrolled in order to demonstrate statistically significant results. The average improvement in survival observed might have been due to a greater than average benefit in some of the patient subgroups, but no precise information is available on the characteristics of patients who actually benefited most from the treatment

used, selecting the infusion rate that decreases the systemic systolic arterial blood pressure by 10–20 mmHg, then gradually adjusting the dose according to the value of the systolic arterial blood pressure. The infusion should be continued for 24 h after the disappearance of chest pain and then tapered gradually in order to avoid rebound effects (see Ch. 19). In such acute conditions, nitrates have advantages over calcium antagonists: because they reduce ventricular preload and, hence, end-diastolic pressure, thus improving subendocardial perfusion and afterload, they are particularly beneficial in patients with left ventricular failure. Correction of anemia and of arterial oxygen desaturation, when required, contributes to improve myocardial oxygen supply.

■ *The greatest absolute benefit is to be expected in patients in classes 2 or 3, who are at high risk. The benefit in class 1 patients, who are at low risk, is much less and cannot easily be quantified.* ■

Myocardial oxygen consumption should be reduced for as long as myocardial ischemia persists. This can be achieved as follows:

a. by slowing the heart rate, unless tachycardia is an essential means of maintaining an adequate cardiac output
b. by reducing preload, unless this is an essential means of maintaining an adequate SV
c. by reducing impedance to ejection, by lowering systemic arterial pressure, unless coronary perfusion pressure becomes too low
d. by reducing β-adrenergic stimulation and contraction velocity, unless this is an essential means of maintaining adequate SV.

Afterload and preload can be reduced by nitrates (see above). When not contraindicated, β-blockers should be given to patients in class 1 and, with careful clinical monitoring, to those in class 2 soon after admission. Atenolol (5 mg i.v.), metoprolol (5 mg i.v., repeated after 5 and 15 minutes if tolerated) or equivalent doses of other selective β-adrenergic receptor-blocking drugs, with no intrinsic sympathomimetic activity, should be given. The intravenous oral doses should be titrated to obtain heart rate values of about 60–70 beats/min (in the absence of side effects).

■ *The most obvious indication for β-blockers is for class 1 patients with a hyperdynamic circulation, but in such a low-risk group the absolute benefit cannot easily be quantified. They produce a detectable reduction of mortality related to VF or cardiac rupture in class 2 patients, who are at a greater risk than class 1 patients, but they are also potentially at risk from the reduction of inotropic support provided by β-adrenergic stimulation.* ■

Limitation of the myocardial damage caused by ischemia and reperfusion has been achieved in animals by pretreatment with calcium antagonists and oxygen free-radical scavengers. Prevention of microvascular damage caused by persistent ischemia or reperfusion can be an additional means of protecting ischemic myocardial cells (see Ch. 7).

The benefits of treatments aimed at protecting ischemic cells have not yet been assessed in adequate clinical trials, but they can only be much smaller than those aimed at recanalizing the infarct-related artery, or at improving collateral blood supply and at reducing myocardial oxygen consumption when the artery cannot be recanalized. Their additional effects on the reduction of mortality can be assessed more readily in high-risk groups.

Demonstrating the benefits of a treatment that reduces infarct size in patients with a small MI without symptoms or signs of recurring ischemia and without severe ventricular dysfunction (typically class 1), requires the recruitment of large numbers of patients, as the absolute reduction of risk (i.e. the number of lives saved per number of patients treated) can only be very small.

22.1.7 Ventricular remodeling

When the loss of myocardium is substantial, remodeling leads to progressive noncompensatory ventricular dilation and hypertrophy with worsening of prognosis.[45] The major known determinant of left ventricular dilation is the hemodynamic load, but the biologic factors that cause a progressive dysfunction of myocardial segments normally contracting in the early post-MI phase are incompletely known. As discussed in Chapter 7, ACE inhibitors were found to improve postinfarction remodeling considerably and to reduce long-term mortality in experimental animals.[46] The long-term beneficial effects of these drugs have been documented in patients (see below) and are discussed in 22.2.3.

The open artery hypothesis

Patients with an "open artery" have a better long-term prognosis than those with a closed artery, but whether the observed relation reflects a lesser degree of myocardial necrosis during the acute phase of the infarction or other mechanisms is not clearly established. It also remains to be demonstrated whether a patent infarct-related artery can favorably affect post-MI ventricular remodeling.[47]

Assessment of the practical relevance of this hypothesis would require the identification of the subset of patients in whom the patency does make a clinically significant difference, independent of whether the MI is complete within the area at risk and, for incomplete MIs, of whether perfusion by collaterals was adequate.

Asymptomatic patients with an EF of more than 50% have, on average, such a good prognosis that it would be difficult to demonstrate a significant improvement by reopening those arteries that are closed. Some patients with incomplete MI, no adequate collateral function, and a low left ventricular EF may have hibernating myocardium (see below), in which case a detectable improvement may be obtained by recanalizing the infarct-related artery.

■ *Prospective randomized trials in carefully defined subgroups of patients are necessary in order to evaluate precisely the specific type of patient to whom this hypothesis applies and in whom late reopening of the artery may clearly improve the course of the disease.* ■

22.1.8 Development of complications

Acute MI can be complicated by rupture of a papillary muscle, interventricular septum, or free wall, by the formation of a ventricular aneurysm, and by intraventricular thrombosis and systemic or (rarely) pulmonary embolism. Venous thrombosis is fairly infrequent now that patients are mobilized at an early stage and it usually occurs only in patients with severe cardiac failure. Mild pericarditis occurs in about 5% of patients in the first few days or weeks.

Rupture of papillary muscles

Rupture of the posteromedial papillary muscle associated with inferior MI is more common than rupture of the anterolateral muscle associated with anterior MI; rupture of the right papillary muscle is very rare. Complete rupture causes massive acute valvular regurgitation and rapid hemodynamic deterioration; it requires emergency surgical repair.

Rupture of the interventricular septum

The severity of the hemodynamic deterioration associated with septal rupture is determined by the size of the septal defect, the consequent decrease in SV attributable to its shunting into the low-impedance right ventricle, and the ability of the right ventricle to cope with the sudden diastolic volume overload. Deterioration of the condition calls for emergency surgical repair by experienced teams.

Rupture of the free ventricular wall

This is the most frequent form of rupture, representing one of the most common causes of hospital death in thrombolyzed patients, reaching 80% in those over 70 years of age (see Ch. 10). It usually occurs during the first few days at the periphery of an anterior or lateral wall MI, is associated with cardiac tamponade, and presents typically with electromechanical dissociation. When gradual and incomplete, rupture may result in a false aneurysm as the adjacent pericardium and thrombosis form a new wall over the rupture.

Ventricular aneurysm

In about 15% of patients who survive infarction, progressive expansion and the thinning of the infarcted ventricular wall over a period of several weeks may result in ballooning of the ventricular wall, which expands during systole. Aneurysm occurs about four times more often in apical, anterior, and lateral MIs than in inferior MIs. The aneurysm can be partially thrombosed and, during the initial 3–4 months, the wall becomes fibrotic. Rupture is the exception after the first week, but long-term mortality seems to be higher in patients with a frank aneurysm than in those without, even when they have comparable values of left ventricular EF.[48]

Intraventricular thrombosis

At autopsy, mural thrombi, attached to the myocardium overlying the infarcted region in the apex, in the anterolateral wall, or situated at the site of aneurysms, were found in over 40% of patients dying from acute MI in the prethrombolytic era.[49] Echocardiographic studies have demonstrated the presence of intraventricular thrombosis in about 50% of extensive anterior and apical MIs within 24–48 h of the onset of symptoms, but rarely in inferior MIs.[50] However, echocardiographically detectable intraventricular thrombi are not usually accompanied by recognizable episodes of arterial embolism.[51] Most thrombi are no longer detectable at the time of discharge, particularly in small and medium-sized infarctions, and in large infarcts a thrombus may splint the infarcted wall, thus protecting it from expansion and rupture.[52] The incidence of peripheral embolism in large thrombolytic trials is less than 1% and there is no definite evidence to suggest that anticoagulants improve prognosis in patients with echocardiographic evidence of intraventricular thrombi.

Venous thrombosis

Venous thrombosis is now seen rarely, and usually only in patients with severe cardiac failure. Similarly, pulmonary embolism was observed at autopsy in about 10% of patients who died from acute MI in the prethrombolytic era.

Pericarditis

Pericardial friction rubs can be heard in about 5% of patients during the first days and weeks. Early pericarditis in transmural MI results from pericardial inflammation caused by necrosis of subepicardial myocardial layers. Late pericarditis can be an expression of the post-MI syndrome described by Dressler,[53] usually occurring 2–10 weeks after the acute episode as a result of an autoimmune antibody response against pericardial and myocardial antigens stimulated by the acute MI. This syndrome usually responds to high doses of non-steroidal anti-inflammatory drugs.

22.2 PREDISCHARGE ASSESSMENT AND RISK STRATIFICATION

There is a growing tendency toward early discharge of patients with uncomplicated MI. This policy is justified by the reduction in both the cost and the inconvenience of hospitalization, but it requires that patients be protected from the risk of reinfarction and death occurring soon after discharge as they may still be in an unstable phase of ischemic heart disease (IHD). Ensuring that each patient be adequately protected requires that their short-term prognosis be assessed on the basis not only of currently available knowledge of the determinants of prognosis but also of the results of predischarge tests, as indicated by symptoms and hospital course.

22.2.1 Determinants of short-term prognosis

Short-term prognosis must be considered separately from long-term prognosis because the mortality rate of post-MI patients is highest immediately after discharge and decreases progressively during the first 6 months. The absolute risk of the occurrence of IHD-related death results from the product of the baseline risk conferred by the severity of left ventricular dysfunction and old age (nonmodifiable determinants) and the additional risk conferred by the instability of IHD, the severity of coronary flow-limiting stenoses, malignant arrhythmias, and cardiac failure (potentially modifiable determinants).

The total mortality and the total number of patients potentially saved by interventions is determined by the relative risk conferred by potentially modifiable determinants of prognosis above that conferred by nonmodifiable determinants at a given time after MI.

For example, a 100% increase in mortality caused by potentially modifiable determinants would result in 20% mortality in a group of patients in whom nonmodifiable determinants cause a 10% baseline mortality, but in only 2% mortality in a group with a 1% baseline mortality. A 50% reduction of mortality would result in 10 patients saved per 100 treated in the first case, but in only one patient saved in the second. The increased mortality conferred by modifiable determinants may be confined to the early postdischarge period or be distributed uniformly during the early and late post-MI period. Thus, for a given relative risk conferred by potentially modifiable determinants, the number of patients saved out of those treated is greatest when the baseline risk conferred by nonmodifiable determinants is high and when interventions cover the time after MI during which modifiable determinants have the greatest effect.

When the prognostic weight of variables (such as age and EF) increases exponentially rather than linearly, it cannot be adequately assessed from linear regression analysis. Furthermore, the prognostic weight of modifiable determinants, such as a positive exercise stress test or reversible defects revealed by myocardial scintigraphy, cannot be adequately assessed from linear regression analysis on the basis only of positive or negative results, as the weight increases with the severity of the alteration.

Studies that include patients enrolled at different times post-MI and followed for varying periods, cannot provide a representative description of the time dependency of risk, as it decreases very rapidly. Studies that include only patients under 65 years of age, or only those with a left ventricular EF above 40%, cannot show the powerful effect of these variables because their effect increases very steeply only after the age of 65 and with values of EF below 40% (see ahead). In studies that also include patients over 65 or with an EF less than 40%, the results of statistical multiple regression analysis would be heavily weighted by the proportion of such patients enrolled in the study group and by the interaction of these prognostic determinants with the others.

The calculated predictive prognostic value of tests is influenced by the severity of the abnormality and by the baseline risk conferred by other prognostic determinants according to the Bayesian theory (which is commonly applied to diagnostic tests) (see Ch 16).

The prognostic predictive value of positive exercise ECG or thallium-201 tests or of flow-limiting coronary stenoses will be much greater in patients with an EF less than 40%, than in those with an EF greater than 50%. An exercise stress test showing 1 mm ST-segment depression, a limited perfusion defect, and a small decrease in EF at a high work load has a smaller prognostic predictive value than a test showing 3 mm ST-segment depression, a large perfusion defect, and a severe drop in EF.

Time dependency of risk

Reliable information on time-dependent post-MI mortality in thrombolyzed and non-thrombolyzed patients, both with and without evidence of reperfusion, is available from the follow-up of patients in the GISSI-1 and GISSI-2 studies.[9,10] These data reflect the average time dependency of mortality of all post-MI patients eligible for thrombolysis that were discharged alive and not submitted to coronary revascularization procedures (less than 2%) (see Figs 22.1 and 22.2). The higher early postdischarge mortality rate may not be influ-

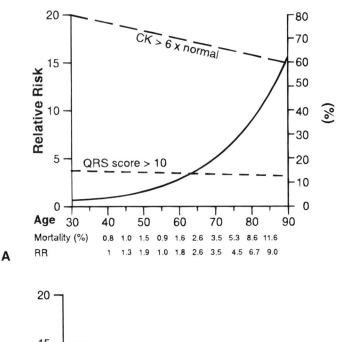

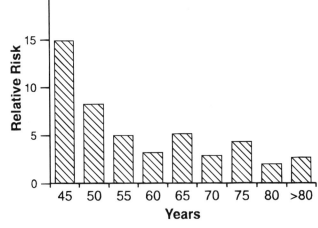

Fig. 22.4 Age-related increase in mortality during the first 6 months post-MI.
The relative risk increases exponentially with age, becoming 9-fold greater in 85-year-old patients compared to 40-year-old patients discharged alive (**A**). This increased mortality rate was similar in men and women and was unrelated to infarct size, as the percentage of patients with values of creatine kinase (CK) 6-times higher than normal and with QRS scores greater than 10 at discharge, tends to decrease with age. The curve describing the absolute risk of death is relatively flat up to the age of 65 (relative risk = 2.5 compared to the age of 40) and then becomes progressively steeper. (Modified from ref. 54.) Compared to age-matched healthy controls (**B**), however, the relative risk of death post-MI is higher in younger patients, in whom IHD becomes the major cause of death, than in older patients, in whom non-IHD-related causes of death also increase exponentially. (From data reported in ref. 55.)

enced by the same prognostic determinants that influence the subsequent lower and fairly constant long-term mortality rate.

Major nonmodifiable determinants of prognosis

The strongest determinants of mortality 6 months after discharge, emerging from the follow-up of patients enrolled in recent megatrials, are age and left ventricular EF.

Age. In patients with their first MI receiving thrombolytic treatment average mortality at 6 months was similar in men and women and was found to increase exponentially from 0.8% in patients under 40 years of age to 11.6% in those over the age of 80. Multiple regression analysis showed that the age-related increase in mortality was independent of other major determinants of prognosis.[54] The rate of increase is relatively slow up to the age of 65, but becomes steeper and steeper thereafter. However, when compared with control age-matched individuals, patients between the ages of 41 and 45 have a 15-fold increase in mortality because their vulnerability to non-IHD-related causes of death is low, whereas patients above the age of 50 have only a sixfold increase because over this age noncardiac causes of death increase exponentially (see Figs 22.4A,B).[55] The causes of this exponential increase in mortality after MI are not precisely known (see Ch. 10).

Left ventricular EF. Angiographic, radionuclide, and echocardiographic studies showed that post-MI mortality increases exponentially with the reduction of EF, independent of other major determinants of prognosis. In a large number of unselected thrombolyzed patients the increase in 6-month mortality was relatively slow down to 40% EF, but became steeper and steeper below this value (see Fig. 22.5).[56]

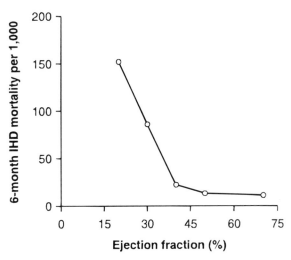

Fig. 22.5 Exponential increase in mortality with the decrease of left ventricular ejection fraction (EF). Predischarge echocardiographic assessment of left ventricular EF is an important nonmodifiable determinant of 6-month mortality. The increased risk is rather small until EF decreases below 40%. The nonmodifiable risk conferred by a reduced EF is a baseline multiplier of potentially modifiable determinants of prognosis. The presence of signs of heart failure doubles the risk for a similar reduction of EF (see Ch. 23). (Modified from ref. 56.)

The predictive value of EF is excellent when it is 50% or more, but, for a similar reduction of EF (i.e. less than 50%), mortality is influenced by the increase of end-systolic volume (see Fig. 22.6)[57] and by the presence of a ventricular aneurysm;[48] for values of EF less than 40%, mortality is also affected by the presence or absence of cardiac failure (see below).

Major potentially modifiable determinants of prognosis

A generally neglected potentially modifiable component of prognosis after MI is represented by psychosocial conditions characterized by stress and social isolation:[58] post-MI mortality was 3% at 3 years (1% per year) in patients with high levels of social support and low levels of stress and 15% (5% per year) in those with high levels of stress and social isolation (see Fig. 22.7). The higher mortality rate in highly stressed, socially isolated patients may be attributable in part to a lower degree of compliance in taking prescribed therapy and to less attention being paid to recurring warning symptoms.

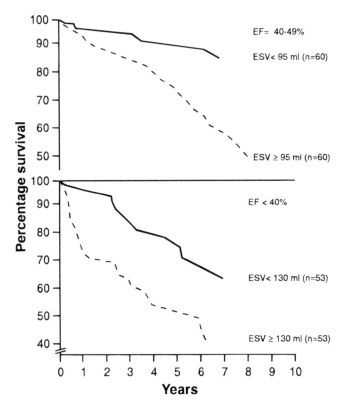

Fig. 22.6 Incremental long-term prognostic value of left ventricular end-systolic volume above ejection fraction (EF). When EF is below 50% a larger end-systolic volume (ESV) increases the long-term risk post-MI. A larger ESV for a similar EF corresponds to either a smaller stroke volume (SV) for a similar end-diastolic volume (EDV) or to a larger EDV for a similar SV. About 75% of IHD-related deaths were sudden. For patients with an EF less than 50%, the measurement of ESV could provide incremental prognostic information, but the underlying causal mechanisms need to be clarified. (Modified from ref. 57.)

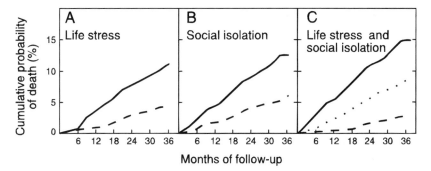

Fig. 22.7 Long-term adverse prognostic effects of stressful life events and social isolation. Stressful life events adversely affect 3 years survival post-MI (——, high stress; ------, low stress) (**A**) to a similar extent to social isolation (——, high; ----, low) (**B**). The effects of stressful life events and social isolation are additive (------, both low-level; ······, one high-level; ——, both high-level) (**C**). Contributory factors may be a reduced compliance to medical treatment and inattention to worsening symptoms in stressed and isolated patients. (Modified from ref. 58.)

The potentially modifiable determinants of short-term prognosis after acute MI are related to each patient's susceptibility to experience new episodes of infarction, malignant arrhythmias, and cardiac failure.

Susceptibility to reinfarction. The risk of new episodes of instability leading to a recurrence of MI is unpredictable because its actual causes are not precisely known. Persisting post-MI angina and ischemia at a distance (i.e. not in the area perfused by the infarct-related vessels)[59] are the most obvious indications of ischemic risk. Additional indications are provided by positive exercise stress tests at low work load, by positive Holter recordings, and by the presence of critical, irregular coronary stenoses in arteries perfusing large areas of noninfarcted segments of the ventricular wall.

Predischarge ECG exercise testing in the prethrombolytic era[60] was found to have a high predictive value, which was not confirmed in thrombolyzed patients.[61,62] In the follow-up of patients enrolled in the GISSI-2 study, the risk ratio conferred by a positive ECG exercise stress test was only 1.6.[56] Smaller studies show that symptom-limited exercise is feasible, without added risk, in eligible patients and is, not surprisingly, positive more often than a submaximal exercise test performed up to 70% of maximal predicted heart rate.[63,64] The response to a mailed questionnaire in 570 centers in the USA indicated that 193 centers performed post-MI exercise testing (147 less than 14 days). The risk of major cardiac complications occurring during symptom-limited exercise was double that associated with submaximal exercise, up to 70% of maximal predicted heart rate but still rather low (0.19% of 28 052 tests versus 0.10% of 99 645 tests).[65] The predictive value of predischarge symptom-limited ECG exercise stress testing up to the end of convalescence (i.e. the initial 2–3 months; see ahead) has not been assessed.

Holter monitoring was found to have a good predictive value for the occurrence of major events in hospital, but not at 6 months after discharge in one study,[66] and a small predictive value for long-term mortality in others.[67,68]

Myocardial scintigraphy, echocardiographic dipyridamole testing, or dobutamine testing were found to have a better predictive accuracy than the ECG,[69–71] but it is not clear in which group of patients.

Finally, ST-segment depression on the resting 12-lead ECG was found to be the most powerful single predictor of prognosis in two large studies of patients with Q-wave and non-Q-wave infarction.[72,73]

In conclusion, the latter finding exemplifies the uncertainties that practising physicians may encounter in the application of a simple, but strong statistical prognostic marker. ST-segment depression on the resting 12-lead ECG may be found in patients with a very broad range of prognosis already indicated by other independent pieces of evidence (large or small MI, good or bad left ventricular function, presence or absence of angina, positive or negative exercise test). Similar uncertainties may apply for any other single prognostic determinant emerging from statistical analysis. This view is supported by the results of Tibbits et al,[74] who found that only the addition of EF values added significantly to the prognostic accuracy derived from clinical variables. Holter monitoring and exercise stress testing failed to provide additional prognostic information (see Fig. 22.8).

The practical application of the varied prognostic markers indicated by various published reports is limited, for the following reasons:

1. There is a wide overlap between modifiable prognostic determinants of myocardium at risk (such as angina, positive Holter monitoring, ECG, thallium and echocardiographic stress tests, coronary arteriographic findings) and between nonmodifiable determinants (previous MI, high peak creatine kinase [CK] values, low EF, ST-segment depression or elevation on the resting ECG). In each study

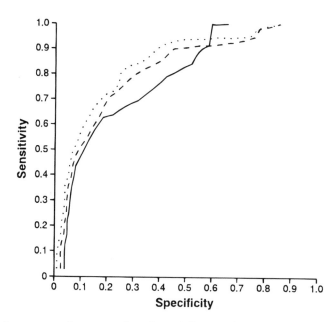

Fig. 22.8 Incremental prognostic value of diagnostic tests above clinical variables (———) post-MI. Only the value of left ventricular EF (-----) increased the prognostic accuracy of diagnostic tests. The addition of exercise stress testing and Holter monitoring (·······) failed to add significant prognostic information, but may do so in some selected groups of patients identified on the basis of clinical variables and routinely available tests. (Modified from ref. 74.)

the significance of any of these determinants is influenced by the variable presence of the others.

2. The average prognostic value of tests reported is influenced by the prevalence of patients with high levels of baseline nonmodifiable risk such as old MI, low EF, and old age, as the predictive values of all tests decreases markedly when a large number of low-risk patients (i.e. with preserved EF, no post-MI angina or arrhythmias) are studied.

3. The results of tests are usually categorized as either positive or negative, with no gradation of the severity of the abnormality (for example, ischemic threshold, extension of ischemia, location, severity, and irregularity of coronary stenoses).

4. There is often no precise information about the time dependency of risk identified by modifiable and baseline prognostic determinants (during convalescence or in the following years). Therefore, the results of early predischarge tests cannot be compared with those performed 4–6 weeks later as a substantial proportion of IHD-related events after acute MI occur during this early period.

■ *The multiplicity of prognostic indicators identified poses practical difficulties for physicians who have no established institutional policy to follow. On the one hand, they may have difficulty in choosing a single test; on the other, when they choose to apply multiple tests, they may have difficulty in interpreting the conflicting results. They should not be tempted to disregard all the clues available from the clinical follow-up and from routine tests in favor of a single test that was shown to be highly predictive in a report published in a major journal, unless it is clear in which specific subgroup of patients and under what conditions it has the prognostic value reported.* ■

Susceptibility to SICD. The risk of SICD is unpredictable because its mechanisms are not precisely known. In general, the risk is highest in patients with a low EF and recurrent malignant arrhythmias and lowest in those with only a slightly reduced EF and very rare premature ventricular contractions (PVCs).

Frequent ventricular ectopy is weakly correlated with prognosis, also independent of the value of left ventricular EF, but the risk increases markedly when patients also have a low EF and cardiac failure.

Episodes of sustained VT (longer than 30 s) after the first 3 days post-MI, usually occurring in patients with extensive infarction, were associated with 50% of deaths occurring in hospital[75] and with 24–83% of deaths occurring over follow-up periods of 8–26 months.[76–78] Nonsustained ventricular arrhythmias (i.e. PVCs), isolated or repetitive, and VT (shorter than 30 s) are also associated with an increased risk of SICD. In one study over a follow-up period of 20 months the risk was 6.6-fold for patients with nonsustained VT and 4.4-fold for those with more than 3 PVCs per hour compared with patients with no ventricular arrhythmias. The risk increased markedly also for nonsustained ventricular arrhythmias in patients with a low left ventricular EF.[35,79]

A comprehensive view of the importance of nonsustained ventricular arrhythmias in unselected patients is provided by the observation of thrombolyzed patients in the GISSI-2 study: the presence of more than 10 PVCs per hour was associated with only 1.6-fold risk of SICD over that of patients with no PVCs.[56] The lower mortality and risk in this study reflects the inclusion of many more uncomplicated patients at low baseline risk, which dilutes the total risk of mortality conferred by arrhythmias in high-risk patients. In the average patient who has an only slightly reduced left ventricular EF, nonsustained ventricular arrhythmias have a very low specificity for identifying their susceptibility to SICD. Late ventricular potentials and reduced heart-rate variability also have a low predictive accuracy when they are applied to unselected patients. Their predictive values increase to about 50% when only patients at high risk are considered.[80]

As discussed in Chapter 10, malignant arrhythmias evolving towards SICD often result from imbalance of either the autonomic nervous system or of the serum electrolytes; this imbalance can occur in a chronic predisposing background for reentry circuits during a potentially reversible ischemic episode, during the very early phase of a new MI, or in the absence of acute ischemia.

■ *The prognostic determinants for these mechanisms of SICD are likely to differ, but no specific information is available because SICD is usually considered as a single endpoint for a very wide range of patients and triggering mechanisms. Furthermore, little information is available on the time dependency of the prognostic determinants of SICD (see Ch. 24).* ■

Susceptibility to cardiac failure. The development of cardiac failure is associated with the doubling of mortality, also for a similar reduction of left ventricular EF, but does not influence the recurrence of acute ischemic events. The presence or absence of the development of cardiac failure for similar values of EF may be due to differences in ESV or to variable hormonal and autonomic nervous system responses to the impairment of cardiac function, which may be potentially modifiable determinants of prognosis above and beyond that related to the reduction of EF.

In the control arm of the two major randomized trials SAVE and AIRE,[42,43] mortality per year was 18.4% in the group with failure (AIRE) and 7.0% in asymptomatic patients with an EF less than 40% (SAVE) (see Table 22.3A). These findings are in agreement with those of the control arm in the SOLVD I (patients with signs of failure) and SOLVD II (patients without failure) trials [81,82] in which mortality was, respectively, 11.6 and 5.1%, in spite of the two groups having a similar average value of left ventricular EF (respectively 25 and 28%) (see Table 22.3B). The presence of clinical signs of cardiac failure failed to affect significantly the average incidence of MI and hospitalization rates for angina which were 12.3% in SOLVD I and 9.1% in SOLVD II for MI, and 18.7% in SOLVD I and 16.8% in SOLVD II for angina, over the 3–4 year follow-up period.

The value of left ventricular EF soon after MI was found to be a good average predictor of the subsequent left ventricular dilation during a 3-year follow-up study,[39] but the reduction of EF may not correlate closely with the increase in ESV. In addition, it may reflect not only the extent of irreversible myocardial loss (a nonmodifiable prognostic determinant), but also the extent of noncontractile, but viable, myocardium (a potentially modifiable prognostic determinant). In patients with a reduced left ventricular EF, with or without signs of left ventricular failure, the possible contribution of viable myocardium that is potentially salvageable by revascularization procedures should be considered (see below).

22.2.2 Indications for predischarge tests

As the risk of reinfarction and of SICD is highest in the period immediately after discharge and decreases sharply during the first few weeks and months, the need for appropriate tests aimed at assessing the short-term prognosis should be considered before discharge.

Table 22.3 Absolute benefit on mortality of ACE-inhibition

A Patients after myocardial infarction

Trial	Number of patients	Follow-up (mean)	Yearly mortality (per 1000)		Lives saved/year (per 1000) (treated group)	Mortality reduction (%)	Statistical significance (P)
			Control group	Treated group			
AIRE (cardiac failure)	2006	15 months	184	132	52	28	0.002
SAVE (asymptomatic)	2231	42 months	70	58	12	17	0.02

B Unselected patients with congestive heart failure

Trial	Number of patients	Follow-up (mean)	Mean EF	Yearly mortality (per 1000)		Lives saved/year (per 1000) (treated group)	Mortality reduction (%)	Statistical significance (P)
				Control group	Treated group			
SOLVD I (cardiac failure)	2569	41 months	25%	116	71	45	39	0.004
SOLVD II (asymptomatic)	4228	37 months	28%	51	48	3	6	0.3

The greatest number of lives saved was observed in the SOLVD I and AIRE trials; 45 lives per 1000 patients treated were saved in the SOLVD I trial, but no significant reduction in mortality was observed in the SOLVD II trial of unselected asymptomatic patients, although average EF was similar in the two trials. The reduction of mortality in asymptomatic patients in the SAVE trial may be related to a reduction of mortality from IHD, as it included only post-MI patients. No precise information is available on the time-dependency of lives saved, i.e. during the first 6 months, 1 year, etc

Persistent angina, malignant arrhythmias, markedly reduced EF, or left ventricular failure are, in themselves, indications that appropriate tests should be performed.

The absence of symptoms, an uncomplicated hospital course, an EF greater than 50%, and age under 65 identify the largest subgroup of post-MI patients who are at a low average risk and in whom the predictive value of any test is very low unless its results are markedly abnormal. Mortality at 6 months post-MI in 60% of patients in the GISSI-2 study[56] who were at low risk was 0.85%. Thus the majority of thrombolyzed patients were at low risk, and among these, a positive ECG exercise test conferred only a small additional risk (see below). In such a group, a negative submaximal ECG exercise stress test should dispense with the need for any other test.

The average rate of mortality of patients after discharge has decreased progressively in the thrombolytic era because patients admitted within a few hours of the onset of symptoms have, on average, small infarcts with only slightly reduced EF and mild or moderate degrees of coronary disease. In the GUSTO trial the average value of left ventricular EF at 5–7 days post-MI was greater than 57% in all treatment groups, and the prevalence of double- and triple-vessel coronary disease was 24 and 14%, respectively. The percentage would probably have been even lower if patients with previous MI (14%) and those with post-MI angina or positive exercise stress tests had been excluded. In the GISSI-2 follow-up study the predictive value of a positive exercise test was quite low (see above).

Predischarge tests should be selected in order to assess the extent of left ventricular dysfunction and to detect the presence of the potentially modifiable short-term adverse determinants of prognosis (myocardium at risk, viable but noncontractile myocardium, and susceptibility to malignant ventricular arrhythmias). The prognostic determinants should be separated according to the baseline nonmodifiable or modifiable alterations that they reveal.

For example, during exercise stress testing a very low effort tolerance, a fall in blood pressure or its failure to increase, a decrease in EF, and an increased thallium-201 uptake in the lungs, indicate severe left ventricular dysfunction, but revascularization procedures are indicated only when left ventricular failure is caused predominantly by transient ischemia or by viable noncontracting myocardium.

Assessment of left ventricular dysfunction

The assessment of the extent of left ventricular dysfunction is the first priority, as all patients should be reclassified before discharge according to their predischarge left ventricular EF (i.e. class 1, $\geq$ 50%; class 2, 40–49%; class 3, 25–39%; class 4, $\leq$ 25%) (see Table 22.4). This is necessary because the initial clinical classification on admission may have been influenced by stimulation of the sympathetic system and ventricular function, which may have deteriorated as a result of infarct extension and of reinfarction or have improved because of resolution of ischemia and stunning.

Patients with an EF greater than 50%, who represent the majority of thrombolyzed patients, can easily be identified by the techniques available, but the difficulty in correctly estimating EF increases with the severity of the dysfunction. Two-dimensional contrast ventriculography is the most accurate technique but, in expert hands, radionuclide angiography and echocardiography can provide reasonable estimates in most cases. Measurements of ESV may provide additional prognostic information in patients with an EF less than 50%, but they are not widely used in clinical practise. The presence of cardiac failure doubles the risk, even for similar values of EF.

Table 22.4 Predischarge left ventricular EF classification

Class	EF (%)
1	>50
2	40–49
3	25–39
4	<25

The usefulness of this classification is suggested by the major prognostic role of the value of left ventricular EF post-MI and by the widely available noninvasive techniques for its assessment. Within each of these classes the incremental prognostic accuracy provided by the presence of cardiac failure, by the measurement of end-systolic left ventricular volume, as well as by the presence of myocardium at risk and of arrhythmias, needs to be assessed in prospective studies. The accuracy of noninvasive techniques in estimating EF values lower than 25% is limited

Assessment of myocardium at risk

During admission, spontaneous episodes of silent myocardial ischemia should be sought by continuous ECG monitoring as they may indicate post-MI unstable angina. The probability of correctly identifying diagnostic ischemic changes of the ST-segment decreases considerably when the resting tracing shows Q waves and persisting ST-segment elevation or other ST-segment or intraventricular conduction abnormalities. A clearly positive Holter recording may dispense with the need for an exercise stress test, as the patient may have unstable angina (see Ch. 19). In patients with no post-MI unstable angina the yield of this test is not precisely known as there are no studies on sufficiently large numbers of unselected patients.

In uncomplicated patients in classes 1 and 2, predischarge tests should be performed on the anti-ischemic therapy on which the patient is being discharged and the exercise test should be submaximal, because in such low-risk patients only markedly positive tests have an important prognostic significance. A submaximal test on anti-ischemic therapy has a lower probability of causing ischemia than a symptom-limited test off therapy, but it identifies those patients in whom predischarge revascularization procedures should be considered (as ischemia cannot be prevented by medical therapy for efforts that could be sustained during ordinary daily life in the convalescent period). The possible average improvement in the assessment of prognosis that can be derived from symptom-limited exercise stress testing is not established.

The tests should try to answer the following questions:

a. is there evidence of spontaneous or inducible myocardial ischemia?
b. what is the ischemic threshold?
c. how extensive is the area at risk?

Assessing the ischemic threshold. An ECG exercise stress test, when positive, is the most informative test because it allows assessment of the work load at which ischemia begins to develop and comparison with the efforts the patient can sustain during ordinary daily life. When performed on full anti-ischemic therapy, the test indicates the residual coronary flow reserve set by fixed coronary stenoses. As discussed above, available studies suggest that a predischarge symptom-limited test is reasonably safe and that it has a greater sensitivity than submaximal tests, with a small increase in risk, but the negative predictive value of ischemic events of a symptom-limited test compared with a submaximal test is not precisely known.

A negative submaximal ECG exercise stress test for a level of effort clearly in excess of that which the patient will perform during convalescence is reassuring, but does not rule out the presence of flow-limiting coronary stenoses that could be assessed further after the initial convalescent phase (see below). Residual coronary flow reserve cannot be assessed precisely by infusion of dobutamine, dipyridamole, or adenosine, although the induction of ischemia by the test identifies myocardium at risk.

A positive exercise stress test at a low work load on full anti-ischemic therapy is a clear indication of a very reduced residual coronary flow reserve and of the need for the assessment of the location and extent of myocardium at risk.

Assessing the extent and location of myocardial ischemia. A drop, or a failure to rise, of systemic blood pressure, or a reduction in EF during the exercise stress test, are usually caused by severe left ventricular dysfunction, which can be due to a critical extension of necrosis, hibernation, or ischemia. The distinction between these components is essential when considering the indications for revascularization procedures. The appearance of transient

ECG ischemic changes is a reliable indication of the onset of ischemia, but not of its location and severity as they may indicate reciprocal changes or be determined by intraventricular conduction disturbances. Myocardial scintigraphy or regional ventricular wall motion studies are necessary to identify more accurately the location and extent of ischemia, of viable noncontractile myocardium, or of post-MI scar tissue (see below).

In patients who cannot exercise before discharge, the presence of myocardium at risk can be sought by intravenous infusion of dobutamine, dipyridamole, or adenosine (see Ch. 16). Ischemia is diagnosed by the appearance of reversible ECG changes, of regional myocardial perfusion defects, or of ventricular contractile dysfunction. Myocardial scintigraphy and studies of left ventricular function have a greater sensitivity for detecting ischemia than ECG stress testing (see Ch. 16).

Viable noncontractile myocardium

Significant amounts of viable noncontractile myocardium are most likely to be found in those patients without previous MI in whom the hospital course suggests a discrepancy between a severe impairment of contractile function and a small elevation of serum CK, a limited development of Q waves, and a limited loss of R waves. Conversely, the likelihood of finding significant amounts of viable noncontractile myocardium is small in patients in whom the hospital course suggests a large extension of myocardial necrosis.

A logical sequence of tests should try to assess the extent to which ventricular dysfunction is caused by scar tissue, by myocardial ischemia, by myocardial stunning, and by myocardial hibernation (see Fig. 22.9).[83]

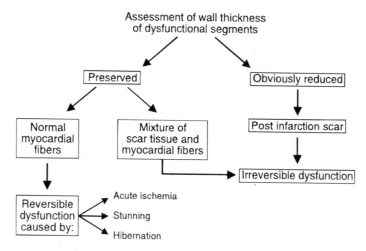

Fig. 22.9 Flow diagram for the practical assessment of noncontractile segments of myocardial wall potentially recoverable by revascularization procedures. An obviously reduced wall thickness is indicative of postinfarction scar. The absence of contractile function in segments of the ventricular wall with preserved wall thickness may be caused by different mechanisms. An acute ischemic cause can be excluded by administration of sublingual nitrates. Stunning can be excluded by repeating the ventricular wall motion study several days after the last ischemic episode. Hibernating myocardium should be distinguished from a mixture of scar tissue and viable myocardial cells.

Myocardial scar tissue should be sought in patients with evidence of previous MI(s). Scar tissue resulting from an old transmural MI is indicated by a markedly reduced thickness of the ventricular wall, and can be identified by echocardiography, nuclear magnetic resonance imaging, and computed tomography. Scar tissue resulting from nontransmural infarction may not be associated with obvious reduction of wall thickness and should be differentiated from viable noncontractile myocardium (see below).

Myocardial ischemia can be responsible for the observed transient ventricular dysfunction only when it occurs at the time of the assessment. As acute ischemia can be precipitated by anxiety about the test and is often silent, ventricular function should always be assessed after administration of sublingual nitrates.

Myocardial stunning with normal perfusion may persist for several days after severe prolonged ischemia; hence, the predischarge assessment of left ventricular EF should be delayed as long as possible after the last episode of myocardial ischemia, which is eventually followed by spontaneous recovery of contractile function (see Ch. 7).

Myocardial hibernation, defined as failure of viable myocardium to contract that is not caused by ischemia or stunning, is associated with chronically reduced perfusion and is potentially reversible by successful revascularization procedures (see Ch. 7). It can be differentiated from ischemia because it is not associated with myocardial lactate production and is not reversible by nitrates. It can be differentiated from stunning because it is associated with reduced myocardial perfusion. It is not easily differentiated from a mixture of viable myocardium and patchy areas of fibrosis in segments of the wall with preserved diastolic thickness (see below).

The diagnostic techniques available for assessing viable noncontractile myocardium include inotropic stimulation, which transiently restores contractile function (both in stunned and in hibernating myocardium) and radionuclide studies, which detect the presence of viable myocardium in noncontractile segments of the left ventricular wall with preserved flow (stunning) or with reduced flow (ischemia or hibernation).

Under optimal conditions, imaging techniques for assessing the transient recovery of regional contractile function have a much greater geometric resolution than radionuclide techniques used to detect viable myocardium. Moreover, the transient recovery of contraction induced by inotropic stimuli is directly indicative of possible recovery following adequate revascularization. Radionuclide techniques may not always be capable of distinguishing viable myocardium interposed within scar tissue in noncontractile segments of the wall with preserved diastolic thickness (see Fig. 22.10).

In expert hands, the techniques available have the potential to demonstrate the presence of noncontractile myocardium that can recover normal contraction following revascularization.[84-87] What remains to be defined is the group of patients in which an improvement in symptoms and prognosis can be expected.

Malignant arrhythmias

Among unselected patients, predischarge tests to detect a patient's susceptibility to malignant arrhythmias are indicated only in those with a complicated hospital course, because the risk of SICD after discharge in unselected patients is quite low. The prognostic predictive value of a positive test is highest in patients with sustained VT or late VF and low left ventricular EF, as their average risk is high; it is lowest in those with nonsustained VT and good EF, because their average risk is low. However, not all patients who had sustained VT or late

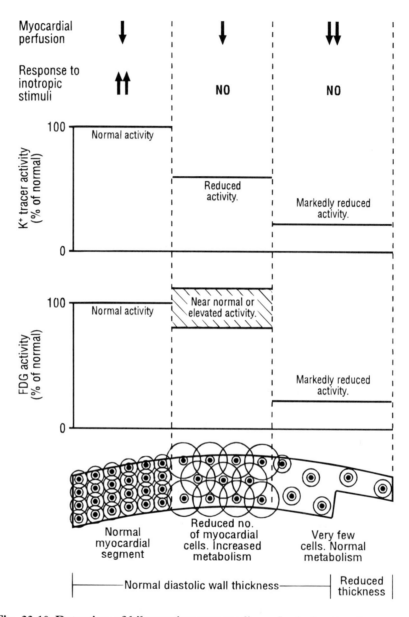

Fig. 22.10 Detection of hibernating myocardium. In dysfunctional segments of the wall with normal thickness and a reduced perfusion, in spite of the administration of sublingual nitrates, the presence of viable myocardium should be distinguished from a mixture of fibrous and normal tissue. A good response to inotropic stimuli and a normal uptake of potassium tracers or water at equilibrium should be considered as reference standards. Increased glucose uptake in ischemic myocardium and inflammatory cells may, in theory, compensate for a reduced uptake in segments of the wall in which myocardial cells have been partially replaced by fibrous scar tissue. (Modified from ref. 83.)

VF and positive tests suffer SICD, yet a tiny minority of those who had nonsustained VT and negative tests may do so.

In patients with recurrent sustained VT, electrophysiologic studies can help to stratify the risk and assist in the selection of antiarrhythmic therapy, but most of the information currently available has been obtained in patients studied after convalescence.[77-79]

In patients with persisting nonsustained VT or with multiple PVCs, Holter monitoring, late potentials on a standard ECG tracing, and heart-rate variability are predictive of an increased risk, particularly when all are positive and particularly in patients with a low left ventricular EF.

No information is available on the time dependency of the predictive value of these tests, yet this information would be essential for considering short-term intense medical therapy during convalescence or early implant of a ventricular defibrillator.

Indications for coronary arteriography

Patients not responding to full medical therapy have absolute indications for predischarge coronary arteriography to assess the possibility of revascularization procedures.

Asymptomatic patients have absolute indications for predischarge coronary arteriography with a view to predischarge revascularization procedures when they have any of the following:

a.   evidence of recurring spontaneous silent ischemic episodes
b.   a positive exercise stress test on anti-ischemic therapy with a critical area of myocardium at risk
c.   a large segment of hibernating myocardium
d.   recurrent malignant arrhythmias during the hospital course.

Major reviews[88,89] suggest that only very markedly positive exercise stress tests or positive tests for ischemia in patients with EF less than 40% represent sufficiently important indications for coronary arteriography with a view to revascularization procedures.

In patients (classes 1 or 2) with an uncomplicated course and negative ECG exercise stress test, the likelihood that arteriography would reveal obstructions that would benefit from revascularization procedures in terms of prognosis, is very low. In such low-risk groups, therefore, indications for coronary arteriography are relative and depend on local practise and the patient's wishes.

22.2.3 Medical therapy on discharge

The treatment prescribed at the time of discharge is intended to correct symptoms and signs of dysfunction, to reduce the unfavorable consequences of MI on cardiac function, and to prevent reinfarction and SICD during convalescence. At the end of convalescence patients should be reassessed for the long-term chronic management strategy discussed in Chapter 13.

At discharge, patients should be advised to concentrate on reducing those risk factors such as smoking and emotional stress, that encourage arrhythmias and thrombosis, as the patient cannot concentrate on too many aspects at the same time. Careful control of arterial hypertension, which is poorly tolerated in the presence of increased ESV and of left ventricular dysfunction, is also mandatory. Those factors that influence long-term prognosis should receive maximal attention at the postconvalescence assessment, as discussed in Chapter 13. Aspirin (75 mg) should be continued indefinitely in all patients with no contraindications. Those with aspirin allergy or gastric intolerance could be continued on ticlopidine while considered to be at high risk.

All patients should be urged to return to the CCU immediately if anginal pain recurs (particularly if it does not immediately respond to nitroglycerin) or if palpitations or paroxysmal dyspnea occur, and to consult their physician if they note the appearance of leg swelling, undue fatigue, and deterioration of effort tolerance. Ideally, they should have the option of contacting a doctor on the management team who is familiar with the course and management of the disease during admission.

For symptomatic patients and for those with positive tests not undergoing predischarge revascularization procedures therapy commenced during hospitalization in order to control symptoms should be continued during convalescence and titrated under careful follow-up. Treatment that relieves failure and recurring ischemia also has beneficial effects on prevention of reinfarction and SICD.

Asymptomatic patients with no evidence of persisting ischemia or of viable noncontractile myocardium are treated only to improve prognosis according to the results of randomized trials, to their hospital course and to their predischarge classification.

Results of randomized trials

Numerous treatment regimens have been shown to produce a statistically significant reduction of mortality in post-MI patients in randomized trials. As in all trials the treatment period extends for several years after MI, they are discussed in the section on the improvement of long-term prognosis in Chapter 13. They included a very broad spectrum of patients, some at high risk because of nonmodifiable or modifiable factors, some requiring treatment because of persistent symptoms or signs, or because they were in the immediate post-MI phase, others at very low risk in the late post-MI phase. In these patients the percentage reduction of mortality ranges from 15 to 20%, but the absolute benefit, i.e. the number of patients saved and the number of non-fatal MIs avoided per 1000 patients treated, was very small. The low absolute benefit derives from the dilution effect caused by the inclusion of low-risk patients and patients who were not susceptible to the risk factor treated, and possibly on the time dependency of risk and of the effect of treatment. For example, the benefit of oral anticoagulants is greatest in the immediate post-MI period;[90] conversely, the reduction in the incidence of infarction and unstable angina produced by ACE inhibitors becomes apparent only about 6 months after MI and the commencement of therapy (see Fig. 22.11A,B).[41]

A statistical meta-analysis of the results of several randomized trials of class I antiarrhythmic drugs in post-MI patients showed a detrimental effect on mortality of the treatment compared with placebo in spite of the favorable effect on the incidence of nonfatal arrhythmias.[91]

■ *Not all patients are likely to benefit from all treatments shown to be beneficial in randomized trials, and the benefit produced by one treatment may not be additive to that produced by the others. The application of these overall results to everyday clinical practise, therefore, cannot be straightforward. It is also unknown to what extent the results of these trials apply to patients treated with thrombolytic drugs and to those treated with aspirin, both of which are now widely used.*

There is, therefore, room to tailor preventive strategies to each individual patient, on the basis of general guidelines. ■

Treatment of asymptomatic low-risk patients

At discharge and throughout the convalescent period, in addition to low dose aspirin (75 mg), β-blockers should be considered for patients who are in either class 1 or class 2 and who had ventricular arrhythmias during the hospital course, and for those who present with

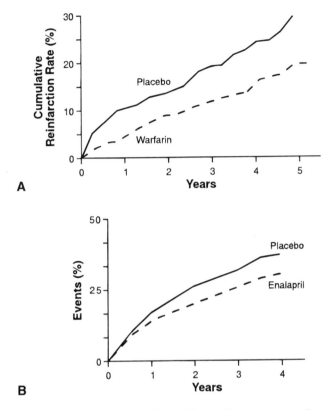

Fig. 22.11 Different time-dependent effects of treatments after acute MI. The effect of oral anticoagulants is greatest within the first 6 months (——, placebo; ----, warfarin) (**A**), whereas the reduction in the number of fatal and nonfatal ischemic events in patients on enalapril (----) begins only after 6 months (**B**). (**A** modified from ref. 90; **B** modified from ref. 41.) The time-dependency of risk and the effects of treatment must be considered when selecting the period of time during which the maximum benefit may be expected.

a heart rate above 70 beats/min (not related to left ventricular failure) and arterial blood pressure above 140/90 mmHg. In general, atenolol (100 mg in the morning) or an equivalent drug should be given. Such patients represent the vast majority of those included in thrombolytic trials, but the type of patient discharged on medical therapy from different institutions is strongly related to referral and local practise. There is ample scope, therefore, for prescribing drugs specific to each individual case.

Diltiazem or verapamil (120 mg retard formulation twice a day) can be considered for patients with evidence of incomplete MI in either class 1 or 2 at discharge, and in those with a low heart rate and low blood pressure who are not eligible for β-blockers or who do not tolerate them.

ACE inhibitors should be considered for patients in classes 2 or 3 even if not required to relieve symptoms or signs of left ventricular failure, with the aim of improving ventricular remodeling and reducing the incidence of cardiac ischemic events. The following dosing regimens can be followed, based on the results of major trials: captopril (starting dose 6.25 mg once a day, up to 50 mg three times a day), enapril (starting dose 2.5 mg once a day, up to 20 mg twice a day) and lisinopril (starting dose 5 mg once a day, up to 40 mg once a day).

22.2.4 Convalescence

The convalescent phase during the initial 2–3 months after MI defines the period in which the trend for ventricular expansion and remodeling becomes established, scar formation in the necrosed myocardium becomes complete, and the acute phase of IHD can be considered to have ended. During convalescence not only does the risk of spontaneous ischemic events decrease rapidly but also the surgical mortality from revascularization procedures in patients with impaired left ventricular function decreases progressively (see Fig. 22.12).[92] Postinfarction scar formation is complete within 2 months in most patients with small or moderate extension of MI and within 3 months in those with large MIs.

For asymptomatic patients the duration of the convalescent period should, therefore, depend on the size of MI. A convalescence of 2 months should be considered reasonable for patients in classes 1 and 2 with negative predischarge tests; a convalescence of 3 months should be considered for those in class 3.

Rehabilitation programs

The occurrence of MI causes considerable psychological trauma in the majority of patients, because of the knowledge of some irreversible damage to their heart and because they suddenly and unexpectedly become aware of their vulnerability to the recurrence of a poten-

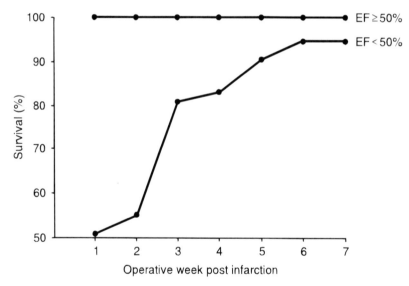

Fig. 22.12 Reduced surgical survival immediately post-MI. Patients with an EF less than 50% have a substantially higher mortality rate in the first 4 weeks post-MI than after about 5 weeks. Conversely, those with a left ventricular EF greater than 50% tolerate cardiac surgery well, even during the first week following acute MI. These results may also indicate that patients in whom surgery could not be deferred for a few weeks are at a higher risk because of their more critical condition. These mortality figures, obtained in an experienced center, cannot be readily applied to other institutions because of the difficulty in relating operative mortality to the severity of a patient's condition. (Modified from ref. 92.)

tially fatal or disabling disease. Thus, particularly for patients without complications, some form of physical and mental rehabilitation becomes an important component of the post-MI convalescence period; for those with complications, the initial emphasis should be on the resolution of the latter.

A 20% reduction in overall mortality over 3 years was reported in a meta-analysis of randomized rehabilitation trials.[93] The mechanisms of this reduction of mortality are certainly varied and are still unclear: the time-dependent increased mortality during convalescence was not specifically explored and the beneficial effect of rehabilitation on social isolation after MI was not adequately assessed.[58] Particularly socially isolated patients are likely to benefit from rehabilitation programs as they are at higher risk (see Fig. 22.7).

The aim of rehabilitation is to bring patients who suffered an acute MI back to or toward normal physical activity, to reduce the risks of reinfarction and SICD and to correct lifestyle when appropriate, and to restore morale.

Physical rehabilitation comprises cardiovascular and muscular retraining (or training) with the intention of allowing the heart to perform its pump function more economically, to make the muscles work more efficiently, and to modify the autonomic nervous system and the metabolic balance of the whole body.

Reducing the risk of reinfarction and SICD can be pursued by giving patients a clear perception of the activities they can engage in and those to be avoided, and by correcting the risk factors that could have contributed to the MI. General aims are to try to improve patients' social adaptation and to encourage them to stop smoking, to follow a healthy diet, to attain an ideal weight, to reduce psychological tension, anxiety, and frustration, and to control hypertension carefully (see Ch. 13).

Restoration of morale is particularly important in some patients, who react with depression, fear, and anxiety to their possible vulnerability to further MI and death. This task is difficult in those who, in spite of their fears, are inclined to persist in the unhealthy lifestyle that they were leading before the MI. They should not be frightened by presenting a gloomy picture of their risk, merely to make them comply with the recommendations for lifestyle modification, as this may increase their anxiety, and thus not only impair the quality of life but possibly also increase the risk.

Rehabilitation after MI can take the form of two or three weekly supervised group sessions lasting between 90 and 120 min, with discussion periods and formal monitored physical training, for 2–3 months. Alternatively, when this arrangement is not available or applicable, a continuing doctor-patient rapport, with discussions about lifestyle, risk factors, and appropriate gradual (unsupervised) resumption of physical activities, is essential. In both options the rehabilitation must be individually tailored, not only with regard to the severity of impairment of left ventricular function but also to risk factors, lifestyle, and personality of the patient.

For patients without complications, the brief stay in hospital causes only a minimal general physical deconditioning (compared with the situation 20–30 years ago, when bed rest was prolonged for 2–3 weeks and hospitalization for 4–8 weeks). Although in such patients the infarction has caused only moderate impairment of ventricular function, there is no rationale for encouraging excessive physical activity soon after discharge.

Exercise testing during rehabilitation should help patients to appreciate the upper levels of activity that they can perform safely during their daily lives. Thus, plans and targets should be tailored carefully to the patients' predischarge assessment and to the level of effort that can be tolerated without the development of dyspnea, fatigue, or signs of ischemia or arrhythmias. This is particularly important when patients do not have supervised group rehabilitation sessions. The desired target level of performance should be attained only at the end of convalescence.

22.2.5 Postconvalescence assessment

Those patients who present recurrences of myocardial ischemia, arrhythmias, or ventricular failure during convalescence should be assessed immediately and treated accordingly. For patients with persistent angina, treatment should be intensified and angiography considered; for patients with malignant arrhythmias, Holter monitoring and electrophysiologic studies should be considered; for patients with evidence of failure, the possibility of mitral valve dysfunction and the presence of potentially viable hypocontractile myocardium should be considered.

Patients who do not present with new episodes of ischemia, ventricular failure, or malignant arrhythmias after a postconvalescence period ranging from 4 to 8 weeks for minor MI and 12–15 weeks for major MI, can be considered to be in a quiescent phase of IHD. Asymptomatic patients should undergo a final assessment in order to decide their long-term management plan.

The absence of symptoms during convalescence may be due to spontaneous adequate compensation of ventricular damage, to healing of the vulnerability to ischemia and arrhythmias, or to the beneficial effects of medical therapy. The postconvalescence assessment is intended to establish the minimal doses of drugs that will maintain this symptom-free state. This can be established empirically by gradually tapering the doses over a period of weeks and by assessing the vulnerability to ischemia after interrupting anti-ischemic therapy and the vulnerability to arrhythmias after interruption of antiarrhythmic therapy (particularly of amiodarone, the protracted use of which can cause side effects); the susceptibility to develop cardiac failure can be assessed by gradually reducing diuretic therapy while monitoring symptoms, body weight, and ventricular function by echocardiography.

Those patients in whom the results of tests are satisfactory and who fail to develop symptoms when therapy is reduced or stopped should be considered to be in a quiescent phase of IHD. They are at very low risk and are eligible for the therapeutic options aimed at improving prognosis that are discussed in Chapter 13.

REFERENCES

1. Antman EM, Braunwald E. Acute MI: Management in the 1990s. Hosp Pract 1990;*15*:73.
2. Davies G, Chierchia S, Maseri A. Prevention of myocardial infarction by very early treatment with intracoronary streptokinase. Some clinical observations. N Engl J Med 1984;*311*:1488.
3. Brush JE, Brand DA, Acampora D et al. Use of the initial electrocardiogram to predict in-hospital complications of acute myocardial infarction. N Engl J Med 1985;*312*:1137.
4. Lee TL, Cook EF, Weisberg M et al. Acute chest pain in the emergency ward: identification and evaluation of low risk patients. Arch Intern Med 1985;*145*:65.
5. Fineberg H, Scadden D, Goldman L. Management of patients with a low probability of acute myocardial infarction: cost-effectiveness of alternatives to coronary care unit admission. N Engl J Med 1984;*310*:1301.
6. Gore JM, Goldberg RJ, Matsumoto AS et al. Validity of serum total cholesterol level obtained within 24 hours of acute myocardial infarction. Am J Cardiol 1984;*54*:722.
7. Gruppo Italiano per lo Studio della Streptochinasi nell'Infarto Miocardico (GISSI). Effectiveness of intravenous thrombolytic treatment in acute myocardial infarction. Lancet 1986;*I*:397.
8. ISIS-2 (Second International Study of Infarct Survival) Collaborative Group. Randomised trial of intravenous streptokinase, oral aspirin, both, or neither among 17 187 cases of suspected acute myocardial infarction. Lancet 1988;*II*:349.
9. Gruppo Italiano per lo Studio della Streptochinasi nell'Infarto Miocardico (GISSI). Long-term effects of intravenous thrombolysis in acute myocardial infarction: final report of the GISSI Study. Lancet 1987;*II*:871.
10. Mauri F, Maggioni AP, Franzosi MG et al for the GISSI-2 Investigators. A simple electrocardio-

graphic predictor of the outcome of patients with acute myocardial infarction treated with a thrombolytic agent. A Gruppo Italiano per lo Studio della Sopravvivenza nell'Infarcto Miocardico (GISSI-2) derived analysis. J Am Coll Cardiol 1994;*24*:600.

11. The European Myocardial Infarction Project Group. Prehospital thrombolytic therapy in patients with suspected acute myocardial infarction. N Engl J Med 1993;*329*:383.

12. Weaver WD, Cerqueira M, Hallstrom AP et al. Prehospital-initiated vs hospital-initiated thrombolytic therapy. The Myocardial Infarction Triage and Intervention Trial. J Am Med Assoc 1993;*270*:1211.

13. Yusuf S, Sleight P, Held P, McMahon S. Routine medical management of acute myocardial infarction. Lessons from overviews of recent randomized controlled trials. Circulation 1990;*82(Suppl. II)*:II-117.

14. The International Study Group. In-hospital mortality and clinical course of 20 891 patients with suspected acute myocardial infarction randomised between alteplase and streptokinase with or without heparin. Lancet 1990;*336*:71.

15. ISIS-3 (Third International Study of Infarct Survival) Collaborative Group. A randomised trial of streptokinase vs tissue plasminogen activator vs anistreplase and of aspirin plus heparin vs aspirin alone among 41 299 cases of suspected acute myocardial infarction. Lancet 1992;*339*:753.

16. The GUSTO Investigators. An international randomized trial comparing four thrombolytic strategies for acute myocardial infarction. N Engl J Med 1993;*329*:673.

17. Topol EJ, Califf RM, Lee KL. More on the GUSTO trial. Letter. New Engl J Med 1994;*331*:277.

18. The GUSTO Angiographic Investigators. The effects of plasminogen activator, streptokinase, or both on coronary-artery patency, ventricular function, and survival after acute myocardial infarction. N Engl J Med 1993;*329*:1615.

19. Grines CD, Browe KF, Marco J et al for the Primary Angioplasty in Myocardial Infarction Study Group. A comparison of immediate angioplasty with thrombolytic therapy for acute myocardial infarction. N Engl J Med 1993;*328*:673.

20. Gibbons RJ, Holmes DR, Reeder GS, Bailey KR, Hopfenspirger MR, Gersh BJ. Immediate angioplasty compared with the administration of a thrombolytic agent followed by conservative treatment for myocardial infarction. N Engl J Med 1993;*328*:685.

21. Zijlstra F, de Boer MJ, Hoorntje JCA, Reiffers S, Reiber JHC, Suryapranata H. A comparison of immediate coronary angioplasty with intravenous streptokinase in acute myocardial infarction. N Engl J Med 1993;*328*:680.

22. Bedotto JB, Kahn JK, Rutherford BD et al. Failed direct coronary angioplasty for acute myocardial infarction: in-hospital outcome and predictors of death. J Am Coll Cardiol 1993;*22*:690.

23. LATE Study Group. Late assessment of thrombolytic efficacy (LATE) study with alteplase 6–24 hours after onset of acute myocardial infarction. Lancet 1993;*II*:759.

24. Meijer A, Verheugt FWA, Werter CJPJ, Lie KI, van der Pol JMJ, van Eeniege MJ. Aspirin versus coumadin in the prevention of reocclusion and recurrent ischemia after successful thrombolysis: a prospective placebo-controlled angiographic study. Results of the APRICOT Study. Circulation 1993;*87*:1524.

25. Maggioni AP, Franzosi MG, Santoro E et al. The risk of stroke in patients with acute myocardial infarction after thrombolytic and antithrombotic treatment. (GISSI-2). N Engl J Med 1992;*327*:1.

26. The TIMI Research Group. Comparison of invasive and conservative strategies after treatment with intravenous tissue plasminogen activator in acute myocardial infarction: Results of the thrombolysis in myocardial infarction (TIMI) phase II trial. N Engl J Med 1989;*320*:618.

27. Kostuk WJ, Beanlands DS. Complete heart block associated with acute myocardial infarction. Am J Cardiol 1970;*26*:380.

28. Rahimtoola SH et al. Left atrial transport function in myocardial infarction. Am J Med 1975;*59*:686.

29. Zoll PM, Zoll RH, Falk RH et al. External noninvasive temporary cardiac pacing: clinical trials. Circulation 1985;*71*:937.

30. ACC/AHA Task Force on Assessment of Diagnostic and Therapeutic Cardiovascular Procedures (Subcommittee on Pacemaker Implantation): Guidelines for permanent cardiac pacemaker implantation. J Am Coll Cardiol 1984;*4*:434.

31. Wilson C, Adgey AAJ. Survival of patients with late ventricular fibrillation after acute myocardial infarction. Lancet 1974;*II:*214.

32. Jensen CVH, Torp-Pedersen C, Kober L et al. Prognosis of late versus early ventricular fibrillation in acute myocardial infarction. Am J Cardiol 1990;*66:*10.

33. Burchart F, Pfisterer M, Kiowski J, Follarth F, Burckardt D. Effect of antiarrhythmic therapy on mortality in survivors of myocardial infarction with asymptomatic complex ventricular arrhythmias. Basel Antiarrhythmic Study of Infarct Survival (BASIS). J Am Coll Cardiol 1990;*16:*1711.

34. Cairns JA, Connolly SJ, Gent M, Roberts R. Post-myocardial infarction mortality in patients with ventricular premature depolarization. Canadian Amiodarone Myocardial Infarction Trial Pilot Study. Circulation 1991;*84:*550.

35. Ceremuzynski L, Kleczar E, Krzeminska-Pakula M et al. Effect of amiodarone on mortality after myocardial infarction: a double-blind, placebo-controlled, pilot study. J Am Coll Cardiol 1992;*20:*1056.

36. Engelstein ED, Lippman N, Stein K, Lerman BB. Mechanism-specific effects of adenosine on atrial tachycardia. Circulation 1994;*89:*2645.

37. Gruppo Italiano per lo Studio della Sopravvivenza nell-Infarto Miocardico (GISSI-3). Effects of lisinopril and transdermal glyceryl trinitrate singly and together on six-week mortality and ventricular function after acute myocardial infarction. Lancet 1994;*343:*1115.

38. ISIS-4 (Fourth International Study of Infarct Survival) Collaborative Group. A randomised factorial trial assessing early oral captopril, oral mononitrate, and intravenous magnesium sulphate in 58 050 patients with suspected acute myocardial infarction. Lancet 1995;*345:*669.

39. Swedberg K, Held P, Kjekshus J et al on behalf of the CONSENSUS II Study Group. Effects of the early administration of enalapril on mortality in patients with acute myocardial infarction. N Engl J Med 1992;*327:*678.

40. Ambrosioni E, Borghi C, Magnani B for the Survival of Myocardial Infarction Long-Term Evaluation (SMILE) Study Investigators. The effect of the angiotensin-converting-enzyme inhibitor Zofenopril on mortality and morbidity after anterior myocardial infarction. New Engl J Med 1995;*332:*80.

41. Yusuf S, Pepine JC, Garges et al. Effect of enalapril on myocardial infarction and unstable angina in patients with low ejection fractions. Lancet 1992;*340:*1173.

42. Pfeffer MA, Braunwal E, Move LA et al on behalf of the SAVE Investigators. Effect of captopril on mortality and morbidity in patients with left ventricular dysfunction after myocardial infarction. N Engl J Med 1992;*327:*669.

43. The Acute Infarction Ramipril Efficacy (AIRE) Study Investigators. Effect of ramipril on mortality and morbidity of survivors of acute myocardial infarction with clinical evidence of heart failure. Lancet 1993;*342:*821.

44. EMIP-FR Pilot Study Group. Free radicals, reperfusion and myocardial infarction therapy: European Myocardial Infarction Project—free radicals pilot study. Eur Heart J 1993;*14:*48.

45. Gaudron P, Eilles C, Kugler I, Ertl G. Progressive left ventricular dysfunction and remodeling after myocardial infarction. Potential mechanisms and early predictors. Circulation 1993;*87:*755.

46. Pfeffer JM, Pfeffer MA, Braunwald E. Influence of chronic captopril therapy on the infarcted left ventricle of the rat. Circ Res 1985;*57:*84.

47. Kim CB, Braunwald E. Potential benefits of late reperfusion of infarcted myocardium. The open artery hypothesis. Circulation 1993;*88:*2426.

48. Meizlish JL, Berger HJ, Plankey M et al. Functional left ventricular aneurysm formation after acute anterior transmural myocardial infarction, incidence, natural history, and prognostic implications. N Engl J Med 1984;*311:*1001.

49. Hellerstein HK, Martin JW. Incidence of thromboembolic lesions accompanying myocardial infarction. Am Heart J 1947;*33:*443.

50. Asinger RW, Mikell F, Elsperger J, Hodges M. Incidence of left ventricular thrombosis after acute transmural myocardial infarction. Serial evaluation of two-dimensional echocardiography. N Engl J Med 1981;*305:*297.

51. Vecchio C, Chiarella F, Lupi G, Bellotti P, Domenicucci S. Left ventricular thrombus in anterior acute myocardial infarction after thrombolysis. A GISSI-2 connected study. Circulation 1991;*84:*512.

52. Nihoyannopoulos P, Smith GC, Maseri A, Foale RA. The natural history of left ventricular thrombus in myocardial infarction: a rationale in support of masterly inactivity. J Am Coll Cardiol 1989;14:902.
53. Lichstein E, Arsura E, Hollander G, Greengart A, Sanders M. Current incidence of postmyocardial infarction (Dressler's) syndrome. Am J Cardiol 1982;50:1269.
54. Maggioni AP, Maseri A, Fresco C et al on behalf of GISSI-2 Investigators. Age-related increase in mortality among patients with first myocardial infarctions treated with thrombolysis. New Engl J Med 1993;329:1442.
55. World Health Organization: World Health Statistics Annual 1990. Geneva, WHO.
56. Gruppo Italiano per lo Studio della Sopravvivenza nell'Infarto Miocardico (GISSI)-2 Data Base. Determinants of 6-month mortality in survivors of myocardial infarction after thrombolysis. Results of the GISSI-2 data base. Circulation 1993;88:416.
57. White HD, Norris RM, Brown MA, Brandt PWT, Whitlock RML, Wild CJ. Left ventricular endsystolic volume as the major determinant of survival after recovery from myocardial infarction. Circulation 1987;76:44.
58. Ruberman W, Weinblatt E, Goldberg JD, Chaudhary BS. Psychosocial influences on mortality after myocardial infarction. N Engl J Med 1984;311:552.
59. Schuster EH, Bulkley BH. Early postinfarction angina. Ischemia at a distance and ischemia in the infarct zone. N Engl J Med 1981;305:1101.
60. Theroux P, Waters DD, Halphen C, Debaisieux JC, Mizgala HF. Prognostic value of exercise testing soon after myocardial infarction. N Engl J Med 1979;310:341.
61. Stevenson R, Umachandran V, Ranjadaylan K, Wilkinson P, Marchant B, Timmis AD. Reassessment of treadmill stress testing for risk stratification in patients with acute myocardial infarction treated by thrombolysis. Br Heart J 1993;70:415.
62. Krone RJ, Dwyer EM Jr, Greenberg H, Miller JP, Gillespie JA. Risk stratification in patients with first non-Q wave infarction: limited value of the early low level exercise test after uncomplicated infarcts. The Multicenter Post-Infarction Research Group. J Am Coll Cardiol 1989;14:31.
63. Juneau M, Colles P, Théroux P et al. Symptom-limited versus low level exercise testing before hospital discharge after myocardial infarction. J Am Coll Cardiol 1992;20:927.
64. Jain A, Myers GH, Sapin PM, O'Rourke R. Comparison of symptom-limited and low level exercise tolerance tests early after myocardial infarction. J Am Coll Cardiol 1993;22:1816.
65. Hamm LF, Crow RS, Stull GA, Hannan P. Safety and characteristics of exercise testing early after acute myocardial infarction. Am J Cardiol 1989;63:1193.
66. Silva P, Galli M, Campolo L for the IRES (Ischemia Residual) Study Group. Prognostic significance of early ischemia after acute myocardial infarction in low-risk patients. Am J Cardiol 1993;71:1142.
67. Langer A, Minkowitz J, Dorian P et al for the Tissue Plasminogen Activator: Toronto (TPAT) Study Group. Pathophysiology and prognostic significance of Holter-detected ST segment depression after myocardial infarction. J Am Coll Cardiol 1992;20:1313.
68. Ruberman W, Crow R, Rosenberg CR et al. Intermittent ST depression and mortality after myocardial infarction. Circulation 1992;85:1440.
69. Brown KA, O'Meara JO, Chambers CE, Plante DA. Ability of dipyridamole–thallium-201 imaging one to four days after acute myocardial infarction to predict inhospital and late recurrent myocardial ischemic events. Am J Cardiol 1990;65:160.
70. Gimple LW, Hutter AM, Guiney TE, Boucher CA. Prognostic utility of predischarge dipyridamole–thallium imaging compared to predischarge submaximal exercise electrocardiography and maximal exercise thallium imaging after uncomplicated acute myocardial infarction. Am J Cardiol 1989;64:1243.
71. Gibson RS, Watson DD, Craddock GB et al. Prediction of cardiac events after uncomplicated myocardial infarction: a prospective study comparing predischarge exercise thallium-201 scintigraphy and coronary angiography. Circulation 1983;68:321.
72. Schechtman KB, Capone RJ, Kleiger RE et al. Risk stratification of patients with non-Q wave myocardial infarction. The critical role of ST segment depression. The Diltiazem Reinfarction Study Research Group. Circulation 1989;80:1148.

73. Moss AJ, Goldstein RE, Hall J et al for the Multicenter Myocardial Ischemia Research Group. Detection and significance of myocardial ischemia in stable patients after recovery from an acute coronary event. J Am Med Asoc 1993;269:2379.

74. Tibbits PA, Evaul JE, Goldstein RE et al and the Multicenter Post-infarction Research Group. Serial acquisition of data to predict one year mortality rate after acute myocardial infarction. Am J Cardiol 1987;60:451.

75. Tofler GH, Stone PH, Muller JE et al. Prognosis after cardiac arrest due to ventricular tachycardia or ventricular fibrillation associated with acute myocardial infarction (The MILIS Study) Am J Cardiol 1987;60:765.

76. Di Marco JP, Lerman BB, Kron IL, Sellers TD. Sustained ventricular tachyarrhythmias within 3 months of acute myocardial infarction: results of medical and surgical therapy in patients resuscitated from the initial episode. J Am Coll Cardiol 1985;6:759.

77. Wellens HJJ, Bar FWH, Vanagt EJDM, Brugada P. Medical treatment of ventricular tachycardia; consideration in the selection of patients for surgical therapy. Am J Cardiol 1982;49:186.

78. Bigger JT Jr, Fleiss JL, Kleiger R, Miller JP, Rolnitzky LM. The Multicenter Post Infarction Research Group. The relationships among ventricular arrhythmias, left ventricular dysfunction and mortality in the 2 years after myocardial infarction. Circulation 1984;69:250.

79. Mukharji J, Rude RE, Pole WK et al for The MILIS Study Group. Risk factors for sudden death after acute myocardial infarction: two-years follow-up. Am J Cardiol 1984;54:31.

80. Farrell TG, Bashir Y, Cripps T et al. Risk stratification for arrhythmic events in postinfarction patients based on heart rate variability, ambulatory electrocardiographic variables and the signal-averaged electrocardiogram. J Am Coll Cardiol 1991;18:687.

81. The SOLVD Investigators. Effect of enalapril on survival in patients with reduced left ventricular ejection fractions and congestive heart failure. N Engl J Med 1991;325:293.

82. The SOLVD Investigators. Effect of enalapril on mortality and the development of heart failure in asymptomatic patients with reduced left ventricular ejection fractions. N Engl J Med 1992;327:685.

83. Maseri A. Viable but noncontractile myocardium: the clinical problem. J Nuc Cardiol 1994;1:S31.

84. de Silva R, Yamamoto Y, Rhodes CG et al. Preoperative prediction of the outcome of coronary revascularization using positron emission tomography. Circulation 1992;86:1738.

85. Perrone-Filardi P, Bacharach SL, Dilsizian V, Maurea S, Frank JA, Bonow RO. Regional left ventricular wall thickening. Relation to regional uptake of [18]fluorodeoxyglucose and ^{201}Tl in patients with chronic coronary artery disease and left ventricular dysfunction. Circulation 1992;86:1125.

86. Dilsizian V, Freedman NMT, Bacharach SL, Perrone-Filardi P, Bonow RO. Regional thallium uptake in irreversible defects. Magnitude of change in thallium activity after reinjection distinguishes viable from nonviable myocardium. Circulation 1992;85:627.

87. Cigarroa CG, deFilippi CR, Brickner E, Alvarez LG, Wait MA, Grayburn PA. Dobutamine stress echocardiography identifies hibernating myocardium and predicts recovery of left ventricular function after coronary revascularization. Circulation 1993;88:430.

88. Moss AJ, Benhorin J. Prognosis and management after a first myocardial infarction. N Engl J Med 1990;322:743.

89. De Busk RF, Blomqvist CG, Kouchoukos NT et al. Identification and treatment of low-risk patients after acute myocardial infarction and coronary-artery bypass graft surgery. N Engl J Med 1986;314:161.

90. Smith P, Arnesen H, Holme L. The effect of warfarin on mortality and reinfarction after myocardial infarction. N Engl J Med 1990;323:147.

91. Hine LK, Laird NM, Hewitt P, Chalmers TC. Meta-analysis of empirical long-term antiarrhythmic therapy after myocardial infarction. J Am Med Ass 1989;262:3037.

92. Hochberg MS, Parsonnet V, Gielchinsky I, Hussain SM, Fisch DA, Norman JC. Timing of coronary revascularization after acute myocardial infarction. Early and late results in patients revascularized within seven weeks. J Thorac Cardiovasc Surg 1984;88:914.

93. O'Connor GT, Buring JE, Yusuf S et al. An overview of randomized trials of rehabilitation with exercise after myocardial infarction. Circulation 1989;80:234.

CHAPTER 23 | Chronic postischemic cardiac failure

INTRODUCTION

The syndrome of chronic postischemic cardiac failure is, by definition, cardiac failure resulting from the loss of a critical mass of myocardial cells through ischemic necrosis. This loss is of such magnitude that it cannot be adequately compensated for by remodeling and hypertrophy of the residual myocardium. Thus, cardiac pump function becomes inadequate with consequent neurohumoral activation and sodium and fluid retention, resulting in lung congestion in chronic left ventricular failure, and in dependent edema in congestive failure. The essential diagnostic criterion is the chronic recurrence of signs of failure whenever diuretic therapy is interrupted. Hence, by definition, patients need chronic diuretic therapy (in addition to therapy specifically aimed at improving ventricular function). Fluid retention, responding to diuretic therapy, is a simple clinical marker of neurohumoral activation which, besides having obvious therapeutic consequences, may have important prognostic implications (see below).

The critical loss of contractile elements may result from only one myocardial infarction (MI), or many. In some patients, failure can be aggravated by potentially correctable conditions such as hypertension, arrhythmias, ischemia, stunning, hibernation, or valvular dysfunction. A differential diagnosis with other forms of cardiomyopathy must be considered for patients with no clear evidence of a large MI or of multiple MIs (see below).

Patients with signs of chronic cardiac failure are particularly vulnerable to new ischemic episodes, to further losses of contractile elements caused by reinfarction and to malignant ventricular arrhythmias because of reduced contractile reserve, and myocardial scarring, but this vulnerability may also be enhanced by associated neurohumoral activation. Therefore, such patients need continuous medical care for the control of symptoms and the improvement of prognosis.

This chapter presents the definition, incidence, pathogenetic components, and classification of the syndrome as a basis for a rational diagnostic, prognostic, and therapeutic approach.

23.1 DEFINITION, INCIDENCE, PATHOGENETIC COMPONENTS, AND CLASSIFICATION

A precise definition of the syndrome with its clinical features, incidence, and pathogenetic components, is useful for selecting rational diagnostic criteria, for assessing the prognostic determinants, and for providing therapeutic guidelines in well-defined groups of patients that are easily recognizable in clinical practise.

23.1.1 Definition

A widely applicable clinical definition of the syndrome is useful for identifying specific forms of clinical presentation with practical prognostic and therapeutic implications.

As indicated in the introduction to this chapter, the essential diagnostic feature of the syndrome is the need for chronic diuretic therapy (in addition to therapy specifically aimed at improving ventricular function) in order for the patient to remain free from left ventricular or congestive cardiac failure or to reduce the severity of these conditions. Cardiac failure results from the combination of a critical irreversible postischemic ventricular dysfunction and the consequent neurohumoral activation.

The introduction of the restrictive definition above was based on several considerations:

a. the lack of a defined value of left ventricular ejection fraction (EF) below which chronic signs of failure develop
b. the unreliability of mild subjective and physical signs of failure
c. the likelihood of detecting clinically an improvement in symptoms and signs with diuretic therapy as a diagnostic aid
d. evidence that patients with cardiac failure have about a twofold greater rate of mortality than patients without failure, in spite of similar levels of left ventricular EF, probably as a result of the associated neurohumoral activation.

This definition excludes patients with a left ventricular EF less than 40%, who have never had signs of cardiac failure or who had an isolated acute episode of failure precipitated by identifiable causes such as myocardial ischemia, uncontrolled systemic hypertension, arrhythmias, anemia, or infection. It also excludes patients treated chronically who display no signs of failure when diuretics are discontinued (see 23.2.1). Such patients, who do not present with chronic neurohumoral activation, are at a lower risk of death than those with no signs of heart failure for a similar reduction of left ventricular EF.

23.1.2 Incidence

The incidence of chronic cardiac failure is high: about 400 000 new cases per year occur in the USA,[1] mostly in elderly individuals, as the incidence of chronic heart failure increases with age. In the Framingham study the number of new cases per year increased from about 3/1000 among men aged 50–59 years to 55/1000 among men aged 85–94 years, and to 85% in women aged 85–94 years.[2] About 50% of cases of failure are related to ischemic heart disease (IHD), associated mostly with hypertension, and about 25% are idiopathic.[3]

The prevalence of chronic cardiac failure is high. It is estimated that 2–3 million Americans suffer from it but, in epidemiologic studies, the estimated prevalence varies considerably according to the diagnostic criteria adopted.[4] Given the high prevalence of both idiopathic congestive failure and IHD, the two conditions may, by chance, coexist in some patients.

After an acute MI only a minority of patients develop chronic cardiac failure. In the Gruppo Italiano per lo Studio della Sopravvivenza nell'Infarto Miocardico-2 (GISSI-2) study,[5] 12% of patients had echocardiographic evidence of severe left ventricular dysfunction (i.e. with an EF less than 40% or with more than 35% of dysfunctional segments) and 9% had signs of failure (some in this group did not have severe left ventricular dysfunction); however, 19% were on diuretics.

Older patients are more vulnerable to the loss of myocardium caused by MI, possibly as a result of both the progressive loss with age of myocytes and their replacement with interstitial tissue,[6] and of the increasing prevalence of systolic hypertension. Thus, in elderly patients, signs of failure may be present after MIs characterized by elevation of total creatine kinase (CK) and by QRS scores not usually associated with the development of heart failure in younger patients.

23.1.3 Pathogenetic components

The development of chronic left ventricular and congestive cardiac failure results from the combination of a critical ventricular hemodynamic dysfunction and a neurohumoral activation leading to sodium and fluid retention, which are not necessarily proportional to the severity of ventricular dysfunction.

In chronic left ventricular failure, limited fluid retention, corresponding to only a 2–3 kg increase in total body weight, may be sufficient to cause a critical elevation of left ventricular filling pressure both at rest and during effort causing, respectively, orthopnea and exertional dyspnea. In congestive failure a much greater fluid retention, corresponding to 3–6 kg, is required in order to become clinically detectable.

Postischemic origin of myocardial dysfunction

In some patients, cardiac failure appears soon after an extensive acute MI; however, in others, signs of failure appear only after some years and are associated with a gradual deterioration of left ventricular function.[7] A dilated ventricle and a reduced left ventricular EF are not necessarily conducive to progressive dilation, as in some patients an EF as low as 25% may not be associated with signs of left or congestive failure and may not deteriorate over several years. Conversely, at the 6-month follow-up examination in the GISSI-2 study,[5] 60% of patients with late-onset left ventricular failure had, predischarge, an EF greater than 40%, or less than 35% of dysfunctional segments.

Chronic postischemic cardiac failure has also been described in patients with no evidence of transmural MI but with very severe diffuse triple-vessel disease.[8] There is, however, no conclusive evidence that repeated episodes of myocardial ischemia can be sufficiently severe to cause patchy necrosis and chronic failure (see 23.2.1).

■ *The precise mechanisms involved in the progressive deterioration of ventricular function post-MI in some patients, but not in others with similar degrees of impairment of left ventricular function soon after MI, are incompletely known.* ■

Variable relationship between severity of left ventricular dysfunction and development of failure

There is no value of left ventricular EF below which chronic left ventricular failure or congestion consistently develop. The clinical observation that some patients with an EF less than 25% may not develop failure for several years, whereas others with an EF of 40% may require chronic diuretic therapy,[5] is supported by the similar average values of left ventricular EF in patients with cardiac failure included in the Studies of Left Ventricular Dysfunction (SOLVD) I trial and in those without cardiac failure included in the SOLVD-II trial (25% in patients with failure and 28% in those without) (see 23.2.2).

In patients with an EF less than 50% the size of left ventricular end-systolic volume was found to influence long-term mortality also for similar values of EF,[9] but the mechanisms of this excess mortality were related predominantly to a higher frequency of sudden ischemic cardiac death (SICD) rather than of heart failure.

Neurohumoral activation

The variable association of cardiac failure with the values of left ventricular EF suggests that neurohumoral activation, which is critical to the development and progression of left ventricular and congestive cardiac failure, can be triggered by varying severities of ventricular dysfunction. Although the components of the neurohumoral activation are more clearly known than their actual triggers, they not only may contribute to the development of symptoms but also may adversely affect the outcome of the syndrome.

Activation of the sympathetic nervous system, possibly related to a basoreceptor dysfunction, is indicated by elevated levels of norepinephrine and by β-receptor downregulation.[10–12]

Systemic and local vascular activation of the renin-angiotensin system are fundamental alterations in cardiac failure. Renin–angiotensin activity is influenced by several factors including reduced renal blood flow, sympathetic activation, basoreceptor dysfunction, and diuretic therapy.[13]

Atrial natriuretic factor (ANF) is released by atrial distension and the increased levels found in congestive failure suggest a diminished response to the hormone, which would counteract the resin–angiotensin system.[14]

Arginine vasopressin levels are elevated in patients with congestive heart failure and may contribute to hyponatremia.[15]

Impairment of vascular endothelium with decreased production of endothelium-derived relaxing factors (EDRF)[16] and increased production of endothelin[17–19] were also found in chronic heart failure.

A common final consequence of neurohumoral activation is intense vasoconstriction resulting from activation of both the sympathetic nervous system and the renin–angiotensin system, as well as from elevated blood levels of arginine vasopressin and endothelin, the reduced response to ANF, and the reduced production of EDRF. Peripheral vasoconstriction and low cardiac output together with physical deconditioning, caused by prolonged physical inactivity, cause skeletal muscle atrophy and altered metabolism.[20]

The extent of neurohumoral activation assessed from plasma levels of norepinephrine, angiotensin II, aldosterone, and ANF was found to be correlated with mortality in the Cooperative North Scandinavian Enalapril Survival Study (CONSENSUS).[21] The mildly elevated levels found in patients with ventricular dysfunction but with no signs of failure enrolled in the SOLVD study[22] suggest that this correlation was causal or a marker of a severe underlying disease.

23.1.4 Classification

The clinical features of the syndrome vary considerably with the severity of left ventricular dysfunction, with the intensity of the neurohumoral activation, and with the involvement of the right ventricle by the MI. Some patients may require only minimal doses of diuretics in order to remain free from failure; in others, signs of failure persist in spite of intensive diuretic therapy. In some, the main complaint is dyspnea due to chronic left ventricular failure, whereas others complain of severe fatigue due to low cardiac output.

The severity of disability caused by cardiac dysfunction is traditionally graded according to the New York Heart Association (NYHA) classification,[23] which is based on the ability of patients to perform "ordinary" daily activities. The advantages of this functional clinical classification are its widespread use, its value in defining the changing physical capacity of an individual patient, and its strong correlation with prognosis. The disadvantage is its rather subjective nature, as "ordinary" physical activity may imply very different levels of activity according to age, coexisting disabilities, and previous levels of physical fitness in each individual patient. Furthermore, the prognostic value of the NYHA classification may be influenced by the underlying severity of ventricular dysfunction. Therefore, given the major, established prognostic importance of left ventricular EF and the increasive availability of techniques for its estimation, the NYHA classification should be applied in association with the post-MI left ventricular EF classification (i.e. class 1: 50% or greater, class 2: 40–49%, class 3: 25–39%, and class 4: below 25%—see Ch. 22). In addition, the need for diuretic therapy may be useful to further subdivide patients in NYHA classes II and III, as fluid retention is an easily recognizable clinical marker of neurohumoral activation, which seems to have additional prognostic implications above those provided by left ventricular EF.

Patients in NYHA class II not requiring diuretic therapy should be reclassified as class IIA, as by definition they do not have chronic cardiac failure. Those requiring chronic diuretic therapy in order to remain in class II should be reclassified as class IIB. (The grad-

Table 23.1 Classification of patients with postischemic cardiac failure

Left ventricular EF classification*	NYHA classification†
2 3 4	IIB: Slight limitation of physical activity: patients are comfortable at rest. Ordinary physical activity results in fatigue, palpitation or dyspnea. No signs of cardiac failure on diuretics
2 3 4	IIIA: Marked limitation of physical activity: although patients are comfortable at rest, less than ordinary activity will lead to symptoms. No signs of cardiac failure on diuretics
2 3 4	IIIB: Marked limitation of physical activity: although patients are comfortable at rest, less than ordinary activity will lead to symptoms. Persisting signs of cardiac failure on diuretics
2 3 4	IV: Inability to carry out any physical activity without discomfort; symptoms of congestive failure are present even at rest. With any physical activity, increased discomfort is experienced

* Patients in EF class 1 do not have sufficient cardiac dysfunction to present chronic postischemic cardiac failure and those in EF class 2 are very unlikely to be in NYHA class IV

† Patients in NYHA class II are unlikely not to respond to diuretic therapy; those in class IV have signs of failure in spite of diuretics

This classification complements the NYHA classification by specifying a patient's post-MI EF classification and the need for diuretic therapy in NYHA class II patients (A = no signs of failure, B = signs of failure in the absence of diuretic therapy) and the response to diuretic therapy in NYHA class III patients (A = disappearance of symptoms of failure on diuretic therapy, B = persistence of symptoms in spite of diuretic therapy). Based on this detailed baseline subdivision, prospective studies are required to define more precisely survival and response to therapeutic intervention, as well as the prognostic value of indices of chronic myocardial vulnerability to arrhythmias such as premature ventricular contractions, heart rate variability, after-potentials, QT prolongation and electrophysiologic studies

ual interruption of diuretic therapy is justified when the failure had been precipitated by an acute corrected cause.)

Patients in NYHA class III generally require diuretic therapy. Those presenting no signs of fluid accumulation in the lungs (see 23.2.1) and no signs of congestive failure as a result of treatment, should be reclassified as class IIIA. Those with persisting signs of failure, in spite of adequate diuretic therapy, should be reclassified as class IIIB.

Therefore, post-MI patients with chronic heart failure should be classified according to the value of postdischarge left ventricular EF, the NYHA classification, and the need for diuretic therapy (see Table 23.1).

For example, a patient with an EF of 24% not taking diuretics and having only a slight limitation of physical activity during ordinary daily life should be classified as class 4–NYHA IIA; a patient with an EF of 35% on diuretics with marked limitation of physical activity during ordinary daily life but with no signs of fluid accumulation should be classified as class 3–NYHA IIIA; finally, a patient with an EF of 20% but unable to carry out any physical activity without suffering discomfort should be classified as class 4–NYHA IV.

Prospective multicentric data collection according to standardized questionnaires is required to assess the prognostic value of this combined classification, compared with those based exclusively on left ventricular EF or exclusively on the NYHA classification.

23.2 DIAGNOSIS, PROGNOSIS, AND THERAPEUTIC GUIDELINES

Diagnosis requires evidence of both cardiac failure and the loss of a critical mass of myocardium as a result of postischemic necrosis. Currently available information on prognosis indicates that the presence of failure has an incremental prognostic value above that conferred by the reduction in the value of EF. Therapy can produce a considerable improvement in symptoms and short-term prognosis, but improvement of long-term prognosis should be based on prevention.

23.2.1 Diagnostic assessment

In patients with a previous history of MI, the demonstration of cardiac failure is the main diagnostic problem. Conversely, in patients with obvious signs of failure but no previous history of MI, the demonstration of an ischemic origin (as opposed to other forms of cardiomyopathy) is the main diagnostic problem. Evaluation of the severity of ventricular dysfunction and of its potentially treatable components is essential for the prognostic assessment and the definition of therapeutic strategy.

Demonstration of cardiac failure

Chronic cardiac failure is rare in patients with an EF between 40 and 49% (class 2). It may occur in patients with an EF of 39–25% (class 3) and is usually present in most patients with an EF less than 25% (class 4). As discussed above, the severity of the signs of failure and the NYHA classification are often, but not always, related to the reduction in the value of left ventricular EF.

Chronic left ventricular cardiac failure. Shortness of breath and, sometimes, cough are common symptoms, but they are fairly nonspecific and, although useful for alerting the patient and physician, should not be interpreted as being due to left ventricular failure and treated as such without confirmatory objective evidence on physical examination. The significance of moist rales should also be confirmed by the finding of an S_3 or S_4 and, whenever possible, either by their disappearance or improvement with diuretic therapy or by signs of interstitial fluid accumulation and upper lobe flow diversion on chest radiography.

Congestive cardiac failure. Diagnosis is based on the combination of raised jugular venous pressure (assessed from the level at which the jugular veins are distended when the supine patient is propped up gradually on pillows to an angle of 45 degrees), hepatomegaly, bilateral ankle edema and increased body weight due to fluid retention (usually at least 3 kg). These signs usually develop in patients with severe left ventricular dysfunction, but may also be the most obvious clinical signs in patients in whom MI involved a large segment of the right ventricle. Signs of congestive failure also disappear or improve and body weight decreases following adequate diuretic therapy.

Demonstration of the postischemic origin of failure

This can pose a problem in patients presenting with obvious signs of failure but with no clear history of MI. The subsequent diagnosis is easy when the resting ECG shows unequivocal signs of a large MI and when echocardiography or ventriculography document akinesia or dyskinesia in the corresponding segment of ventricular wall, with good contraction of the unaffected segments. A postischemic origin cannot be established easily when no segmental abnormalities of motion of the left ventricular wall can be demonstrated, and is unlikely when right ventricular dilation and hypokinesia are out of proportion to those of the left ventricle.

The finding of flow-limiting stenoses at coronary arteriography does not necessarily provide diagnostic evidence as, on the one hand, a proximal occlusion leading to a large MI may recanalize and leave no significant stenosis and, on the other, the presence of coronary stenoses is not, in itself, proof that they were the cause of failure, because idiopathic cardiomyopathy is also a common cause of cardiac failure and the two conditions may coexist in the same patient. This possibility is suggested by a global hypokinesis of the left and right ventricles.

Initial assessment of the severity of impaired ventricular function

A reference baseline assessment of each patient's cardiovascular condition is required when they are in a chronic stable phase. At baseline and during each follow-up visit, body weight, heart rate, blood pressure and jugular venous pressure should be measured and recorded. The presence of S_3 or S_4 signs of mitral and tricuspid regurgitation should also be specifically sought. Baseline information should include standard chest radiography in posteroanterior and lateral projections and a quantitative echocardiogram providing at least semiquantitative measurements of left ventricular EF and of the four chambers.

This objective baseline information is necessary in order to detect the subclinical evolutive tendency of cardiac dysfunction over the following months and years and should be systematically correlated with symptoms, levels of effort tolerance, body weight, and physical signs. Worsening symptoms, with cardiovascular findings unchanged from baseline, suggest noncardiovascular causes.

Periodic reassessment

Patients should be reassessed every 3–6 months if symptoms remain stable and if failure is mild, and more frequently when failure is severe. All patients should keep a chart of their body weight and report back whenever their weight increases steadily over a period of a few days.

Whenever patients with predominantly left-sided failure deteriorate they should be promptly reassessed clinically and with chest radiography, watching for changes in body weight, physical signs of failure, upper lobe lung flow diversion, interstitial fluid accumulation in the lungs, and further cardiac enlargement. A repeated echocardiographic study is desirable in order to assess changes in the size of the cardiac chambers and in values of left ventricular EF.

For patients with congestive cardiac failure, changes in body weight are a fundamental element when assessing objectively changes in cardiac function and in the response to diuretic therapy. Excessive fluid depletion may cause a critical reduction in ventricular filling pressure, in stroke volume (SV), and in cardiac output with consequent symptoms of severe fatigue (see 23.2.3).

■ *Sequential changes during follow-up should be systematically noted in order to evaluate trends. Whenever possible, the patient should be seen by the same physician or team and assessed in the same noninvasive laboratory, comparing the results of the latest tests with those obtained previously.* ■

Assessment of potentially treatable conditions

Further assessment should focus on the possible existence of noncardiovascular or potentially treatable cardiovascular conditions that are responsible for, or contribute to, chronic cardiac failure.

Noncardiovascular causes. Infections are the most common cause of worsening signs of cardiac failure, chest infections in particular for chronic left ventricular failure. Fever, increased sedimentation rates, and cough with yellowish-green sputum are suggestive of a chest infection. Conditions that increase the work load of the heart, such as anemia, hyperthyroidism, or excessive physical activity, may exacerbate heart failure.

Arrhythmias. The onset of atrial fibrillation can exacerbate heart failure because of both the loss of atrial contribution to diastolic filling and the variable diastolic periods.

Acute ischemia. Acute ischemic episodes, painful or painless, can cause a sudden worsening of failure. The diagnosis has important practical implications, as increased diuretic therapy need not be continued after acute fluid retention has been eliminated and body weight returned to the baseline level. When ischemic episodes are painless, the diagnosis can be inferred only by the exclusion of noncardiac causes and of other acute cardiac causes such as arrhythmias and acute hypertension. Prevention of acute episodes of worsening heart failure caused by ischemia requires the elimination of ischemic episodes rather than the intensification of diuretic therapy.

Systemic hypertension. Neither diastolic nor systolic hypertension are well tolerated by a dilated, dysfunctional left ventricle because the wall tension required to generate a given pressure is increased and the wall stress at the borders of the infarcted segment is abnormally distributed. Control of diastolic and systolic hypertension and reduction of impedance to left ventricular ejection may prevent the exacerbation of cardiac failure and limit the progressive deterioration of left ventricular function; moreover, acute episodes of hypertension can cause rapidly worsening cardiac failure that could be prevented by better control of hypertension.

Mitral regurgitation and reversible hypocontractility. The search for contributory causes of chronic cardiac failure is particularly important for patients in whom signs of failure are disproportionate to the size of MI, as assessed from increased concentrations of CK during the acute phase and from extension of Q waves on the ECG. Whenever there is a suspicion that the extent of cardiac failure is disproportionate to the estimated extent of myocardial necrosis, it is appropriate that tests are performed in order to establish whether mitral regurgitation (not detectable clinically) or potentially reversible myocardial hypocontractility (see Ch. 22) are contributing to left ventricular failure.

23.2.2 Prognostic assessment

In the Framingham study the clinical diagnosis of heart failure was associated with mortality rates of 40 and 30% in men and women, respectively, at 2 years, and with mortality rates of 80 and 60%, respectively, at 8 years.[24] Mortality rates increase very steeply with the severity of the NYHA functional classification, both in unselected patients with mixed causes of heart failure and in selected patients with heart failure after acute MI. The increase in post-MI mortality associated with the presence of failure is additive to that associated with the reduction of left ventricular EF, but no precise data are yet available on the specific mortality of patients in each class 1–4 after MI (as determined by their EF) according to their NYHA functional classification and to the need for diuretic therapy.

Mortality and NYHA classification

Mortality rates increase several-fold in class IV patients compared with those in classes II and III.

In unselected patients in NYHA classes II and III included in the placebo control arm of the SOLVD-I trial[25] and the Vasodilator–Heart Failure Trial-I (V-HeFT),[26] with average left ventricular EF values of 25 and 29%, respectively, annual mortality was 11.6 and 15.2%, respectively, but reached 52% in patients in class IV enrolled in the CONSENSUS trial.[27]

Mortality, left ventricular EF, and neurohumoral activation

In patients with cardiac failure, mortality is about double that of those without failure, even when the average values of left ventricular EF are similar.

In the prevention arm of the SOLVD trial,[28] mortality in patients without failure was 5.1% per year whereas in those with failure enrolled in the treatment arm[25] it was 11.6% per year, although the values of left ventricular EF were respectively, 28 and 25%. Mortality in patients without failure in the prevention arm of the SOLVD trial was similar to that observed in the control arm of the Survival and Ventricular Enlargement (SAVE) study of asymptomatic postacute MI patients with an EF less than 40% (7.0%).[29] The incidence of unstable angina and reinfarction was only slightly higher in the SOLVD-I[25] (patients with signs of failure) than in the SOLVD-II[28] (asymptomatic patients) trials (see Ch. 22). Thus, the increased rate of mortality in patients with signs of failure must be due largely to primary arrhythmias and/or to an unfavorable cardiac response to new ischemic insults.

These observations lend support to the view that neurohumoral activation can be deleterious to the long-term outcome of patients with heart failure,[22,30] rather than being merely a marker of the severity of cardiac dysfunction.[31]

Conclusions

The reduction of left ventricular EF, the degree of limitation of effort tolerance indicated by the NYHA classification, and the presence of cardiac failure are the main determinants of prognosis in patients with chronic postischemic cardiac failure. Within each subgroup defined by the NYHA classification, by the presence of cardiac failure, and by the EF value, the extent to which prognosis is modulated by the presence of ventricular arrhythmias is not precisely known. The relative prognostic importance of each component is influenced strongly not only by its prevalence and range of variation but also by the prevalence and range of variation of the other determinants of prognosis in the population studied.

23.2.3 Therapeutic guidelines

Patients with chronic postischemic cardiac failure require intensive therapy, not only because they are symptomatic but also because mortality increases with the limitation of functional capacity as they progress from NYHA class II to class IV.

Correction of the neurohumoral activation can improve symptoms and prognosis, and correction of physical deconditioning can improve effort tolerance. However, only by improving cardiac pump function can the fatal outcome of the syndrome be prevented.

The immediate benefits of some treatments, such as diuretic therapy on fluid retention and vasodilator and inotropic drugs on intracardiac pressures and volumes, are easily demonstrable, but reliable information on the long-term effects of therapy on prognosis can be derived only from prospective randomized clinical trials.

Results of randomized trials

Several drugs have been shown to cause a significant reduction in mortality over follow-up periods ranging from 6 to 36 months and, as expected, the most significant reduction in mortality occurred in patients with a poor prognosis and with the highest baseline mortality in the control groups (see Fig. 23.1).

Survival benefits were observed for some vasodilator drugs and demonstrated repeatedly for angiotensin-converting enzyme (ACE) inhibitors, but not for digitalis and β-blockers. The increased life expectancy of patients saved during follow-up is not known. Treatments that reduced mortality also improved symptoms and reduced hospitalization rates.

Vasodilator drugs. A significant reduction in long-term mortality was first demonstrated in a mixed group of patients with moderately severe heart failure treated with a combination of hydralazine and isosorbide dinitrate (ISDN), compared with those treated with prazosin, an α-adrenergic blocking drug, or placebo. The reasons for the lack of beneficial effect of prazosin, which was the only treatment that actually lowered systemic blood pressure, are unknown.[26]

The long-term effect of nitrates on prognosis are not clearly established,[32,33] although their short-term beneficial effects (as long as the development of tolerance can be avoided)

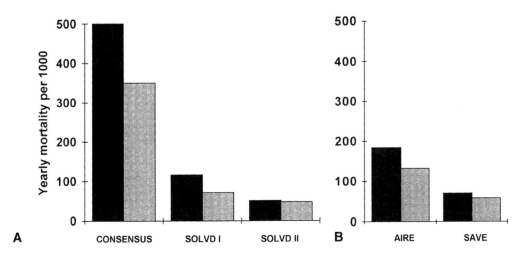

Fig. 23.1 Number of lives saved by treatment with ACE inhibitors is proportional to the severity of disease. In unselected patients (A), and in post-MI patients (B), the total number of lives saved was related to the baseline risk and was highest in patients in NYHA class IV included in the Cooperative North Scandinavian Enalapril Survival Study (CONSENSUS)-I trial (▇, mortality in treated group; ▇, mortality in the control group; SOLVD, Studies of Left Ventricular Dysfunction; AIRE, Acute Infarction Ramipril Efficacy; SAVE, Survival and Ventricular Enlargement). (Modified from data in refs 25, 27–29, and 38.)

have been documented convincingly.[34] The failure of nitrates to influence 6-week survival in the unselected post-MI patients with an average low risk, enrolled in the GISSI-3[35] and International Study of Infarct Survival (ISIS) 4[36] studies, may be related to the dilution effect introduced by very large numbers of patients with good ventricular function. These studies do not, therefore, exclude benefits from long-term treatment in selected patients with failure, in whom possible benefits would be more easily detectable because of their greater absolute baseline risk.

ACE inhibitors. In an unselected group of patients with multiple causes of failure in NYHA class IV, a significant reduction in mortality was demonstrated by the CONSENSUS trial[27] and in a mixed group of patients with cardiac failure in NYHA classes II and III by the SOLVD-I trial.[25] No survival benefits were observed in the prevention arm of the same study (SOLVD-II) in patients with a left ventricular EF less than 35% but no signs of failure,[28] or in the CONSENSUS-II trial.[37]

In a selected group comprising only postacute MI patients with signs of cardiac failure enrolled in the Acute Infarction Ramipril Efficacy (AIRE) study,[38] ramipril caused a significant reduction of mortality over a follow-up period of 15 months; however, a significant reduction of mortality was also produced by captopril in the SAVE study,[29] which included only post-MI asymptomatic patients with an EF less than 40%. The reduction of reinfarction observed in the SOLVD-I and II trials[39] suggests that at least part of the reduction in the late mortality in post-MI patients was due to a decreased incidence of reinfarction. The prevalence of this mechanism is expected to be higher in the SAVE trial, in which only post-MI patients were enrolled.

In treatment studies in patients following acute MI with a reduced EF and signs of failure, ACE inhibitors significantly reduced symptoms and hospitalization rates for heart failure, and in prevention studies they reduced the development of heart failure (as well as of MI and unstable angina—see Ch. 22). The results of a comparison between enalapril and the combination of hydralazine and ISDN in patients with a mean EF of 28% in NYHA classes II and III showed a 28% reduction in mortality in patients treated with the ACE inhibitor.[40]

Digitalis and other inotropic agents. Although the role of inotropic agents in acute heart failure is undisputed, that in patients with chronic stable heart failure is still unknown. Thus, the role of digitalis in the long-term treatment of patients with postischemic cardiac failure is still debated.[41] The conflicting findings probably reflect heterogeneous groups of patients with differing causes and differing degrees of severity of heart failure, and a wide range of doses, some too high, some too low. The increased mortality observed in post-MI patients on digoxin[42] was not confirmed in subsequent studies.[43] Double-blind randomized placebo controlled trials have shown that digoxin is superior to placebo in improving left ventricular EF, that it increases exercise capacity, and that it prevents the worsening of heart failure.[43-46] Discontinuation of digoxin in stable patients receiving constant doses of diuretics and ACE inhibitors was followed by a decrease in exercise tolerance, in values of EF, and in cardiac dilation.[47] The additional beneficial effects of digoxin over that of ACE inhibitors is currently being assessed in a large trial. It is hoped that such a study will provide clinically useful indications on which specific types of patients are likely to benefit from the addition of digoxin.

The chronic use of phosphodiesterase inhibitors and also intermittent home infusion of dobutamine were shown to increase mortality rates compared with placebo, largely owing to fatal arrhythmias.[48-50] Thus, in unselected patients with heart failure, the assumption that the long-term improvement of myocardial contractility would improve survival was not substantiated by clinical trials,[51-53] but these negative findings do not exclude the possibility that some specific types of patient at specific stages of their disease may benefit from some inotropic support.

Prevention of arrhythmias. Although the presence of arrhythmias is associated with increased mortality, the beneficial effects of antiarrhythmic drug therapy seems proven for amiodarone and for drugs selected on the basis of electrophysiologic studies, whereas Class I antiarrhythmic drugs were shown actually to increase mortality (see Ch. 22). Amiodarone, shown to reduce mortality in post-MI patients (see Ch. 22), is the drug of first choice for NYHA class IV patients because of their very poor prognosis, as its side effects do not usually appear before 6 months of continuous therapy. In patients with malignant ventricular arrhythmias, mortality can be reduced by implantable defibrillators, but the resulting increase in life expectancy in high-risk patients has yet to be assessed (see Ch. 24).

β-Blockers. In patients with heart failure, β-blockers were shown to improve their functional classification, exercise tolerance, and EF[54,55] in association with a trend toward reduced mortality.[56,57] However, these trials included only limited numbers of patients and clinical recommendations must await the results of appropriate large studies on carefully defined homogeneous groups of patients.

Prevention of worsening left ventricular dysfunction. The large reduction of mortality in class IV patients treated with ACE inhibitors is unlikely to increase life expectancy considerably, because of the severity of the underlying ventricular dysfunction; prevention of left ventricular dysfunction is, therefore, the most desirable goal. The reduced incidence of heart failure in prevention trials suggests a possible beneficial preventative effect of ACE inhibitors, possibly resulting from their effect on left ventricular remodeling (see Ch. 22). However, a better understanding of the determinants of progression of ventricular dysfunction and of the triggers of neurohumoral activation is necessary in order to develop more specifically targeted preventive treatments.

Physical activity. In acute heart failure, physical activity must be kept to a minimum, but congestive heart failure is also often considered to be an absolute contraindication to exercise or rehabilitation programs.[58] In chronic stable patients there is no evidence to justify this belief; on the contrary, such patients may benefit from an appropriate cardiac rehabilitation program because even a small increase in exercise performance may have a profound beneficial effect on the quality of life of these severely limited patients.[59] In a small but well-controlled study, a low-level home-based bicycle training program lasting 8 weeks improved effort tolerance in a group of patients with chronic postischemic heart failure and an average EF of 19%.[60] Although large clinical trials are necessary in order to evaluate the practical feasibility and actual benefits to be gained by formal rehabilitation training programs, the evidence available suggests that stable patients in NYHA classes III and IV should not be ordered to reduce their daily physical activities unnecessarily, as this may contribute to their further rapid deconditioning.

Management of symptoms

In addition to ACE inhibitors and vasodilator therapy shown to improve prognosis, patients should be treated with drugs that contribute to the improvement of both symptoms and the quality of life according to each individual patient's response. Diuretics are, by definition, the cornerstone of symptomatic therapy. Chlorothiazide and derivatives in mild cases, and loop diuretics (such as furosemide and ethacrynic acid) in more severe cases, should be combined with potassium-sparing diuretics such as aldosterone antagonists or direct inhibitors of collecting-duct sodium conductance (such as amiloride or triamterene) whenever plasma potassium levels decrease below 4.0 mEq/L.

The response to chronic diuretic therapy should be judged on the changes that occur in body weight as well as on the basis of improved symptoms, physical signs, and results of tests.

In patients in whom excessive fluid retention has been totally eliminated, the chronic maintenance dose of diuretics should be the lowest sufficient to maintain the "dry" weight reached at the end of the initial intensive phase. In patients in whom additional drug therapy is not strictly required by the inadequate response to diuretic therapy, the benefits should be judged on the basis of the improvement in symptoms obtained in each patient.

In patients with persisting excess fluid retention in spite of intense diuretic therapy, or in those in whom maximal fluid depletion is associated with the exacerbation of symptoms of severe fatigue, there is an obvious need to increase the doses of nitrates (up to 60 mg ISDN early in the morning and at lunch time) or transdermal nitroglycerin patches (up to 60 mg from early morning to evening) in order to reduce preload during the most active periods of the day and to introduce digoxin (in doses that achieve plasma levels of about 1.5 ng/ml).

Patients should be instructed to keep a weight chart recording the results of measurements taken in the morning in standardized conditions; every day for patients in classes IV and IIIB and at least twice a week for those in classes IIIA and IIB. Diuretic therapy should be increased whenever symptoms, physical signs, and results of tests worsen as body weight increases steadily by 1–2 kg in successive measurements.

Some patients in classes III or IV, when adequately treated with diuretics, may present with severe fatigue as their chief complaint (owing to chronic reduction of cardiac output and peripheral hypoperfusion) rather than with dyspnea.

When low cardiac output occurs in the presence of a reasonably preserved left ventricular function but is associated with severe impairment of the right ventricle caused by MI, intensive diuretic therapy may cause a decrease in right ventricular filling pressure and a fall in SV, with corresponding chronic peripheral hypoperfusion and severe fatigue. These patients may feel better if the fluid retention is not eliminated completely.

When the low cardiac output is due to very severe left ventricular dysfunction, the elevated left ventricular filling pressure required to maintain SV causes pulmonary venous congestion and dyspnea, but the reduction of left ventricular filling pressure required to reduce dyspnea may cause a fall in SV, a reduced cardiac output, and severe fatigue; a greater reduction of afterload and inotropic drugs are, therefore, the only available options.

In stable patients with severe symptoms, the response to the addition of new drugs and to changes in doses can usually be judged from both physical signs and test results. Subjective assessment of the patient's quality of life should be evaluated carefully in order to separate the components related to the actual inadequacy of the circulatory function from those related to the psychological depression commonly associated with the condition.

Conclusions

The results of the clinical prospective, placebo-controlled randomized studies reported above suggest that ACE inhibitors should be considered for all patients with postischemic cardiac failure. The greatest absolute beneficial effect (i.e. the number of lives saved per number of patients treated per year) is to be expected in patients in class IV during the initial 6 months of therapy. Patients not eligible for, or intolerant of, ACE inhibitors should be treated with a combination of hydralazine and ISDN. The smallest absolute benefit in terms of mortality is to be expected in patients with no signs of failure, as they are at a much lower risk (see Ch. 22). Treatment should be continued indefinitely, as the improvement in survival achieved during the initial 6 months in class IV patients was maintained to 1 year and the benefit increased progressively up to 12–18 months in patients in NYHA classes II and III.

Nitrates, β-blockers, and digoxin, for which no convincing effects on prognosis are yet available, should be used only in those patients in whom they appear to improve symptoms. Phosphodiesterase inhibitors should not be used as they increase mortality rates. Patients in classes III and IV should be encouraged to perform low-level physical activity appropriate to their condition in order to avoid physical deconditioning.

REFERENCES

1. Ghali JK, Cooper R, Fort E. Trends in hospitalization rates for heart failure in the United States, 1973–1986: evidence for increasing population prevalence. Arch Intern Med 1990;150:769.
2. Ho KKL, Pinski JL, Kannel WB, Levy D. The epidemiology of heart failure: the Framingham Study. J Am Coll Cardiol 1993;22(Suppl A):6A.
3. Teerlink JR, Godhaber SZ, Pfeffer MA. An overview of contemporary etiologies of congestive heart failure. Am Heart J 1991;121:1852.
4. Remes J, Miettinen H, Reunamen A, Pyorala K. Validity of clinical diagnosis, mortality and morbidity and related factors in Finland. Eur Heart J 1991;12:315.
5. Gruppo Italiano per lo Studio della Sopravvivenza nell'Infarto Miocardico (GISSI)-2 Data Base. Determinants of 6-month mortality in survivors of myocardial infarction after thrombolysis. Results of the GISSI-2 data base. Circulation 1993;88:416.
6. Olivetti G, Melissari M, Capasso JM, Anversa P. Cardiomyopathy of the ageing human heart. Myocyte loss and reactive cellular hypertrophy. Circ Res 1991;68:1560.
7. Gaudron P, Eilles C, Kugler I, Ertl G. Progressive left ventricular dysfunction and remodeling after myocardial infarction. Potential mechanisms and early predictors. Circulation 1993;87:755.

8. Schuster EH, Bulkley BH. Ischemic cardiomyopathy: a clinicopathologic study of fourteen patients. Am Heart J 1980;*100:*506.

9. White HD, Norris RM, Brown MA, Brandt PWT, Whitlock RML, Wild CJ. Left ventricular end-systolic volume as the major determinant of survival after recovery from myocardial infarction. Circulation 1987;*76:*44.

10. Viquerat CE, Daly P, Swedberg K et al. Endogenous catecholamine levels in chronic heart failure: relation to the severity of hemodynamic abnormalities. Am J Med 1985;*78:*455.

11. Kluger J, Cody RJ, Laragh JH. The contributions of sympathetic tone and the renin angiotensin system to severe chronic congestive heart failure: response to specific inhibitors (prazosin and captopril). Am J Cardiol 1982;*49:*1667.

12. Kubo SH. Neurohormonal activation and the response to converting enzyme inhibitors in congestive heart failure. Circulation 1990;*81 (Suppl. III):*107.

13. Cody RJ, Laragh JH. The renin angiotensin aldosterone system in chronic heart failure: pathophysiology and implications for treatment. In: Cohn JN (ed) Drug Treatment of Heart Failure. Secaucus, New Jersey: Adv Ther Comm Int, 1988:*79.*

14. Laragh JH. Atrial natriuretic hormone, the renin–aldosterone axis and blood pressure–electrolyte homeostasis. N Engl J Med 1985;*313:*1330.

15. Schrier RW. Pathogenesis of sodium and water retention in high-output and low-output cardiac failure, nephrotic syndrome, cirrhosis, and pregnancy. N Engl J Med 1988;*319:*1065.

16. Kubo SH, Rector TS, Bank AJ, Williams RE, Heifetz SM. Endothelium-dependent vasodilation is attenuated in patients with heart failure. Circulation 1991;*84:*1589.

17. Cody RJ, Haas GJ, Binkley PF, Capers Q, Kelley R. Plasma endothelin correlates with the extent of pulmonary hypertension in patients with chronic congestive heart failure. Circulation 1992;*85:*504.

18. Stewart DJ, Cernacek P, Costello KB, Rouleau JL. Elevated endothelin-1 heart failure and loss of normal response to postural change. Circulation 1992;*85:*510.

19. McMurray JJ, Ray SG, Abdullah I, Dargie HJ, Morton JJ. Plasma endothelin in chronic heart failure. Circulation 1992;*85:*1374.

20. Mancini DM, Walter G, Reichek N et al. Contribution of skeletal muscle atrophy to exercise intolerance and altered muscle metabolism in heart failure. Circulation 1992;*85:*1364.

21. Swedberg K, Eneroth P, Kjekshus J, Wilhelmsen L for the CONSENSUS Trial Study Group. Hormones regulating cardiovascular function in patients with severe congestive heart failure and their relation to mortality. Circulation 1990;*82:*1730.

22. Francis GS, Benedict C, Johnstone DE et al, for the SOLVD Investigators. Comparison of neuroendocrine activation in patients with left ventricular dysfunction with and without congestive heart failure. A substudy of the Studies of Left Ventricular Dysfunction (SOLVD). Circulation 1990;*82:*1724.

23. The Criteria Committee of the New York Heart Association: Diseases of the Heart and Blood Vessels; Nomenclature and Criteria for Diagnosis. 6th edition. Little, Brown and Co., Boston, 1964.

24. Ho KKL, Anderson KM, Kannel WB, Grossman W, Levy D. Survival after the onset of congestive heart failure in Framingham Heart Study Subjects. Circulation 1993;*88:*107.

25. The SOLVD Investigators. Effect of enalapril vs survival in patients with reduced left ventricular ejection fractions and congestive heart failure. N Engl J Med 1991;*325:*293.

26. Cohn JN, Archibald DG, Ziesche S et al. Effect of vasodilator therapy on mortality in chronic congestive heart failure: Results of a Veterans Administration Cooperative Study. N Engl J Med 1986;*314:*1547.

27. The CONSENSUS Trial Study Group. Effects of enalapril on mortality in severe congestive heart failure: results of the Cooperative North Scandinavian Enalapril Survival Study. N Engl J Med 1987;*316:*1429.

28. The SOLVD Investigators. Effect of enalapril on mortality and the development of heart failure in asymptomatic patients with reduced left ventricular ejection fractions. N Engl J Med 1992;*327:*685.

29. Pfeffer MA, Braunwald E, Move LA et al on behalf of the SAVE Investigators. Effect of captopril

on mortality and morbidity in patients with left ventricular dysfunction after myocardial infarction. N Engl J Med 1992;*327*:669.

30. Swedberg K. Is neurohormonal activation deleterious to the long-term outcome of patients with heart failure? II. Protagonists' viewpoint. J Am Coll Cardiol 1988;*12*:550.

31. Cohn JN. Is neurohormonal activation deleterious to the long-term outcome of patients with heart failure? III. Antagonists' viewpoint. J Am Coll Cardiol 1988;*12*:554.

32. Cohn JN. Nitrates are effective in the treatment of chronic congestive heart failure: the protagonist's view. Am J Cardiol 1990;*66*:444.

33. Packer M. Are nitrates effective in the treatment of chronic heart failure? Antagonist's viewpoint. Am J Cardiol 1990;*66*:458.

34. Abrams J. Nitrates and nitrate tolerance in congestive heart failure. Cor Art Dis 1993;*4*:27.

35. Gruppo Italiano per lo Studio della Sopravvivenza nell-Infarto Miocardico (GISSI-3). Effects of lisinopril and transdermal glyceryl trinitrate singly and together on six-week mortality and ventricular function after acute myocardial infarction. Lancet 1994;*343*:1115.

36. ISIS-4 (Fourth International Study of Infarct Survival) Collaborative Group. A randomised factorial trial assessing early oral captopril, oral mononitrate, and intravenous magnesium sulphate in 58 050 patients with suspected acute myocardial infarction. Lancet 1995;*345*:669.

37. Swedberg K, Held P, Kjekshus J et al on behalf of the CONSENSUS II Study Group. Effects of the early administration of enalapril on mortality in patients with acute myocardial infarction. N Engl J Med 1992;*327*:678.

38. The Acute Infarction Ramipril Efficacy (AIRE) Study Investigators. Effect of ramipril on mortality and morbidity of survivors of acute myocardial infarction with clinical evidence of heart failure. Lancet 1993;*342*:821.

39. Yusuf S, Pepine JC, Garces C et al. Effect of enalapril on myocardial infarction and unstable angina in patients with low ejection fractions. Lancet 1992;*340*:1173.

40. Cohn JN, Johnson G, Ziesche S et al. A comparison of enalapril with hydralazine–isosorbide dinitrate in the treatment of chronic congestive heart failure. N Engl J Med 1991;*325*:303.

41. Jaeschke R, Oxman AD, Guyatt GH. To what extent do congestive heart failure patients in sinus rhythm benefit from digoxin therapy: a systematic overview and meta-analysis. Am J Med 1990;*88*:279.

42. Moss AJ, Davis HT, Conrad DL, DeCamilla KK, Odoroff CL. Digitalis-associated cardiac mortality after myocardial infarction. Circulation 1981;*64*:1150.

43. Smith JR, Gheorghiade M, Goldstein S. The current role of digoxin in the treatment of heart failure. Cor Art Dis 1993;*4*:16.

44. Lee DC-S, Johnson RA, Bingham JB et al. Heart failure in out-patients. A randomized trial of digoxin versus placebo. N Engl J Med 1982;*306*:699.

45. The Captopril–Digoxin Multicenter Research Group. Comparative effects of therapy with captopril and digoxin in patients with mild to moderate heart failure. J Am Med Assoc 1988;*259*:539.

46. The German and Austrian Xamoterol Study Group. Double-blind placebo-controlled comparison of digoxin and xamoterol in chronic heart failure. Lancet 1988;*I*:489.

47. Packer M, Gheorghiade M, Young JB et al. Withdrawal of digoxin from patients with chronic heart failure treated with converting-enzyme inhibitors. N Engl J Med 1993;*329*:1.

48. Packer M, Carver JR, Rodeheffer RJ et al. Effect of oral milrinone on mortality in severe chronic heart failure. N Engl J Med 1991;*325*:1468.

49. Uretsky BF, Jessup M, Konstam MA et al. Multicenter trial of oral enoximone in patients with moderate to moderately severe congestive heart failure: lack of benefit compared with placebo. Circulation 1990;*82*:774.

50. Dies F, Krell MJ, Whitlow P et al. Intermittent dobutamine in ambulatory outpatients with chronic cardiac failure (abstract). Circulation 1986;*74(Suppl. III)*:175.

51. Curfman GD. Inotropic therapy for heart failure—an unfulfilled promise (Editorial). N Engl J Med 1991;*325*:1509.

52. Katz AM. Potential deleterious effect of inotropic agents in the therapy of chronic heart failure. Circulation 1986;*73(Suppl. III)*:184.

53. Lejemtel TH, Sonnenblick EH. Should the failing heart be stimulated? (Editorial) N Engl J Med 1984;*310*:1384.

54. Waagstein F, Hjalmarson A, Varnauskas E, Wallentin I. Effect of chronic beta-adrenergic receptor blockade in congestive cardiomyopathy. Br Heart J 1975;*37:*1022.
55. Engelmeier RS, O'Connel JB, Walsh R, Rad N, Scanslon PJ, Gunnar RM. Improvement in symptoms and exercise tolerance by metoprolol in patients with dilated cardiomyopathy: a double-blind, randomized, placebo-controlled trial. Circulation 1985;*72:*536.
56. Swedberg K, Hjalmarson A, Waagstein F, Wallentin I. Prolongation of survival in congestive cardiomyopathy. Am J Cardiol 1985;*55:*471.
57. Anderson JL, Lutz JR, Gilbert EM et al. A randomized trial of low dose beta-blockade therapy for idiopathic dilated cardiomyopathy. Am J Cardiol 1985;*55:*471.
58. McHenry MM. Medical screening of patients with coronary heart disease: criteria for entry into exercise conditioning programs. Am J Cardiol 1974;*33:*752.
59. Sullivan MJ, Higginbotham MB, Cobb FR. Exercise training in patients with chronic heart failure delays ventilatory anaerobic threshold and improves submaximal exercise performance. Circulation 1989;*79:*324.
60. Coats AJS, Adamopoulos S, Meyer TE, Conway J, Sleight P. Effects of physical training in chronic heart failure. Lancet 1990;*335:*63.

Sudden ischemic cardiac death and fatal arrythmias

INTRODUCTION

Sudden ischemic cardiac death (SICD) is defined as unexpected, natural cardiac death occurring as a result of some of the consequences of either acute myocardial ischemia and necrosis or of postinfarction scarring, hypertrophy, and cardiac failure. The current definition of SICD is based on time from the onset of symptoms to death, and on some evidence of ischemic heart disease (IHD). Witnessed death within 1 h of the onset of symptoms has now become a standard definition for classifying sudden death in epidemiologic studies.[1]

In adults, SICD represents by far the largest proportion of cases of sudden death in the community; about 50% of cases occur in individuals without known IHD, and the other 50% occur in patients with known IHD, about 75% with a history of myocardial infarction (MI) and about 50% with a history of heart failure (see Ch. 13). The incidence of SICD increases markedly in the successive classes of the New York Heart Association (NYHA) functional classification of symptoms, but the percentage of cardiac deaths represented by SICD is, on average, about 50% in each of the four classes.[2] About 50% of patients with stable or unstable angina or with a history of MI die suddenly out of hospital. Furthermore, patients with acute MI dying within 1 h from the onset of symptoms are defined as having died from SICD. About 40% of patients resuscitated from cardiac arrest out of hospital deny any symptoms before the arrest, and about 30% of witnessed cases of sudden death in patients with a recent MI, occur instantaneously.[3]

The dramatic problem of SICD is seen from different angles by epidemiologists, pathologists, clinical investigators, and practising physicians.

Epidemiologists are interested in the description of the phenomenon and in its correlation with parameters and risk factors that can easily be assessed in population studies. The need to have sufficiently large numbers of cases for statistical analysis often leads to broad inclusion criteria: for example, patients with different ischemic syndromes can be considered with individuals with no known IHD, and patients presenting with severe continuous chest pain of 50 min duration (suggestive of acute MI) can be considered with patients dying suddenly in the absence of any preceding discomfort (suggestive of a primary arrhythmia).

Pathologists are interested in finding a plausible organic cause of death such as coronary flow-limiting stenosis, thrombosis, plaque fissure, myocardial necrosis, or post-MI scarring.

Thus, patients dying at the very onset of an acute MI but with no signs of either necrosis or flow-limiting stenosis, and those dying during a potentially reversible ischemic episode caused by occlusive coronary artery spasm but with no flow-limiting stenosis, would not be classified as SICD. When the clinical history and symptoms immediately preceding death are not carefully collated, individuals with continuous chest pain, suggestive of acute MI, can be considered with patients with variant angina and also with an old MI and a primary arrhythmia.

Clinical investigators are interested in the specific predisposing and precipitating mechanisms of the fatal event, but the prevalence of such mechanisms varies in each group of patients. For example, data obtained during Holter monitoring is often used to infer the incidence of ischemia-induced fatal arrhythmias, but nonischemia-related arrhythmias are the most likely cause of death in patients during Holter monitoring applied because of arrthymias. Conversely, patients with acute MI dying within the first few hours of the onset of chest pain probably die from acute necrosis-induced arrhythmias and those with variant angina probably die from arrhythmias induced by potentially reversible epicardial coronary artery spasm.

Practising physicians are interested in the specific risks and causes of SICD in the individual patients, with each of the specific clinical ischemic syndromes, encountered during the course of their practise. They need to know the likelihood of typical patients, with each syndrome, dying suddenly with no time to seek medical attention, and whether the risk is more likely to be reduced by the prevention of ischemic episodes, of MI, or of the development of primary malignant arrhythmias. They also need to know, for each specific type of patient, the reduction in life expectancy that may result from SICD.

This chapter defines the pathogenetic mechanisms, the diagnostic criteria, and a classification that would be useful for clinical identification of the risk and of the most prevalent causes of SICD in easily recognizable groups of patients. Finally, it outlines the general principles involved in the prevention of SICD in clinical practise.

24.1 PATHOGENETIC MECHANISMS, DIAGNOSIS, AND CLASSIFICATION

Sudden ischemic cardiac death is caused by an abrupt, irreversible disturbance of cardiac function that is incompatible with the maintenance of adequate cerebral blood flow. Unless the disturbance is reversed (either spontaneously or by cardiopulmonary resuscitation) within 2–6 min, irreversible brain damage occurs and biologic death follows. It can be preceded by prodromal nonspecific symptoms (such as dyspnea, palpitations, fatigue, and vital exhaustion) occurring over periods of days or weeks. In the vast majority of cases the sudden inability of the heart to maintain adequate cerebral blood flow is caused either by primary arrhythmias developing in the presence of postinfarction scarring but in the absence of acute ischemia or of necrosis, or by a fatal arrhythmia developing during acute myocardial ischemia or necrosis. In both cases, SICD is influenced to varying degrees by autonomic nervous system imbalance, and by neurohumoral activation associated with acute ischemia, necrosis, heart failure, or electrolyte disturbance.

Precise diagnosis of the actual cause of SICD is necessary in order to define the prevalence of its various predisposing and precipitating causes and the consequent reduction of life expectancy in each of the identifiable homogeneous groups of patients defined in 23.1.3.

24.1.1 Pathogenetic mechanisms of SICD

In individuals without known IHD and in patients with known IHD, the most common cause of SICD is cardiac arrest due to either ventricular tachycardia (VT) or ventricular fibrillation (VF), and, more rarely, to severe bradyarrhythmias. Less than 10% of cases are caused by SICD attributable to ischemia or MI causing hyperacute left ventricular cardiac failure, electromechanical dissociation, or cardiac rupture,[4] as they are usually preceded by symptoms persisting for periods longer than 1 h.

In cases of SICD examined at autopsy, the prevalence both of fresh thrombi, suggestive of acute ischemia, and of necrosis is much higher than the prevalence of acute ischemic ST-segment changes in patients suffering SICD during Holter monitoring, but is comparable to the prevalence of acute MI or persistent ST T-wave changes suggestive of severe ischemia in survivors resuscitated out of hospital. Most mural thrombi do not occlude the lumen completely.

Data from patients resuscitated from out-of-hospital cardiac arrest

An ischemic origin is the most common, transient ischemic episodes and acute MI occurring in about equal proportions. Ventricular tachyarrhythmias were found in most individuals successfully treated by a resuscitating team (VF in about 60% and VT in 10%). Ventricular bradyarrhythmias were found in the remaining 30%, mainly in patients with the most severe pre-existing left ventricular dysfunction.[3,5,6]

Holter recordings

Findings in patients dying suddenly during Holter monitoring reflect the bias introduced by the clinical indications for the test. In these patients, VF secondary to either VT (50%) or torsades de pointe (19%) and, less often, primary VF (12%), appear to be the major triggering mechanisms of SICD, with bradyarrhythmias accounting for only 20% of cases. Ischemic ST-segment depression prior to the onset of the fatal arrhythmia was rare (13%) and ST-segment elevation was exceptional.[5,6]

Postmortem findings

In unselected victims of SICD, autopsy findings are the same as those in unselected patients with IHD. Although most studies emphasize the very common finding of extensive, severe coronary atherosclerosis being the pathologic hallmark of SICD, all report also a small percentage of cases with mild or minimal coronary stenoses.[7] The degree of coronary atherosclerosis was found to be small in cases of SICD (with no known IHD) occurring within 1 h of the onset of symptoms[8] (see Chs. 8 and 9). In a classic study of sudden death within 6 h, Davies and Thomas exclude from their definition of SICD all cases with a less than 75% area stenosis.[9] They found plaque fissure in 90% of patients dying as a result of SICD; it was associated with large thrombi in over 40% of cases and with small mural thrombi in 30%. About 32% of large thrombi were located at the site of plaques and these reduced the lumen by less than 50% (30% diameter stenosis); 10% of mural thrombi had no plaque fissure. The rarity of *occlusive* thrombi suggests that thrombi may undergo rapid lysis, that coronary vasoconstriction may contribute to the fatal ischemic episode, or that platelet microemboli may precipitate the fatal arrhythmia. When caused by a primary arrhthymia, as opposed to an arrhythmia associated with ischemia or necrosis, SICD is more likely to occur in patients with old myocardial scarring and no evidence of recently formed coronary thrombi.[10]

Precipitating factors

There is increasing evidence that the most common causes of SICD (i.e. VT and VF) may result from a combination of acute or chronic myocardial alterations favoring the disorganization of the sequence of electric activation and multiple reentrant circuits, and premature ventricular impulses. Thus, frequent and complex premature ventricular contractions (PVCs) may be innocuous in the absence of myocardial vulnerability.

The distinction between an acute (ischemia or necrosis related) and chronic (scar related) myocardial arrhythmogenic substrate is important, because the former can be prevented by anti-ischemic therapy, whereas the latter requires specific antiarrhythmic therapy. The practical importance of this distinction is supported by the good long-term prognosis of patients who develop VF in the first few hours following an acute MI, and of survivors of cardiac arrest attributable to acute MI, compared with that of patients with late VF and with survivors of cardiac arrest with no evidence of acute MI. Both acute and chronic electric instability of the myocardium are enhanced by myocardial hypertrophy,[11] and modulated by neural, humoral, and hemodynamic factors that contribute both to the genesis of arrhythmias and to their fatal outcome (see Ch. 10).

Predisposing factors

The predisposing causes of the final event that leads to SICD are scarcely known. About 40% of patients dying suddenly out of hospital had consulted a doctor in the previous 4 weeks;[12] in less than 25% of cases this was because of angina, the usual cause being fatigue. A similar finding was reported in patients who had been resuscitated from cardiac arrest.[13-16]

Predictive value of tests

In low-risk patients the predictive accuracy of tests is low, according to the Bayesian theory. In high-risk patients a high predictive value was provided by heart failure, reduced ejection fraction (EF), prolongation of the QT interval, frequent PVCs (more than 10/h), reduced heart rate variability, and ventricular after-potentials, but most of these variables are interrelated and their interdependence and incremental pathogenetic roles need to be clearly established. For example, the presence of frequent PVCs was found to have an incremental predictive value above that provided by the reduction of left ventricular EF,[17] but the prevalence of PVCs could have been associated with heart failure.

24.1.2 Diagnosis

The diagnosis of SICD requires evidence of the presence of either acute ischemia or necrosis (which are the acute substrates for fatal arrhythmias and hyperacute cardiac failure), or of post-MI scarring (which is the chronic substrate for electric vulnerability). It also requires the exclusion of nonischemic causes of fatal arrhythmias and noncardiac causes.

The *clinical diagnosis* of SICD and of its ischemic or nonischemic nature can be established easily when death occurs suddenly soon after the onset of either ischemic cardiac pain or ischemic ST-segment changes during a Holter recording, or in patients with a history of MI and frequent malignant arrhythmias, or in patients with known IHD and a fatal arrhythmia not preceded by ischemic changes on a Holter recording. The diagnosis can be inferred in patients with known IHD who die instantaneously with no symptoms, but they may have suffered a primary fatal arrhythmia, a painless ischemic episode, or a painless MI.

The *postmortem diagnosis* in individuals dying suddenly can be made with certainty when a fresh MI or a fresh intracoronary thrombus is detected, but the diagnosis can only be inferred when old postinfarction scarring or chronic critical atherosclerotic obstructions are found. In witnessed deaths preceded by chest pain, lack of postmortem evidence does not exclude an ischemic cause, as ischemia may have been caused by an occlusive spasm or an occlusive thrombus that subsequently lysed, even in the absence of coronary flow-limiting stenosis or post-MI scarring.

The *differential diagnosis* should consider nonatherosclerotic and nonischemic causes of SICD, which can also be caused by coronary embolism, arteritis, or congenital malformations (i.e. not by coronary atherosclerosis). Conversely, sudden death may not necessarily be ischemic, even when occurring in the presence of coronary atherosclerosis, which is sufficiently common in individuals with no detectable evidence of myocardial ischemia.

The following principal diseases and disorders (other than myocardial ischemia) account for about 15% of cases of SICD in adults:

a.   myocardial alterations: cardiac failure, cardiomyopathies, myocarditis, myocardial hypertrophy
b.   valvular and endocardial alterations: aortic stenosis, endomyocardial fibrosis
c.   electrophysiologic alterations: electrolyte imbalance, drug treatment, Wolff–Parkinson–White syndrome, long QT syndrome, disease of the specific conduction system and complete A–V block
d.   miscellaneous: massive pulmonary embolism, aortic dissection
e.   in about 5% of cases, sudden death occurs in the absence of identifiable extra-cardiac causes and of heart disease detectable at autopsy.

Specific causes of SICD

For clinical purposes it would be important to establish in each subgroup of patients classified below, not only the frequency with which SICD is caused by VT, VF, or bradyarrhythmias related to either a chronic or an acute myocardial arrhythmogenic substrate, but also the contributory role of neurohumoral activation or altered concentrations of plasma electrolytes. It would also be useful to establish the value of specific markers of risk in each subgroup.

24.1.3 Clinical classification of SICD

The distinction of SICD in terms of time from onset of symptoms (instantaneous or within 1 h) is useful to physicians because only death occurring within 1 h could give patients sufficient time to seek medical assistance. Obviously, prevention strategies differ in patients at risk of primary VT and VF, or of bradyarrhythmias, and in those in whom the risk of SICD is predominantly related to the development of either new episodes of ischemia (as in patients with variant angina) or of necrosis.

A classification of out-of-hospital, unexpected SICD that would be useful for clinical practise should cover three aspects:

a.   the time of occurrence after the onset of symptoms
b.   the specific causes that should be prevented
c.   the clinical condition in which it may develop.

The time potentially available for patients to seek medical attention after the onset of symptoms is defined by the criteria of instantaneous death or death occurring within 1 h of the onset of symptoms.

The type of fatal event that should be prevented (see 21.1.2) is defined by the relative frequency of the following:

a.   anginal pain and its duration before cardiac arrest, indicative of acute ischemia or MI
b.   the frequency of primary VT or VF (in the absence of acute ischemia or necrosis)
c.   the presence of bradyarrhythmias or asystole.

Finally, the average risk in an individual patient with a given clinical ischemic syndrome is defined by the frequency with which SICD occurs in that syndrome.

The following clinical conditions can be recognized easily by any practising physician:

a.   no previously known IHD (see Ch. 13)
   • high levels of risk factors
   • normal levels of risk factors
b.   quiescent phase of IHD (see Ch. 10)
   • old MI (>6 months, EF ≥40% or <40%)
   • resolved unstable angina
   • resolved chronic stable angina
c.   chronic stable angina (see Ch. 17)
   • without previous MI
   • with previous MI (EF ≥40% or <40%)
d.   resolved unstable angina (see Ch. 19)
   • without previous MI
   • with previous MI (EF ≥40% or <40%)
e.   variant angina (see Ch. 20)
   • without flow-limiting coronary stenosis
   • with flow-limiting coronary stenosis
f.   recent MI (<6 months) (see Ch. 22)
   • EF ≥40%
   • EF <40%
g.   chronic postischemic cardiac failure (see Ch. 23)
   • EF ≥25–39% (plus NYHA classification)
   • EF <25% (plus NYHA classification).

In these groups, specific information concerning the most prevalent causes of SICD, the resulting reduction in life expectancy, and the predictive value of prognostic markers of SICD is scarce. Thus, appropriate prospective multicentric data collection in a common clinical database would be desirable.

24.2 ASSESSMENT OF RISK AND PREVENTION OF SICD

Although SICD is a most dramatic event, its occurrence in patients with chronic ischemic syndromes is rare in the absence of severe impairment of left ventricular function, signs of heart failure, or ventricular arrhythmias, and is even less frequent in individuals without known IHD (see Fig. 13.1).

On average, the risk of SICD is about half that of total IHD mortality, as in each ischemic syndrome about 50% of deaths are sudden. However, identification of the 50% who are likely to die suddenly is difficult, particularly in patients at low risk in whom the predictive accuracy of any test is low according to the Bayesian theory (see Fig. 16.2). In those at high risk of ischemic death the predictive accuracy of tests for SICD is higher but, in such patients, the further reduction of life expectancy caused by SICD is much smaller than in those at low risk because prognosis is determined largely by the severity of the underlying condition.[16]

24.2.1 Assessment of risk of SICD

The Framingham study showed that only about 50% of cases of sudden death in adults occurs within that 10% of the population with an identifiable risk, with a gradient for men from about 0.2% per year in the lowest decile of risk, to 6.5% per year in the upper decile, and from 0.04 to 3.0% for women.[2] The multivariate analysis that produced this remarkably wide gradient of risk largely reflects the relative statistical strength and prevalence of the multiple variables considered which, besides modifiable risk factors, included body weight and vital capacity as well as age (a nonmodifiable risk factor) and ECG abnormalities (possible signs of preexisting IHD). Thus, this stratification is more useful for identifying patients at risk than for assessing the importance of specific causal factors, that can be targeted by preventive strategies.

General predictors of SICD

Known risk factors are unable to distinguish between patients who will suffer SICD and those in whom other manifestations of IHD will occur, nor can angiography reveal which patients had previously been resuscitated from a cardiac arrest.[17] No information is available on risk factors for an acute myocardial arrhythmogenic background.

No precise information is available on the risk of SICD in patients who either have chronic stable angina or are in a quiescent phase of IHD, and the risk can be assessed only in the light of their overall prognosis (see Chs 13 and 17). In patients with chronic stable angina, SICD seems to be slightly less common than in patients who had suffered an MI, possibly because of the development of extensive collateral vessels.[18] In patients resuscitated from cardiac arrest, ventricular dysfunction and NYHA classification were stronger predictors of mortality than ventricular arrhythmias detected during Holter monitoring.[19]

Specific predictors of a chronic myocardial arrhythmogenic background

Most studies have concentrated on the detection of specific indicators of risk in patients after acute MI, but insufficient information is available on the time dependency of risk (see Ch. 13). The most significant findings are summarized below:

1. Primary VF in the very early phase of infarction is not associated with increased long-term risk. Conversely, the development of VT or VF outside the acute phase, and the appearance of intraventricular conduction defects or bundle branch block, are associated with a higher incidence of SICD, also when ventricular dysfunction is mild.

2. Specific types of arrhythmias carry a high risk of SICD. There is evidence that frequent or complex ventricular ectopics are associated with an independent increased risk of SICD. The risk is particularly great when such ectopics occur in

patients with severe impairment of ventricular function,[17] but it is not clear whether an additional risk is conferred by the presence of cardiac failure.

3. Late potentials in postinfarction patients are a reasonably sensitive indicator of the risk of SICD, but they have a low specificity, as about 50% of post-MI patients who present late potentials do not develop malignant ventricular arrhythmias or suffer SICD.[20,21]

4. Prolongation of the QT interval was reported to be associated with an increased incidence of SICD by some investigators,[22] but not by others.[23]

5. The induction of malignant ventricular arrhythmias during electrophysiologic studies by programed stimulation in unselected patients after MI does not appear to be a sufficiently valuable independent predictor of SICD, although it may help in the selection of antiarrhythmic drugs.[24-26]

The specific additional risk conferred by after-potentials, prolonged QT, and positive electrophysiologic studies, over and above the basal risk conferred by age, the severity of impairment of ventricular dysfunction, the presence of heart failure, and the spontaneous occurrence of arrhythmias, needs to be more precisely assessed in well-defined groups of patients (as indicated in 24.1.3).

24.2.2 General guidelines for the prevention of SICD

The notion that ventricular tachyarrhythmias are the most common cause of SICD, and its more frequent occurrence in patients presenting with arrhythmias, have led to the use of antiarrhythmic drugs in patients presenting with frequent PVCs. However, antiarrhythmic drug therapy may increase, rather than decrease, the risk of SICD. The Coronary Artery Surgery Study (CASS) showed a threefold increase in mortality rates following MI in patients with a mean left ventricular EF of 40% and frequent PVCs treated with encainide and flecainide.[27] Antiarrhythmic drugs should, therefore, be used only in those circumstances in which they have been shown to prolong survival.

In selected groups of patients with malignant ventricular arrhythmias, antiarrhythmic therapy was found to reduce the mortality rate. In these studies, drugs and doses were chosen and evaluated empirically on the basis of the acute response to the drug, electrophysiologic studies, and plasma levels. These studies, although uncontrolled, suggest that in some patients antiarrhythmic drugs are effective in preventing SICD.[28-30]

At present, however, it is not clear how patients can be distinguished: acute drug tests can be performed only in patients with frequent arrhythmias; electrophysiologic studies are too complex for routine use and their results are not always applicable to long-term therapy.[31] A recent report has suggested that the 1-year mortality rate in patients treated with metoprolol without electrophysiologic studies was similar to that of patients in whom antiarrhythmic therapy was chosen on the basis of electrophysiologic studies.[32]

Interventional therapy with implantable devices should be considered for patients who neither respond to nor tolerate full medical therapy and for those not eligible for cardiac surgery.[33] Evaluation of the reduction in mortality achievable by implantable defibrillators, in patients with no history of malignant arrhythmias but judged to be at high risk, is still in progress.

In patients *without* a clinically detectable chronic myocardial arrhythmogenic substrate (even after resuscitation from cardiac arrest), reduction of global IHD mortality according to the general strategies presented in Chapters 13, 17, 19, 20, and 22 remains the only available option until the mechanisms responsible for the development of fatal arrhythmias during acute ischemia or necrosis are eliminated and specific markers of risk are identified.[34] The average incidence of SICD during a 5-year follow-up study was 2% in surgically treated patients in the CASS study compared with 6% in the medically treated group. The difference was much larger in the subgroup at high risk (i.e. patients with triple vessel disease and a history of heart failure), than in that at low risk (i.e. those with single or double vessel disease and no history of heart failure).[35] However, treatments that reduce reinfarction may not reduce the incidence of SICD, as was observed in the Aspirin Myocardial Infarction study.[36]

In patients *with* a clinically detectable chronic myocardial arrhythmogenic substrate, in whom fatal arrhythmias may develop even in the absence of acute ischemia or necrosis (see 24.2.1), specific antiarrhythmic therapy is required. The therapeutic strategy should vary, not only according to whether they are in a subacute phase of IHD, have recently suffered a cardiac arrest (as their risk decreases progressively with time), or are in a chronic stable phase (in which case the risk is likely to remain constant in time), but also according to the estimated reduction in life expectancy caused by the underlying severity of the disease. In patients presenting with life-threatening arrhythmias in the early phases after MI or unstable angina, antiarrhythmic therapy may be required for only a few months as, subsequently, the risk decreases considerably. Patients with a very reduced life expectancy, such as those in class IV and, in general, those with a very low left ventricular EF, may require antiarrhythmic therapy for only short periods, as other causes of death are likely to supervene. Both groups of patients are, therefore, also eligible for drugs such as amiodarone, that have side effects only when used for long periods.[37,38]

Patients with a clinically detectable chronic myocardial arrhythmogenic substrate, but otherwise with a good short-term life expectancy, require long-term protection based on sustained antiarrhythmic drug therapy (empirical or guided by electrophysiologic studies), and on the use of implantable devices or cardiac surgical techniques. Until prospective randomized studies are performed on homogeneous groups of patients classified as indicated above, the choice between these options is influenced largely by the availability of electrophysiologic laboratories, of surgical expertise, and of the financial resources needed for implantable devices.

■ *Conclusive evidence concerning the increase in survival and life expectancy produced by pharmacologic and interventional antiarrhythmic treatment, can come only from the results of randomized controlled trials, conducted in carefully defined homogeneous groups of patients.* ■

REFERENCES

1. Goldstein S. The necessity of a uniform definition of sudden coronary death: witnessed death within 1 hour of the onset of acute symptoms. Am Heart J 1982;*103:*156.
2. Kannel WB, Thomas HE. Sudden coronary death: the Framingham study. Ann NY Acad Sci 1982;*382:*3.
3. Goldstein S, Landis JR, Leighton R et al. Characteristics of the resuscitated out-of-hospital cardiac arrest victim with coronary heart disease. Circulation 1981;*64:*977.
4. Hinkle LE, Thaler HT. Clinical classification of cardiac deaths. Circulation 1982;*65:*457.
5. Panidis IP, Morganroth J. Holter monitoring and sudden cardiac death. Cardiovasc Rev 1984;*5:*283.
6. Bayes de Luna A, Coumel P, Leclercq JF. Ambulatory sudden death: mechanisms of production of fatal arrhythmia on the basis of data from 157 cases. Am Heart J 1989;*117:*154.
7. Perper JA, Kuller LH, Cooper M. Arteriosclerosis of coronary arteries in sudden unexpected deaths. Circulation 1975;*52(Suppl.3):*27.

8. Baroldi G, Falzi G, Mariani F. Sudden coronary death: a post-mortem study in 208 selected cases compared to 97 "control" subjects. Am Heart J 1979;98:20.

9. Davies MJ, Thomas A. Thrombosis and acute coronary artery lesions in sudden cardiac ischemic death. N Engl J Med 1984;310:1137.

10. Davies MJ, Bland JM, Hangartner JRW, Angelini A, Thomas AC. Factors influencing the presence or absence of acute coronary artery thrombi in sudden ischaemic death. Eur Heart J 1989;10:203.

11. Anderson KP. Sudden death, hypertension and hypertrophy. J Cardiovasc Pharmacol 1984;6(Suppl.3):S498.

12. Fulton M, Lutz W, Donald KW et al. Natural history of unstable angina. Lancet 1972;1:860.

13. Feinlieb M, Simon AB, Gillum JR, Margolis JR. Prodromal symptoms and signs of sudden death. Circulation 1975;52(Suppl.3):155.

14. Kuller LH. Prodromata of sudden death and myocardial infarction. Adv Cardiol 1978;25:61.

15. Liberthson RR, Nagel EL, Hirschman JC, Nussenfeld SR. Prehospital ventricular fibrillation: prognosis and follow-up course. N Engl J Med 1974;291:317.

16. Goldstein S, Landis JR, Leighton R et al. Predictive survival models for resuscitated victims of out-of-hospital cardiac arrest with coronary heart disease. Circulation 1985;71:873.

17. Weaver WD, Lorch GS, Alvarez HA, Cobb LA. Angiographic findings and prognostic indicators in patients resuscitated from sudden cardiac death. Circulation 1976;54:895.

18. Epstein SE, Quyyumi AA, Bonow RO. Sudden cardiac death without warning. Possible mechanisms and implications for screening asymptomatic populations. New Engl J Med 1989;321:320.

19. Bigger JT. Relation between left ventricular dysfunction and ventricular arrhythmias after myocardial infarction. Am J Cardiol 1986;57:8B.

20. Tofler GH, Stone PH, Muller JE et al. Prognosis after cardiac arrest due to ventricular tachycardia or ventricular fibrillation associated with acute myocardial infarction (The MILIS Study). Am J Cardiol 1987;60:765.

21. Simson MB. Noninvasive identification of patients at high risk for sudden cardiac death. Signal-averaged electrocardiography. Circulation 1992;85(Suppl.I):I-145.

22. Schwartz PJ, Wolf S. QT interval prolongation as predictor of sudden death in patients with myocardial infarction. Circulation 1978;57:1074.

23. Vedin A, Wilhelmsen L, Wedel H et al. Predictor of cardiovascular deaths and non-fatal reinfarctions after myocardial infarction. Acta Med Scand 1977;201:309.

24. Wellens HJJ, Bar FWH, Vanagt EJDM, Brugada P. Medical treatment of ventricular tachycardia; consideration in the selection of patients for surgical therapy. Am J Cardiol 1982;49:186.

25. Bigger JT Jr, Fleiss JL, Kleiger R, Miller JP, Rolnitzky LM. The Multicenter Post Infarction Research Group. The relationships among ventricular arrhythmias, left ventricular dysfunction and mortality in the 2 years after myocardial infarction. Circulation 1984;69:250.

26. Mukharji J, Rude RE, Pole WK et al for The MILIS Study Group. Risk factors for sudden death after acute myocardial infarction: two-years follow-up. Am J Cardiol 1984;54:31.

27. The Cardiac Arrhythmia Suppression Trial (CAST) Investigators. Preliminary report. Effect of encainide and flecainide on mortality in a randomized trial of arrhythmia suppression after myocardial infarction. N Engl J Med 1989;321:406.

28. Di Marco JP, Lerman BB, Kron IL, Sellers TD. Sustained ventricular tachyarrhythmias within 3 months of acute myocardial infarction: results of medical and surgical therapy in patients resuscitated from the initial episode. J Am Coll Cardiol 1985;6:759.

29. Wellens HJJ, Bar FWH, Vanagt EJDM, Brugada P. Medical treatment of ventricular tachycardia; consideration in the selection of patients for surgical therapy. Am J Cardiol 1982;49:186.

30. Marchlinski FE, Waxman HL, Buxton AE, Josephson ME. Sustained ventricular tachyarrhythmias during the early postinfarction period: electrophysiologic findings and prognosis for survival. J Am Coll Cardiol 1983;2:240.

31. Myerburg RJ, Kessler KM. Management of patients who survive cardiac arrest. Mod Concepts Cardiovasc Dis 1986;55:61.

32. Steinbeck G, Andresen D, Bach P et al. A comparison of electrophysiologically guided antiarrhythmic drug therapy with beta-blocker therapy in patients with symptomatic, sustained ven-

tricular tachyarrhythmias. New Engl J Med 1992;*327:*987.

33. Myerburg RJ et al. In: Zipes DP, Jalipe J (eds). Cardiac Electrophysiology: From Cell to Bedside. Philadelphia, WB Saunders, 1990;666.

34. Morady F, DiCarlo L, Winston S et al. Clinical features and prognosis of patients with out-of-hospital cardiac arrest and a normal electrophysiologic study. J Am Coll Cardiol 1984;*4:*39.

35. Holmes DR, Davis KB, Moch MB et al. The effect of medical and surgical treatment on subsequent sudden cardiac death in patients with coronary artery disease: a report from the Coronary Artery Surgery Study. Circulation 1986;*73:*1254.

36. Aspirin Myocardial Study Research Group: a randomized controlled trial of aspirin in persons recovered from myocardial infarction. J Am Med Ass 1980;*243:*661.

37. Cairns JA, Connolly SJ, Gent M, Roberts R. Post-myocardial infarction mortality in patients with ventricular premature depolarization. Canadian Amiodarone Myocardial Infarction Trial Pilot Study. Circulation 1991;*84:*550.

38. Ceremuzynski L, Kleczar E, Krzeminska-Pakula M et al. Effect of amiodarone on mortality after myocardial infarction: a double-blind, placebo-controlled, pilot study. J Am Coll Cardiol 1992;*20:*1056.

Doctor–patient relationship and general philosophy of clinical research in IHD

A thorough understanding of the relationship between doctor and patient is the basis of good clinical practise. Clinical research is necessary to discover the genetically and environmentally determined causes of both the multiple manifestations of the disease and the varying responses of different individuals, as well as to assess objectively the benefits of new forms of treatment. When dealing with ischemic heart disease (IHD), both aspects have some important peculiarities, because myocardial infarction (MI) and sudden ischemic cardiac death (SICD) may develop totally unheralded in individuals with mild or no symptoms as a result of multiple predisposing and precipitating factors still incompletely known.

DOCTOR–PATIENT RELATIONSHIP

In all diseases, during acute or severely symptomatic phases, the major concerns of both patients and physicians are the improvement of symptoms and of short-term prognosis. Also, in the field of IHD sick patients need abundant sympathy and encouragement, as well as appropriate treatment, the benefits of which are soon apparent.

When acute or severely symptomatic phases have subsided and when symptoms are mild or absent, the doctor–patient relationship in the field of IHD is dominated by anxiety about the possible occurrence of unheralded catastrophic events, but the benefits of preventive treatment cannot be easily assessed. Patients seek reassurance, and doctors know only too well that they could be blamed by patients and relatives for not having predicted and prevented an event, even when the patient was at very low risk. Doctors are naturally concerned about possible allegations of not having been strict enough with, or not having prescribed a more aggressive form of therapy for, patients when dramatic events occur. This concern may lead them to advise the restriction of holiday trips, recreational sporting activities, or journeys unnecessarily. It may also lead to interventions and forms of therapy that, although of proven benefit in high-risk patients or in those who are severely symptomatic, have not been proven beneficial in low-risk patients with mild or even no symptoms.

In phases of the disease with an average risk of dramatic events of about 1% per year, and often much lower, such as those that are quiescent and mildly symptomatic, patients who are likely to suffer an event cannot be identified with confidence, even by the most sophisticated tests presently available, according to the Bayesian theorem. Moreover, both doctors and patients should be aware that when the risk of events is as low as 1% per year, therapy capable of reducing the average event rate by as much as 50% will prevent only one event for every 200 patients treated, so that 199 patients will have been subjected to treatment that produced no benefit. As discussed in Chapter 13, the reduction of IHD-related events can improve life expectancy significantly only when such events represent a very substantial proportion of all possible causes of death in the age-group considered, as the individuals spared will then be exposed to other non-IHD-related causes of death. This awareness should bring doctors and patients to consider not only the fear of an uncertain, rather distant, future, but also the quality of life in the present and more immediate future. In patients free from limiting symptoms, the quality of life is influenced by two contrasting aspects:

a.   feeling free from medical constraints as much as possible
b.   being free from anxiety about possible future unheralded events.

Deciding how to deal with mildly symptomatic or asymptomatic patients who may suffer MI or SICD at some point in the future, but who are at low risk, is quite common in clinical practise. There are no specific rules or standardized approaches to such a typically individual problem but, according to my experience, a series of steps should be followed.

1. *Inform patients about their absolute risk.* Patients should be apprised of their average estimated risk by informing them how many, among 100 patients having exactly the same clinical features, will be well at 1 and 5 years, and ideally, by how much their life expectancy is likely to be reduced by disease.
2. *Inform patients of the absolute reduction of risk obtainable from available therapeutic options.* Patients should be informed of the number of patients having the same clinical features, out of 100 treated, who would benefit from each form of treatment at 1 and 5 years, and, whenever possible, also about the average improvement in life expectancy offered by the various possible options.
3. *Adapt accepted therapeutic options to each individual patient.* Quantifying a patient's average absolute risk and its possible reduction by treatment requires competence. Applying this information to the best possible management strategy requires that doctors have a perceptive understanding of the personalities of their individual patients, as only this understanding will allow them to optimize the available strategies in order to reduce the risk of future events, while at the same time providing reassurance and not interfering unnecessarily with life-style.

Patients should not be scared by their doctors painting a gloomy picture of their risk in order to make them more compliant with preventive strategies, as fear and anxiety about the future could impair the quality of life for the rest of their lives. As a Tuscan proverb says "che serve vivere da malati per morire da sani?" This translates roughly to "What is the use of living as a sick person only to die healthy?" This concept is an aspect of the "tyranny of health," discussed recently.[1]

A thorough discussion with patients and their relatives can eliminate misunderstandings, allow the patient to make responsible, informed decisions,[2] and reduce inappropriate anxieties. Some patients wish to make their own informed decisions, while others prefer to leave it to the doctor. For some patients, anxiety about the future is so dominant that they wish "something" to be done, others fear interventions or feel "diminished" by having to alter their life styles or take drugs. Reassurance is mandatory, as a patient's quality of life begins to deteriorate as soon as they learn they have or may develop IHD. This "labelling effect" is associated with anxiety or depression and the quality of life may deteriorate even further after the initiation of drug therapy, as observed in the treatment of hypertension.[3]

Alternatively, anxiety can be reduced in patients who, although informed of the low risk, are particularly concerned about their prognosis, by the awareness that they are receiving the most advanced available established forms of treatment, often in the hope that this will dispense with the need to modify their life styles by losing weight, working less, increasing recreational physical activity, and living a more serene life. Thus, it is essential that sufficient time be spent communicating with patients not only about their estimated risk, but also about life style changes, medications,[4] and quality of life. Patients should be encouraged to live a full life, as long as they are not limited by symptoms and as long as this does not increase their absolute risk to any measurable extent; but it should, at the same time, be explained that no one is entirely free from risk, no matter how intensely one tries to minimize it.

Reassurance, based on balanced explanations, is the most beneficial and least costly medicine available to improve the quality of life in most individuals. It should be given abundantly and appropriately at every check-up visit.

GENERAL PHILOSOPHY OF CLINICAL RESEARCH IN IHD

Scientific communities are built around accepted paradigms that determine major lines of research, influence the chances of obtaining grant support or publishing results and establish standards of therapy.[5,6] In the field of IHD, the paradigms that were established in the 1950s and 1960s on the basis of the evidence then available, still largely dominate the scientific scenario.

Once a paradigm becomes established, it is very difficult to change, just like criminal cases are hard to reopen once a culprit has been blamed, and it monopolizes research. First, there is no longer the incentive to pursue the investigation, and second, there is strong resistance to the acceptance of newly discovered evidence. In the past, clinical studies have, at times, provided compelling new evidence that has succeeded in changing established paradigms and, thus, has influenced lines of research and standards of practise.

This last point is illustrated by three selected examples.

1. In the 1950s nitroglycerin was thought to act by increasing coronary blood flow (CBF) because that effect had been observed in animal studies. Such a paradigm was so well established that dypridamole and carbochromene were marketed as antianginal drugs just because they markedly increased CBF in animals. However, in patients, catheterization of the coronary sinus showed that nitroglycerin did not increase CBF at doses effective in relieving angina.[7] This invasive clinical study oriented research toward investigation of the peripheral effects of nitrates and other ways of allowing the heart to work more economically. Also, the evidence that nitroglycerin dilated coronary stenoses[8] and prevented or reduced ischemia by direct coronary and peripheral blood pooling effects[9] could only come from clinical studies.

2. Until the mid-1970s, coronary artery spasm had long been considered a resort of the diagnostically destitute.[10] This was because at autopsy coronary atherosclerosis was such an obvious and readily identifiable culprit, whereas spasm was invisible. The demonstration of the pathogenetic role of coronary artery spasm could only come from clinical studies[11] because there was no incentive to develop animal models. The revival of this concept not only opened up new lines of research on epicardial coronary artery vasomotor tone, but also pro-

vided a rationale for the use of calcium antagonists as anti-ischemic drugs, and nitrates as dilators of epicardial coronary arteries.[12]

3. Until the late 1970s, thrombolytic therapy, although available, had not been used clinically in cases of acute MI. Coronary arteriographic studies, daringly performed in the very early hours after the onset of chest pain, demonstrated convincingly the presence of coronary thrombosis[13] and led to its widespread use.

Has clinical pathophysiologic research now identified all the most important causes that predispose to, and trigger, myocardial ischemia, and produce necrosis, fatal arrhythmias, and cardiac failure in humans? Or does it still have a role in rearranging the priority list for the application of cellular and molecular biology techniques, a role that cannot be replaced by the further study of accepted mechanisms in animal models or at the cellular and molecular levels?

To what extent does the last generation of multicentric trials and consensus conferences allow the best available management of individual patients?

Pathophysiologic and etiologic components of ischemic cardiac syndromes

In IHD, the fundamental pathophysiologic question should concern the actual causes of myocardial ischemia, without which no ischemic syndromes would exist. However, just as the causes of chronic stable, unstable, variant, and microvascular angina can be multiple, the causes responsible for the sudden development of MI and of fatal arrhythmias can also be multiple. Two additional questions concern the nature of the predisposing background alterations that favor the occurrence of ischemic stimuli, and the determinants of the heart's response to the ischemic insult in terms of myocardial necrosis, fatal arrhythmias, and cardiac failure. Both can result from multiple environmentally and genetically determined etiologic components and from protective components. However, these latter questions would become irrelevant in the absence of ischemic stimuli. The search for the actual nature and cause of such stimuli is difficult because the same, ultimate pathogenetic mechanism, such as coronary artery thrombosis, occlusive spasm, or microvascular dysfunction, can have multiple and varied etiologic components. The search for the determinants of the heart's response to ischemic insult is also difficult because they are multiple and varied and because patients respond in ways that cannot be mimicked by the ischemic response of healthy experimental animals. Thus, the atherosclerotic background is the most widely studied because it is the most easily detectable and because, in the search for a single denominator of myocardial ischemic syndromes, it stands out as the most obvious correlate of angina, MI, and SICD. In the impetus to find a clearly identifiable culprit, the paradigm that the fundamental cause of IHD is represented by gradually forming atherosclerosis, developing largely as a result of altered lipid metabolism, has monopolized research on its causes and prevention.

The explosion of knowledge in the fields of cellular and molecular biology provides the intellectual and technical background for studying in greater and greater depth mechanisms of disease that are considered fundamental on the basis of existing knowledge, i.e. the molecular causes of altered blood lipid levels, smooth muscle proliferation, endothelial dysfunction, and myocardial hypertrophy.[14] However, only the potential mechanisms of disease already identified can be studied in depth. Isolated studies of the molecular alterations of those selected components of disease that can be reproduced in tissue cultures and animal models are unlikely to provide, by themselves, a comprehensive understanding of the various missing pathogenetic and etiologic components of human ischemic syndromes.[15]

For example, the causes of restenosis or the failure to achieve prompt recanalization of occluded coronary arteries in acute MI are more likely to be discovered in patients than in experimental animals. Causative and protective mechanisms may be varied and are not likely to be present in experimental models. Patients who are "protected" from restenosis, in spite of unfavorable plaque morphology, represent a valuable model in which to investigate protective mechanisms. Conversely, the effects of local stenosis and of procedure-related restenosis are best studied in patients who have undergone multi-vessel PTCA. Patients who fail to achieve prompt coronary recanalization in spite of appropriate, very early thrombolytic therapy, represent a key model for investigation. Patients with unstable angina who are refractory to maximal medical therapy, represent another unique clinical model for investigation of the unknown mechanisms of acute persistent coronary occlusion.

Choosing a research project

Research may be undertaken as a learning experience, or to obtain some publications that may prove useful on a curriculum vitae when applying for a desirable job, or it may be the fruit of a natural curiosity. When research is a long-term commitment, choosing a research project is a critical decision. Ideally, it should ask important questions, the answers to which may lead to a seminal observation and novel ways of thinking which set the stage for subsequent research. As Kahn[16] recently recognized, work leading to seminal observations frequently "goes counter to existing dogma," thus making peers skeptical and funding and publication difficult. In turn, this restricts innovation and leads to investigators following the prevailing lines of research in major journals, and to repeating, in patients, studies already performed in experimental animals.

Exposure to the varied presentations of individual clinical cases provides a continuous stimulus for inquisitive doctors, as long as they do not limit themselves to identifying the minimal diagnostic criteria that allow patients to be classified into one of the generally accepted syndromes. When doctors consider a case in greater detail with an open mind, they will observe deviations from standard paradigms. When these deviations are very considerable they may suggest a research project. This was, after all, the way that clinical syndromes were identified about a century ago by the clinicians whose names they bear. This approach may also lead to seminal observations and to a previously unoccupied research niche and may allow the investigator to build up a theme, as long as he or she is prepared to focus and pursue the project to any depths necessary.[16] The results of investigations that suggest different hypotheses from those tested are also very useful, as they are the least likely to be biased by preconceived ideas and may open up a new line of research.

Individual investigators may chose projects when the "cue" comes along, as used to be the case. However, a more systematic means of gathering homogeneous groups of patients with similar pathogenetic and etiologic components is represented by the prospective collection of cases in a computerized database that groups patients not only according to the similarities that allow them to be classified into a given syndrome, but also according to the deviations from standard paradigms.[17] The consequent dispersion of patients within each syndrome into many subgroups too small for statistical analysis, can be compensated for by pooling the data from multiple centers. This approach could also be used in randomized clinical trials on homogeneous groups of patients.

Randomized clinical therapeutic trials

The availability of therapeutic options poses practical questions: Is interventional therapy better than medical therapy? Is one thrombolytic drug better than another? Do antiarrhythmic drugs reduce mortality? Does reduction of plasma cholesterol improve longevity? Providing the answers to these questions usually demands large-scale trials involving several thousand patients. This implies one of two caveats when applying the results to clinical practise. If the patient group enrolled is homogeneous, the larger the trial needed to prove a reduction of the relative risk, the smaller the reduction of the absolute risk to be expected in the individual patient (unless the inclusion of a large number of low-risk patients "dilutes" the greater absolute beneficial effect in high-risk patients). If the group is heterogeneous, some patients may experience a large benefit, or none at all, or even deleterious effects from a treatment that, on average, was found to be statistically beneficial to the group as a whole.

The organization of large double-blind trials has become remarkably efficient. Statisticians have become extremely meticulous in the application of appropriate tests for evaluating the statistical significance of the effects of treatments. But, in the effort to enrol, within a short period, large numbers of patients, the entry criteria adopted in most large trials are quite broad. Statisticians have no way of assessing whether the patients enrolled represent an homogeneous group in terms of absolute risk and of pathogenetic mechanisms. Indeed, as indicated in Chapter 13, heterogenous responses to the same treatment among patients who met the entry criteria were detected by retrospective subgroup analysis in several studies.

The application of the results of very large trials to clinical practise poses no problem when a small absolute reduction of risk is produced by a low-cost drug with a known low incidence of side-effects, such as for example, low-dose aspirin. However, given the multiplicity of pathogenetic and etiologic components of each clinical ischemic syndrome and the variability of individual responses to treatment, it would be desirable to obtain quantitative information on the beneficial effects on groups of patients as homogeneous as possible, selected prospectively from a common database. The search for markers of specific pathogenetic mechanisms (for example, in hematology, hypochromic red cells are markers of iron deficiency anemia and megalocytes are markers of vitamin B_{12} or folic acid deficiency anemias) would represent the basis not only for more rationale therapeutic strategies, but also for focused pathogenetic and etiologic studies. This novel approach to IHD is certainly difficult, but the battles less likely to be won are those that never start.

REFERENCES

1. Fitzgerald FT. The tyranny of heath. New Engl J Med 1994;*331*:196.
2. Kassirer JP. Incorporating patients' preferences into medical decisions. New Engl J Med 1994;*330*:1895.
3. Oparil S. Antihypertensive therapy—efficacy and quality of life. New Engl J Med 1993;*328*:959.
4. Kessler DA. Communicating with patients about their medications. New Engl J Med 1991;*325*:1650.
5. Kuhn TS. The Structure of Scientific Revolutions. Chicago, University of Chicago Press. 1970.
6. Romanucci-Ross L, Moerman DE. The extraneous factor in western medicine. Ethos 1988;*16*:146.
7. Gorlin R, Brachfeld N, MacLeod C, Bopp P. Effect of nitroglycerin on the coronary circulation in patients with coronary artery disease or increased left ventricular work. Circulation 1959;*19*;705.
8. Brown BG, Bolson E, Petersen RB, Pierce CD, Dodge HT. The mechanisms of nitroglycerin

action: stenosis vasodilatation as a major component of the drug response. Circulation 1981;*64*:1089.

9. De Coster PM, Chierchia S, Davies GJ, Hackett D, Fragasso G, Maseri A. Combined effects of nitrates on the coronary and peripheral circulation in exercise-induced ischemia. Circulation 1990;*81*:1881.

10. Pickering GW. Vascular spasm. Lancet 1951;*2*:845.

11. MacAlpin RN. Coronary arterial spasm: a historical perspective. J Hist Med Allied Sci 1980;*35*:288.

12. Maseri A. The revival of coronary spasm. Am J Med 1981;*70*:752.

13. De Wood MA, Spores J, Notske R et al. Prevalence of total coronary occlusion during the early hours of transmural myocardial infarction. N Engl J Med 1980;*303*:897.

14. Hathaway DR, March KL. Molecular cardiology: new avenues for the diagnosis and treatment of cardiovascular disease. J Am Coll Cardiol 1989;*13*:265.

15. Maseri A. Integration of cellular and molecular biology with clinical research in cardiology. New Engl J Med. Letter to the Editor, 1993;*328*:447.

16. Kahn CR. Picking a research problem. The critical decision. New Engl J Med 1994;*330*:1530.

17. Cianflone D, Carandente O, Chierchia SL. Structure of a multidimensional relational database optimized for daily clinical use and decision support in cardiology departments. Computers in Cardiology. IEEE Comp. Society Press 2. 1991, p. 565.

Index

Numbers followed by *f* indicate figures; those followed by *t* indicate tables.

693